W9-CCY-707

Reperfusion Therapy for Acute Myocardial Infarction

FUNDAMENTAL AND CLINICAL CARDIOLOGY

Editor-in-Chief

Samuel Z. Goldhaber, M.D.
*Harvard Medical School and Brigham
and Women's Hospital Boston,
Massachusetts, U.S.A.*

Reperfusion Therapy for Acute Myocardial Infarction

Edited by

Eric R. Bates
University of Michigan Medical Center
Ann Arbor, Michigan, USA

informa
healthcare

New York London

Informa Healthcare USA, Inc.
52 Vanderbilt Avenue
New York, NY 10017

© 2008 by Informa Healthcare USA, Inc.
Informa Healthcare is an Informa business

No claim to original U.S. Government works
Printed in the United States of America on acid-free paper
10 9 8 7 6 5 4 3 2 1

International Standard Book Number-10: 0-8493-4358-5 (Hardcover)
International Standard Book Number-13: 978-0-8493-4358-2 (Hardcover)

Library of Congress Cataloging-in-Publication Data

Reperfusion therapy for acute myocardial infarction / edited by Eric R. Bates.
    p. ; cm. — (Fundamental and clinical cardiology ; v. 64)
  Includes bibliographical references and index.
  ISBN-13: 978-0-8493-4358-2 (hardcover : alk. paper)
  ISBN-10: 0-8493-4358-5 (hardcover : alk. paper)
    1. Myocardial infarction—Treatment. 2. Myocardial reperfusion.
  I. Bates, Eric R. II. Series.
    [DNLM: 1. Myocardial Infarction—therapy. 2. Reperfusion—methods.
  W1 FU538TD v.64 2008 / WG 300 R4255 2008]
  RC685.I6R45 2008
  616.1'23706—dc22

                             2007047358

For Corporate Sales and Reprint Permissions call 212-520-2700 or write to: Sales Department, 52 Vanderbilt Avenue, 16th floor, New York, NY 10017.

Visit the Informa Web site at
www.informa.com

and the Informa Healthcare Web site at
www.informahealthcare.com

Series Introduction

Informa Healthcare has developed various series of beautifully produced books in different branches of medicine. These series have facilitated the integration of rapidly advancing information for both the clinical specialist and the researcher, especially in the area of cardiovascular medicine.

Eric R. Bates, MD, has compiled and edited a new masterpiece on the management of the developed world's number one killer: acute myocardial infarction. The revolution in treatment began three decades ago with emergency reperfusion therapy. Restoring blood flow to the thrombosed coronary artery became standard of care, rather than a maverick procedure stigmatized by little evidence to prove its success. In fact, reperfusion therapy has saved millions of lives and has changed the landscape of cardiology. Immediate death from heart attack has become much less common than chronic illness from advanced heart failure among survivors of myocardial infarction afflicted with "ischemic cardiomyopathy."

Dr. Bates, an interventional cardiologist with legendary technical skills, has advanced the field with his academic contributions in fibrinolytic reperfusion, mechanical reperfusion, and adjunctive therapy for reperfusion. In this gem of a textbook, he has summoned the world's All Stars to provide updated accounts in their areas of reperfusion expertise. The authors constitute a Who's Who in the field of myocardial infarction treatment. Eugene Braunwald, MD, writes the first chapter on historical milestones while Elliott M. Antman, MD, concludes with future perspectives. Dr. Bates includes an appendix with the most recent reperfusion guidelines issued by the world's three leading cardiology organizations.

My goal as an editor-in-chief of the Fundamental and Clinical Cardiology Series is to assemble the talents of world-renowned authorities to discuss virtually every area of cardiovascular medicine. We have achieved this objective with *Reperfusion Therapy for Acute Myocardial Infarction*. Future contributions to this series will include books on molecular biology, interventional cardiology, and clinical management of such problems as chronic coronary artery disease, venous thromboembolism, peripheral vascular disease, and cardiac arrhythmias.

Samuel Z. Goldhaber, MD
Boston, Massachusetts, U.S.A.

Preface

Reperfusion therapy for ST-segment elevation myocardial infarction (STEMI) has been an important clinical focus for 25 years. Impressive reductions in morbidity and mortality rates have been achieved in STEMI, but with a growing and aging population, STEMI remains a major public health problem. Moreover, many eligible patients are not receiving recommended therapies.

Enormous strides have been made in understanding the pathophysiology of atherosclerosis and plaque rupture, the usual inciting factor in STEMI, and new interventions have been developed to treat thrombosis and inflammation. Numerous clinical trials and registries have clarified the epidemiology of STEMI. Subgroup analyses have resulted in the ability to accurately predict individual patient risk.

The achievement of successful myocardial reperfusion has evolved from infarct artery patency to infarct artery flow to microvascular reperfusion. The administration of fibrinolytic therapy has become easier as intravenous therapy replaced intracoronary administration, and bolus therapy replaced infusion therapy, but a ceiling of reperfusion success rates of approximately 75% has limited further advances. Catheter-based reperfusion achieves higher infarct artery patency rates, but access has been limited to a minority of patients and treatment delays may diminish some of its advantage. The combination of pharmacological therapy and catheter-based therapy as a rescue or facilitated percutaneous coronary intervention (PCI) strategy has been studied with the hope that better outcomes can be achieved. Others are performing PCI at hospitals without on-site cardiac surgery or establishing rapid transfer policies in an attempt to decrease door-to-balloon times.

The results of reperfusion therapy with fibrinolytics and PCI have been improved with adjunctive antiplatelet and antithrombotic agents. New pharmacological and mechanical interventions are under investigation to reduce the impact of reperfusion injury and thrombus embolization on myocardial infarct size.

Major limitations in delivering care to patients with STEMI are systems problems in organizing pre-hospital and emergency department diagnosis and treatment plans. Quality improvement initiatives and critical pathway development can reduce logistical barriers, improve times-to-treatment, and ensure that appropriate medications are administered.

Complications associated with STEMI and its treatment remain challenging. However, new interventions and the possibility of myocyte regeneration offer the opportunity of even better therapies in the future.

The goal of this book is to review the past, present, and future of reperfusion therapy for STEMI. An internationally known group of leading authorities in this field have contributed their expertise to this effort. We hope that this book will be a useful resource for all of the health professionals who care for patients with STEMI.

Eric R. Bates

Contents

Background

Fibrinolytic Reperfusion

Catheter-based Reperfusion

Adjunctive Therapy

Challenges and Opportunities

Appendix

Contributors

Sameer Amin   Atherosclerosis Research Center, Division of Cardiology, Department of Medicine, Burns and Allen Research Institute, Cedars Sinai Medical Center and David Geffen School of Medicine at UCLA, Los Angeles, California, U.S.A.

Elliott M. Antman   Cardiovascular Division, TIMI Study Group, Brigham and Women's Hospital, Harvard Medical School, Boston, Massachusetts, U.S.A.

Paul W. Armstrong   Division of Cardiology, University of Alberta, Edmonton, Alberta, Canada

Eric R. Bates   Department of Internal Medicine, Division of Cardiovascular Diseases, University of Michigan, Ann Arbor, Michigan, U.S.A.

Farzin Beygui   Institut de Cardiologie, Pitié-Salpêtrière University Hospital, Paris, France

Eugene Braunwald   Department of Medicine, Brigham and Women's Hospital, Harvard Medical School, Boston, Massachusetts, U.S.A.

Mauricio G. Cohen   Division of Cardiology, Department of Medicine, The University of North Carolina at Chapel Hill, Chapel Hill, North Carolina, U.S.A.

Eduardo I. de Oliveira   Hospital de Santa Maria and Faculdade de Medicina de Lisboa, Lisbon, Portugal

Simon R. Dixon   Division of Cardiology, William Beaumont Hospital, Royal Oak, Michigan, U.S.A.

Stephen G. Ellis   Department of Cardiovascular Medicine, Cleveland Clinic, Cleveland, Ohio, U.S.A.

David Faxon   Department of Medicine, Brigham and Women's Hospital, Harvard Medical School, Boston, Massachusetts, U.S.A.

Anthony H. Gershlick   Department of Cardiology, University Hospitals of Leicester, Glenfield Hospital, Leicester, United Kingdom

C. Michael Gibson   Department of Cardiology, Beth Israel-Deaconess Medical Center, Boston, Massachusetts, U.S.A.

Christopher B. Granger   Duke Clinical Research Institute and Duke University Medical Center, Durham, North Carolina, U.S.A.

Claudia P. Hochberg   Department of Cardiology, Beth Israel-Deaconess Medical Center, Boston, Massachusetts, U.S.A.

Judd E. Hollander   Department of Emergency Medicine, Hospital of the University of Pennsylvania, Philadelphia, Pennsylvania, U.S.A.

Steven M. Hollenberg   Division of Cardiology, Cooper University Hospital, Camden, New Jersey, U.S.A.

E. Marc Jolicoeur   Duke Clinical Research Institute and Duke University Medical Center, Durham, North Carolina, U.S.A.

Damian J. Kelly   Department of Cardiology, University Hospitals of Leicester, Glenfield Hospital, Leicester, United Kingdom

Nestor Mercado   Division of Cardiovascular Diseases, Scripps Clinic, La Jolla, California, U.S.A.

Gilles Montalescot   Institut de Cardiologie, Pitié-Salpêtrière University Hospital, Paris, France

Brahmajee K. Nallamothu   Department of Internal Medicine, Division of Cardiovascular Medicine, University of Michigan, Ann Arbor, Michigan, U.S.A.

William W. O'Neill   Division of Cardiology, Department of Internal Medicine, University of Miami, Miller School of Medicine, Miami, Florida, U.S.A.

E. Magnus Ohman   Division of Cardiovascular Medicine, Duke University Medical Center, Duke Clinical Research Institute, Durham, North Carolina, U.S.A.

Sanjeevan Pasupati   Division of Cardiology, St. Paul's Hospital, University of British Columbia, Vancouver, Canada

Prediman K. Shah   Atherosclerosis Research Center, Division of Cardiology, Department of Medicine, Burns and Allen Research Institute, Cedars Sinai Medical Center and David Geffen School of Medicine at UCLA, Los Angeles, California, U.S.A.

Peter R. Sinnaeve   Department of Cardiology, Gasthuisberg University Hospital, University of Leuven, Leuven, Belgium

Frans J. Van de Werf   Department of Cardiology, Gasthuisberg University Hospital, University of Leuven, Leuven, Belgium

John G. Webb   Division of Cardiology, St. Paul's Hospital, University of British Columbia, Vancouver, Canada

Robert C. Welsh   Division of Cardiology, University of Alberta, Edmonton, Alberta, Canada

Thomas P. Wharton   Section of Cardiology and Cardiac Catheterization Laboratory, Exeter Hospital, Exeter, New Hampshire, U.S.A.

1 Historical Milestones in Reperfusion Therapy for Myocardial Infarction

Eugene Braunwald

Department of Medicine, Brigham and Women's Hospital, Harvard Medical School, Boston, Massachusetts, U.S.A.

INTRODUCTION

Acute myocardial infarction (AMI) remains one of the world's most common life-threatening illnesses. In the United States alone, approximately 850,000 cases occur each year. The clinical syndrome of AMI was described in the earliest years of the 20th century. Once considered a medical curiosity, by midcentury it was recognized as the most common cause of death in the industrialized world. The second half of the 20th century saw a massive attack on this serious public health problem, an attack that proved on the whole to be quite successful, with an estimated early mortality rate declining from approximately 30% to 7% in patients who are now treated using approved guidelines.

Reperfusion of the infarcting myocardium, one of the cornerstones of AMI therapy, has evolved from the convergence of four major research efforts: (1) elucidation of the role of thrombosis in the development of AMI, (2) demonstration that infarcting myocardium can be salvaged by early reperfusion, (3) development of fibrinolytic agents and their use in myocardial reperfusion, and (4) development of primary percutaneous coronary intervention to provide optimal blood flow to infarcting myocardium.

CORONARY THROMBOSIS IN THE PATHOGENESIS OF MYOCARDIAL INFARCTION

In the 19th century it was demonstrated in animal experiments that ligation of a major coronary artery usually caused sudden death; pathological observations in patients also led to the conclusion that sudden occlusion of these arteries was immediately fatal. In his classic text, *The Principles and Practice of Medicine*, William Osler stated: "The blocking of one of these vessels [coronary arteries] by a thrombus or an embolus leads to a condition which is known as anaemic necrosis, or white infarct. This is most commonly seen in the left ventricle and in the septum, in the territory of distribution of [left] anterior coronary [descending] artery" (1). Thus was established the link between coronary artery thrombosis and AMI. In 1901, Krehl, a German physician, speculated that coronary thrombosis may not always cause sudden death (2).

Although William Herrick is usually credited with the description of the clinical syndrome of AMI, in 1910 two Russian physicians, Obraztsov and Strazhesko, described five patients with MI, in three of whom coronary thrombosis was found at autopsy (3). They concluded that coronary thrombosis is not always immediately fatal but that it can also produce a nonfatal clinical syndrome. Two years later, Herrick described two patients with AMI, one of whom was found to have coronary thrombosis at postmortem examination (4). Herrick's observation of coronary thrombosis as the cause of AMI was so widely accepted that the terms "coronary thrombosis" and "myocardial infarction" were considered to be synonymous for a number of years. In a statement that anticipated reperfusion therapy by many decades, Herrick concluded: "The hope for the damaged myocardium lies in the direction of securing a blood supply from friendly neighboring vessels so as to restore so far as possible its functional integrity" (4). By the second decade of the 20th century, AMI was recognized as a clinical syndrome, albeit one with a very high mortality.

Although Herrick's paper had profound impact on Western medicine, autopsy studies in patients with MI during the following six decades revealed many instances of AMI in which severe atherosclerosis was evident but without coronary thrombosis. In 1939 Friedberg and Horn, two eminent American cardiologists, summarized the beliefs of that era as follows: "It is well-known that the clinical and electrocardiographic features of coronary thrombosis may be observed in patients in whom a coronary artery thrombus is subsequently *not* found at necropsy. In such patients the clinical picture may have been caused by a myocardial infarction in the absence of coronary artery occlusion" (5). European pathologists took a similar position. Indeed, Branwood and Montgomery concluded that coronary thrombosis is the *result* of rather than the *cause* of AMI (6). In 1974, Roberts, an experienced cardiac pathologist stated: "There is substantial evidence that acute thrombus formation does not precipitate acute fatal ischemic heart disease. The major problem is diffuse generalized coronary atherosclerosis with (>75%) luminal narrowing of at least two of the three major coronary arteries" (7). Thus, for a half century (1930 to 1980), the pendulum of opinion had swung in the direction opposite to where Osler, Obraztsov, Strazhesko, and Herrick had initially pushed it (8). Nevertheless, a vocal minority clung firmly to what was termed the "Herrick school of thought," which led to early efforts to lyse presumptive coronary thrombi (see below).

The issue was finally resolved in 1979, when Rentrop et al. (9), reported total occlusion of the infarct-related artery in 74% of 35 patients with AMI studied by coronary arteriography. This was followed a year later by De Wood's report on the coronary arteriographic findings in 517 patients with AMI; nearly 90% of those studied within the first four hours had occlusive coronary thrombi, but this figure fell to approximately 60% in patients studied between 12 and 24 hours after the onset of symptoms (10) (Fig. 1). These observations, subsequently amply confirmed, provided the strongest evidence that coronary thrombosis was indeed the proximate cause of MI. The lower percentage of thrombi in patients studied more than 12 hours after the onset of symptoms by De Wood et al. (10) was presumably related to endogenous lysis of previously occlusive thrombi. The latter process also explained the absence of coronary thrombi at necropsy in many patients with AMI, especially those who died after the first few hours. A thrombotic origin of AMI was even more strongly suggested by Rentrop's demonstration of reperfusion with the intracoronary administration of streptokinase (11) (see below). By 1980, the pendulum had swung back to where it had started at the beginning of the century and the overriding questions became: (1) Can infarct size be limited by reestablishing myocardial perfusion? and (2) if it can be, how is reperfusion best accomplished?

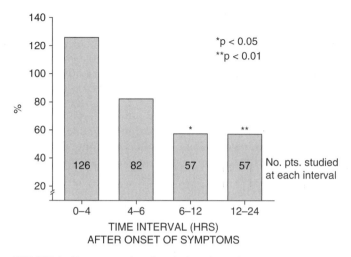

FIGURE 1 Frequency of total occlusion shown by coronary arteriography at various time intervals after onset of symptoms. There is a significant decrease in total occlusion in both the 6- to 12-hour group and the 12- to 24-hour group as compared with the group studied 0 to 4 hours after the onset of symptoms. *Source*: From Ref. 10.

SALVAGE OF JEOPARDIZED MYOCARDIUM

Although the idea of reperfusing infarcting myocardium in the management of AMI was developed in the early 1970s, it had its roots much earlier. In 1935 Tennant and Wiggers (12) demonstrated that immediately after occlusion of a major coronary artery, contraction of the myocardium perfused by the occluded artery became impaired, resulting in systolic bulging of the affected segment within a few seconds. In their words, "occlusion of a main coronary branch is followed by ... progressive enfeeblement of contraction." Reversal of these changes occurred when the ischemic myocardium was reperfused by removing the clamp on the artery. Although determination of the duration of ischemia compatible with myocardial survival was not the principal purpose of their study, Tennant and Wiggers did note that when occlusions were maintained for 23 minutes or longer, recovery of function an hour later was partial at best. While Tennant and Wiggers used a physiologic approach, Blumgart et al. employed pathologic techniques to study the consequences of coronary occlusion. In 1941 they reported that no infarction was noted by gross or microscopic examination in dogs in which reperfusion was carried out up to 20 minutes following occlusion and that beyond that temporal threshold the size of the infarct was roughly proportional to the duration of the occlusion (13). Although these investigators did not consider reperfusion to be a potential therapeutic intervention, both approaches—the physiologic and the pathologic—supported the idea that myocardial damage could be prevented by early reperfusion.

By the middle of the 20th century, it was clear that there were two major causes of early deaths in patients with AMI-primary arrhythmias and failure of the cardiac pump. The incidence of early arrhythmic deaths was markedly reduced when the coronary care unit was developed in the early 1960s (14), resulting in a halving of early mortality. However, despite this notable therapeutic advance, the mortality in AMI secondary to cardiac pump failure remained unacceptably high, approximately 15%, and attention turned to prevention of this complication. Pathologic studies showed that cardiogenic shock and pulmonary edema, the principal manifestations of pump failure, were caused by large infarctions and loss of substantial quantities of functioning myocardium. In addition to the high initial mortality associated with early cardiac failure, patients who survived large infarctions had impaired left ventricular function, and their morbidity and mortality following hospital discharge was much higher than in patients who survived with small infarcts. Given the adverse consequences of large infarction, interest in reducing the extent of MI developed.

In 1969, my colleagues (Maroko, Ross, Sobel, Covell, and Libby) and I proposed that limiting the quantity of myocardium that becomes necrotic after the onset of AMI could prevent the development of cardiac pump failure (15). We began experiments in open-chest anesthetized dogs that showed that ischemic damage secondary to coronary occlusion could be modified (16). Interventions that we had shown in earlier physiologic experiments (17) to augment myocardial oxygen demand, such as β-adrenergic stimulation or those that reduced collateral blood flow, expanded myocardial damage, whereas interventions that lowered oxygen demand, such as β-adrenergic blockade, reduced damage. From our experiments we concluded:

> Of greatest interest, from the clinical point of view, is the finding that the severity and extent of myocardial ischemic injury resulting from coronary occlusion could be radically altered not only by pretreatment of the animal but also by an appropriate intervention as late as 3 hr after the coronary occlusion. This suggests that measures designed for reduction of myocardial oxygen demands and improvement of coronary perfusion, when effected promptly after a patient has been brought to a hospital, might potentially reduce the ultimate size of the infarction. (16)

Early reperfusion was clearly the most potent of the salutary interventions studied. Our group observed that coronary artery reperfusion carried out as late as three hours after occlusion resulted in less pathologic evidence of myocardial necrosis, less myocardial CK depletion, and improved cardiac function than when the occlusion was sustained (18,19) (Fig. 2). In subsequent elegant experiments in dogs in which reperfusion was carried out at varying intervals following coronary occlusion, Reimer et al. showed that infarction followed a "wavefront," commencing with the subendocardium and proceeding to the epicardium (20). Reperfusion within four hours salvaged jeopardized myocardium. By four hours, infarcts were transmural and no myocardial salvage occurred. Clearly, as had been shown earlier by Blumgart et al. (13), the extent of infarction was related inversely to the duration of the ischemia. By 1979, at the time of Rentrop's seminal paper (11), the idea of salvaging jeopardized myocardium by early reperfusion was firmly grounded and ready for clinical testing. Fortunately, by that time the means to do so were at hand.

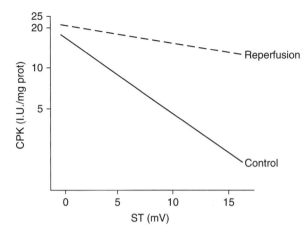

FIGURE 2 ST segment elevation 15 minutes after coronary occlusion (an index of the severity of ischemia) and CPK activity (a marker of myocardial viability) 24 hours later at the same sites. (*Lower line*): Relationship in the control (unreperfused) group. (*Upper line*): Relationship in group with reperfusion 3 hours after occlusion. The slopes of the two are statistically different, showing less CPK depression, i.e. less myocyte necrosis at any given severity of ischemia consequent to reperfusion 3 hours after reocclusion, signifying salvage of jeopardized myocardium. *Abbreviation*: CPK, creatine phosphokinase. *Source*: Modified from Ref. 19.

DEVELOPMENT AND APPLICATIONS OF THROMBOLYTIC AGENTS

In 1933, three years before the above-mentioned experiments of Tennant and Wiggers (12), Tillet and Garner isolated a substance from group A β-hemolytic streptococci that could liquefy plasma clots (21). It was later named streptokinase (SK) and found to activate plasminogen. In 1950, when I was a student at the New York University School of Medicine, Tillet was chair of medicine and I had the opportunity to observe him and his coworker, Sherry, administer purified SK to lyse fibrinous pleural adhesions in patients with empyema (22). Tillett et al. then infused SK intravenously into patients (23). SK was also shown to lyse experimental thrombi when it was infused into rabbits. It then seemed logical to study this agent in patients with AMI. In 1959, Fletcher et al. reported the first randomized trial of intravenous SK versus controls in a total of 30 patients with AMI (24). Although fewer treated than control patients died, the difference was not statistically significant, perhaps because of the trial's small size. Thus, almost a quarter of a century before the critical role of coronary thrombi in the pathogenesis of AMI was settled by Rentrop's (9) and DeWood's (10) angiographic observations, efforts to lyse coronary thrombi in patients had already begun. Fletcher's trial was followed by a number of other small- and intermediate-sized trials with diverse results (25). It was not at all clear from these early trials whether SK actually lysed coronary thrombi. In 1979, in a controlled trial involving 315 patients, a prolonged intravenous infusion of SK was found to reduce the mortality by half (26). It was felt that SK-induced reduction in peripheral resistance and improvement of the microcirculation were responsible, at least in part, for its salutary effect.

Reperfusion of RCA

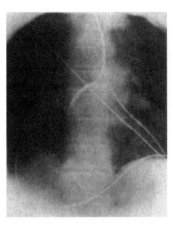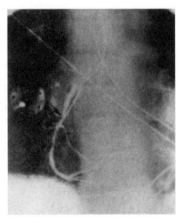

FIGURE 3   (*Left*): Catheter in ostium of occluded right coronary artery. (*Right*): Coronary angiogram showing reperfusion following intracoronary SK. *Source*: From Ref. 27.

It seemed desirable to deliver high concentrations of SK to the region of the presumed thrombus in order to maximize the drug's effectiveness. Accordingly, in 1976, a Soviet team led by Chazov infused SK directly into occluded coronary arteries in two patients with AMI (27). Coronary patency, as established by arteriography, was restored in one patient in whom the duration of occlusion was less than 4 hours (Fig. 3) but not in the other in whom it was 10 hours. For the first time there was direct evidence for early reperfusion. However, this important study, published in Russian, did not gain the attention of Western investigators for several years. In 1979, Rentrop et al. (11) reported successful fibrinolysis in four of five patients by means of intracoronary SK. They laid to rest the question of the thrombotic etiology of AMI when they stated in a follow-up paper in 1981: "Rapid revascularization of occluded vessels and improvement of lumen at the site of high-degree lesions during intracoronary SK infusion imply that fresh thrombotic material was present at the site of obstruction in 21 of 29 patients" (28). In 1981, our group showed that in patients using intracoronary [201]Thallium, the restoration of coronary patency with intracoronary SK actually salvaged jeopardized myocardium (29). Thus, with the use of intracoronary SK, a means to reduce the size of myocardial infarctions in patients was established. In 1982, the FDA approved SK for intracoronary infusion in patients with evolving myocardial infarction.

By 1985, 944 patients had been studied in 9 randomized trials of intracoronary SK (25). Patency was restored in about 75% of patients. Although meta-analysis showed an 18% reduction in mortality, this was not statistically significant, again because of inadequate sample size. It was also recognized that the need for the intracoronary administration of a fibrinolytic, carried out on an emergent basis, would present a logistical obstacle to the widespread application of coronary fibrinolysis and that intravenous administration would be far more preferable. Also, SK had a number of disadvantages: Its potency varied from lot to lot, apparently depending on the method of production. SK was antigenic, and despite efforts at purification, it occasionally caused febrile reactions; hypofibrinogenemia and bleeding also occurred. Therefore, a search for a superior fibrinolytic began.

Human tissue-type plasminogen activator (tPA), a naturally occurring direct activator of fibrinolysis, was isolated from a melanoma tissue culture by Rijken and Collen in 1982 (30). This relatively fibrin-specific fibrinolytic lysed coronary thrombi in dogs without depleting circulating fibrinogen to the extent that SK did. Van de Werf et al. then reported successful lysis of coronary artery thrombi by the intracoronary injection of this melanoma cell–derived tPA in six of seven patients with evolving MI (31). The gene responsible for the synthesis of human tPA was cloned (32), and expressed in Chinese hamster ovary cells, providing enough drug for the intracoronary, and then the intravenous, administration of this agent. Recombinant (rt-PA) was one of the first drugs that emanated from the emerging biotechnology industry.

In 1983, the National Institutes of Health established the Thrombolysis in Myocardial Infarction (TIMI) Study Group. In the first TIMI trial, we compared the effects on coronary patency of the intravenous administration of SK and rt-PA in patients with occluded coronary arteries (33). rt-PA was found to be clearly superior to SK. Sixty-two percent of patients treated with rt-PA achieved coronary patency, compared with only 31% with SK. In patients in whom early reperfusion was achieved, left ventricular ejection fraction and wall motion improved (34) and mortality was reduced (35). The finding in TIMI 1 that coronary arterial patency could be restored in almost two-thirds of patients with AMI by intravenous rt-PA encouraged the use of this route of administration. The shift from intracoronary to intravenously administered fibrinolytic occurred rapidly and was largely complete a decade after Chazov's paper (27). Indeed, despite its great historic importance to the concept of reperfusion of occluded coronary arteries in patients with AMI, intracoronary fibrinolytic therapy was employed for only a relatively brief period.

While intravenous fibrinolytic therapy had been demonstrated to restore arterial patency (33), and early arterial patency to salvage jeopardized myocardium (29), what remained to be shown was that this therapy could actually reduce mortality in patients with AMI. This was strongly suggested by a meta-analysis of 24 randomized trials of intravenous fibrinolytic therapy of approximately 6000 patients that demonstrated a significant 22% reduction of mortality (25). However, what was really needed was a single, adequately sized trial with unambiguous results. The results of such a trial was provided in 1986, when the Gruppo Italiano per lo Studio della Streptochinasi nell'Infarto Miocardico (GISSI) investigators reported a highly significant 18% relative improvement in 21-day mortality among 11,712 subjects who received 1.5 million units of SK intravenously, compared with controls (36). The 47% mortality reduction in patients treated within the first hour of the symptom onset, later termed "the golden hour," was especially dramatic. Remarkably, the initial benefits of SK were sustained after 10 years of follow-up (37). The GISSI trial was the first of many megatrials of fibrinolysis, i.e., trials involving more than 10,000 subjects. These numbers were unheard of in clinical trials in any field and were required to demonstrate mortality differences.

The results of GISSI were soon verified and extended importantly by the International Study of Infarct Survival (ISIS)-2 Collaborative Group (38). These investigators randomized 17,187 subjects with suspected AMI to one of four study arms: SK alone, aspirin alone, combined SK and aspirin, and placebo. The SK and aspirin arms individually showed robust reductions in mortality when compared with placebo, with an additive effect when they were combined (Fig. 4). Indeed, the combination was associated with a 42% reduction in mortality. Thus, by 1988 the benefit of antiplatelet therapy with aspirin as an adjunct to fibrinolytic therapy had

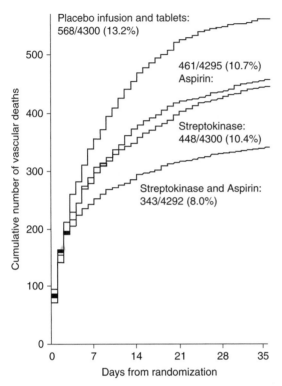

FIGURE 4 Cumulative vascular mortality (deaths from cardiac, cerebral, hemorrhagic, or other known vascular disease) in days 0 to 35 of the ISIS-2. The four curves describe mortality for patients allocated (1) active streptokinase only, (2) active aspirin only, (3) both active treatments, (4) neither. Note that individually, aspirin and streptokinase have a favorable effect of similar magnitudes, and that together the benefits appear additive. *Source*: From Ref. 38.

been firmly established, and aspirin has been used routinely as "foundation therapy" in all subsequent trials of myocardial reperfusion with a lytic or by means of percutaneous intervention. In 1994, the Fibrinolytic Therapy Trialists' (FTT) Collaborative Group published a meta-analysis of 58,600 patients with AMI in randomized trials of fibrinolytic therapy (39). A highly significant 25% mortality reduction in the subset of 45,000 patients with ST-segment elevation MI or bundle branch block was reported. In addition, fibrinolytic therapy reduced left ventricular failure, malignant arrhythmias, cardiogenic shock, and septal rupture.

While TIMI 1 had demonstrated the superiority of intravenous rt-PA compared with SK for opening occluded coronary arteries, there was, at first, considerable debate whether this superiority would translate into a clinical benefit. Accordingly, the first Global Utilization of Streptokinase and Tissue Plasminogen Activator for Occluded Coronary Arteries (GUSTO) trial compared fibrinolytic strategies in more than 41,000 patients with AMI (40). The combination of rt-PA (administered on an accelerated basis to enhance reperfusion) and heparin (to reduce reocclusion) was associated with a relative reduction of 14% in 30-day mortality compared with SK ($P = 0.001$). However, the rt-PA-heparin regimen was associated with two additional intracranial hemorrhages per 1000 patients treated. Nevertheless, the combined outcome of death and nonfatal disabling stroke was still significantly lower with rt-PA than with SK. An important angiographic substudy of GUSTO correlated improved survival with early, more complete vascular patency and improved ventricular function (41).

By the early 1990s, with intravenous fibrinolytic therapy firmly established as routine treatment for patients with AMI, and with a clear-cut enhancement of benefits with earlier treatment, attention turned to reducing the "door-to-needle" time in the emergency department, or commencing therapy even earlier, in the ambulance, or even in the home. The recognition that "time is muscle" was rooted firmly in the experiments of Blumgart et al. (13) in the 1940s, of Reimer and Jennings (20) in the 1970s, and subsequently in numerous clinical trials (36–40). The Myocardial Infarction Triage and Intervention (MITI) trial (42) reemphasized this very important concept. When fibrinolytic therapy was begun within 70 minutes of symptom onset, left ventricular function was better preserved and the mortality was significantly lower than when it was started after 70 minutes. The European Myocardial Infarction Project (EMIP) Group showed that prehospital treatment resulted in a significant 16% reduction in cardiovascular mortality (43).

The search for improved lytic regimens continued. Several new fibrinolytic agents, molecular variants of tPA, with longer half-lives and differing degrees of fibrin specificity, were developed. Two of these, tenecteplase and reteplase, have been approved and are now widely used. Although they have not been shown to reduce mortality when compared with rt-PA, their longer half-lives allows them to be administered as a single or double bolus, thereby greatly facilitating their use, especially under emergency conditions. In addition, there has been considerable effort to enhance adjunctive therapy. The thienopyridine clopidogrel, when added to aspirin, has been shown to sustain fibrinolytic reperfusion in the CLARITY-TIMI 28 trial (44) and to reduce mortality in the COMMIT trial (45), while enoxaparin appears to be superior to unfractionated heparin in STEMI patients receiving fibrinolytic therapy (46).

SURGICAL REPERFUSION

In the 1970s, as coronary bypass surgery became more widely employed, some intrepid surgeons reported emergency surgical revascularization of AMI, with varying results (47,48). With the growing appreciation of the importance of immediate reperfusion, because of time constraints, surgical revascularization was never widely adopted, except in a small minority of patients with AMI who also required emergency surgical repair of ruptured papillary muscle or interventricular septum. Other candidates for this procedure include patients who experienced an infarction in the course of diagnostic catheterization or percutaneous coronary intervention (PCI), as well as those with persistent or recurrent ischemia despite fibrinolysis or PCI.

PERCUTANEOUS PRIMARY CORONARY INTERVENTION

As described above, intravenous fibrinolytic therapy established, without doubt, that early reperfusion favorably influenced the clinical course of AMI. An advantage of this therapy was that it could be administered almost anywhere by virtually any medical practitioner and that no special facilities or equipment were required, except for an electrocardiogram to aid in the diagnosis of ST-elevation MI. However, several deficiencies with this therapy were clearly evident. Patency could be achieved in only about 80% of patients, and full perfusion, i.e., TIMI 3 flow, in only about 60%, even with fibrin-specific lytics. Reocclusion occurred in 5–10% of the arteries in which patency had been achieved. Furthermore, there was the small

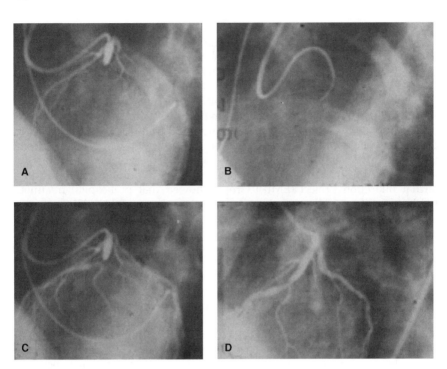

FIGURE 5 Transluminal recanalization with a guidewire. Left coronary artery in LAO half-axis projection. (**A**) Subselective injection into the totally occluded LAD via a Shirey end-hole catheter, (**B**) advancement of a special 0.38″ guidewire beyond the total occlusion, (**C**) visualization of the distal LAD after transluminal recanalization, (**D**) control angiogram of the left coronary artery after five months, showing patency left obstructive lesions in both branches. *Abbreviations*: LAO, left anterior oblique; LAD, left anterior descending. *Source*: From Ref. 11.

but ever-present risk of serious bleeding, including disabling intracerebral hemorrhage.

In 1978, Gruntzig (49) described percutaneous transluminal (balloon) coronary angioplasty (PTCA). The initial goal of this procedure was to relieve coronary arterial narrowing in patients with chronic angina, and it proved to be quite successful in this regard. Long-standing total coronary occlusions in patients with chronic coronary artery disease were difficult to cross with a balloon-tipped catheter. In 1979, Rentrop and coworkers (50) restored patency in the acutely occluded coronary arteries in 7 of 13 patients by passing a guidewire through the thrombus, thereby disrupting it. This was the first example of primary coronary intervention for AMI (Fig. 5). These investigators recognized the potential importance of their observations, stating, "Results of this pilot study suggest that transluminal recanalization in the early phase of acute myocardial infarction might result in limitation of myocardial injury" (50).

In the early 1980s, it was reported that wire-guided balloon angioplasty could achieve more complete reperfusion than intravenous fibrinolytic therapy—even with accelerated rt-PA, heparin, and aspirin. Soon after its introduction, balloon angioplasty was used after failed intracoronary fibrinolysis (rescue angioplasty) (51). This was soon extended to "primary balloon angioplasty" carried out in lieu of fibrinolysis (52).

An obvious disadvantage of primary PCI[a] was that, as in intracoronary fibrinolytic therapy a few years earlier, the great majority of patients did not have access to facilities in which the procedure could be carried out by an experienced team led by an expert operator and conducted on an emergent basis. However, in the 1990s, as elective PCI became more widespread when operators became more skilled, as the equipment improved, and as simple balloon angioplasty made way for stents that were used with aspirin, a thienopyridine and/or a glycoprotein IIb/IIIa inhibitor, each of which improved outcome, primary PCI was employed with increasing frequency. The major advantages of primary PCI were its ability to achieve full reperfusion (TIMI 3 flow) in more than 90% of patients, and to achieve this without incurring the risk of early reocclusion and serious bleeding, especially intracranial hemorrhage. Two important trials that showed the superiority of primary PCI compared with fibrinolysis were the Primary Angioplasty in Myocardial Infarction (PAMI) trial (53) and the GUSTO IIb trial. (54). These provided the stimulus for further investigation and application of this mode of reperfusion therapy.

In 2003, Keeley et al. (55) published a meta-analysis that compared primary PCI with fibrinolysis in 7437 patients in 23 randomized trials. Significant reductions in death, reinfarction, stroke, and hemorrhagic stroke with PCI were noted. This influential meta-analysis underscored the superiority of mechanical versus pharmacological reperfusion, continued the movement to this approach, and led to the development of PCI teams on standby 24 hours a day and 7 days a week. Catheterization facilities were constructed in many community hospitals. Another meta-analysis showed superior results of coronary stenting compared with balloon angioplasty with respect to the need for later revascularization (56). Several trials then compared interhospital transfer for primary PCI with on-site fibrinolysis. Pooled analysis of 2307 patients in four trials showed a significant reduction (6.8 vs. 9.6) in 30-day mortality with PCI following interhospital transfer (57).

Clearly PCI, when it can be carried out quickly after the onset of symptoms by a skilled team, is the reperfusion therapy of choice in AMI patients, especially those presenting more than two or three hours after the onset of symptoms (58). PCI has also been employed frequently to achieve coronary reperfusion when fibrinolysis fails (rescue PCI) or when the patient develops ischemia at rest or with exertion (adjunctive PCI).

CONCLUDING COMMENTS

Current investigations on reperfusion therapy focus on the improvement of systems to provide restoration of blood flow to infarcting myocardium at the earliest possible time, irrespective of whether reperfusion is carried out by fibrinolysis or PCI. There is continuing search for more effective, yet safe, adjunctive pharmacologic agents for both modes of reperfusion, including drugs to reduce reperfusion injury as well as to improve microvascular perfusion. Interventional cardiologists and engineers are seeking ever more easily deliverable stents, and drug-eluting stents are gradually replacing bare metal stents in order to minimize late restenosis.

In retrospect, it is interesting to note that the elucidation of thrombosis in the pathogenesis of AMI, the demonstration that jeopardized myocardium can be salvaged by reperfusion, the discovery and development of fibrinolytic agents, and

---

[a]As coronary stenting replaced balloon angioplasty, the term percutaneous coronary intervention (PCI) replaced percutaneous transluminal balloon angioplasty (PTCA).

the application of PCI to patients with AMI were carried out largely independently of one another. Each of these four areas of investigation may be considered analogous to a separate building block. These four blocks have been assembled to create a "therapeutic structure" that has contributed importantly to the greatly improved management of one of humankind's most serious illnesses.

REFERENCES

1. Osler W. The Principles and Practice of Medicine. New York: D. Appleton, 1892.
2. Krehl L. Die Ekrankungen des Herzmuskels und die Nervosen Herzkrankheiten. Vienna: Alfred Holder, 1901.
3. Obraztov VP, Strazhesko ND. Simptomatiologii I diagnostike tromboza venecchinikh arteril cerdtsa. In: Vorobeva VA, Konchalovski MP, eds. Trudi pervogo sesda rossushkikh terapevtov. Vol 10. Moscow: Tovareschejestvo Tepografre, A.E. Mamontov, 1910:26–43 (Russian).
4. Herrick JB. Clinical features of sudden obstruction of the coronary arteries. JAMA 1912; 59:2015–2022.
5. Friedberg K, Horn H. Acute myocardial infarction not due to coronary artery occlusion. JAMA 1939; 112:1675–1679.
6. Branwood AW, Montgomery GL. Observations on the morbid anatomy of coronary artery disease. Scot Med J 1956; 1:367–375.
7. Roberts WC. Coronary thrombosis and fatal myocardial ischemia. Circulation 1974; 49:1–3.
8. Rentrop KP. Development and pathophysiological basis of thrombolytic therapy in acute myocardial infarction: Part I. 1912–1977—The controversy over the pathogenetic role of thrombus in acute myocardial infarction. J Intervent Cardiol 1998; 11:255–263.
9. Rentrop KP, Blanke H, Karsch KR, et al. Koronarmorphologie und linksventrikulaere. Pumpfunktion im akuten Infarktstadium und ihre Aenderungen im chronischem Stadium. Z Kardiol 1979; 68:335–350.
10. DeWood M, Spores J, Notske R, et al. Prevalence of total coronary occlusion during the early hours of transmural myocardial infarction. N Engl J Med 1980; 303:898–902.
11. Rentrop KP, Blanke H, Wiegand V, et al. Acute myocardial infarction: Intracoronary application of nitroglycerin and streptokinase in combination with transluminal recanalization. Clin Cardiol 1979; 2:354–363.
12. Tennant R, Wiggers CJ. The effect of coronary occlusion on myocardial contraction. Am J Physiol 1935; 112:351–361.
13. Blumgart L, Gilligan R, Schlesinger MJ. Experimental studies on the effect of temporary occlusion of coronary arteries. II. The production of myocardial infarction. Am Heart J 1941; 22:374–389.
14. Julian DG. Treatment of cardiac arrest in acute myocardial ischemia and infarction. Lancet 1961; 11:840–844.
15. Braunwald E, Covell JW, Maroko PR, Ross J Jr. Effect of drugs and of counterpulsation on myocardial oxygen consumption. Circulation 1969; 40(suppl 4):220–228.
16. Maroko PR, Kjekshus JK, Sobel E, et al. Factors influencing infarct size following experimental coronary artery occlusion. Circulation 1971; 43:67–82.
17. Braunwald E. Control of myocardial oxygen consumption: Physiologic and clinical considerations. Am J Cardiol 1971; 27:416–432.
18. Ginks WR, Sybers PR, Maroko PR, et al. Coronary artery reperfusion. II. Reduction of myocardial infarct size at one week after the coronary occlusion. J Clin Invest 1972; 51:2717–2723.
19. Maroko PR, Braunwald E. Modification of myocardial infarction size after coronary occlusion. Ann Intern Med 1973; 79:720–733.
20. Reimer KA, Lower JE, Rasmussen MM, et al. The wavefront phenomenon of ischemic cell death. I. Myocardial infarct size vs. duration of coronary occlusion in dogs. Circulation 1977; 56:786–794.

21. Tillet W, Garner R. The fibrinolytic activity of hemolytic streptococci. J Exp Med 1933; 58:485–502.
22. Tillet W, Sherry S, Read C. The use of streptokinase-streptodornase in the treatment of chronic empyema. J Thorac Surg 1951; 21:325–341.
23. Tillett WS, Johnson AJ, McCarty WR. The intravenous infusion of the streptococcal fibrinolytic principle (streptokinase) into patients. J Clin Invest 1955; 34:169–185.
24. Fletcher AP, Sherry S, Alkjaersig H, et al. The maintenance of a sustained thrombolytic state in man. II. Clinical observations on patients with myocardial infarction and other thromboembolic disorders. J Clin Invest 1959; 38:1111–1119.
25. Yusuf S, Collins R, Peto R, et al. Intravenous and intracoronary fibrinolytic therapy in acute myocardial infarction: overview of results on mortality, reinfarction and side-effects from 33 randomized controlled trials. Eur Heart J 1985; 6:556–585.
26. European Cooperative Study Group. Streptokinase in acute myocardial infarction. N Engl J Med 1979; 301:797–802.
27. Chazov EI, Mateeva LS, Mazaev AV. Intracoronary administration of fibrinolysin in acute myocardial infarction. Ter Arkh 1976; 48:8–19.
28. Rentrop P, Blanke H., Karsch KR, et al. Selective intracoronary thrombolysis in acute myocardial infarction and unstable angina pectoris. Circulation 1981; 63:307–317.
29. Markis JE, Malagold M, Parker JA, et al. Myocardial salvage after intracoronary thrombolysis with streptokinase in acute myocardial infarction: assessment of intra-coronary thallium-201. N Engl J Med 1981; 305:777–782.
30. Rijken DC, Collen D. Purification and characterization of the plasminogen activator secreted by human melanoma cells in culture. J Biol Chem 1981; 256:7035–7041.
31. Van de Werf F, Ludbrook PA, Berhmann SR, et al. Coronary thrombolysis with tissue-type plasminogen activator in patients with evolving myocardial infarction. N Engl J Med 1984; 310:609–613.
32. Pennica D, Holmes WE, Kohr WJ, et al. Cloning and expression of human tissue-type plasminogen activator cDNA in *E. coli*. Nature 1983; 301:214–221.
33. The TIMI Study Group. The thrombolysis in myocardial infarction (TIMI) trial. Phase I findings. N Engl J Med 1985; 312:932–936.
34. Sheehan FH, Braunwald E, Canner P, et al. The effect of intravenous thrombolytic therapy on left ventricular function: A report on tissue-type plasminogen activator and streptokinase from the Thrombolysis in Myocardial Infarction (TIMI Phase I) Trial. Circulation 1987; 75:817–829.
35. Dalen JE, Gore JM, Braunwald E, et al. Six and twelve-month follow-up of the Phase I Thrombolysis in Myocardial Infarction (TIMI) Trial. Am J Cardiol 1988; 62:179–185.
36. Gruppo Italiano per lo Studio della Streptochinasi nell'Infarto Miocardico (GISSI). Effectiveness of intravenous thrombolytic treatment in acute myocardial infarction. Lancet 1986; 1:397–402.
37. Fanzosi MG, Santoro E, De Vita C, et al. Ten-year follow-up of the first megatrial testing thrombolytic therapy in patients with acute myocardial infarction: results of the Gruppo Italiano per lo Studio della Sobrevivenza nell'Infarto-1 Study. Circulation 1998; 98: 2659–2665.
38. ISIS-2 Collaborative Group. Randomized trial of intravenous streptokinase, oral aspirin, both, or neither among 17,187 cases of suspected acute myocardial infarction: ISIS-2. Lancet 1988; 1:349–360.
39. Fibrinolytic Therapy Trialists' (FTT) Collaborative Group. Indications for fibrinolytic therapy in suspected acute myocardial infarction: collaborative overview of early mortality and major morbidity results from all randomized trials of more than 1000 patients. Lancet 1994; 343:311–322.
40. The GUSTO investigators. An international randomized trial comparing four throm-bolytic strategies for acute myocardial infarction. N Engl J Med 1993; 329:673–682.
41. The GUSTO Angiographic Investigators. The comparative effects of tissue plasmi-nogen activator, streptokinase, or both on coronary artery patency, ventricular function and survival after acute myocardial infarction. N Engl J Med 1993; 329:1615–1622.

42. Weaver WD, Cerqueira M, Hallstrom AP, et al. Prehospital-initiated vs. hospital-initiated thrombolytic therapy. The Myocardial Infarction Triage and Intervention Trial. JAMA 1993; 270:1211–1216.
43. The European Myocardial Infarction Project Group. Prehospital thrombolytic therapy in patients with suspected acute myocardial infarction. N Engl J Med 1993; 329:383–389.
44. Sabatine MS, Cannon CP, Gibson CM, et al. Addition of clopidogrel to aspirin and fibrinolytic therapy for myocardial infarction with ST-segment elevation. N Engl J Med 2005; 352:1179–1189.
45. Chen ZM, Jiang LX, Chen YP, et al. Addition of clopidogrel to aspirin in 45,852 patients with acute myocardial infarction: randomised placebo-controlled trial. Lancet 2005; 366:1607–1621.
46. Sabatine MS, Morrow DA, Montalescot G, et al. Angiographic and clinical outcomes in patients receiving low-molecular weight heparin versus unfractionated heparin in ST-elevation myocardial infarction treated with fibrinolytics in the CLARITY-TIMI 28 trial. Circulation 2005; 112:3846–3854.
47. Cheanvechai C, Effler DB, Loop FD, et al. Emergency myocardial revascularization. Am J Cardiol 1973; 32:901–908.
48. Berg R, Everhart FJ, Duvoisin G, et al. Operation for acute coronary occlusion. Am Surg 1976; 42:517–521.
49. Gruntzig A. Transluminal dilatation of coronary artery stenosis. Lancet 1978; 1:263.
50. Rentrop KP, Blanke H, Karsch KR, et al. Initial experience with transluminal recanalization of the recently occluded infarct-related coronary artery in acute myocardial infarction—comparison with conventionally treated patients. Clin Cardiol 1979; 2:92–105.
51. Meyer J, Merx W, Dorr R, et al. Successful treatment of acute myocardial infarction shock by combined percutaneous transluminal coronary revascularization (PTCR) and percutaneous coronary angioplasty (PTCA). Am Heart J 1982; 103:132–134.
52. Papapietro SE, MacLean WAH, Stanley AWH Jr, et al. Percutaneous transluminal coronary angioplasty in acute myocardial infarction. J Am Coll Cardiol 1983; 1:580.
53. Grines CL, Browne KF, Marco J, et al. A comparison of immediate angioplasty with thrombolytic therapy for acute myocardial infarction. The Primary Angioplasty in Myocardial Infarction Group. N Engl J Med 1993; 328:673–679.
54. GUSTO IIb Angioplasty Substudy Investigators. A clinical trial comparing primary coronary angioplasty with tissue plasminogen activator for acute myocardial infarction. The Global Use of Strategies to open Occluded Coronary Arteries in Acute Coronary Syndromes (GUSTO IIb) Angioplasty Substudy Investigators. N Engl J Med 1997; 336:1621–1628.
55. Keeley EC, Boura JA, Grines CL. Primary angioplasty versus intravenous thrombolytic therapy for acute myocardial infarction: A quantitative review of 23 randomized trials. Lancet 2003; 361:13–20.
56. Zhu MM, Feit A, Chadow H, et al. Primary stent implantation compared with primary balloon angioplasty for acute myocardial infarction. A meta analysis of randomized clinical trials. Am J Cardiol 2001; 88:297–301.
57. Lane GE, Holmes DR Jr. Primary percutaneous coronary intervention in the management of acute myocardial infarction. In: Zipes DR, Libby P, Bonow RO, et al., eds. Braunwald's Heart Disease. 7th ed. Philadelphia: WB Saunders, 2005:1227–1240.
58. Antman EM, Anbe DT, Armstrong P.W, et al. ACC/AHA guidelines for the management of patients with ST-elevation myocardial infarction—executive summary. A report of the American College of Cardiology/American Heart Association Task Force on Practice Guidelines. J Am Coll Cardiol 2004; 44:671–719.

2 Pathophysiology of Myocardial Infarction

Sameer Amin and Prediman K. Shah
Atherosclerosis Research Center, Division of Cardiology, Department of Medicine, Burns and Allen Research Institute, Cedars Sinai Medical Center and David Geffen School of Medicine at UCLA, Los Angeles, California, U.S.A.

INTRODUCTION

Acute myocardial infarction (AMI) is the most common cause of death in the industrialized world, responsible for between 500,000 and 700,000 deaths per year in the United States alone. Nearly one-half of these deaths occur in the prehospital setting. Several studies have shown that in 40% to 60% of cases, the first clinical manifestation of coronary artery disease is AMI or sudden death. With a few exceptions (such as vasculitis, dissection, embolism, spasm), AMI results from an abrupt occlusion of an epicardial coronary artery; this occlusion is due to a disrupted atherosclerotic plaque with a superimposed thrombus. Downstream embolization of the epicardial coronary artery thrombus into the microcirculation may also contribute to myocyte necrosis, especially in patients with subtotal occlusion.

Following abrupt coronary artery occlusion, myocyte necrosis begins within 20 to 30 minutes, starting in the subendocardium, where metabolic needs are high and collateral flow is inadequate. With continued coronary occlusion, a wavefront of myocyte necrosis advances toward the epicardium in a time-dependent fashion. Unless coronary blood flow to the threatened myocardial segment is restored, transmural necrosis may be completed within three to six hours.

CORONARY THROMBOSIS WITHOUT PLAQUE RUPTURE

Necropsy studies have demonstrated that a vast majority of coronary thrombi overlie atherosclerotic plaques with a fissured or ruptured fibrous cap; however, in 20% to 40% of instances, cap rupture is not found (1–5). In these cases, superficial endothelial erosion of the plaque surface can often be detected underneath the thrombus. These superficial plaque erosions are most common in smokers, women, and young victims of sudden death. Although the exact trigger for thrombosis under these circumstances has not been discovered, there are fundamental differences between such plaques and those seen in rupture. The lesions associated with erosion tend to have a proteoglycan-rich matrix instead of the thrombogenic lipid core found in most ruptured plaques. In addition, there is a lesser degree of inflammation associated with these atheromas.

Currently, there are three probable, not necessarily mutually exclusive, explanations for thrombosis over superficial erosions. The most evident contributing factor is the already established increased systemic likelihood of thrombosis in women and smokers. It is possible that patients who suffer from myocardial infarction (MI) without rupture have enhanced platelet adhesion or aggregation, protein C deficiency or dysfunction, an increased level of tissue factor, or another similar preexisting thrombogenic state predisposing them to thrombosis with even simple erosion (5,6). Also, plaque erosions themselves may contribute to thrombosis, since endothelial apoptosis has been noted to cause increased local thrombogenicity. Another explanation implicates activated circulating leukocytes. By shedding microparticles, activated leukocytes may transfer tissue factor to adherent platelets, thus acting as mobile sources of tissue factor. This would allow atherosclerotic plaques lacking a large lipid core (and therefore a vast pool of tissue factor) to thrombose over simple erosion (7,8).

In addition to superficial erosions causing acute MI, there are reports of erosions in calcified nodules within atherosclerotic lesions triggering thrombosis and subsequent arterial lumen blockage. This, however, is a relatively rare cause of acute thrombosis.

DETERMINANTS OF PLAQUE RUPTURE AND THROMBOSIS: STENOSIS, PLAQUE COMPOSITION, MORPHOLOGICAL FEATURES

Stenosis

Traditionally, cardiology teachings preached progressive stenosis as a main determinant of thrombosis and AMI. Without a full understanding of inflammation's key role in atherosclerotic rupture, an intuitive hypothesis would equate a bulky plaque to a vulnerable plaque. Multiple analyses over the last 20 years have diminished the role of luminal narrowing in plaque vulnerability. Retrospective studies of serial angiograms and prospective angiographic data indicate that two-thirds of patients suffering an AMI had a less than 70% diameter stenosis (frequently <50% diameter stenosis) at the culprit site, in the months leading up to the event (5,9–17). Stress testing in patients with stable angina has also contributed to mounting evidence; surprisingly, stress myocardial perfusion scintigraphy does not accurately predict the future site of AMI (18).

There are a number of reasons why atherosclerotic rupture and thrombosis occur more often in arteries shown to have only mild to moderate stenosis on previous angiography. However, three contributors to this paradox can be considered confounding factors. Because there are a larger number of mild to moderate regions of narrowing in comparison with areas of severe stenoses, one would expect there to be a larger number of ruptures associated with minor stenoses. For every 5 to 10 minor stenoses in a coronary artery disease patient, on average, only one severe stenosis is found. It is possible that the shear number of minor stenoses, and therefore ruptures, masks a higher likelihood of rupture in severe stenosis (19). In addition to the inadequacy of raw numbers, underestimations inherent to angiography may also contribute to the confusion. Since angiography compares an alleged diseased segment of artery to supposed normal caliber segments, this test assumes that there is no atherosclerotic narrowing in the reference segment. In many cases, patients have diffuse atherosclerotic disease, invalidating the assumption of a normal reference and thus leading to an underestimation of the degree of stenosis (19). Yet another underestimation may occur when likening plaque rupture to clinical events. Because a minor stenosis does not necessitate the creation of collaterals to supply chronically ischemic tissue, an abrupt rupture would most certainly cause infarction. On the other hand, rupture of a chronically severe stenosis may not cause an acute clinical event due to continued perfusion from collateral vessels. It is possible that despite having similar or greater rates of rupture, plaque rupture in severe stenosis is missed because of clinical silence (19).

Though there may be a few confounding factors, an explanation for the association of a higher rate of rupture with mild to moderate stenosis can be sought by examining the plaques themselves. Mild to moderately narrow lesions tend to have more characteristics of a vulnerable plaque than those that more completely block the artery; generally, such atherosclerotic plaques have a larger lipid core as well as a greater degree of inflammation (19). In addition, vulnerable plaques are more likely to grow by positive remodeling, an outward adventitial expansion that does not cause a significant decrease in lumen diameter with further enlargement (20). Intravascular studies have corroborated this observation by demonstrating outward expansion sites responsible for unstable angina and inward or negative remodeling in association with patients suffering from stable angina (21,22).

While the plaque itself gives us vital insight into the relationship between stenosis and the likelihood of rupture, the physics of blood flow also produces compelling logic. Laplace's law states that a comparably higher luminal diameter produces more wall stress. The larger lumen allowed by a mild to moderately narrowed artery subjects the plaque to a stronger circumferential stress. This increased stress may add to the likelihood of fibrous cap rupture (23).

Plaque Composition

Whereas the role of stenosis as a determinant of plaque rupture can be debated, there is a definitive collection of attributes that create a propensity for rupture. This set of traits allows a clear distinction between stable atherosclerosis and vulnerable plaques. The characteristics can best be divided into those involving composition and those relating to the morphology of the lesion.

One main element of composition that defines a vulnerable lesion is the acellular lipid-rich core. It has been known for some time that a lipid core contains multiple factors promoting thrombosis. The extracellular lipids, a mixture of free cholesterol, cholesterol crystals, and cholesterol esters, are bathed in prothrombotic factors including tissue factor. Further still, oxidized lipids themselves promote platelet activation (24–28). Aside from contributing to thrombosis and infarction once the plaque has ruptured, the lipid core also makes the atheroma more friable. This can be demonstrated through computer modeling (23,29–32). A large atheroma, made unwieldy by an eccentric lipid core, redistributes wall stress to the shoulders of the lesion. This change in blood flow by the luminal irregularity translates to a greater likelihood of rupture, as breaks in the fibrous cap occur preferentially (in up to 60% of cases) in the shoulder regions.

Atheromas with a core bulky enough to produce such irregularity are created by the extracellular lipid's tendency to support its own expansion. Macrophage apoptosis is the main contributor to expulsion of additional cholesterol into the extracellular lipid core. Since foam cells are regulated by a caspase-based apoptotic system spurred by cholesterol, the larger the core grows the more the apoptosis, which in turn causes cholesterol release (33,34). It has also been suggested that red blood cell membranes promote the release of cholesterol into extracellular space (35). This implies that subocclusive lesions undergoing repeated cap rupture and thrombosis might actually bolster their own vulnerability through intraplaque hemorrhage. Additionally, larger plaques likely support lipid core growth via an intensification of vasculogenesis, leading to wider exposure to red blood cells. Such self-propelling vulnerability sets up a vicious cycle that can only end in occlusive thrombus: the larger and more lipid-rich the core, the more likely it is to expand; with greater expansion, the plaque is more likely to rupture.

In addition to forces exerted on the core, composition of the atheroma's exterior also dictates plaque vulnerability. The fibrous cap undergoes significant change, as the plaque grows unstable. Of the modifications, reduction in collagen content is perhaps the key alteration. After years of study, researchers have redefined the fibrous cap as a dynamic structure with a finely tuned balance of extracellular matrix (36). Since interstitial collagen provides the main scaffolding for the fibrous cap, collagen shelters the thrombogenic lipid core. The depletion of fibrillar collagens is an important event in creation of a vulnerable plaque. An imbalance in synthesis and degradation is the proximal cause of cap thinning. This imbalance is created by a decrease in the rate of collagen synthesis and a concurrent increase in the rate of collagen breakdown (5).

Matrix synthesis is slowed in vulnerable plaques through two main mechanisms: increased smooth muscle cell (SMC) death and release of cytokines by activated inflammatory cells. Because SMCs are the main factories for the production of collagen, elastin, and proteoglycans, the fibrous cap's structure is maintained by the presence and activity of SMCs. Vulnerable plaques are unusual because they contain few SMCs, limiting the atheroma's ability to replete matrix (37,38). The likely reason for this anomaly is increased SMC death via apoptosis. There are several arguments bolstering this hypothesis. Recent studies have identified significant players of the apoptotic pathway within atherosclerotic plaques (39–50). Investigators have also determined that oxidized lipids, epidermal growth factor–like domain of tenascin-C (secreted by macrophages and exposed by metalloproteinases), and apo C1–enriched HDL have the ability to stimulate SMC apoptosis (51,52). This indicates that vulnerable plaques contain the constituents of cell death signaling and are stimulated to proceed down the apoptotic pathway by factors that grow in intensity as the plaque spirals deeper toward rupture. Aside from reducing the number of SMCs available for collagen production, activated T-cells also affect matrix synthesis by producing interferon gamma. In vitro studies have shown decreased expression of the collagen gene with interferon gamma treatment (48). Additional studies in mice have shown similar evidence of a connection between interferon gamma and synthesis modulation. Mice, genetically engineered to be especially susceptible to atherosclerosis, with an inactivated interferon gamma receptor, accumulate collagen in their atherosclerotic plaques (53). Thus, the SMCs that are able to evade apoptosis in a vulnerable plaque may have difficulty maintaining their collagen backbone of fibrous caps.

While matrix synthesis is decelerated, breakdown of the collagen scaffold is hastened in vulnerable plaques. Normally, a delicate balance is struck between matrix-degrading metalloproteinases (MMPs) and tissue inhibitors of metalloproteinases (TIMPs), which ensures a healthy turnover of collagen. Atherosclerotic plaques create a unique environment for matrix metabolism; inflammatory cells within the lesion drive breakdown of the fibrous cap through a multitude of proteases such as cysteine and aspartate proteases, proteinases including cathepsins, tryptase, chymase, and the primary modulator, a family of MMPs (54,55). The effect of these enzymes can be influenced at several points, anywhere from formation to action. Using MMPs as an example, initial regulation occurs through alteration of gene transcription. Inflammation and oxidative stress are the chief processes affecting gene expression. Oxidized lipids, reactive oxygen species, chlamydial heat shock protein, CD-40 ligand, inflammatory cytokines, tenascin-C, and hemodynamic stress are just a few of the transcription-modulating factors recruited to increase production of MMPs (56–69). Consequently, these factors are abundant in vulnerable plaques. After transcription, the next major step of regulation is extracellular activation. MMPs are secreted by macrophages, foam cells, and SMCs (minor contributor) in a zymogen form (56–58,70–77). This inactive enzyme can be activated by a myriad of chemokines, including urokinase-type plasminogen activator (uPA), trypsin, and chymase. As is the pattern, the activating substances are secreted by inflammatory cells (uPA by macrophages and trypsin and chymase by mast cells) and are found in the highest concentration in vulnerable plaques. Yet another point of regulation is the inhibition of metalloproteinase. TIMP is secreted to moderate the activity of MMP (61). In the environment of escalating inflammation, collagen destruction, and consequent vulnerability, TIMP activity is pathologically diminished.

The confluent effect of upregulated matrix degradation and downregulated matrix synthesis leads to a thinned fibrous cap. This, in addition to a large, soft, acellular lipid-rich core (often over 40% of plaque volume), is a principal characteristic of plaques susceptible to rupture and thrombosis. The other major element of plaque composition, which defines vulnerable atherosclerotic lesions, is increased inflammation. A plaque on the brink of rupture tends to have increased macrophage density and activity in its fragile fibrous cap, elevated overall activated T-cell infiltration, and macrophage, T-cell, and mast cell permeation of the adventitia (1,5,9,37,78–83). Penetration of atheroma with inflammatory cells, observed by pathologists and confirmed by clinical studies, has firmly solidified inflammation at the forefront of AMI pathophysiology.

Evidence has emerged that relates circulating lipopolysaccharide, a systemic pro-inflammatory substance, to the development of atherosclerosis (84–86). Toll-like receptor (TLR) signaling is thought to be the link between stimulus and response. TLRs are a family of pathogen-recognizing receptors found on immunocompetent cells like macrophages, dendritic cells, neutrophils, and endothelial cells. After binding a ligand (such as an epitope on oxidized lipids or *Chlamydia pneumoniae*), the TLRs activate a phosphorylation cascade, leading to increased expression of immune-responsive genes capable of spurring inflammation (87). The transcribed proteins range from vascular adhesion molecule-1 (VCAM-1) to chemokines like monocyte chemoattractant protein-1 (MCP-1) and cytokines like colony-stimulating factor (M-CSF) (88). The current synthesis of inflammation's role in plaque vulnerability tells a compelling story. Endothelial cells and local monocytes bind pathogen-like patterns on passing inflammatory substances, triggering TLR activation and transcription of molecules such as VCAM-1 and MCP-1. MCP-1 attracts additional inflammatory cells, while VCAM-1 provides them an avenue for entry into the vascular wall. At this point, monocytes are activated by M-CSF, prompting them to secrete enzymes such as MMPs, tryptase, and chymase. As explained above, the proteinases thin the fibrous cap and lead to plaque rupture. Consequently, high levels of inflammatory cells are often found near sites of fibrous cap rupture, the lipid core, and areas of adventitial neovascularization (89–94). This is just one possible pathway demonstrating a method by which inflammation can lead to plaque rupture. With the discovery of new methods of inflammation-mediated lesion destabilization, recent laboratory and clinical evidence suggests that inflammatory and immune mechanisms are key characteristics of atheroma vulnerability.

Plaque Morphology

Although the composition of atherosclerotic plaques plays an important role in driving the lesion toward rupture and thrombosis, a description of the vulnerable plaque is not complete without a discussion of its morphological features. One of the first characteristics noted by histopathologists is the relatively large volume of the plaques that tend to rupture. Paradoxically, these bulkier atheromas do not cause greater luminal narrowing. Vulnerable plaques tend to produce less luminal stenosis. Through outward (positive) remodeling, unstable lesions can minimize arterial blockage despite growing to a larger volume than stable plaques (20). Instead of causing vessel contraction (negative inward remodeling), unstable lesions are defined by their adventitial expansion. This observation has prompted scientists to look beyond degree of stenosis for identification of at-risk patients.

Another morphological feature found in vulnerable plaques is adventitial neovascularization. The process of neovascularization is likely intertwined with inflammation and chemokine release. Culprit lesions tend to show increased vascularity of the adventitial tissue, perhaps providing an additional route for inflammatory cell entry into the plaque (5,90–96). Rupture of the newly formed vessels exposes the interior of the atheroma to red blood cell membranes, perhaps increasing accumulation of extracellular lipid in the plaque's core. As described earlier, a richer lipid core pushes the atheroma toward rupture. Greater neovascularity may also lead to atherosclerotic hemorrhage, a process that can prompt plaque rupture and thrombosis.

In the past decade, scientists have shown that a stable plaque is fundamentally different from a vulnerable lesion. An unstable plaque can be described on the basis of composition and morphology. With regard to composition, the plaque contains a large lipid-rich core, is covered by a thin fibrous cap with reduced collagen content, and demonstrates a higher degree of inflammation with greater macrophage activity in the cap, increased activated T-cell infiltration, and adventitial invasion by inflammatory cells. Morphologically, the vulnerable plaque is characterized by a large volume, outward remodeling, and increased adventitial neovascularity (5,9,78,95).

TRIGGERS FOR PLAQUE RUPTURE AND SUBSEQUENT THROMBOSIS

With the description of vulnerable plaques complete, a proper discussion of MI pathophysiology must turn to the inciting factors propelling rupture. Some of these triggers have already become ingrained in the public conscious; either a period of unaccustomed physical activity, sudden severe emotional trauma, illicit drugs like cocaine and amphetamines, or sexual activity may be the event that finally pushes a vulnerable plaque to rupture. Other provocations may not be as intuitive. Exposures to cold temperatures and acute infection have both been implicated in MI as associated occurrences. Though a myriad of triggers have been documented, most times, sudden rupture occurs spontaneously (97–105).

Regardless of how plaque rupture arises, the clinical significance is often based on the process of thrombosis. While a clinically silent rupture is known to occur, the rate at which it does is somewhat surprising. In 40% to 80% of MIs, clinically insignificant plaque ruptures have been found in addition to the rupture responsible for the infarction (106). Just as certain characteristics describe an atherosclerotic lesion that is more likely to rupture, there are traits that increase the likelihood a ruptured plaque will thrombose. Similar to atherogenesis and plaque rupture, inflammation is critical in promoting thrombogenicity. Apoptosis of macrophages and platelet activation are just a few of the notable results of inflammation. Atheromas with lipid-rich cores tend to accumulate tissue factor, a substance that often produces thrombosis when coupled with activated platelets (28). Another noteworthy contributor to thrombosis is smoking. Smokers have a higher risk of MI due to promotion of inflammation and tissue factor accumulation (107).

PLAQUE STABILIZATION VS. REGRESSION

At the time of MI, effective treatments for reversal of ischemia are limited to reperfusion. During this acute period, focus is placed on stenotic arteries and the need to reperfuse dying muscle. Our new understanding of plaque vulnerability will hopefully afford the opportunity to attack specific points of pathophysiology, thus averting the need to treat stenosis acutely. The true goal of treatment should be to target the traits leading to plaque instability, instead of seeking regression of any and all atheromas. Plaque stabilization, bolstering the plaque against rupture and thrombosis, may be the key to future prevention of MI and may also explain many of the benefits seen from current treatments.

Multiple studies have shown lipid-lowering therapies to cause a decrease in mortality and morbidity that is disproportionate to the associated increase in luminal diameter (108). Such findings have inspired a search for alternate sources of benefit. One explanation for the discordance may be a link between lipid lowering and the degree of inflammation. Animal studies have shown that low-lipid diets produce diminished MMP-1 expression, increased collagen, and reduced macrophage accumulation, thus stabilizing the vulnerable plaque (109–111). Treatment of rabbits with statins and inhibitors of acyl-CoA cholesterol acyl-transferase has demonstrated atheromas with less MMPs, tissue factor, and macrophages (112–114). Statins may also decrease the chance of thrombosis after plaque rupture by affecting endothelial cell function. By promoting nitric oxide synthesis and shifting the balance between tissue plasminogen activator and plasminogen activator inhibitor, statins may be able to prevent thrombus and encourage clot lysis when plaques rupture (115–118).

Recent advances in cardiology have altered the way stenosis is viewed. The focus has changed from ridding vessels of atherosclerosis to stabilizing atheromas that are already present. By attacking factors that contribute to vulnerability, calls for regression can be muted. The phenotypes of a plaque at risk (the large acellular lipid core, thin fibrous cap, positive remodeling, inflammatory cell infiltration, and increased neovascularity) have already been targeted, with the goal of converting unstable plaques into secure lesions. Angiographic evidence suggests that this strategy has been utilized, oddly enough, without foresight. Though unanticipated, statins seem to reduce the level of inflammation, thus bracing lesions against rupture. Evidence shows that statins have an anti-inflammatory effect on even nonvascular disease processes such as multiple sclerosis and Alzheimer's disease. Just like statins, fibric acid derivatives also have secondary repercussions outside of inhibiting triglyceride synthesis. Anti-inflammatory benefits are produced via direct activation of peroxismal proliferation activating receptor (PPAR-α) (119–122).

NOVEL THERAPEUTICS: APOLIPOPROTEIN ADMINISTRATION AND VACCINATION

As our understanding of the pathophysiology of MI grows, the sophistication of drug targeting and efficacy increases. Though the effectiveness of statin therapy cannot be denied, the reduction in incidence of acute coronary syndrome has not eliminated AMI. Sixty to seventy percent of morbidity and mortality from coronary artery disease still remains despite modern lipid-lowering therapy. New interventions, based on pathophysiology, aim to bolster our armamentarium.

Key characteristics of the vulnerable plaque are the fibrous cap collagen content and lipid-rich core (which can compose up to 40% of the plaque volume). Since high-density lipoprotein (HDL) is a moderator of fatty streak formation, the HDL is a logical choice to reduce the content of lipid within a plaque. By promoting cholesterol efflux, HDL elevation is a potential boon to atherosclerosis management. Aside from observational studies showing a relationship between high levels of HDL and lower incidence of acute coronary syndromes, an abundance of experimental evidence outlines how HDL may stabilize an atherosclerotic plaque (123,124). HDL has a potent anti-oxidant and anti-inflammatory effect that decreases SMC apoptosis, thus stabilizing the fibrous cap (125,126). In particular, apolipoprotein A-1, which recovers cholesterol from vessels, lowers macrophage content and reduces plaque cholesterol in animal experiments (127–129). Studies have also discovered routes of inflammation inhibition; it is possible that HDL encourages plaque stability by reducing the quantity of cytokine-induced monocyte adhesion receptors and decreasing tumor necrosis factor release (125,130,131). Novel therapeutics will soon bring this benchwork to the bedside. Experimental ideas include direct parenteral administration of the apolipoprotein A-1 component of HDL and injection of recombinant apo A-1$_{milano}$-phospholipid complex. Apo A-1$_{milano}$ is a naturally occurring mutant, with an Arg-173 to Cys substitution, present in populations blessed with a low incidence of MI. This variant of apolipoprotein A-1 has been shown to reduce plaque cholesterol by 40% and macrophage content by 46% with parenteral administration to apo E knockout mice (127). Of perhaps even greater import, apo A-1$_{milano}$ can theoretically be used as an acute treatment to lower lipid and macrophage content, stabilizing vulnerable plaques during acute MI (129).

Apolipoprotein treatment represents just one possibility for future atheroprotection. Vaccination has also garnered a great deal of attention as a new treatment. Autoantigens, such as oxidized low-density lipoproteins, β2 glycoprotein 1, and heat shock protein 60, incite an atherogenic immune response in both human and animal studies (132). Identification of apolipoprotein B antigens that trigger immunotolerance may allow future modulation of inflammation in the vulnerable plaque. Recently, scientists have generated mucosal immunity to heat shock protein 65/60 and β2 glycoprotein 1, demonstrating atheroprotection through immune modulation (132). Similar adaptive responses have been shown with oxidized low-density lipoprotein–related epitopes (132). Such data suggest that a vaccination approach to atherosclerosis may be a valuable therapeutic paradigm.

CONCLUSION

MI is the leading cause of death in the industrialized world. As our understanding of the disease continues to expand, we come closer to using pathophysiology to target treatment. Concepts such as plaque rupture and "vulnerability" have slowly replaced those of inert atherosclerosis and gradual stenosis. The expansive activities of endothelial cells, SMCs, and monocytes have transformed the image of atheroma into that of an active lesion, with multiple junctures susceptible to intervention. Cardiologists have now outlined a likely course of acute coronary syndrome (ACS): creation of a vulnerable atherosclerotic plaque, plaque rupture, coronary thrombosis superimposed on the lesion, and extension of thrombosis into the plaque with upstream propagation. By focusing on stabilizing lesions, the ultimate goal of eliminating MI in the modern world may yet be attainable.

REFERENCES

1. Virmani R, Burke AP, Farb A. Plaque rupture and plaque erosion. Thromb Haemost 1999; 82(suppl 1):1–3.
2. Davies MJ, Thomas A. Thrombosis and acute coronary-artery lesions in sudden cardiac ischemic death. N Engl J Med 1984; 310:1137–1140.
3. Burke AP, Farb A, Malcom GT, et al. Coronary risk factors and plaque morphology in men with coronary disease who died suddenly. N Engl J Med 1997; 336:1276–1282.
4. Farb A, Burke AP, Tang AL, et al. Coronary plaque erosion without rupture into a lipid core. A frequent cause of coronary thrombosis in sudden coronary death. Circulation 1996; 93:1354–1363.
5. Shah PK. Pathophysiology of coronary thrombosis: role of plaque rupture and erosion. Prog Cardiovasc Dis 2002; 44:357–368.
6. Laszik ZG, Zhou XJ, Ferrell GL, et al. Down-regulation of endothelial expression of endothelial cell protein C receptor and thrombomodulin in coronary atherosclerosis. Am J Pathol 2001; 159:797–802.
7. Rauch U, Bonderman D, Bohrmann B, et al. Transfer of tissue factor from leukocytes to platelets is mediated by CD15 and tissue factor. Blood 2000; 96:170–175.
8. Mallat Z, Benamer H, Hugel B, et al. Elevated levels of shed membrane microparticles with procoagulant potential in the peripheral circulating blood of patients with acute coronary syndromes. Circulation 2000; 101:841–843.
9. Falk E, Shah PK, Fuster V. Coronary plaque disruption. Circulation 1995; 92:657–671.
10. Ambrose JA, Winters SL, Stern A, et al. Angiographic morphology and the pathogenesis of unstable angina pectoris. J Am Coll Cardiol 1985; 5:609–616.
11. Ambrose JA, Winters SL, Arora RR, et al. Coronary angiographic morphology in myocardial infarction: a link between the pathogenesis of unstable angina and myocardial infarction. J Am Coll Cardiol 1985; 6:1233–1238.
12. Ambrose JA, Winters SL, Arora RR, et al. Angiographic evolution of coronary artery morphology in unstable angina. J Am Coll Cardiol 1986; 7:472–478.
13. Ambrose JA, Monsen C. Significance of intraluminal filling defects in unstable angina. Am J Cardiol 1986; 57:1003–1004.
14. Little WC, Constantinescu M, Applegate RJ, et al. Can coronary angiography predict the site of a subsequent myocardial infarction in patients with mild-to-moderate coronary artery disease? Circulation 1988; 78:1157–1166.
15. Hackett D, Davies G, Maseri A. Pre-existing coronary stenoses in patients with first myocardial infarction are not necessarily severe. Eur Heart J 1988; 9:1317–1323.
16. Giroud D, Li JM, Urban P, et al. Relation of the site of acute myocardial infarction to the most severe coronary arterial stenosis at prior angiography. Am J Cardiol 1992; 69:729–732.
17. Brown G, Albers JJ, Fisher LD, et al. Regression of coronary artery disease as a result of intensive lipid-lowering therapy in men with high levels of apolipoprotein B. N Engl J Med 1990; 323:1289–1298.
18. Naqvi TZ, Hachamovitch R, Berman D, et al. Does the presence and site of myocardial ischemia on perfusion scintigraphy predict the occurrence and site of future myocardial infarction in patients with stable coronary artery disease? Am J Cardiol 1997; 79: 1521–1524.
19. Shah PK. Pathophysiology of plaque rupture and the concept of plaque stabilization. Cardiol Clin 1996; 14:17–29.
20. Shah PK. Plaque size, vessel size and plaque vulnerability: bigger may not be better. J Am Coll Cardiol 1998; 32:663–664.
21. Schoenhagen P, Ziada KM, Kapadia SR, et al. Extent and direction of arterial remodeling in stable versus unstable coronary syndromes: an intravascular ultrasound study. Circulation 2000; 101:598–603.

22. von Birgelen C, Klinkhart W, Mintz GS, et al. Plaque distribution and vascular remodeling of ruptured and nonruptured coronary plaques in the same vessel: an intravascular ultrasound study in vivo. J Am Coll Cardiol 2001; 37:1864–1870.
23. Loree HM, Kamm RD, Stringfellow RG, et al. Effects of fibrous cap thickness on peak circumferential stress in model atherosclerotic vessels. Circ Res 1992; 71:850–858.
24. Essler M, Retzer M, Bauer M, et al. Stimulation of platelets and endothelial cells by mildly oxidized LDL proceeds through activation of lysophosphatidic acid receptors and the Rho/Rho-kinase pathway. Inhibition by lovastatin. Ann N Y Acad Sci 2000; 905:282–286.
25. Toschi V, Gallo R, Lettino M, et al. Tissue factor modulates the thrombogenicity of human atherosclerotic plaques. Circulation 1997; 95:594–599.
26. Mallat Z, Hugel B, Ohan J, et al. Shed membrane microparticles with procoagulant potential in human atherosclerotic plaques: a role for apoptosis in plaque thrombogenicity. Circulation 1999; 99:348–353.
27. Badimon JJ, Lettino M, Toschi V, et al. Local inhibition of tissue factor reduces the thrombogenicity of disrupted human atherosclerotic plaques: effects of tissue factor pathway inhibitor on plaque thrombogenicity under flow conditions. Circulation 1999; 99:1780–1787.
28. Fernandez-Ortiz A, Badimon JJ, Falk E, et al. Characterization of the relative thrombogenicity of atherosclerotic plaque components: implications for consequences of plaque rupture. J Am Coll Cardiol 1994; 23:1562–1569.
29. Richardson PD, Davies MJ, Born GV. Influence of plaque configuration and stress distribution on fissuring of coronary atherosclerotic plaques. Lancet 1989; 2:941–944.
30. Cheng GC, Loree HM, Kamm RD, et al. Distribution of circumferential stress in ruptured and stable atherosclerotic lesions. A structural analysis with histopathological correlation. Circulation 1993; 87:1179–1187.
31. Loree HM, Tobias BJ, Gibson LJ, et al. Mechanical properties of model atherosclerotic lesion lipid pools. Arterioscler Thromb 1994; 14:230–234.
32. Huang H, Virmani R, Younis H, et al. The impact of calcification on the biomechanical stability of atherosclerotic plaques. Circulation 2001; 103:1051–1056.
33. Guyton JR, Klemp KF. Development of the lipid-rich core in human atherosclerosis. Arterioscler Thromb Vasc Biol 1996; 16:4–11.
34. Feng B, Yao PM, Li Y, et al. The endoplasmic reticulum is the site of cholesterol-induced cytotoxicity in macrophages. Nat Cell Biol 2003; 5:781–792.
35. Kolodgie FD, Gold HK, Burke AP, et al. Intraplaque hemorrhage and progression of coronary atheroma. N Engl J Med 2003; 349:2316–2325.
36. Libby P, Aikawa M. Stabilization of atherosclerotic plaques: new mechanisms and clinical targets. Nat Med 2002; 8:1257–1262.
37. Felton CV, Crook D, Davies MJ, et al. Relation of plaque lipid composition and morphology to the stability of human aortic plaques. Arterioscler Thromb Vasc Biol 1997; 17:1337–1345.
38. Burleigh MC, Briggs AD, Lendon CL. Collagen types I and III, collagen content, GAGs and mechanical strength of human atherosclerotic plaque caps: span-wise variations. Atherosclerosis 1992; 96:71–81.
39. Bennett MR, Evan GI, Schwartz SM. Apoptosis of human vascular smooth muscle cells derived from normal vessels and coronary atherosclerotic plaques. J Clin Invest 1995; 95:2266–2274.
40. Bjorkerud S, Bjorkerud B. Apoptosis is abundant in human atherosclerotic lesions, especially in inflammatory cells (macrophages and T cells), and may contribute to the accumulation of gruel and plaque instability. Am J Pathol 1996; 149:367–380.
41. Kockx MM, Knaapen MW. The role of apoptosis in vascular disease. J Pathol 2000; 190:267–280.
42. Ihling C, Haendeler J, Menzel G, et al. Co-expression of p53 and MDM2 in human atherosclerosis: implications for the regulation of cellularity of atherosclerotic lesions. J Pathol 1998; 185:303–312.
43. Crisby M, Kallin B, Thyberg J, et al. Cell death in human atherosclerotic plaques involves both oncosis and apoptosis. Atherosclerosis 1997; 130:17–27.
44. Bennett MR. Apoptosis of vascular smooth muscle cells in vascular remodeling and atherosclerotic plaque rupture. Cardiovasc Res 1999; 41:361–368.

45. Galle J, Heermeier K, Wanner C. Atherogenic lipoproteins, oxidative stress, and cell death. Kidney Int Suppl 1999; 71:S62–S65.
46. Vieira O, Escargueil-Blanc I, Jurgens G, et al. Oxidized LDLs alter the activity of the ubiquitin-proteasome pathway: potential role in oxidized LDL-induced apoptosis. FASEB J 2000; 14:532–542.
47. Rossig L, Dimmeler S, Zeiher AM. Apoptosis in the vascular wall and atherosclerosis. Basic Res Cardiol 2001; 96:11–22.
48. Geng YJ, Wu Q, Muszynski M, et al. Apoptosis of vascular smooth muscle cells induced by in vitro stimulation with interferon-gamma, tumor necrosis factor-alpha, and interleukin-1 beta. Arterioscler Thromb Vasc Biol 1996; 16:19–27.
49. Geng YJ, Henderson LE, Levesque EB, et al. Fas is expressed in human atherosclerotic intima and promotes apoptosis of cytokine-primed human vascular smooth muscle cells. Arterioscler Thromb Vasc Biol 1997; 17:2200–2208.
50. Mallat Z, Tedgui A. Apoptosis in the vasculature: mechanisms and functional importance. Br J Pharmacol 2000; 130:947–962.
51. Wallner K, Li C, Shah PK, et al. EGF-like domain of tenascin-C is proapoptotic for cultured smooth muscle cells. Arterioscler Thromb Vasc Biol 2004; 24:1416–1421.
52. Kolmakova A, Kwiterovich P, Virgil D, et al. Apolipoprotein C-I induces apoptosis in human aortic smooth muscle cells via recruiting neutral sphingomyelinase. Arterioscler Thromb Vasc Biol 2004; 24:264–269.
53. Gupta S, Pablo AM, Jiang X, et al. IFN-γ potentiates atherosclerosis in ApoE knock-out mice. J Clin Invest 1997; 99:2752–2761.
54. Sukhova GK, Shi GP, Simon DI, et al. Expression of the elastolytic cathepsins S and K in human atheroma and regulation of their production in smooth muscle cells. J Clin Invest 1998; 102:576–583.
55. Shi GP, Sukhova GK, Grubb A, et al. Cystatin C deficiency in human atherosclerosis and aortic aneurysms. J Clin Invest 1999; 104:1191–1197.
56. Xu XP, Meisel SR, Ong JM, et al. Oxidized low-density lipoprotein regulates matrix metalloproteinase-9 and its tissue inhibitor in human monocyte-derived macrophages. Circulation 1999; 99:993–998.
57. Rajavashisth TB, Xu XP, Jovinge S, et al. Membrane type 1 matrix metalloproteinase expression in human atherosclerotic plaques: evidence for activation by proinflammatory mediators. Circulation 1999; 99:3103–3109.
58. Shah PK, Falk E, Badimon JJ, et al. Human monocyte-derived macrophages induce collagen breakdown in fibrous caps of atherosclerotic plaques. Potential role of matrix-degrading metalloproteinases and implications for plaque rupture. Circulation 1995; 92:1565–1569.
59. Uzai H, Harpf A, Liu M, et al. Increased expression of membrane type 3 matrix metalloproteinase in human atherosclerotic plaques: role of activated macrophages and inflammatory cytokines. Circulation 2002; 106:3024–3030.
60. Shah PK. Role of inflammation and metalloproteinases in plaque disruption and thrombosis. Vasc Med 1998; 3:199–206.
61. Doherty TM, Asotra K, Pei D, et al. Therapeutic developments in matrix metalloproteinase inhibition. Expert Opin Ther Pat 2002; 12:665–707.
62. Sukhova GK, Schonbeck U, Rabkin E, et al. Evidence for increased collagenolysis by interstitial collagenases-1 and -3 in vulnerable human atheromatous plaques. Circulation 1999; 99:2503–2509.
63. Lee RT, Schoen FJ, Loree HM, et al. Circumferential stress and matrix metalloproteinase 1 in human coronary atherosclerosis. Implications for plaque rupture. Arterioscler Thromb Vasc Biol 1996; 16:1070–1073.
64. Galis ZS, Muszynski M, Sukhova GK, et al. Enhanced expression of vascular matrix metalloproteinases induced in vitro by cytokines and in regions of human atherosclerotic lesions. Ann N Y Acad Sci 1995; 748:501–507.
65. Galis ZS, Sukhova GK, Kranzhofer R, et al. Macrophage foam cells from experimental atheroma constitutively produce matrix-degrading proteinases. Proc Natl Acad Sci U S A 1995; 92:402–406.

66. Kol A, Sukhova GK, Lichtman AH, et al. Chlamydial heat shock protein 60 localizes in human atheroma and regulates macrophage tumor necrosis factor-alpha and matrix metalloproteinase expression. Circulation 1998; 98:300–307.
67. Mach F, Schonbeck U, Fabunmi RP, et al. T lymphocytes induce endothelial cell matrix metalloproteinase expression by a CD40L-dependent mechanism: implications for tubule formation. Am J Pathol 1999; 154:229–238.
68. Schonbeck U, Mach F, Sukhova GK, et al. Regulation of matrix metalloproteinase expression in human vascular smooth muscle cells by T lymphocytes: a role for CD40 signaling in plaque rupture? Circ Res 1997; 81:448–454.
69. Wallner K, Li C, Shah PK, et al. Tenascin-C is expressed in macrophage-rich human coronary atherosclerotic plaque. Circulation 1999; 99:1284–1289.
70. Henney AM, Wakeley PR, Davies MJ, et al. Localization of stromelysin gene expression in atherosclerotic plaques by in situ hybridization. Proc Natl Acad Sci U S A 1991; 88:8154–8158.
71. Galis ZS, Sukhova GK, Lark MW, et al. Increased expression of matrix metalloproteinases and matrix degrading activity in vulnerable regions of human atherosclerotic plaques. J Clin Invest 1994; 94:2493–2503.
72. Brown DL, Hibbs MS, Kearney M, et al. Identification of 92-kD gelatinase in human coronary atherosclerotic lesions. Association of active enzyme synthesis with unstable angina. Circulation 1995; 91:2125–2131.
73. Nikkari ST, O'Brien KD, Ferguson M, et al. Interstitial collagenase (MMP-1) expression in human carotid atherosclerosis. Circulation 1995; 92:1393–1398.
74. Li Z, Li L, Zielke HR, et al. Increased expression of 72-kd type IV collagenase (MMP-2) in human aortic atherosclerotic lesions. Am J Pathol 1996; 148:121–128.
75. Galis ZS, Sukhova GK, Libby P. Microscopic localization of active proteases by in situ zymography: detection of matrix metalloproteinase activity in vascular tissue. FASEB J 1995; 9:974–980.
76. Rajavashisth TB, Liao JK, Galis ZS, et al. Inflammatory cytokines and oxidized low density lipoproteins increase endothelial cell expression of membrane type 1-matrix metalloproteinase. J Biol Chem 1999; 274:11924–11929.
77. Herman MP, Sukhova GK, Libby P, et al. Expression of neutrophil collagenase (matrix metalloproteinase-8) in human atheroma: a novel collagenolytic pathway suggested by transcriptional profiling. Circulation 2001; 104:1899–1904.
78. Davies MJ. The pathophysiology of acute coronary syndromes. Heart 2000; 83:361–366.
79. van der Wal AC, Becker AE, van der Loos CM, et al. Site of intimal rupture or erosion of thrombosed coronary atherosclerotic plaques is characterized by an inflammatory process irrespective of the dominant plaque morphology. Circulation 1994; 89:36–44.
80. Kovanen PT. The mast cell–a potential link between inflammation and cellular cholesterol deposition in atherogenesis. Eur Heart J 1993; 14(suppl K):105–117.
81. Kovanen PT, Kaartinen M, Paavonen T. Infiltrates of activated mast cells at the site of coronary atheromatous erosion or rupture in myocardial infarction. Circulation 1995; 92:1084–1088.
82. Kaartinen M, van der Wal AC, van der Loos CM, et al. Mast cell infiltration in acute coronary syndromes: implications for plaque rupture. J Am Coll Cardiol 1998; 32: 606–612.
83. Laine P, Kaartinen M, Penttila A, et al. Association between myocardial infarction and the mast cells in the adventitia of the infarct-related coronary artery. Circulation 1999; 99:361–369.
84. Wiedermann CJS, Kiechl S, Dunzendorfer P, et al. Association of endotoxemia with carotid atherosclerosis and cardiovascular disease: prospective results from the Bruneck Study. J Am Coll Cardiol 1999; 34:1975.
85. Kiechl S, Egger G, Mayr M, et al. Chronic infections and the risk of carotid atherosclerosis: prospective results from a large population study. Circulation 2001; 103:1064.
86. Lehr HA, Sagban TA, Ihling C, et al. Immunopathogenesis of atherosclerosis: endotoxin accelerates atherosclerosis in rabbits on hypercholesterolemic diet. Circulation 2001; 104:914.
87. Akira S. Toll-like receptor signaling. J Biol Chem 2003; 278:38105.
88. Libby P. Inflammation in atherosclerosis. Nature 2002; 420:868–874.

89. Barger AC, Beeuwkes R 3rd, Lainey LL, et al. Hypothesis: vasa vasorum and neo-vascularization of human coronary arteries. A possible role in the pathophysiology of atherosclerosis. N Engl J Med 1984; 310:175–177.
90. Kamat BR, Galli SJ, Barger AC, et al. Neovascularization and coronary atherosclerotic plaque: cinematographic localization and quantitative histologic analysis. Hum Pathol 1987; 18:1036–1042.
91. Barger AC, Beeuwkes R 3rd. Rupture of coronary vasa vasorum as a trigger of acute myocardial infarction. Am J Cardiol 1990; 66:41G–43G.
92. Heistad DD, Armstrong ML. Blood flow through vasa vasorum of coronary arteries in atherosclerotic monkeys. Arteriosclerosis 1986; 6:326–331.
93. Williams JK, Heistad DD. The vasa vasorum of the arteries. J Mal Vasc 1996; 21:266–269.
94. Kwon HM, Sangiorgi G, Ritman EL, et al. Enhanced coronary vasa vasorum neo-vascularization in experimental hypercholesterolemia. J Clin Invest 1998; 101:1551–1556.
95. Depre C, Havaux X, Wijns W. Neovascularization in human coronary atherosclerotic lesions. Cathet Cardiovasc Diagn 1996; 39:215–220.
96. Tenaglia AN, Peters KG, Sketch MH Jr., et al. Neovascularization in atherectomy specimens from patients with unstable angina: implications for pathogenesis of unstable angina. Am Heart J 1998; 135:10–14.
97. Muller JE, Tofler GH, Stone PH. Circadian variation and triggers of onset of acute cardiovascular disease. Circulation 1989; 79:733–743.
98. Muller JE. Morning increase of onset of myocardial infarction. Implications concerning triggering events. Cardiology 1989; 76:96–104.
99. Muller JE, Tofler GH. Triggering and hourly variation of onset of arterial thrombosis. Ann Epidemiol 1992; 2:393–405.
100. Willich SN, Jimenez AH, Tofler GH, et al. Pathophysiology and triggers of acute myocardial infarction: clinical implications. Clin Investig 1992; 70:S73–S78.
101. Willich SN, Maclure M, Mittleman M, et al. Sudden cardiac death. Support for a role of triggering in causation. Circulation 1993; 87:1442–1450.
102. Peters A, Dockery DW, Muller JE, et al. Increased particulate air pollution and the triggering of myocardial infarction. Circulation 2001; 103:2810–2815.
103. Mittleman MA, Lewis RA, Maclure M, et al. Triggering myocardial infarction by marijuana. Circulation 2001; 103:2805–2809.
104. Muller JE. Circadian variation and triggering of acute coronary events. Am Heart J 1999; 137:S1–S8.
105. Muller JE. Triggering of cardiac events by sexual activity: findings from a case-crossover analysis. Am J Cardiol 2000; 86:14F–18F.
106. Goldstein JA, Demetriou D, Grines CL, et al. Multiple complex coronary plaques in patients with acute myocardial infarction. N Engl J Med 2000; 343:915–922.
107. Matetzky S, Tani S, Kangavari S, et al. Smoking increases tissue factor expression in atherosclerotic plaques: implications for plaque thrombogenicity. Circulation 2000; 102:602–604.
108. Blankenhorn DH, Hodis HN. Arterial imaging and atherosclerosis reversal. Arterioscler Thromb 1994; 14:177.
109. Aikawa M, Rabkin E, Okada Y, et al. Lipid lowering by diet reduces matrix metal-loproteinase activity and increases collagen content of rabbit atheroma: A potential mechanism of lesion stabilization. Circulation 1998; 97:2433–2444.
110. Aikawa M, Sugiyama S, Hill CC, et al. Lipid lowering reduces oxidative stress and endothelial cell activation in rabbit atheroma. Circulation 2002; 106:1390–1396.
111. Kockx MM, De Meyer GR, Buyssens N, et al. Cell composition, replication, and apoptosis in atherosclerotic plaques after 6 months of cholesterol withdrawal. Circ Res 1998; 83:378–387.
112. Bustos C, Hernández-Presa MA, Ortego M, et al. HMG-CoA reductase inhibition by atorvastatin reduces neointimal inflammation in a rabbit model of atherosclerosis. J Am Coll Cardiol 1998; 32:2057–2064.
113. Aikawa M, Rabkin E, Sugiyama S, et al. An HMG-CoA reductase inhibitor, cerivastatin, suppresses growth of macrophages expressing matrix metalloproteinases and tissue factor in vivo and in vitro. Circulation 2001; 103:276–283.

114. Bocan TM, Krause BR, Rosebury WS, et al. The ACAT inhibitor avasimibe reduces macrophages and matrix metalloproteinase expression in atherosclerotic lesions of hypercholesterolemic rabbits. Arterioscler Thromb Vasc Biol 2000; 20:70–79.
115. Laufs U, La Fata V, Plutzky J, et al. Upregulation of endothelial nitric oxide synthase by HMG CoA reductase inhibitors. Circulation 1998; 97:1129–1135.
116. Hernandez-Perera O, Pérez-Sala D, Navarro-Antolín J, et al. Effects of the 3-hydroxy-3-methylglutaryl-CoA reductase inhibitors, atorvastatin and simvastatin, on the expression of endothelin-1 and endothelial nitric oxide synthase in vascular endothelial cells. J Clin Invest 1998; 101:2711–2719.
117. Bourcier T, Libby P. HMG CoA reductase inhibitors reduce plasminogen activator inhibitor-1 expression by human vascular smooth muscle and endothelial cells. Arterioscler Thromb Vasc Biol 2000; 20:556–562.
118. Lopez S, Peiretti F, Bonardo B, et al. Effect of atorvastatin and fluvastatin on the expression of plasminogen activator inhibitor type-1 in cultured human endothelial cells. Atherosclerosis 2000; 152:359–366.
119. Marx N, Sukhova GK, Collins T, et al. PPARα activators inhibit cytokine-induced vascular cell adhesion molecule-1 expression in human endothelial cells. Circulation 1999; 99:3125–3131.
120. Marx N, Mackman N, Schönbeck U, et al. PPARα activators inhibit tissue factor expression and activity in human monocytes. Circulation 2001; 103:213–219.
121. Neve BP, Corseaux D, Chinetti G, et al. PPARα agonists inhibit tissue factor expression in human monocytes and macrophages. Circulation 2001; 103:207–212.
122. Marx N, Kehrle B, Kohlhammer K, et al. PPAR activators as antiinflammatory mediators in human T lymphocytes: Implications for atherosclerosis and transplantation-associated arteriosclerosis. Circ Res 2002; 90:703–710.
123. Price MJ, Shah PK. New strategies in managing and preventing atherosclerosis: focus on HDL. Rev Cardiovasc Med 2002; 3:129–137.
124. Shah PK, Kaul S, Nilsson J, et al. Exploiting the vascular protective effects of high-density lipoprotein and its apolipoproteins: an idea whose time for testing is coming, part II. Circulation 2001; 104:2498–2502.
125. Barter PJ. Inhibition of endothelial cell adhesion molecule expression by high density lipoproteins. Clin Exp Pharmacol Physiol 1997; 24:286–287.
126. Nilsson J, Dahlgren B, Ares M, et al. Lipoprotein-like phospholipid particles inhibit the smooth muscle cell cytotoxicity of lysophosphatidylcholine and platelet-activating factor. Arterioscler Thromb Vasc Biol 1998; 18:13–19.
127. Shah PK. Plaque disruption and thrombosis: potential role of inflammation and infection. Cardiol Rev 2000; 8:31–39.
128. Rong JX, Li J, Reis ED, et al. Elevating high-density lipoprotein cholesterol in apolipoprotein E-deficient mice remodels advanced atherosclerotic lesions by decreasing macrophage and increasing smooth muscle cell content. Circulation 2001; 104: 2447–2452.
129. Shah PK, Yano J, Reyes O, et al. High–dose recombinant apolipoprotein A-1(milano) mobilizes tissue cholesterol and rapidly reduces plaque lipid and macrophage content in apolipoprotein e-deficient mice. Potential implications for acute plaque stabilization. Circulation 2001; 103:3047–3050.
130. Cockerill GW, Rye KA, Gamble JR, et al. High-density lipoproteins inhibit cytokine-induced expression of endothelial cell adhesion molecules. Arterioscler Thromb Vasc Biol 1995; 15:1987–1994.
131. Dimayuga P, Zhu J, Oguchi S, et al. Reconstituted HDL containing human apolipoprotein A-1 reduces VCAM-1 expression and neointima formation following peri-adventitial cuff-induced carotid injury apoE null mice. Biochem Biophys Res Commun 1999; 264:465–468.
132. Shah PK, Chyu KY, Fredrikson GN, et al. Immunomodulation of atherosclerosis with a vaccine. Nat Clin Pract Cardiovasc Med 2005; 2:639–646.

3 Successful Myocardial Reperfusion

Claudia P. Hochberg and C. Michael Gibson
Department of Cardiology, Beth Israel-Deaconess Medical Center, Boston, Massachusetts, U.S.A.

INTRODUCTION

Epicardial coronary artery patency has been the primary outcome measure of coronary angiography and intervention in patients with ST-segment acute myocardial infarction (STEMI). Strategies to improve the effectiveness of both fibrinolytic and percutaneous interventional therapies have relied on this angiographic measure to assess treatment efficacy and outcome. Despite the reliance on epicardial patency, there is still significant variability in morbidity and mortality among patients with full restoration of coronary artery blood flow or Thrombolysis in Myocardial Infarction (TIMI) grade 3 flow. The realization that restoration of epicardial flow is necessary, but not sufficient, has led to the evaluation of the myocardial vasculature and reperfusion downstream at the level of the capillary bed as a more accurate predictor of clinical outcome and treatment efficacy (1–8). The goal of this chapter is to review the methods used to evaluate myocardial perfusion and their association with clinical outcomes.

TIMI Flow Grade

For the past 20 years, the TIMI flow grade (TFG) classification scheme has been used to evaluate coronary blood flow in acute coronary syndromes (Table 1) (1). It has been widely used in trials to compare angiographic outcomes of epicardial reperfusion strategies, and the association of TFG with clinical outcomes and mortality has been well documented (2–8).

High rates of TIMI grade 3 flow approaching 100% after primary percutaneous intervention (PCI) have been reported when a "3 cardiac cycles to fill the artery" definition is applied (9). However, when assessed more rigorously, rates of TIMI grade 3 flow may be substantially lower at approximately 80% (10). The persistence of abnormal epicardial blood flow after PCI is unlikely because of residual stenosis, but rather related to increased vascular resistance in the downstream vessels. Persistent slowing of flow after PCI despite relief of stenosis is associated with an increase in mortality rate from 0.8% to 9.7% (11).

Confounding by other variables makes the use of TIMI grade 3 flow as the sole correlate of mortality problematic. Infarct location is one such confounder. For example, the majority of TIMI grade 3 flow is observed in the right coronary artery (RCA), while the majority of TIMI grade 2 flow is observed in the left anterior descending artery (LAD) territory (7). The differential between the mortality rate of inferior myocardial infarction and anterior myocardial infarction may therefore account for some of the improved outcomes among patients with TIMI grade 3 flow (7). Use of more precise angiographic measures, such as the TIMI frame count, supports the notion that improved epicardial flow is associated with improved clinical outcomes. However, the magnitude of the clinical improvement associated with TIMI grade 3 flow may have been overestimated. An additional variable that

TABLE 1 Definitions of the TFG and TMPG Systems

Grade	Characteristics
TFG, a grading system for epicardial coronary flow	
0	No perfusion; no antegrade flow beyond the point of occlusion
1	Penetration without perfusion; the contrast material passes beyond the area of obstruction but "hangs up" and fails to opacify the entire coronary bed distal to the obstruction for the duration of the cine run
2	Partial reperfusion; the contrast material passes across the obstruction and opacifies the coronary bed distal to the obstruction. However, the rate of entry of contrast into the vessel distal to the obstruction and/or its rate of clearance from the distal bed is perceptibly slower than its entry into and/or clearance from comparable areas not perfused by the culprit vessel (e.g., the opposite coronary artery or coronary bed proximal to the obstruction)
3	Complete perfusion; antegrade flow into the bed distal to the obstruction occurs as promptly as into the bed proximal to the obstruction and clearance of the contrast material from the involved bed is as rapid as from an uninvolved bed in the same vessel or the opposite artery
TMPG, a grading system for myocardial perfusion	
0	Dye fails to enter the microvasculature; there is either minimal or no ground glass appearance ("blush") or opacification of the myocardium in the distribution of the culprit artery indicating lack of tissue level perfusion
1	Dye slowly enters but fails to exit the microvasculature; there is the ground glass appearance ("blush") or opacification of the myocardium in the distribution of the culprit lesion that fails to clear from the microvasculature, and dye staining is present on the next injection (approximately 30 sec between injections)
2	Delayed entry and exit of dye from the microvasculature; there is the ground glass appearance ("blush") or opacification of the myocardium in the distribution of the culprit lesion that is strongly persistent at the end of the washout phase (i.e., dye is strongly persistent after 3 cardiac cycles of the washout phase and either does not diminish or only minimally diminishes in intensity during washout)
3	Normal entry and exit of dye from the microvasculature; there is the ground glass appearance ("blush") or opacification of the myocardium in the distribution of the culprit lesion that clears normally, and it is either gone or only mildly/moderately persistent at the end of the washout phase (i.e., dye is gone or only mildly/moderately persistent after 3 cardiac cycles of the washout phase and noticeably diminishes in intensity during washout phase), similar to that in an uninvolved artery; blush that is of only mild intensity throughout the washout phase but fades minimally is also classified as grade 3

Abbreviations: TFG, TIMI flow grade; TMPG, TIMI myocardial perfusion grade.
Source: From Ref. 35.

complicates the association of TFG with mortality is the nonlinearity of TFG. Far greater clinical improvement is seen with reestablishment of TIMI grade 2 flow from TIMI grade 0/1 flow than is seen in progress from grade 2 to grade 3 flow.

Restoration of epicardial flow does not necessarily lead to restoration of tissue level or microvascular perfusion (12,13), suggesting that "not all TIMI grade 3 flow is created equally." Impaired tissue perfusion can be present despite restoration of normal epicardial flow, and its assessment can provide important diagnostic and prognostic information. Perfusion of the myocardium can be assessed indirectly by quantitative measurements of epicardial flow rates with use of the corrected TIMI frame count (CTFC), can be inferred from ongoing electrocardiographic injury, or can be assessed by the TIMI myocardial perfusion grade (TMPG), myocardial blush grade (MBG), or digital subtraction angiography. Beyond epicardial flow, myocardial perfusion has been shown to be an independent predictor of outcome (14).

METHODS OF MEASURING MYOCARDIAL PERFUSION

Indirect Measures

The Corrected TIMI Frame Count

The TFG classification has been extraordinarily useful in assessing the success of reperfusion strategies and identifying patients at higher risk for poor outcomes in acute coronary syndromes for the past two decades. Despite its widespread use, it is not without limitations (7). A more objective and precise index of coronary blood flow, the CTFC, can be used to overcome some of the limitations of TFG. To use CTFC, the number of cine frames required for dye to reach standardized distal landmarks is counted (Fig. 1) (7,8,14). In the first frame used for TIMI frame counting, a column of dye touches both borders of the coronary artery and moves forward (Fig. 1) (7). In the last frame, the dye begins to enter (but does not necessarily fill) a standard distal landmark in the artery. These standard distal landmarks are as follows: in the RCA, the first branch of the posterolateral artery; in the

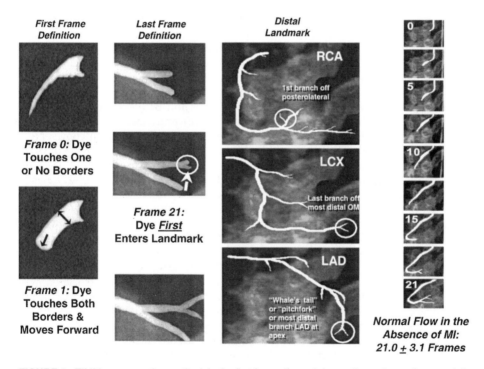

FIGURE 1 TIMI frame-counting method. In the first frame (*lower left panel*), a column of near or fully concentrated dye touches both borders of the coronary artery and moves forward. In the last frame (*second column*), dye begins to enter (but does not necessarily fill) a standard distal landmark in the artery. These standard distal landmarks are as follows: the first branch of the posterolateral artery in the RCA (*third column, top panel*); in the circumflex system, the most distal branch of the obtuse marginal branch that includes the culprit lesion in the dye path (*third column, middle panel*); and in the LAD the distal bifurcation, which is also known as the moustache, pitchfork, or whale's tail (*third column, bottom panel*). *Abbreviations*: RCA, right coronary artery; LCX, left circumflex coronary artery; LAD, left anterior descending artery. *Source*: From Ref. 35.

circumflex artery, the most distal branch of the obtuse marginal branch that includes the culprit lesion in the dye path; and in the LAD, the distal bifurcation, also known as the "moustache," "pitchfork," or "whale's tail" (Fig. 1). These frame counts are corrected for the longer length of the LAD by dividing by 1.7 to arrive at the CTFC (7). By knowing the time for the dye to go down the artery from the CTFC (CTFC/30 seconds) and length of the artery (either from an angioplasty guidewire or by planimetry), dye velocity (cm/sec) can be calculated in a more accurate fashion (15), which then allows calculation of the velocity proximal and distal to the lesion (15).

The CTFC is a quantitative measurement of epicardial flow, rather than a qualitative assessment, and it is highly reproducible (7). It should be noted that if an epicardial artery is occluded, then a frame count of 100 is imputed. A normal CTFC is 21 frames, and despite extensive physiologic variability and operator technique, there is only a 3.1-frame standard deviation among patients with normal flow. The 95% confidence interval extends from >14 frames to <28 frames (7). Faster than normal flow is defined as CTFC <14 frames and constitutes what we now term "TIMI grade 4 flow" (7). Several variables, both technical and physiologic, do impact the CTFC. The use of a power injector, dye injection at the beginning of diastole, and increasing the heart rate by 20 beats/min all significantly decrease the CTFC, whereas nitrate administration increases it (16,17).

The CTFC is related to a variety of clinical outcomes (7,8,14). Flow in the infarct-related artery in survivors is significantly faster than in patients who die, and mortality rates increase by 0.7% for every 10-frame rise in CTFC ($P < 0.001$) (8). Likewise, in patients with unstable angina (UA) or non–ST elevation MI (NSTEMI), the post-PCI culprit flow among survivors is significantly faster than among those patients who die (23). Rapid flow is associated with good clinical outcomes. None of the patients in the TIMI studies who have had a CTFC <14 died by 30 days (8). Multiple studies have now documented an association between the CTFC and clinical outcomes among patients treated with primary PCI as well (18–22). Lastly, the CTFC is associated with lower restenosis rates (23).

Until recently, it was assumed that flow in nonculprit arteries in the setting of acute coronary syndromes was "normal." However, the CTFC in uninvolved arteries in acute STEMI (30.5 frames) is 40% slower than normal (21 frames, $P < 0.001$) (7,24,25). In STEMI, adjunctive and rescue PCI restores flow in culprit arteries. This flow is nearly identical to that in nonculprit arteries, but remains slower than normal (24). The PCI of the culprit lesion is also associated with improvements in nonculprit artery flow after the intervention in both STEMI and UA/NSTEMI (24,25). Importantly, slower flow throughout all three arteries in STEMI is associated with a higher risk of adverse outcomes, poorer wall motion in remote territories, poorer tissue perfusion on digital subtraction angiography (DSA), and a greater magnitude of ST-segment depression in remote territories on the ECG (24–26). Poorer flow in nonculprit arteries may be the result of more extensive necrosis in shared microvasculature or a result of vasoconstriction mediated through either a local neurohumoral or paracrine mechanism leading to an overall worse outcome (35).

Delayed flow after fibrinolysis has been assumed to be secondary to residual stenosis. However, even after adjunctive PCI and relief of stenoses, flow remains persistently delayed to 26 frames post-stent, and 34% of stented vessels have abnormal flow with a CTFC ≥ 28 (10). This persistence of slow flow is probably not due to the residual stenosis or an intraluminal obstruction, but rather to other factors that influence epicardial flow. These include symptom duration prior to arrival, the presence of collaterals, the percent diameter stenosis, the presence of pulsatile flow, the presence of thrombus in the artery, and the involvement of the LAD as the culprit artery (10). For instance, prolonged symptom-to-treatment times in patients with ST-segment elevation MI are associated with impaired myocardial perfusion grades. Patients who experience a delay of >4 hours in symptom onset to treatment have a higher CTFC at 60 minutes [42.9 frames vs. 38.2 frames; $P = 0.001$] (27). Even in patients with TIMI grade 3 flow, the CTFC at 60 minutes tended to be higher among patients with symptom onset-to-treatment time >4 hours (27).

The Electrocardiogram

The electrocardiogram (ECG) is another useful clinical marker of myocardial perfusion. All clinicians have seen patients with a patent artery following primary PCI and persistent ST-segment elevation. Greater ST-segment resolution on ECG correlates with TIMI grade 3 flow, TMPG 3, smaller infarct sizes, and improved survival (28–30). Although the ECG and the TMPG are associated, they provide independent prognostic information about infarct size (31). Two additional studies have now documented the complementary prognostic information provided by the ECG (degree of ST-segment resolution) and the angiographic blush, with failure to achieve ST-segment resolution and myocardial perfusion on angiography following primary PCI that carried a particularly poor prognosis (32,33). These data suggest a potential electromechanical dissociation; the angiogram may reflect mechanical patency of the microvasculature and the integrity of the endothelium, while the electrocardiogram may reflect the functional status of the supplied myocardium (31). Measures of both processes appear to be independent and complementary in their prognostic significance. Finally, restoration of normal (TMPG 3) myocardial perfusion is associated not only with complete ST-segment resolution but also with earlier ST-segment resolution with continuous ST-segment monitoring (34).

Direct Measures
The TIMI Myocardial Perfusion Grade and Myocardial Blush Grade

As previously mentioned, impaired tissue perfusion may be present despite restoration of normal epicardial flow and direct measurement of myocardial perfusion provides important diagnostic and prognostic information. Two methods of direct measurement of myocardial perfusion are the TMPG and the myocardial blush grade (MBG). In the TMPG system (Table 1), TMPG 0 represents minimal or no myocardial blush; in TMPG 1, dye stains the myocardium, and this stain persists on the next injection; in TMPG 2, the dye enters the myocardium, but washes out slowly, so that the dye is strongly persistent at the end of the injection; and in TMPG 3, there is normal entrance and exit of the dye in the myocardium (Fig. 2) (35). Another method of assessing myocardial perfusion on the angiogram is the MBG, developed by van 't Hof et al. (36). A grade of 0 (no blush) and a grade of 3 (normal blush) are the same in the TMPG and MBG systems. An MBG grade 1 or 2 represents diminished intensity in the myocardium and corresponds to a value of 0.5 in the expanded TMPG grading system. A TMPG of 1 or a stain in the TIMI

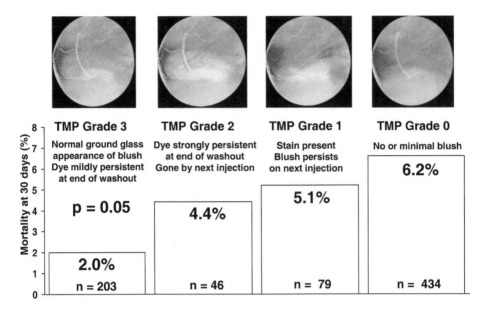

FIGURE 2 The TMPG assesses tissue level perfusion using the angiogram and is a multivariate predictor of mortality in acute MI. The TMPG permits risk stratification even within epicardial TIMI grade 3 flow. Despite achieving epicardial patency with normal TIMI grade 3 flow, those patients whose microvasculature fails to open (TMPG 0/1) have a persistently elevated mortality of 5.4% at 30 days. In contrast, those patients with both TIMI grade 3 flow in the epicardial artery and TMPG 3 have a mortality under 1% [0.7% (1/137) vs. 4.7% (15/318); $P = 0.05$ using Fisher's exact test for TMPG 3 vs. grades 0, 1, and 2]. *Abbreviations*: TMPG, MI. *Source*: From Ref. 35.

system is subsumed within the value of 0 in the MBG system. Thus, normal perfusion in the myocardium carries a score of 3 in both the TMPG and MBG systems, and closed myocardium carries a score of 0 in both systems (35).

TMPG has been shown to be a multivariate predictor of mortality in acute STEMI independent of flow in the epicardial artery, age, blood pressure, and heart rate (14). TIMI grade 2/3 flow, reduced CTFC, and an open microvasculature (TMPG 2/3) were all associated with an improved 2-year survival (14). Thus, the TMPG adds additional long-term prognostic information to the conventional epicardial TFG and CTFC. Compared with patients who achieve both TIMI grade 3 flow and TMPG 3, patients in whom epicardial flow is restored (TIMI grade 3 flow) and whose microvasculature fails to open (TMPG 0/1) have a sevenfold increase in mortality. Achievement of TIMI grade 3 flow in both the artery and the myocardium is associated with mortality under 1% (Fig. 2) (14). In a recent analysis of the PROTECT-TIMI 30 study, an abnormal post-PCI TMPG was the strongest correlate of death, MI, or an ischemic event within 48 hours in patients with NSTEMI undergoing PCI (37).

Analysis of angiograms from patients enrolled in the CLARITY-TIMI 28 trial after fibrinolytic therapy for STEMI demonstrated that residual thrombus was associated with more frequent TIMI grade 2 flow, higher corrected TIMI frame counts, and a lower incidence of normal TMPG (38). The association between thrombus and impaired TMPG remained even after further adjustment for CTFC or

TFG, suggesting that residual thrombus following fibrinolytic therapy is associated with impaired myocardial perfusion, independent of TFG (38).

Impaired myocardial perfusion on the angiogram has also been associated with higher left ventricular end diastolic pressure (40) and the presence of overt congestive heart failure on presentation. Among patients presenting with cardiogenic shock, a restoration of normal myocardial perfusion is associated with improved survival (41).

Similar to what has been observed in STEMI, TMPG 0/1 flow in UA/NSTEMI is associated with elevated troponin T and I (both pre- and post-PCI), and levels were higher among patients with TMPG 0/1 compared with TMPG 2/3 (11). TMPG 0/1 was independently associated with elevations of cardiac troponin, independent of the epicardial TFG, the severity of the stenosis, or the presence of thrombus in the artery. Importantly, TMPG 0/1 was associated with increased risk of death or MI at 6 months (11). Similarly, TMPG 0/1/2 perfusion following PCI is associated with a nearly 10-fold rise in the risk of creatine kinase (CK)–MB elevations in patients with UA/NSTEMI, as well as a higher risk of adverse clinical outcomes at one year (42). These findings implicate a pathophysiologic link between impaired myocardial perfusion, the release of markers of myonecrosis (both pre- and post-PCI), and adverse clinical outcomes.

Digital Subtraction Angiography

To quantitatively characterize the kinetics of dye entering the myocardium using the angiogram, digital subtraction angiography (DSA) has been utilized to estimate the rate of brightness (gray/sec) and the rate of growth of blush (cm/sec). DSA is performed at end diastole by aligning cine frame images before dye fills the myocardium with those at the peak of myocardial filling to subtract spine, ribs, diaphragm, and epicardial artery (Fig. 3). A representative region of the myocardium is sampled that is free of overlap by epicardial arterial branches to determine the increase in the gray-scale brightness of the myocardium at peak intensity. The circumference of the myocardial blush is measured using a handheld planimeter. The number of frames required for the myocardium to reach peak brightness is converted into time by dividing the frame count by 30 (35). In patients with UA/NSTEMI treated with PCI, treatment with the glycoprotein IIb/IIIa (GPIIb/IIIa) inhibitor eptifibatide improves the rate at which the dye enters the myocardium (44).

The Angiographic Perfusion Score

A simplified, broadly applicable angiographic metric that integrates epicardial and myocardial perfusion assessments is needed. The Angiographic Perfusion Score (APS) is the sum of the TFG (0 to 3) added to the TMPG (0 to 3) before and after PCI (total possible grade of 0 to 12) (45). Failed perfusion can be defined as an APS of 0 to 3; partial perfusion, 4 to 9; and full perfusion, 10 to 12 (45). Among STEMI patients, the APS is associated with larger SPECT infarct sizes and with the incidence of death or MI. The integration of epicardial and tissue level perfusion to arrive at a single angiographic variable that is associated with infarct size and 30-day death or MI may prove valuable in clinical risk stratification.

Other Angiographic Factors Associated with Outcomes

Other factors seen on angiography that are associated with poorer outcomes include lesion location, lesion complexity, and the presence of pulsatile flow in the

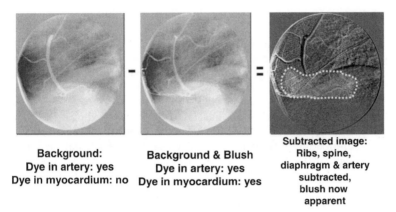

<table>
<tr><td>Background:
Dye in artery: yes
Dye in myocardium: no</td><td>Background & Blush
Dye in artery: yes
Dye in myocardium: yes</td><td>Subtracted image:
Ribs, spine,
diaphragm & artery
subtracted,
blush now
apparent</td></tr>
</table>

FIGURE 3 DSA was developed to quantitatively characterize the kinetics of dye entering the myocardium using the angiogram. DSA is performed at end diastole by aligning cine frame images before dye fills the myocardium with those at the peak of myocardial filling to subtract spine, ribs, diaphragm, and epicardial artery. A representative region of the myocardium is sampled that is free of overlap by epicardial arterial branches to determine the increase in the gray-scale brightness of the myocardium when it first reached its peak intensity. The circumference of the myocardial blush is measured using a handheld planimeter. The number of frames required for the myocardium to first reach its peak brightness is converted into time (sec) by dividing the frame count by 30. In this way, the rate of rise in brightness (gray/sec) and the rate of growth of blush (cm/sec) can be calculated. *Abbreviation*: DSA, digital subtraction angiography. *Source*: From Ref. 35.

artery. More proximal stenoses are associated with higher mortality, poorer ST-segment resolution, and larger infarct sizes, particularly in the LAD distribution (46). Reversal of systolic flow on myocardial contrast echocardiography has been associated with impaired tissue perfusion in patients with STEMI. Angiographic evidence of systolic flow reversal is also associated with higher CTFC, impaired TMPG, less complete ($\geq$70%) ST-segment resolution, and a higher risk of death or reinfarction at 30 days independent of the velocity of antegrade flow in the epicardial artery (47). Lastly, lesion complexity is associated with poorer PCI results and poorer myocardial perfusion, pre- and post-PCI, in patients with STEMI (48,49).

THERAPIES TO IMPROVE MYOCARDIAL PERFUSION

Vasodilators

There are few randomized trials looking at the efficacy of vasodilator therapy in improving myocardial perfusion. One small trial evaluated high dose intracoronary adenosine (100 µg during each intracoronary injection) and demonstrated that adenosine was associated with improved echocardiographic and clinical outcomes (50). Adenosine administration may be associated with bradycardia, and the placement of a temporary pacing wire should be considered (Table 2). In the randomized Vasodilator Prevention of No-Reflow (VAPOR) trial, intragraft verapamil (200 µg IC) was associated with a reduction in no reflow during saphenous vein graft PCI. Care must be taken in administration, as verapamil administration can be associated with decreased contractility and bradycardia (51). A more recent

TABLE 2 Agents Used To Treat Impaired Myocardial Perfusion[a]

	Dose	Side effects
Adenosine	100 μg IC to a total dose of 4000 μg Half-life is 6 sec. Adenosine can be repeatedly administered when pulse and blood pressure normalize	Bradycardia, hypotension, difficulty breathing
Verapamil	200 μg IC as a single dose to a total of 1000 μg (1 mg)	Bradycardia, hypotension
Diltiazem	200 μg IC as a single dose to a total dose of 1000 μg (1 mg) IC	Bradycardia, hypotension
Nicardipine	200 μg IC as a single dose to a total dose of 1000 μg (1 mg) IC	Lower incidence of bradycardia, hypotension with this vasoselective agent
Nitroprusside[b]	100 μg IC as a single dose to a total dose of 1000 μg (1 mg) IC	Lower incidence of bradycardia, hypotension

[a]Administration of these agents is not listed as an approved indication in the package insert (i.e., off label use).
[b]Median dose was 200 μg IC in the Hillegass study (53).
Source: From Ref. 56.

study looking at intracoronary verapamil (50–100 μg) in patients with acute MI showed a significant improvement in post-PCI TMPG in patients treated with intracoronary verapamil (52). Intracoronary nitroprusside administration at a median dose of 200 μg produces improved CTFC among patients with no reflow and may also be associated with a lower incidence of hypotension and bradycardia (53).

GPIIb/IIIa Inhibitors
A substudy of the Intergrillin and Tenecteplase in Acute Myocardial Infarction (INTEGRITI) trial looking at the impact of combination reperfusion therapy with reduced dose tenecteplase plus eptifibatide compared with full-dose lytic on ST-segment recovery and angiographic measures of reperfusion demonstrated a trend toward improvement in TFG, TMPG, and CTFC across the dosing regimens compared with full-dose tenecteplase (54). Another substudy of INTEGRITI looking at the association between platelet receptor occupancy after eptifibatide and myocardial perfusion in patients with STEMI showed a higher percent receptor occupancy in patients with TMPG 2/3 than those with delayed or no perfusion (TMPG 0/1) (55). These results taken cumulatively suggest that combination reperfusion with fibrinolysis and GPIIb/IIIa inhibitors are associated with improved angiographic measures of myocardial perfusion.

FUTURE DIRECTIONS
While the last 25 years have been the era of the "open artery hypothesis," there is growing recognition that epicardial artery patency is necessary, but not sufficient, to assure good clinical outcomes. There is gaining recognition of the "open muscle hypothesis," which asserts that the best outcomes are present when both epicardial and myocardial perfusion are restored. We must now incorporate the evaluation of myocardial perfusion into our clinical practice as both a measure of treatment efficacy and as a predictor of clinical outcome. We must shift the paradigm away from relying solely on "coronary angiography" toward the emerging technique of "myocardial angiography," where we assess both epicardial and myocardial perfusion.

REFERENCES

1. The Thrombolysis in Myocardial Infarction (TIMI) trial. Phase I findings. TIMI Study Group. N Engl J Med 1985; 312:932–936.
2. Simes RJ, Topol EJ, Holmes DR, Jr., et al. Link between the angiographic substudy and mortality outcomes in a large randomized trial of myocardial reperfusion. Importance of early and complete infarct artery reperfusion. GUSTO-I Investigators. Circulation 1995; 91:1923–1928.
3. The effects of tissue plasminogen activator, streptokinase, or both on coronary-artery patency, ventricular function, and survival after acute myocardial infarction. The GUSTO Angiographic Investigators. N Engl J Med 1993; 329:1615–1622.
4. Vogt A, von Essen R, Tebbe U, et al. Impact of early perfusion status of the infarct-related artery on short-term mortality after thrombolysis for acute myocardial infarction: retrospective analysis of four German multicenter studies. J Am Coll Cardiol 1993; 21:1391–1395.
5. Karagounis L, Sorensen SG, Menlove RL, et al. Does thrombolysis in myocardial infarction (TIMI) perfusion grade 2 represent a mostly patent artery or a mostly occluded artery? Enzymatic and electrocardiographic evidence from the TEAM-2 study. Second Multicenter Thrombolysis Trial of Eminase in Acute Myocardial Infarction. J Am Coll Cardiol 1992; 19:1–10.
6. Anderson JL, Karagounis LA, Becker LC, et al. TIMI perfusion grade 3 but not grade 2 results in improved outcome after thrombolysis for myocardial infarction. Ventriculographic, enzymatic, and electrocardiographic evidence from the TEAM-3 Study. Circulation 1993; 87:1829–1839.
7. Gibson CM, Cannon CP, Daley WL, et al. TIMI frame count: a quantitative method of assessing coronary artery flow. Circulation 1996; 93:879–888.
8. Gibson CM, Murphy SA, Rizzo MJ, et al. Relationship between TIMI frame count and clinical outcomes after thrombolytic administration. Thrombolysis In Myocardial Infarction (TIMI) Study Group. Circulation 1999; 99:1945–1950.
9. Gibson CM, Ryan KA, Kelley M, et al. Methodologic drift in the assessment of TIMI grade 3 flow and its implications with respect to the reporting of angiographic trial results. The TIMI Study Group. Am Heart J 1999; 137:1179–1184.
10. Gibson CM, Murphy S, Menown IB, et al. Determinants of coronary blood flow after thrombolytic administration. TIMI Study Group. Thrombolysis in Myocardial Infarction. J Am Coll Cardiol 1999; 34:1403–1412.
11. Wong GC, Morrow DA, Murphy S, et al. Elevations in troponin T and I are associated with abnormal tissue level perfusion: a TACTICS-TIMI 18 substudy. Treat angina with aggrastat and determine cost of therapy with an invasive or conservative strategy-thrombolysis in myocardial infarction. Circulation 2002; 106:202–207.
12. Ito H, Tomooka T, Sakai N, et al. Lack of myocardial perfusion immediately after successful thrombolysis. A predictor of poor recovery of left ventricular function in anterior myocardial infarction. Circulation 1992; 85:1699–1705.
13. Ito H, Maruyama A, Iwakura K, et al. Clinical implications of the 'no reflow' phenomenon. A predictor of complications and left ventricular remodeling in reperfused anterior wall myocardial infarction. Circulation 1996; 93:223–228.
14. Gibson CM, Cannon CP, Murphy SA, et al. Relationship of the TIMI myocardial perfusion grades, flow grades, frame count, and percutaneous coronary intervention to long-term outcomes after thrombolytic administration in acute myocardial infarction. Circulation 2002; 105:1909–1913.
15. Gibson CM, Dodge JT, Jr., Goel M, et al. Angioplasty guidewire velocity: a new simple method to calculate absolute coronary blood velocity and flow. Am J Cardiol 1997; 80:1536–1539.
16. Abaci A, Oguzhan A, Eryol NK, et al. Effect of potential confounding factors on the thrombolysis in myocardial infarction (TIMI) trial frame count and its reproducibility. Circulation 1999; 100:2219–2223.
17. Dodge JT Jr., Rizzo M, Nykiel M, et al. Impact of injection rate on the Thrombolysis in Myocardial Infarction (TIMI) trial frame count. Am J Cardiol 1998; 81:1268–1270.

18. Edep ME, Guarneri EM, Teirstein PS, et al. Differences in TIMI frame count following successful reperfusion with stenting or percutaneous transluminal coronary angioplasty for acute myocardial infarction. Am J Cardiol 1999; 83:1326–1329.
19. Vrachatis AD, Alpert MA, Georgulas VP, et al. Comparative efficacy of primary angioplasty with stent implantation and thrombolysis in restoring basal coronary artery flow in acute ST segment elevation myocardial infarction: quantitative assessment using the corrected TIMI frame count. Angiology 2001; 52:161–166.
20. Hamada S, Nishiue T, Nakamura S, et al. TIMI frame count immediately after primary coronary angioplasty as a predictor of functional recovery in patients with TIMI 3 reperfused acute myocardial infarction. J Am Coll Cardiol 2001; 38:666–671.
21. Capozzolo C, Piscione F, De Luca G, et al. Direct coronary stenting: effect on coronary blood flow, immediate and late clinical results. Catheter Cardiovasc Interv 2001; 53: 464–473.
22. Bickel C, Rupprecht HJ, Maimaitiming A, et al. The superiority of TIMI frame count in detecting coronary flow changes after coronary stenting compared to TIMI Flow Classification. J Invasive Cardiol 2002; 14:590–596.
23. Gibson CM, Dotani MI, Murphy SA, et al. Correlates of coronary blood flow before and after percutaneous coronary intervention and their relationship to angiographic and clinical outcomes in the RESTORE trial. Randomized Efficacy Study of Tirofiban for Outcomes and REstenosis. Am Heart J 2002; 144:130–135.
24. Gibson CM, Ryan KA, Murphy SA, et al. Impaired coronary blood flow in nonculprit arteries in the setting of acute myocardial infarction. The TIMI Study Group. Thrombolysis in myocardial infarction. J Am Coll Cardiol 1999; 34:974–982.
25. Gibson CM, Goel M, Murphy SA, et al. Global impairment of coronary blood flow in the setting of acute coronary syndromes (a RESTORE substudy). Randomized Efficacy Study of Tirofiban for Outcomes and Restenosis. Am J Cardiol 2000; 86:1375–1377 (abstr).
26. Gibson RS, Crampton RS, Watson DD, et al. Precordial ST-segment depression during acute inferior myocardial infarction: clinical, scintigraphic and angiographic correlations. Circulation 1982; 66:732–741.
27. Gibson CM, Murphy SA, Kirtane AJ, et al. Association of duration of symptoms at presentation with angiographic and clinical outcomes after fibrinolytic therapy in patients with ST-segment elevation myocardial infarction. J Am Coll Cardiol 2004; 44:980–987.
28. Schroder R, Dissmann R, Bruggemann T, et al. Extent of early ST segment elevation resolution: a simple but strong predictor of outcome in patients with acute myocardial infarction. J Am Coll Cardiol 1994; 24:384–391.
29. van 't Hof AW, Liem A, de Boer MJ, et al. Clinical value of 12-lead electrocardiogram after successful reperfusion therapy for acute myocardial infarction. Zwolle Myocardial infarction Study Group. Lancet 1997; 350:615–619.
30. Krucoff MW, Croll MA, Pope JE, et al. Continuous 12-lead ST-segment recovery analysis in the TAMI 7 study. Performance of a noninvasive method for real-time detection of failed myocardial reperfusion. Circulation 1993; 88:437–446.
31. Angeja BG, Gunda M, Murphy SA, et al. TIMI myocardial perfusion grade and ST segment resolution: association with infarct size as assessed by single photon emission computed tomography imaging. Circulation 2002; 105:282–285.
32. Haager PK, Christott P, Heussen N, et al. Prediction of clinical outcome after mechanical revascularization in acute myocardial infarction by markers of myocardial reperfusion. J Am Coll Cardiol 2003; 41:532–538.
33. Poli A, Fetiveau R, Vandoni P, et al. Integrated analysis of myocardial blush and ST-segment elevation recovery after successful primary angioplasty: real-time grading of microvascular reperfusion and prediction of early and late recovery of left ventricular function. Circulation 2002; 106:313–318.
34. Gibson CM, Karha J, Giugliano RP, et al. Association of the timing of ST-segment resolution with TIMI myocardial perfusion grade in acute myocardial infarction. Am Heart J 2004; 147:847–852.

35. Gibson CM, Schomig A. Coronary and myocardial angiography: angiographic assessment of both epicardial and myocardial perfusion. Circulation 2004; 109:3096–3105.

36. van 't Hof AW, Liem A, Suryapranata H, et al. Angiographic assessment of myocardial reperfusion in patients treated with primary angioplasty for acute myocardial infarction: myocardial blush grade. Zwolle Myocardial Infarction Study Group. Circulation 1998; 97:2302–2306.

37. Gibson CM, Kirtane AJ, Morrow DA, et al. Association between thrombolysis in myocardial infarction myocardial perfusion grade, biomarkers, and clinical outcomes among patients with moderate- to high-risk acute coronary syndromes: observations from the randomized trial to evaluate the relative PROTECTion against post-PCI microvascular dysfunction and post-PCI ischemia among antiplatelet and antithrombotic agents-Thrombolysis In Myocardial Infarction 30 (PROTECT-TIMI 30). Am Heart J 2006; 152:756–761.

38. Kirtane AJ, Vafai JJ, Murphy SA, et al. Angiographically evident thrombus following fibrinolytic therapy is associated with impaired myocardial perfusion in STEMI: a CLARITY-TIMI 28 substudy. Eur Heart J 2006; 27:2040–2045.

39. De Luca G, Suryapranata H, Zijlstra F, et al. Symptom-onset-to-balloon time and mortality in patients with acute myocardial infarction treated by primary angioplasty. J Am Coll Cardiol 2003; 42:991–997.

40. Kirtane AJ, Bui A, Murphy SA, et al. Association of epicardial and tissue-level reperfusion with left ventricular end-diastolic pressures in ST-elevation myocardial infarction. J Thromb Thrombolysis 2004; 17:177–184.

41. Tarantini G, Ramondo A, Napodano M, et al. Myocardial perfusion grade and survival after percutaneous transluminal coronary angioplasty in patients with cardiogenic shock. Am J Cardiol 2004; 93:1081–1085.

42. Gibson CM, Murphy SA, Marble SJ, et al. Relationship of creatine kinase-myocardial band release to thrombolysis in myocardial infarction perfusion grade after intracoronary stent placement: an ESPRIT substudy. Am Heart J 2002; 143:106–110.

43. Gibson CM, de Lemos JA, Murphy SA, et al. Methodologic and clinical validation of the TIMI myocardial perfusion grade in acute myocardial infarction. J Thromb Thrombolysis 2002; 14:233–237.

44. Gibson CM, Cohen DJ, Cohen EA, et al. Effect of eptifibatide on coronary flow reserve following coronary stent implantation (an ESPRIT substudy). Enhanced Suppression of the Platelet IIb/IIIa Receptor with Integrilin Therapy. Am J Cardiol 2001; 87:1293–1295.

45. Gibson CM, Murphy SA, Morrow DA, et al. Angiographic perfusion score: an angiographic variable that integrates both epicardial and tissue level perfusion before and after facilitated percutaneous coronary intervention in acute myocardial infarction. Am Heart J 2004; 148:336–340.

46. Karha J, Murphy SA, Kirtane AJ, et al. Evaluation of the association of proximal coronary culprit artery lesion location with clinical outcomes in acute myocardial infarction. Am J Cardiol 2003; 92:913–918.

47. Gibson CM, Karha J, Murphy SA, et al. Association of a pulsatile blood flow pattern on coronary arteriography and short-term clinical outcomes in acute myocardial infarction. J Am Coll Cardiol 2004; 43:1170–1176.

48. Ryan TJ, Faxon DP, Gunnar RM, et al. Guidelines for percutaneous transluminal coronary angioplasty. A report of the American College of Cardiology/American Heart Association Task Force on Assessment of Diagnostic and Therapeutic Cardiovascular Procedures (Subcommittee on Percutaneous Transluminal Coronary Angioplasty). Circulation 1988; 78:486–502.

49. Ellis SG, Vandormael MG, Cowley MJ, et al. Coronary morphologic and clinical determinants of procedural outcome with angioplasty for multivessel coronary disease. Implications for patient selection. Multivessel Angioplasty Prognosis Study Group. Circulation 1990; 82:1193–1202.

50. Marzilli M, Orsini E, Marraccini P, et al. Beneficial effects of intracoronary adenosine as an adjunct to primary angioplasty in acute myocardial infarction. Circulation 2000; 101:2154–2159.

51. Michaels AD, Appleby M, Otten MH, et al. Pretreatment with intragraft verapamil prior to percutaneous coronary intervention of saphenous vein graft lesions: results of the randomized, controlled vasodilator prevention on no-reflow (VAPOR) trial. J Invasive Cardiol 2002; 14:299–302.
52. Hang CL, Wang CP, Yip HK, et al. Early administration of intracoronary verapamil improves myocardial perfusion during percutaneous coronary interventions for acute myocardial infarction. Chest 2005; 128:2593–2598.
53. Hillegass WB, Dean NA, Liao L, et al. Treatment of no-reflow and impaired flow with the nitric oxide donor nitroprusside following percutaneous coronary interventions: initial human clinical experience. J Am Coll Cardiol 2001; 37:1335–1343.
54. Roe MT, Green CL, Giugliano RP, et al. Improved speed and stability of ST-segment recovery with reduced-dose tenecteplase and eptifibatide compared with full-dose tenecteplase for acute ST-segment elevation myocardial infarction. J Am Coll Cardiol 2004; 43:549–556.
55. Gibson CM, Jennings LK, Murphy SA, et al. Association between platelet receptor occupancy after eptifibatide (integrilin) therapy and patency, myocardial perfusion, and ST-segment resolution among patients with ST-segment-elevation myocardial infarction: an INTEGRITI (Integrilin and Tenecteplase in Acute Myocardial Infarction) substudy. Circulation 2004; 110:679–684.
56. Gibson CM. Has my patient achieved adequate myocardial reperfusion? Circulation 2003; 108:504–507.

4 Infusion Fibrinolytic Therapy

Eric R. Bates

Department of Internal Medicine, Division of Cardiovascular Diseases, University of Michigan, Ann Arbor, Michigan, U.S.A.

INTRODUCTION

ST-elevation myocardial infarction (STEMI) is a major cause of cardiovascular morbidity and mortality. Fibrinolytic therapy is recommended in STEMI patients with (*i*) symptom onset within 12 hours, (*ii*) greater than 0.1 mV ST-segment elevation in at least two contiguous ECG leads or new left bundle branch block, and (*iii*) low bleeding risk (1). It restores infarct artery patency, reduces infarct size, preserves left ventricular function, and decreases mortality in patients with STEMI. Three seminal events ushered in the "fibrinolytic era." First, DeWood and colleagues (2) performed acute coronary angiography in patients with STEMI and showed that 87% had thrombotic coronary artery occlusion within 4 hours of symptom onset, but only 54% did 12 to 24 hours after onset. Coronary thrombosis had previously been thought to be a postmortem finding. Second, Rentrop and coworkers (3) demonstrated that occluded infarct arteries could acutely be reperfused with an intracoronary streptokinase infusion. Third, Reimer et al. (4) demonstrated in a dog model that myocardial necrosis after coronary artery occlusion spread from the endocardial surface to the epicardial surface over a period of hours. Restoration of arterial patency before three hours preserved an epicardial rim of viable muscle, establishing the anatomical justification for reperfusion therapy to modify infarct size.

This chapter summarizes information on the infusion fibrinolytic agents, including streptokinase, alteplase, duteplase, anistreplase, urokinase, and saruplase. Characteristics of the two infusion and two bolus fibrinolytic agents available in the United States for treating STEMI are shown in Table 1.

STREPTOKINASE

In 1933, Tillet and Garner (5) discovered that a filtrate of b-hemolytic strains of Streptococcus could dissolve human thrombus. Streptokinase is a single-chain nonenzyme protein that forms a 1:1 stoichiometric complex with plasminogen. The streptokinase-plasminogen activator complex then converts plasminogen to plasmin, which initiates fibrinolysis. Intravenous streptokinase was initially used in the late 1950s for STEMI (6) and was tested in several multicenter trials in the 1960s and 1970s (7). Unfortunately, improvement in left ventricular function and mortality were inconsistently found because of inadequate doses and late implementation of therapy. Immediate arteriographic recanalization following intracoronary injection of streptokinase during STEMI was first reported by Chazov (8) and later in the English literature by Rentrop et al (3). These observations legitimized fibrinolytic therapy for STEMI and initiated the angiographic evaluation of mechanisms and clinical benefit. More easily administered intravenous therapy allowed greater access to therapy and shorter time to treatment.

TABLE 1 Comparison of Approved Fibrinolytic Agents

	Streptokinase	Alteplase	Reteplase	TNK-t-PA
Dose	1.5 MU over 30–60 min	Up to 100 mg in 90 min (based on weight)[a]	10 U × 2 each over 2 min	30–50 mg based on weight[b]
Bolus administration	No	No	Yes	Yes
Antigenic	Yes	No	No	No
Allergic reactions (hypotension most common)	Yes	No	No	No
Systemic fibrinogen depletion	Marked	Mild	Moderate	Minimal
90-min patency rates (%)	~50	~75	~75	~75
TIMI grade 3 flow (%)	32	54	60	63
Cost per dose (U.S.) (3)	$613	$2974	$2750	$2833 for 50 mg

TIMI indicates Thrombolysis in Myocardial Infarction.
[a]Bolus 15 mg, infusion 0.75 mg/kg times 30 minutes (maximum 50 mg), then 0.5 mg/kg not to exceed 35 mg over the next 60 minutes to an overall maximum of 100 mg.
[b]30 mg for less than 60 kg; 35 mg for 60 to 69 kg; 40 mg for 70 to 79 mg; 45 mg for 80 to 89 kg; 50 mg for greater than or equal to 90 kg.
Source: From Ref. 1.

TABLE 2 Infarct Artery Patency Results[a]

Time	Control	Streptokinase	Alteplase (3 hr)	Alteplase (90 min)	Anistreplase	Urokinase
60 min	15 (6–24)	48 (41–56)	57 (52–61)	74 (70–77)	61 (55–67)	–
90 min	21 (11–31)	51 (48–55)	70 (68–72)	84 (82–87)	70 (66–74)	60 (55–64)
2–3 hr	24 (14–35)	70 (65–75)	73 (65–80)	–	74 (68–80)	58 (48–68)
1 day	21 (9–32)	86 (82–89)	84 (82–86)	86 (82–90)	80 (77–83)	–
3–21 days	61 (57–64)	73 (70–78)	80 (78–81)	89 (85–94)	85 (81–89)	72 (63–81)

[a]Percent (95% CI).
Source: From Ref. 10.

Coronary Patency, Infarct Size, and Left Ventricular Function

The conventional dose of 1.5 million units over 60 minutes for intravenous streptokinase was derived empirically by Schroeder and colleagues (9). Sixty- and 90-minute patency rates are approximately 50%, and two- to three-hour patency rates are 70% (10) (Table 2).

Enzymatic estimation of infarct size in the Netherlands Interuniversity Cardiology Institute study (11) of intracoronary streptokinase demonstrated a 51% decrease in infarct size in patients treated within one hour of onset of symptoms, 31% in those treated between one and two hours, and 13% in those treated between two and four hours. The Intravenous Streptokinase in Acute Myocardial infarction (ISAM) trial (12) measured a lower enzymatic infarct size in patients treated within three hours after onset of pain, but found no difference in patients treated later. Likewise, early treatment is associated with preservation of approximately six ejection fraction points (13,14). End-systolic volume measurements are smaller in treated patients (13,15).

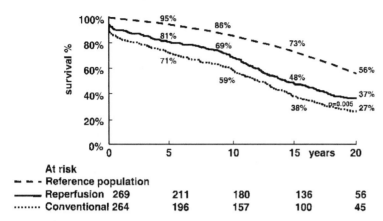

FIGURE 1 Twenty-year survival in the Interuniversity Cardiology Institute of the Netherlands trial. *Source*: From Ref. 23.

Effects of Streptokinase on Mortality

The Western Washington intracoronary streptokinase trial (16,17) randomized 134 patients to streptokinase and 116 patients to control a mean of 4.7 hours after symptom onset. Recanalization was achieved in 68% of the streptokinase-treated group. The 30-day mortality rate was significantly reduced (3.7% vs. 11.2%, $p < 0.02$) and the one-year mortality rate was also lower (8.2% vs. 14.7%). The mortality rate was 2.5% with complete reperfusion, 23.1% with partial reperfusion, and 14.6% with no reperfusion, establishing the importance of successful reperfusion. The Western Washington intravenous streptokinase trial randomized 368 patients to intravenous streptokinase or standard therapy (18). At 14 days, there was an insignificant difference in mortality (6.3% vs. 9.6%), with survival benefit in anterior MI but not in inferior MI. Survival benefit in these two trials was not maintained at five years (80% vs. 76%) (19). The results were limited by delayed time to treatment and low reperfusion rates.

The Netherlands Interuniversity Cardiology Institute trial (11,20–23) allocated 264 patients to conventional treatment and 269 to intracoronary streptokinase, the last 117 of whom were first treated with 500,000 units of intravenous streptokinase. The time to treatment was 80 minutes faster than in the Western Washington intracoronary trial (16), and the recanalization rate was higher (79%). The 30-day mortality was significantly reduced with streptokinase (6.5% vs. 11.8%). The cumulative 10-, 15-, and 20-year survival rates were 59%, 38%, and 27% in the conventional therapy group and 69%, 48%, and 37% in the streptokinase group, respectively. Thus, the absolute 10% 1-year survival benefit with reperfusion therapy was sustained throughout 20 years (Fig. 1). Overall, there was an absolute benefit of 105 lives saved per 1000 treated patients and an increase in life expectancy of 2.8 years. Even better results were achieved in patients with extensive ST-segment elevation, anterior infarct location, or treatment within two hours of symptom onset.

The Registry of the Society for Cardiac Angiography (24) included 1029 patients from 35 institutions who were treated with intracoronary streptokinase 240 ± 413 minutes after symptom onset. The reperfusion rate was 71% and the in-hospital mortality rate was 8.2%. The mortality rate was lower with successful reperfusion (5.5%) than with unsuccessful reperfusion (14.7%).

The ISAM trial (12,25) randomized 1741 patients to intravenous streptokinase or placebo within six hours of symptom onset. Mortality at 21 days (6.3% vs. 7.1%) was lower than expected in the control group, rendering the trial underpowered to detect a treatment difference. At 21 months, the mortality rate was 14.4% with streptokinase and 16.1% with placebo.

The Gruppo Italiano per lo Studio della Streptochinasi nell'infarto Miocardico (GISSI)-1 (26) and International Study of Infarct Survival (ISIS)-2 (27) trials were the first properly powered trials to demonstrate the mortality advantage of intravenous fibrinolytic therapy. In the GISSI-1 trial (26,28,29), 11,712 patients were randomized to either intravenous streptokinase or control within 12 hours of symptom onset. Only 21% of patients received anticoagulation therapy, and only 14% received antiplatelet therapy. Mortality at 21 days was 10.7% in the streptokinase group versus 13% in the control group, an 18% risk reduction. The extent of the benefit was time dependent, with relative reductions in in-hospital mortality of 47% within one hour of symptom onset, 23% within three hours, and 21% within six hours, but no benefit after six hours. The benefit was maintained after hospital discharge up to 10 years, but there was no further improvement (45.0% vs. 46.9%). The ISIS-2 trial (27,30) randomized 17,187 patients within 24 hours of the onset of symptoms of suspected MI to streptokinase, aspirin, both, or neither. Streptokinase alone reduced the five-week vascular mortality (9.2% vs. 12%), a 23% risk reduction, and the combination of aspirin plus streptokinase additionally reduced mortality (8% vs. 13.2%), a 39% risk reduction. Again, the benefit was maintained for 10 years, but did not change after 35 days (chap. 1, Fig. 4).

The Estudio Multicentrico Estreptoquinasa Republicas de America del Sur (EMERAS) trial (31) found an insignificant 14% reduction (11.7% vs. 13.2%) in hospital mortality in 2080 patients randomized to streptokinase or placebo 6 to 12 hours after symptom onset, but no benefit in patients presenting after 13 to 24 hours.

ALTEPLASE

Tissue plasminogen activator is a naturally occurring single-chain serine protease normally secreted by vascular endothelium. It was first obtained from the Bowes melanoma cell line and is now produced by recombinant DNA technology. Native tissue-type plasminogen activator (t-PA) and alteplase (rt-PA) have a binding site for fibrin, which causes a great affinity for attaching to thrombus and preferentially lysing it, although systemic plasminogen activation occurs at clinical doses. The first clinical trial with alteplase was reported in 1984 (32).

Coronary Patency, Infarct Size, and Left Ventricular Function

The Thrombolysis in Myocardial Infarction (TIMI)-I (33) and European Cooperative Study Group (ECSG)-1 (34) studies established higher 90-minute patency rates for rt-PA than streptokinase. The TIMI-II trial (35) began with a dose of 150 mg over six hours, but this was reduced to 100 mg over three hours because of an unacceptable rate of intracerebral hemorrhage. Numerous studies established a 90-minute patency rate of 70% with this dose (10), a success rate equal to that achieved with streptokinase two to three hours after initiation of therapy (Table 2). Neuhaus and colleagues (36) accelerated the dosing, infusing the total dose of 100 mg before the 90-minute angiogram and achieved a 90-minute patency rate of 91%. Purvis and coworkers (37) tested double-bolus (two 50-mg injections 30 minutes apart) alteplase and demonstrated a 93% patency rate at 90 minutes. Subsequent testing has established that a weight-adjusted accelerated or front-loaded dose (15 mg bolus, 0.75 mg/kg over 30 minutes, 0.5 mg/kg over 60 minutes) is superior to double-bolus dosing and achieves 90-minute patency rates of approximately 82% (10,38).

The ECSG-5 trial (39) was a double-blind placebo-controlled trial in 721 patients treated within five hours of symptom onset. The cumulative myocardial enzyme release over 72 hours was 20% lower in patients treated with alteplase. Three small trials (40–42) had previously revealed a 6% to 7% higher ejection fraction in patients treated with alteplase. The ECSG-5 (39) trial measured a 2.2% higher ejection fraction and lower end-diastolic and end-systolic volumes in patients randomized to alteplase.

The TAMI Trials

The Thrombolysis and Angioplasty in Myocardial Infarction (TAMI) Study Group completed 10 studies (43–52) of various therapeutic regimens in STEMI with alteplase and urokinase, focusing on dosing and adjunctive therapies. Angiography was used to assess infarct artery patency and left ventricular function. Ten different doses of alteplase were given, with an accelerated dose similar to that used by Neuhaus et al. (36) having the highest patency rate (50). Treating patients 6 to 24 hours after symptom onset improved early patency (65% vs. 27%) and preserved end-diastolic volume (49). The strategy of immediate PTCA after successful fibrinolysis offered no clinical benefit (43), but acute angiography and rescue PTCA as necessary were feasible and potentially useful (43,48). Immediate heparin administration did not facilitate fibrinolysis (45), as suggested in animal studies, but more potent platelet inhibition with a monoclonal antibody directed against the platelet GP IIb/IIIa receptor did improve patency rates (51). Preclinical studies suggesting that prostacyclin and fluosol decreased reperfusion injury, by inhibiting free radicals and neutrophil activity, and improved left ventricular function were not confirmed in the TAMI-4 (46) and TAMI-9 (52) studies, respectively. Furthermore, the TAMI data set was analyzed in a number of publications to examine patient selection, clinical outcomes, and prognosis (53).

The TIMI Trials

In parallel with the TAMI investigators, the TIMI investigators were also studying fibrinolysis with streptokinase and alteplase (33,35,54–64). After demonstrating superior recanalization rates for rt-PA compared with streptokinase in TIMI-1 (33), the TIMI-II (35,54) trial showed no advantage for PTCA immediately or 18 to 48 hours after thrombolysis versus a selective strategy of treating postinfarction ischemia. The TIMI-III trial (55,56) examined patients with unstable angina and NSTEMI. Patients treated with alteplase instead of placebo had a higher rate of MI (8.3% vs. 4.6%) and a 0.55% risk of intracerebral hemorrhage. An early invasive strategy with angiography rather than an early conservative strategy with routine medical care and risk stratification was associated with no difference in death or MI, but fewer patients were rehospitalized or taking antianginal medications at six weeks. In TIMI-4 (57), accelerated alteplase had higher earlier patency rates and improved clinical benefit compared with anistreplase or combination thrombolytic therapy. Hirudin, a direct thrombin inhibitor, achieved a more consistent level of anticoagulation than heparin when tested with alteplase in TIMI-5 (58) and streptokinase in TIMI-6 (59). Clinical end points were also improved. However, a high dose was associated with an unacceptable rate of intracerebral hemorrhage in TIMI-9 (60), and a lower dose had no survival advantage (61). The TIMI-10B trial (62) showed equivalent patency rates with accelerated alteplase and tenecteplase. Coadministration of abciximab with reduced-dose alteplase or reteplase increased patency rates in TIMI-14 (63). There was no mortality difference between accelerated alteplase and lanoteplase in TIMI-17 (64), but intracerebral hemorrhage rates were higher with lanoteplase. The TIMI data set has also produced a number of important publications (65).

Effects of Alteplase on Mortality

The Anglo-Scandinavian Study of Early Thrombolysis (ASSET) (66,67) was the first large randomized clinical trial to evaluate mortality as an end point. A total of 5013 patients with less than five hours of symptoms were randomized to alteplase or placebo. Although patients received intravenous heparin, aspirin was not given. At one month, mortality was reduced by 26% with alteplase (7.2% vs. 9.8%). At six months, the rates were 10.4% with alteplase and 13.1% with placebo. The effect was similar for anterior (15.6% vs. 21.2%) and inferior (7.7% vs. 12.8%) myocardial infarction. The ECSG-5 trial (39) randomized 721 patients with less than five hours of symptoms to alteplase or placebo. Despite only small differences in ejection fraction, the 14-day mortality was reduced with alteplase (2.8% vs. 5.7%). The Late Assessment of Thrombolytic Efficacy (LATE) study (68) randomized 5711 patients with symptoms between 6 and 24 hours from onset to alteplase or placebo. A significant 26% reduction in 35-day mortality (8.9% vs. 12%) was found in the 6- to 12-hour group, but no difference was seen between 12 and 24 hours.

There have been two comparative trials of standard-dose alteplase versus streptokinase (Table 3). The GISSI-2 trial (69) tested a three-hour alteplase infusion and found no treatment advantage. The 12,490 patients from GISSI-2 were added to 8401 recruited elsewhere to form the International Study (70), with no mortality difference between alteplase and streptokinase (8.9% vs. 8.5%). Streptokinase was associated with fewer strokes and more allergic reactions and transfusions compared with alteplase.

In contrast, the Global Utilization of Streptokinase and Tissue Plasminogen Activator for Occluded Coronary Arteries (GUSTO)-I trial (71) tested the accelerated dose (two-thirds of the dose administered by 30 minutes instead of by 90 minutes) combined with intravenous heparin against streptokinase and found a significant mortality reduction (6.3% vs. 7.3%) with alteplase. Also, there were significantly

TABLE 3 Study Design of Thrombolytic Megatrials

	International (70)[a]	ISIS-3 (75)	GUSTO-1 (71)
Sample size	20,891	41,299	41,021
Thrombolytic regimen	1. Streptokinase	1. Streptokinase	1. Streptokinase
	2. Alteplase (3 hr)	2. Duteplase (4 hr)	2. Alteplase (90 min)
		3. Anistreplase	3. Streptokinase/Alteplase
Heparin regimen	12,500 IU SQ b.i.d.	12,500 IU SQ b.i.d.	12,500 IU SQ b.i.d.
	or placebo	or placebo	or 1,000–1,200 IU/hr
Delay in heparin Rx	12 hr	4 hr	4 hr SQ
			0 hr IV

[a]Includes 12,490 patients from GISSI-2 trial.

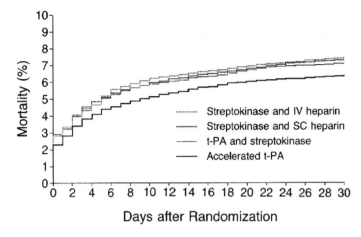

FIGURE 2 Thirty-day mortality in the Global Utilization of Streptokinase and Tissue Plasminogen Activator for Occluded Coronary Arteries (GUSTO)-I trial. *Source*: From Ref. 71.

lower rates of heart failure, cardiogenic shock, sustained hypotension, asystole, atrioventricular block, atrial arrhythmias, and ventricular arrhythmias. There were two excess hemorrhagic strokes per 1000 patients treated with alteplase, but the 30-day mortality or disabling stroke rate was lower with alteplase than streptokinase (6.9% vs. 7.8%) (Fig. 2) (71). No real differences in bleeding were noted. At one year, the mortality advantage with alteplase was maintained (9.1% vs. 10.1%) (72).

Finally, the Continuous Infusion Vs. Double Bolus Administration of Alteplase (COBALT) trial (73), comparing double bolus dosing with the accelerated dose in 7169 patients, was prematurely stopped when no mortality benefit (8.0% vs. 7.5%) was seen during an interim analysis.

DUTEPLASE

Duteplase is a nearly pure two-chain form of rt-PA. It differs from alteplase only in the substitution of methionine for valine at position 245 in the amino acid sequence in the kringle 2 region. Duteplase produced a 90-minute patency rate of 69% in 488 patients when given over four hours, with 0.4 megaunits/kg given in the first hour (including a 10% bolus) and 0.2 megaunits/kg given over the subsequent three hours (74). As with the conventional alteplase dose of 100 mg over three hours used in the GISSI-2 trial (69), two-thirds the dose was administered by 90 minutes. This dose was used in the ISIS-3 trial (75), where no mortality difference was seen between streptokinase (10.6%), duteplase (10.3%), and anistreplase (10.5%), and lower stroke rates were seen with streptokinase (Table 3). Patency results and the mortality data from GISSI-2 and ISIS-3 suggest that duteplase and alteplase are clinically equivalent. Duteplase was withdrawn from further development after the loss of a patent infringement legal suit to the manufacturer of alteplase.

ANISTREPLASE

Anistreplase (anisoylated plasminogen streptokinase activator complex, APSAC) is a stoichiometric combination of streptokinase and human Lys-plasminogen. An anisoyl group reversibly bound to the catalytic center of the plasminogen moiety slowly undergoes deacylation prior to direct plasminogen activation. The delayed onset of action permits the agent to be administered over a few minutes.

Coronary Patency, Infarct Size, and Left Ventricular Function
A dose of 30 mg injected over five minutes contains approximately 1 million units of streptokinase. The 70% 90-minute patency rate is equivalent to the three-hour alteplase dose (10).

The APSAC Multicenter Trial Group (76) found no difference in peak creatine kinase activity, although the time to peak activity was shorter with anistreplase versus placebo. In contrast, Bassand et al. (77) demonstrated a 31% decrease in infarct size measured by single photon emission computed tomography. Similarly, the former trial (76) showed no difference in left ventricular function, whereas the latter trial (77) found a 6% higher mean left ventricular ejection fraction with anistreplase.

Mortality Trials
The APSAC Intervention Mortality Study (AIMS) (78) randomized 1258 patients to anistreplase or placebo within six hours from symptom onset. They were also treated with unfractionated heparin and three months of warfarin, but not aspirin. The trial was stopped prematurely because of the 47% mortality reduction seen with anistreplase (6.4% vs. 12.1%). The one-year mortality rate was 11.1% with anistreplase and 17.8% with placebo (79).

There have been five trials comparing anistreplase with streptokinase and rt-PA. The Second Thrombolytic Trial of Eminase in Acute Myocardial Infarction (TEAM-2) (80) compared anistreplase and streptokinase, showing comparable patency and mortality (5.9% vs. 7.1%) results in 370 patients. The TEAM-3 trial (81) documented equivalent patency rates and mortality (6.2% vs. 7.9%) between anistreplase and standard alteplase in 325 patients. The ISIS-3 study (75) showed no difference in mortality between streptokinase, duteplase, and anistreplase. The rt-PA-APSAC Patency Study (TAPS) (82) showed higher patency and lower mortality (2.4% vs. 8.1%) for accelerated alteplase versus anistreplase in 435 patients. Similarly, TIMI-4 (57) showed the same mortality advantage (2.2% vs. 8.8%) for accelerated alteplase compared with anistreplase in 382 patients. Anistreplase was withdrawn from the U.S. market in 2000.

UROKINASE

Urokinase is a double-chain serine protease derived initially from urine and subsequently from neonatal renal parenchymal cell cultures. It directly activates plasminogen without forming an activator complex, like alteplase, but like streptokinase, it is not specific for fibrin-bound thrombus.

Urokinase can be given as a bolus, like alteplase, or infused over 60 to 90 minutes. Mathey and coworkers (83) injected a bolus of 2 million units and documented a 60% patency rate at 60 minutes in 50 patients. Four other trials had similar patency rates at 90 minutes with 3 million unit infusion protocols (47,48,84,85). Mortality trials have not been performed, and the Food and Drug Administration has not approved intravenous urokinase for use in STEMI.

Urokinase has been used in combination with alteplase (44,48,50,86), producing an improved 90-minute patency rate of 72% and low reocclusion rates. However, other trials (57,71) of combination thrombolytic therapy have not demonstrated clinical benefit, and there may be an increased risk of intracerebral hemorrhage.

SARUPLASE

Saruplase is a recombinant unglycosylated form of single-chain urokinase (pro-urokinase). It exhibits relative fibrin specificity, a short half-life, and concomitant need for adjunctive heparin infusion. Saruplase has generally been administered as a 20-mg bolus and a 60-mg infusion over 60 minutes. In the Pro-Urokinase in Myocardial Infarction (PRIMI) trial (87), saruplase patency rates were superior to streptokinase and equivalent to those seen with standard alteplase and anistreplase. The Comparative Trial of Saruplase versus Streptokinase (COMPASS) (88) showed that 30-day mortality rates were at least as low with saruplase as with streptokinase (5.7% vs. 6.7%). The Study in Europe of Saruplase and Alteplase in Myocardial Infarction (SESAM) (89) found equivalent patency, reocclusion, and complication rates compared with standard alteplase.

COMPLICATIONS

The major complication of fibrinolytic therapy is bleeding. Although fibrin-specific agents were expected to result in fewer bleeding complications, the large comparative trials found no difference in bleeding or transfusion rates (69,71,75). The true incidence of bleeding has been difficult to determine because of underreporting in larger trials of streptokinase, the subjective nature of the events, different definitions for bleeding, and the variable use of invasive procedures. In GUSTO-I (71), the transfusion rate was 10%. Concomitant use of heparin increases bleeding risk, particularly when the aPTT exceeds 100 seconds (90). Therefore, therapeutic heparin was not recommended with the longer-acting agents streptokinase and anistreplase, although it was given with alteplase and saruplase to prevent infarct artery reocclusion. Many patients have conditions that increase the risk of serious bleeding and are absolute or relative contraindications for fibrinolytic therapy (Table 4) (1).

When life-threatening bleeding occurs, heparin should be discontinued. Therapeutic interventions include protamine to normalize the aPTT, cryoprecipitate to increase fibrinogen levels, fresh frozen plasma to replace clotting factors, platelet transfusions if the bleeding time is prolonged, and packed red blood cells to restore hemoglobin mass (91). A computerized tomographic scan of the head should be performed to document suspected intracranial hemorrhage.

The most devastating complication of fibrinolytic therapy is intracerebral hemorrhage. Data from clinical trials and unselected populations suggest that the risk is 0.5% to 1% (92). At least half the patients die, and severe disability occurs in an additional 25%. Increased risk is associated with age greater than 65 years, hypertension, and low body weight (93). More potent fibrinolytic agents increase risk. It is important to note, however, that fibrinolytic therapy decreases late, presumably thrombotic, stroke so there is no overall excess in stroke.

Streptokinase and anistreplase are antigenic because they are foreign proteins. Because of antibody formation, retreatment should not be given after four

TABLE 4 Contraindications and Cautions for Fibrinolytic Use in STEMI[a]

Absolute contraindications

- Any prior intracranial hemorrhage (ICH)
- Known structural cerebral vascular lesion (e.g., AVM)
- Known malignant intracranial neoplasm (primary or metastatic)
- Ischemic stroke within 3 mo EXCEPT acute ischemic stroke within 3 hr
- Suspected aortic dissection
- Active bleeding or bleeding diathesis (excluding menses)
- Significant closed head or facial trauma within 3 mo

Relative contraindications

- History of chronic severe poorly controlled hypertension
- Severe uncontrolled hypertension on presentation (SBP greater than 180 Hg or DBP greater than 110 Hg)[b]
- History of prior ischemic stroke greater than 3 mo, dementia, or known intracranial pathology not covered in contraindications
- Traumatic or prolonged (greater than 10 min) CPR or major surgery (less than 3 wk)
- Recent (within 2–4 wk) internal bleeding
- Noncompressible vascular punctures
- For streptokinase/anistreplase: prior exposure (especially within 5 days–2 yr) or prior allergic reaction to these agents
- Pregnancy
- Active peptic ulcer
- Current use of anticoagulants: the higher the INR, the higher the risk of bleeding

[a]Viewed as advisory for clinical decision making and may not be all-inclusive or definitive.
[b]Could be an absolute contraindication in low-risk patients with myocardial infarction (see Section 6.3.1.6.3.2).
Abbreviations: INR, international normalized ratio; CPR, cardiopulmonary resuscitation; SBP, systolic blood pressure; DBP, diastolic blood pressure.
Source: From Ref. 1.

days of the initial exposure to avoid neutralization of streptokinase activity (94). Moreover, mild allergic reactions (fever, rash, rigor, bronchospasm) occur in 5% of patients, including anaphylactic shock in 0.2%, and release of bradykinin produces hypotension in 5% to 10% (27).

Early reports suggested that reocclusion rates were higher with alteplase (14%) than with streptokinase, anistreplase, or urokinase (8%) (92). However, no differences were seen in GUSTO-I (38), perhaps because of the use of monitored intravenous heparin and aspirin with alteplase. Additionally, there does not appear to be any difference between agents in rates of recurrent ischemia (20%) or reinfarction (4%).

CONCLUSION

First-generation fibrinolytics including streptokinase, anistreplase, and urokinase are not fibrin specific and activate plasminogen systemically. Second-generation fibrinolytics including alteplase, duteplase, and saruplase preferentially activate plasminogen at the fibrin clot. Accelerated or front-loaded alteplase administered with intravenous heparin for 24 to 48 hours has proven to be as good as any fibrinolytic strategy tested to date. Its superior ability to restore early normal blood flow to the infarct artery has been associated with improved left ventricular function and lower mortality and morbidity rates than the first-generation agents. Bolus administration of alteplase and combination therapy with alteplase and streptokinase, anistreplase, or urokinase have not proven to be superior strategies. The standard three-hour infusion of alteplase appears to produce clinical outcomes similar to those of streptokinase, anistreplase, and saruplase. Anistreplase is the easiest to administer, and streptokinase is the least expensive agent. Long-term follow-up demonstrates that the short-term reduction in mortality is maintained for at least one year (28,67,72,79).

The link between normal infarct artery blood flow, preserved left ventricular function, and mortality reduction documented in GUSTO-I (38,71) has stimulated new efforts to develop superior lytic agents and new adjunctive strategies. However, the major reductions in clinical events over the past two decades with improved therapies have made it increasingly difficult to show incremental benefit with any new agent. The next major reduction in adverse events will probably come from organizing better systems of care that allow more patients to receive reperfusion therapy with faster times to treatment.

REFERENCES

1. Antman EM, Anbe DT, Armstrong PW, et al. ACC/AHA guidelines for the management of patients with ST-elevation myocardial infarction—executive summary: a report of the American College of Cardiology/American Heart Association Task Force on Practice Guidelines (Writing Committee to Revise the 1999 Guidelines for the Management of Patients with Acute Myocardial Infarction). Circulation 2004; 110:588–636.
2. DeWood MA, Spores J, Notske R, et al. Prevalence of total coronary occlusion during the early hours of transmural infarction. N Engl J Med 1980; 303:897–902.
3. Rentrop KT, Blanke H, Karsch KR, et al. Acute myocardial infarction: intracoronary application of nitroglycerine and streptokinase. Clin Cardiol 1979; 2:354–363.
4. Reimer KA, Lowe JE, Rasmussen MM, et al. The wave-front phenomenon of ischemic death. I. Myocardial infarct size vs. duration of coronary occlusion in dogs. Circulation 1977; 56:786–794.
5. Tillet WS, Garner RI. The fibrinolytic activity of hemolytic streptococci. J Experimental Med 1933; 58:485–502.
6. Fletcher AP, Alkjaersig N, Smyrniotis FE, et al. The treatment of patients suffering from early myocardial infarction with massive and prolonged streptokinase therapy. Trans Assoc Am Physicians 1958; 71:287–296.
7. Yusuf S, Collins R, Peto R, et al. Intravenous and intracoronary fibrinolytic therapy in acute myocardial infarction: overview of results on mortality, reinfarction, and side-effects from 33 randomized controlled trials. Eur Heart J 1985; 6:556–585.
8. Chazov EI, Mateeva LS, Mazaev AV, et al. Intracoronary administration of fibrinolysis in acute myocardial infarction. Ter Arkh 1976; 48:8–19.
9. Schröder, Biamino G, von Leitner ER, et al. Intravenous short-term infusion of streptokinase in acute myocardial infarction. Circulation 1983; 67:536–548.
10. Granger CB, White H, Bates ER, et al. Patency profiles and left ventricular function after intravenous thrombolysis: A pooled analysis. Am J Cardiol 1994; 74:1220–1228.
11. Simoons ML, Serruys PW, van den Brand M, et al. Early thrombolysis in acute myocardial infarction: limitation of infarct size and improved survival. J Am Coll Cardiol 1986; 7:717–728.
12. ISAM Study Group. A prospective trial of intravenous streptokinase in acute myocardial infarction (I.S.A.M.). Mortality, morbidity and infarct size at 21 days. N Engl J Med 1986; 314:1465–1471.
13. Serruys PW, Simoons ML, Suryapranata H, et al. Preservation of global and regional left ventricular function after early thrombolysis in acute myocardial infarction. J Am Coll Cardiol 1986; 7:729–742.

14. White HD, Norris RM, Brown MA, et al. Effect of intravenous streptokinase on left ventricular function and early survival after acute myocardial infarction. N Engl J Med 1987; 317:850–855.
15. White HD, Norris RM, Brown MA, et al. Left ventricular end-systolic volume as the major determinant of survival after recovery from myocardial infarction. Circulation 1987; 76:41–51.
16. Kennedy JW, Ritchie JL, Davis KB, et al. Western Washington randomized trial of intracoronary streptokinase in acute myocardial infarction. N Engl J Med 1983; 309: 1477–1482.
17. Kennedy JW, Ritchie JL, Davis KB, et al. The Western Washington randomized trial of intracoronary streptokinase in acute myocardial infarction. A 12-month follow-up report. N Engl J Med 1985; 312:1073–1078.
18. Kennedy JW, Martin GV, Davis KB, et al. The Western Washington intravenous streptokinase in acute myocardial infarction randomized trial. Circulation 1988; 77: 345–352.
19. Cerqueira MD, Maynard C, Ritchie JL, et al. Long-term survival in 618 patients from the Western Washington streptokinase in myocardial infarction trials. J Am Coll Cardiol 1992; 20:1452–1459.
20. Simoons ML, Serruys PW, Van den Brand M, et al. Improved survival after early thrombolysis in acute myocardial infarction: a randomized trial of the Interuniversity Cardiology Institute in the Netherlands. Lancet 1985; 2:578–582.
21. Simoons ML, Vos J, Tijssen JGP, et al. Long-term benefit of early thrombolytic therapy in patients with acute myocardial infarction: 5 year follow-up of a trial conducted by the Interuniversity Cardiology Institute of the Netherlands. J Am Coll Cardiol 1989; 14:1609–1615.
22. Maas ACP, van Domburg RT, Deckers JW, et al. Sustained benefit at 10–14 years follow-up after thrombolytic therapy in myocardial infarction. Eur Heart J 1999; 20:819–826.
23. Van Domburg RT, Sonnenschein K, Nieuwlaat R, et al. Sustained benefit 20 years after reperfusion therapy in acute myocardial infarction. J Am Coll Cardiol 2005; 46:15–20.
24. Kennedy JW, Gensini GG, Timmis GC, et al. Acute myocardial infarction treated with intracoronary streptokinase: a report of the Society for Cardiac Angiography. Am J Cardiol 1985; 55:871–877.
25. Schroder R, Neuhaus KL, Leizorovicz A, et al. A prospective placebo-controlled double-blind multicenter trial of intravenous streptokinase in acute myocardial infarction (ISAM): long-term mortality and morbidity. J Am Coll Cardiol 1987; 9:197–203.
26. Gruppo Italiano per lo Studio della Streptochinasi nell'infarto Miocardico (GISSI). Effectiveness of intravenous thrombolytic treatment in acute myocardial infarction. Lancet 1986; 1:397–401.
27. ISIS-2 (Second International Study of Infarct Survival) Collaborative Group. Randomised trial of intravenous streptokinase, oral aspirin, both, or neither among 17,187 cases of suspected acute myocardial infarction: ISIS-2. Lancet 1988; 2:349–360.
28. Gruppo Italiano per lo Studio della Streptochinasi nell'infarto Miocardico (GISSI). Long-term effects of intravenous thrombolysis in acute myocardial infarction: final report of the GISI study. Lancet 1987; 2:871–874.
29. Franzosi MG, Santoro E, De Vita C, et al. Ten-year follow-up of the first megatrial testing thrombolytic therapy in patients with acute myocardial infarction; results of the Gruppo Italiano per lo Studio della Sopravvivenza nell'infarto–1 study. The GISSI Investigators. Circulation 1998; 98:2659–2665.
30. Baigent C, Collins R, Appleby P, et al. ISIS-2: 10 year survival among patients with suspected acute myocardial infarction in randomized comparison of intravenous streptokinase, oral aspirin, both, or neither. BMJ 1998; 316:1337–1343.
31. EMERAS (Estudio Multicentrico Estreptoquinasa Republica de America de Sur) Collaborative Group. Randomised trial of late thrombolysis in patients with suspected acute myocardial infarction. Lancet 1993; 342:767–772.
32. Collen D, Topol EJ, Tiefenbrunn AJ, et al. Coronary thrombolysis with recombinant human tissue-type plasminogen activator: a prospective, randomized, placebo-controlled trial. Circulation 1984; 70:1012–1017.

33. The TIMI Study Group. The Thrombolysis in Myocardial Infarction (TIMI) Trial. Phase 1 findings. N Engl J Med 1985; 312:932–936.
34. Verstraete M, Bernard R, Bory M, et al. Randomised trial of intravenous recombinant tissue-type plasminogen activator versus intravenous streptokinase in acute myocardial infarction. Lancet 1985; 1:842–847.
35. TIMI Study Group. Comparison of invasive and conservative strategies after treatment with intravenous tissue plasminogen activator in acute myocardial infarction. Results of the Thrombolysis in Myocardial Infarction (TIMI) Phase II Trial. N Engl J Med 1989; 320:618–627.
36. Neuhaus K-L, Feuerer W, Jeep-Tebbe S, et al. Improved thrombolysis with a modified dose regimen of recombinant tissue-type plasminogen activator. J Am Coll Cardiol 1989; 14:1556–1559.
37. Purvis JA, McNeill AJ, Rizwan A, et al. Efficacy of 100 mg of double-bolus alteplase in achieving complete perfusion in the treatment of acute myocardial infarction. J Am Coll Cardiol 1994; 23:6–10.
38. The GUSTO Angiographic Investigators. The effects of tissue plasminogen activator, streptokinase, or both on coronary-artery patency, ventricular function, and survival after acute myocardial infarction. N Engl J Med 1993; 329:1615–1622.
39. Van de Werf F, Arnold AER. Intravenous tissue plasminogen activator and size of infarct, left ventricular function, and survival in acute myocardial infarction. Br Med J 1988; 297:1374–1379.
40. Guerci AD, Gerstenblith G, Brinker JA, et al. A randomized trial of intravenous tissue plasminogen activator for acute myocardial infarction with subsequent randomization to elective coronary angioplasty. N Engl J Med 1987; 317:1613–1618.
41. O'Rourke M, Baron D, Keogh A, et al. Limitation of myocardial infarction by early infusion of recombinant tissue-type plasminogen activator. Circulation 1988; 77:1311–1315.
42. National Heart Foundation of Australia Coronary Thrombolysis Group. Coronary thrombolysis and myocardial salvage by tissue plasminogen activator given up to 4 hours after onset of myocardial infarction. Lancet 1988; 1:203–207.
43. Topol EJ, Califf RM, George BS, et al. A randomized trial of immediate versus delayed elective angioplasty after intravenous tissue plasminogen activator in acute myocardial infarction. N Engl J Med 1987; 317:581–588.
44. Topol EJ, Califf RM, George BS, et al. Coronary arterial thrombolysis with combined infusion of recombinant tissue-type plasminogen activator and urokinase in patients with acute myocardial infarction. Circulation 1988; 77:1100–1107.
45. Topol EJ, George BS, Kereiakes DJ, et al. A randomized controlled trial of intravenous tissue plasminogen activator and early intravenous heparin in acute myocardial infarction. Circulation 1989; 79:281–286.
46. Topol EJ, Ellis SG, Califf RM, et al. Combined tissue-type plasminogen activator and prostacyclin therapy for acute myocardial infarction. J Am Coll Cardiol 1989; 14:877–884.
47. Wall TC, Phillips HR, Stack RS, et al. Results of high dose intravenous urokinase for acute myocardial infarction. Am J Cardiol 1990; 65:124–131.
48. Califf RM, Topol EJ, Stack RS, et al. Evaluation of combination thrombolytic therapy and timing of cardiac catheterization in acute myocardial infarction. Results of Thrombolysis and Angioplasty in Myocardial Infarction - Phase 5 randomized trial. Circulation 1991; 83:1543–1556.
49. Topol EJ, Califf RM, Vandormael M, et al. A randomized trial of late reperfusion therapy for acute myocardial infarction. Circulation 1992; 85:2090–2099.
50. Wall TC, Califf RM, George BS, et al. Accelerated plasminogen activator dose regimens for coronary thrombolysis. J Am Coll Cardiol 1992; 19:482–489.
51. Kleiman NS, Ohman EM, Califf RM, et al. Profound inhibition of platelet aggregation with monoclonal antibody 7E3 fab after thrombolytic therapy: results of the Thrombolysis and Angioplasty in Myocardial Infarction (TAMI) 8 pilot study. J Am Coll Cardiol 1993; 22:381–389.
52. Wall TC, Califf RM, Blankenship J, et al. Intravenous fluosol in the treatment of acute myocardial infarction: results of the Thrombolysis and Angioplasty in Myocardial Infarction 9 trial. Circulation 1994; 90:114–120.

53. Barseness GW, Ohman EM, Califf RM, et al. The Thrombolysis and Angioplasty in Myocardial Infarction (TAMI) trials: A decade of reperfusion strategies. J Interv Cardiol 1996; 9:89–115.
54. Rogers WJ, Baim DS, Gore JM, et al. Comparison of immediate invasive, delayed invasive, and conservative strategies after tissue-type plasminogen activator. Results of the Thrombolysis in Myocardial Infarction (TIMI) Phase II-A Trial. Circulation 1990; 81:1457–1476.
55. The TIMI IIIA Investigators. Early effects of tissue-type plasminogen activator added to conventional therapy on the culprit lesion in patients presenting with ischemic cardiac pain at rest. Results of the Thrombolysis in Myocardial Ischemia (TIMI-IIIA) Trial. Circulation 1993; 87:38–52.
56. The TIMI IIIB Investigators. Effects of tissue plasminogen activator and a comparison of early invasive and conservative strategies in unstable angina and non-Q-wave myocardial infarction: results of the TIMI IIIB Trial. Circulation 1994; 89:1545–1556.
57. Cannon CP, McCabe CH., Diver DJ, et al. Comparison of front-loaded recombinant tissue-type plasminogen activator, anistreplase and combination thrombolytic therapy for acute myocardial infarction: results of the Thrombolysis in Myocardial Infarction (TIMI) 4 trial. J Am Coll Cardiol 1994; 24:1602–1610.
58. Cannon CP, McCabe CH, Henry TD, et al. A pilot trial of recombinant desulfatohirudin compared with tissue-type plasminogen activator and aspirin for acute myocardial infarction: results of the Thrombolysis in Myocardial Infarction (TIMI) 5 trial. J Am Coll Cardiol 1994; 23:993–1003.
59. Lee LV. Initial experience with hirudin and streptokinase in acute myocardial infarction: results of the Thrombolysis in Myocardial Infarction (TIMI) 6 trial. Am J Cardiol 1995; 75:7–13.
60. Antman EM. Hirudin in acute myocardial infarction: safety report from the Thrombolysis and Thrombin Inhibition in Myocardial Infarction (TIMI) 9A trial. Circulation 1994; 90:1624–1630.
61. Antman EM. Hirudin in acute myocardial infarction. Thrombolysis and Thrombin Inhibition in Myocardial Infarction (TIMI) 9B Trial. Circulation 1996; 94:911–921.
62. Cannon CP, Gibson CM, McCabe CH, et al. TNK-tissue plasminogen activator compared with front-loaded alteplase in acute myocardial infarction: results of the TIMI 10B trial. Circulation 1998; 98:2805–2814.
63. Antman EM, Giugliano RP, Gibson CM, et al. Abciximab facilitates the rate and extent of thrombolysis: results of the thrombolysis in myocardial infarction (TIMI) 14 trial. Circulation 1999; 99:2720–2732.
64. INTIME-II Investigators. Intravenous NPA for the treatment of myocardium infracting early; INTIME-II, a double-blind comparison of single-bolus lanateplase vs accelerated alteplase for the treatment of patients with acute myocardial infarction. Eur Heart J 2000; 21:2005–2013.
65. Cannon CP, Braunwald E, McCabe CH, et al. The Thrombolysis in Myocardial Infarction (TIMI) trials: The first decade. J Interv Cardiol 1995; 8:117–135.
66. Wilcox RG, von der Lippe G, Olsson CG, et al. Trial of tissue plasminogen activator for mortality reduction in acute myocardial infarction: The Anglo-Scandinavian Study of Early Thrombolysis (ASSET). Lancet 1988; 2:525–530.
67. Wilcox RG, von der Lippe G, Olsson CG, et al. Effects of alteplase in acute myocardial infarction: 6-month results from the ASSET study. Lancet 190; 335: 1175–1178.
68. LATE Study Group. Late assessment of thrombolytic efficacy (LATE) study with alteplase 6-12 hours after onset of acute myocardial infarction. Lancet 1993; 342:759–766.
69. Gruppo Italiano per lo Studio Della Sopravvivenza nell'infarto Miocardico. GISSI-2: a factorial randomised trial of alteplase versus streptokinase and heparin versus no heparin among 12,490 patients with acute myocardial infarction. Lancet 1990; 336:65–71.
70. International Study Group. In-hospital mortality and clinical course of 20,891 patients with suspected acute myocardial infarction randomized between alteplase and streptokinase with or without heparin. Lancet 1990; 336:71–75.
71. The GUSTO Investigators: An international randomized trial comparing four thrombolytic strategies for acute myocardial infarction. N Engl J Med 1993; 329:673–682.

72. Califf RM, White HD, van de Werf F, et al. One-year results from the Global Utilization of Streptokinase and TPA for Occluded Coronary Arteries (GUSTO-1) Trial. Circulation 1996; 94:1233–1238.
73. The COBALT Investigators. A comparison of continuous infusion of alteplase with double-bolus administration for acute myocardial infarction. The continuous infusion versus double bolus administration of alteplase (rt-PA): the COBALT trial. N Engl J Med 1997; 337:1124–1130.
74. Kalbfleisch JM, Kurnik PB, Thadani U, et al. Myocardial infarct artery patency and reocclusion rates after treatment with duteplase at the dose used in the International Study of Infarct Survival–3. Am J Cardiol 1993; 71:386–392.
75. ISIS-3 (Third International Study of Infarct Survival) Collaborative Group. ISIS-3: a randomized comparison of streptokinase vs tissue plasminogen activator vs anistreplase and of aspirin plus heparin vs aspirin alone among 41,299 cases of suspected acute myocardial infarction. Lancet 1992; 339:753–770.
76. Meinertz T, Kasper W, Schumacher M, et al. The German multicenter trial of anisoylated plasminogen streptokinase activator complex versus heparin for acute myocardial infarction. Am J Cardiol 1988; 62:347–351.
77. Bassand JP, Machecourt J, Cassagnes J, et al. Multicenter trial of intravenous anisoylated plasminogen streptokinase activator complex (APSAC) in acute myocardial infarction: effects on infarct size and left ventricular function. J Am Coll Cardiol 1989; 13:988–997.
78. AIMS Trial Study Group: Effect of intravenous APSAC on mortality after acute myocardial infarction: preliminary report of a placebo-controlled clinical trial. Lancet 1988; 1:545–549.
79. AIMS Trial Study Group: Long-term effects of intravenous anistreplase in acute myocardial infarction: final report of the AIMS study. Lancet 1990; 335:427–431.
80. Anderson JL, Sorenson S, Moreno F, et al. Multicenter patency trial of intravenous APSAC compared with streptokinase in acute myocardial infarction. Circulation 1991; 88:126–140.
81. Anderson JL, Becker LC, Sorenson SG, et al. APSAC versus alteplase in acute myocardial infarction: comparative effects on left ventricular function, morbidity and 1-day coronary artery patency. J Am Coll Cardiol 1992; 20:753–766.
82. Neuhaus K-L, Von Essen R, Tebbe U, et al. Improved thrombolysis in acute myocardial infarction with front-loaded administration of alteplase: results of the rt-PA-APSAC Patency Study (TAPS). J Am Coll Cardiol 1992; 19:885–891.
83. Mathey DG, Schofer J, Sheehan FH, et al. Intravenous urokinase in acute myocardial infarction. Am J Cardiol 1985; 55:878–882.
84. Neuhaus KL, Tebbe U, Gotwik M, et al. Intravenous recombinant tissue plasminogen activator (rt-PA) and urokinase in acute myocardial infarction: results of the German Activator Urokinase Study (GAUS). J Am Coll Cardiol 1988; 12:581–587.
85. Whitlow PL, Bashore TM. Catheterization/Rescue Angioplasty Following Thrombolysis (CRAFT) study: acute myocardial infarction treated with recombinant tissue plasminogen activator versus urokinase (abstr). J Am Coll Cardiol 1991; 17:276A.
86. Urokinase and Alteplase in Myocardial Infarction Collaborative Group (URALMI). Combination of urokinase and alteplase in the treatment of myocardial infarction. Coron Artery Dis 1991; 2:225–235.
87. PRIMI Trial Study Group: Randomized double-blind trial of recombinant prourokinase against streptokinase in acute myocardial infarction. Lancet 1989; 1:863–868.
88. Tebbe U, Michels R, Adgey J, et al. Randomized, double-blind study comparing saruplase with streptokinase therapy in acute myocardial infarction: the COMPASS equivalence trial. J Am Coll Cardiol 1998; 31:487–493.
89. Bär FW, Meyer J, Vermeer F, et al. Comparison of saruplase and alteplase in acute myocardial infarction. Am J Cardiol 1997; 79:727–732.
90. Granger CB, Hirsh J, Califf RM, et al. Activated partial thromboplastin time and outcome after thrombolytic therapy for acute myocardial infarction. Results from the GUSTO-I trial. Circulation 1996; 93:870–878.
91. Sane DC, Califf RM, Topol EJ, et al. Bleeding during thrombolytic therapy for acute myocardial infarction: mechanisms and management. Ann Intern Med 1989; 111:1010–1022.

92. Granger CB, Califf RM, Topol EJ. Thrombolytic therapy for acute myocardial infarction. Drugs 1992; 44:293–325.
93. Simoons ML, Maggioni AP, Knatterud G, et al. Individual risk assessment for intracranial hemorrhage during thrombolytic therapy. Lancet 1993; 342:1523–1528.
94. White HD. Thrombolytic treatment for recurrent myocardial infarction. Avoid repeating streptokinase or anistreplase. Br Med J 1991; 302:429–430.

Bolus Fibrinolytic Therapy

Peter R. Sinnaeve and Frans J. Van de Werf
Department of Cardiology, Gasthuisberg University Hospital, University of Leuven,
Leuven, Belgium

INTRODUCTION

Acute ST-elevation myocardial infarction (STEMI) remains the leading cause of death in industrialized countries. Numerous studies during the past decades have firmly established the paradigm of achieving early, complete, and sustained infarct-related artery patency, resulting in a reduction in average 30-day mortality from 18% in the prefibrinolytic era to less than 6% in the context of contemporary clinical trials (1). Because primary percutaneous coronary intervention (PCI) achieves higher patency rates and is associated with fewer intracranial bleeding complications, current guidelines recommend primary PCI if the procedure can be performed by an experienced team within 90 minutes after initial medical contact. Nevertheless, fibrinolytic therapy is still used for STEMI in the majority of centers worldwide. First-generation fibrinolytic regimens, including streptokinase and tissue-type plasminogen activator (t-PA; alteplase), required continuous intravenous infusion. Although initial attempts at bolus administration of these agents were disappointing (2,3), second- and third-generation fibrinolytics are administered by intravenous bolus injection.

BOLUS FIBRINOLYTICS VS. CONVENTIONAL INFUSION FIBRINOLYTIC THERAPY

There are several important benefits associated with bolus administration of fibrinolytic agents. Foremost, bolus fibrinolytics are easier to administer. This reduces the risk of dosing error but also reduces treatment delays and facilitates prehospital treatment.

Dosing Errors

Emergency and coronary care personnel are increasingly confronted with complicated therapeutic strategies for patients presenting with an acute coronary syndrome. Prior fibrinolytic agents, such as the accelerated alteplase regimen, required preparation of three different infusions, which substantially increases the risk of dosing errors. Indeed, inappropriately high doses appear to be more common with continuous infusion of alteplase than with bolus fibrinolytics, and this has been associated with an increased risk of intracranial hemorrhage (4). Appropriate dosing or dose adjustments also decrease the risk of serious bleeding complications in clinical trials (5–7). Bolus fibrinolytics are generally much easier to prepare and only require administration of a single or double bolus. This reduces the risk of inappropriately high doses and hence might reduce the risk of bleeding complications.

Time To Treatment and Prehospital Fibrinolysis

Bolus administration greatly facilitates the preparation of fibrinolytic agents. In a community hospital, tenecteplase took 10.5 minutes less to prepare compared with standard fibrinolytics requiring a continuous infusion (8). This resulted in a

significantly higher percentage of patients receiving fibrinolytic therapy within
30 minutes after presentation (76% vs. 58% using conventional therapy). Because
every minute lost between identifying a patient and treatment initiation affects
outcome, easier administration of bolus fibrinolytics might improve outcome.

Time lost between symptom onset and treatment initiation remains a crucial
contributor to treatment delay in STEMI. Since mortality rates in randomized
fibrinolytic trials are consistently lower when patients are treated within two hours
of symptom onset, early prehospital detection and treatment might be an attractive
approach to improve outcome in STEMI. A meta-analysis of six trials including
6434 patients showed that the time gained with prehospital treatment resulted in a
significant 17% mortality reduction compared with in-hospital fibrinolysis (9).
Bolus fibrinolytic agents undoubtedly facilitate prehospital reperfusion protocols.
Less complicated fibrinolytic regimens might also facilitate initiation of prehospital
fibrinolytic treatment by trained paramedical staff. Indeed, in the Assessment of
the Safety and Efficacy of a New Thrombolytic (ASSENT)-3 PLUS prehospital
study, the administration of a bolus fibrinolytic by paramedical ambulance staff
did not influence efficacy and safety (10).

Bolus Fibrinolytics in Pharmacoinvasive Strategies

Bolus fibrinolytics also facilitate strategies combining fibrinolysis with early-planned
PCI, especially in the prehospital setting. Earlier studies using infusion fibrinolytics
showed that this approach was both effective and safe (11,12). More recently,
pharmacoinvasive strategies using bolus fibrinolytics have been examined in the
GRACIA-2 study (13) and in ASSENT-4 PCI trial (14). In GRACIA-2[13], tenecteplase
led to a higher incidence of infarct artery patency and more complete ST-segment
resolution at six hours, resulting in similar left ventricular size and function as those
treated with primary PCI. In the ASSENT-4 PCI trial (14), patients presenting with
STEMI were randomized to tenecteplase followed by early-planned PCI or primary
PCI alone. Randomization was allowed in non-PCI centers, PCI centers, or in the
ambulance. Unfortunately, the study was halted prematurely because of excess
mortality in the facilitated arm. Still, further studies comparing prehospital bolus
fibrinolytic versus transport to a PCI center for primary intervention are being
planned.

Bolus Fibrinolysis During Refractory CPR

As STEMI is often the cause of sudden death, bolus fibrinolytics have also been
studied in refractory cardiopulmonary resuscitation. Earlier pilot trials using
infusion fibrinolytics in this setting have shown promising results (15,16). Recently,
however, a large international trial examining the safety and efficacy of a bolus
fibrinolytic given during CPR for cardiac arrest has been halted prematurely
because of futility (17).

SAFETY AND BOLUS FIBRINOLYTICS

Intracranial hemorrhage is the most serious side effect of fibrinolysis. In the past
decade, several interventions to reduce the risk of intracranial bleeding complications have been studied, including dose reduction of concomitant antithrombotic
agents (18), improved monitoring (19), and weight-adjusted dosing (7). Results
from individual trials showed no significantly higher risk of intracranial bleeding

complications with bolus versus infusion fibrinolytics (20,21). Much controversy arose when a meta-analysis showed increased risk of intracerebral hemorrhage with bolus administration of fibrinolytic drugs (22). This meta-analysis included all phase 3 trials comparing bolus administration versus continuous infusion of fibrinolytic agents. Agents administered via bolus included anistreplase (ISIS-3) (23), reteplase (INJECT, GUSTO III) (20,24), alteplase (COBALT) (2), tenecteplase (ASSENT-2) (25), saruplase (BASE) (26), and lanoteplase (InTIME-II) (27). The authors concluded that the overall odds ratio for intracranial hemorrhage (ICH) after bolus compared with infusion administration was 1.25 (95% CI 1.08–1.45, $p = 0.003$). However, the inclusion of different bolus fibrinolytic agents or different dosing regimens has raised questions about the conclusions drawn from this meta-analysis. A similar meta-analysis comparing bolus versus infusion administration in phase 2 trials even showed a nonsignificant *lower* risk of ICH for bolus agents (28). Part of this discrepancy between findings in phase 2 and 3 trials might be explained by a lower rate of high-risk patients randomized in phase 2 trials (28). Also, when taking only GUSTO III (reteplase) (20) and ASSENT-2 (tenecteplase) (25) data, the analysis showed an odds ratio of 1.01 for ICH after bolus administration. Moreover, the different agents included in the analysis all have unique profiles as to fibrin specificity and pharmacodynamic profiles. Also, different antithrombin strategies have been used in the trials included in this meta-analysis, while bolus fibrinolytic studies subsequent to those included in the analysis have incorporated a more conservative antithrombotic approach. Furthermore, only two trials included compared the very same agent in bolus versus continuous administration. Thus, given the ease of administration of bolus fibrinolytics and subsequent possibilities for prehospital treatment and reduction of dosing errors, these agents have been accepted for standard fibrinolytic therapy.

BOLUS FIBRINOLYTIC AGENTS

In the past decade, several bolus fibrinolytics have been developed (Table 1) (29). Most of these are mutants of alteplase with reduced plasma clearance, while staphylokinase has been derivatized with a maleimide-polyethylene glycol (PEG) residue to increase plasma half-life. Many mutants also have additional modifications to improve fibrin specificity and resistance to plasminogen activator inhibitor 1 (PAI-1).

Reteplase

Reteplase, a second-generation fibrinolytic agent, was a first attempt to improve on the shortcomings of alteplase (Table 2). It is a mutant of alteplase in which the

TABLE 1 Bolus Fibrinolytic Agents

Fibrinolytic	Half-life (min)	Fibrin specificity	PAI-1 resistance
Reteplase	15–18	↓	N
Tenecteplase	20–24	↑↑	↑
Lanoteplase	30–45	↓	↑
Pamiteplase	30–47	↑	N
Monteplase	23	↑	↑
Amediplase	12	n	N
PEG-staphylokinase	13	↑↑↑	N

Abbreviations: n, neutral; PAI, plasminogen activator inhibitor; PEG, maleimide-polyethylene glycol.

TABLE 2 Dosing of Commercially Available Bolus Fibrinolytic Agents

Fibrinolytic (bolus)	Dosing regimen
Tenecteplase	Weight-adjusted single bolus 30 mg if <60 kg 35 mg if 60–69 kg 40 mg if 70–79 kg 45 mg if 80–89 kg 50 mg if ≥90 kg
Reteplase	Initial bolus of 10 U, followed by second 10 U bolus 30 min later

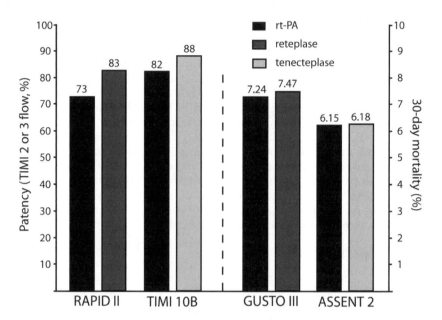

FIGURE 1 Patency and 30-day mortality rates for alteplase, reteplase, and tenecteplase. Patency rates (TIMI grade 2 or 3 flow) were higher with either reteplase or tenecteplase when compared to alteplase, but this benefit was not translated in lower mortality rates.

finger, the kringle 1 domain, and epidermal growth factor domains were removed, resulting in decreased plasma clearance. In contrast with alteplase, which requires a continuous 90-minute infusion, reteplase can be given as a double bolus. Unfortunately, the removal of the finger domain reduces fibrin specificity (30), although inactivation by PAI-1 remains similar to alteplase. In an open-label randomized pilot trial, TIMI-3 flow rates were higher with reteplase than with front-loaded alteplase (31).

In two open-label randomized pilot trials, different doses of reteplase were evaluated in patients with STEMI. In RAPID I (32), patients treated with two boluses of 10 MU reteplase given 30 minutes apart had a significantly higher rate of TIMI-3 flow (63%) compared with patients treated with 100-mg alteplase over three hours (49%). In RAPID II (31), the same dose of reteplase was compared against 90-minute front-loaded alteplase in 324 patients. Again, reteplase achieved significantly higher TIMI-3 flow rates at 90 minutes than alteplase (60% vs. 45%) (Fig. 1). Total patency, defined as TIMI flow grade 2 or 3 rate, was also significantly higher in patients treated with reteplase (83% vs. 73% for alteplase).

Double-bolus reteplase was also compared with streptokinase in the double-blind INJECT trial (24); 6010 patients with STEMI within 12 hours of symptom onset were randomized to either double-bolus reteplase (10 U), given 30 minutes apart, or 1.5-MU streptokinase over 60 minutes. Double-bolus reteplase was shown to be at least equivalent to streptokinase (35-day mortality, 9.0% vs. 9.5%; 95% CI 0.96–1.98).

In the GUSTO III trial (20), which was designed as a superiority trial, 15,059 patients were randomized to double-bolus reteplase (10 MU), given 30 minutes apart, or front-loaded alteplase. Mortality at 30 days was again similar in both treatment arms (7.47% vs. 7.24%) (Fig. 1), as was the incidence of hemorrhagic stroke or other major bleeding complications. Similar mortality rates were maintained for both treatment groups at one-year follow-up (33). Thus, higher TIMI-3 rates at 90 minutes with reteplase, as seen in pilot studies, were not associated with lower short-term mortality rates. This might be explained in part by increased platelet activation and surface receptor expression with reteplase compared with alteplase (34).

The effect of low-dose reteplase with abciximab on early reperfusion was tested in 528 patients in the SPEED trial (35). TIMI grade 3 flow rate was only 27% when abciximab was used in monotherapy and 47% with full-dose reteplase (10 U + 10 U) alone. The highest TIMI-3 flow rate (61%) was observed in the group that received reduced double-bolus reteplase (5 U + 5 U) in combination with abciximab and 60 U/kg heparin. Unfortunately, this benefit was at the expense of a substantial increase in major bleeding (36). The effect of half-dose reteplase plus abciximab on outcome was further studied in the GUSTO-V trial; 16,588 patients were randomized to either reteplase, administered in two boluses of 10 U 30 minutes apart, or half-dose reteplase (two boluses of 5 U 30 minutes apart) with weight-adjusted abciximab (37). The combination of half-dose reteplase and abciximab was shown to induce less prothrombin activation than full-dose reteplase (38). Thirty-day mortality rates were 5.9% for reteplase and 5.6% for the combined reteplase-abciximab group, thus fulfilling the criteria for noninferiority. Ischemic complications after STEMI were significantly reduced with the combination therapy. Intracranial hemorrhage rates were equal (0.6%) for both treatment arms, although in patients above 75 years of age the rate of intracranial bleeding was almost twice as high in the combination treatment arm (2.1% vs. 1.1% for standard dose reteplase).

Tenecteplase

Tenecteplase (TNK-t-PA) is also derived from alteplase. Mutations at three places (**T**103, **N**117, **K**HRR296-299) increase the plasma half-life, fibrin binding and specificity, and resistance to PAI-1. Its slower clearance allows convenient single-bolus administration (Table 2). The efficiency of tenecteplase to activate plasminogen is reduced in the presence of fibrinogen and fibrin degradation products, while efficiency in the presence of fibrin remains equivalent, explaining its improved fibrin specificity (39). Tenecteplase also has higher fibrinolytic potency than its parent molecule (40) and lanoteplase (41). As a consequence, tenecteplase leads to faster recanalization compared with alteplase (42).

Efficacy for clot lysis was evaluated in the TIMI-10A (43) and TIMI-10B trials (6). In the TIMI-10A trial (43), 113 patients with evolving STEMI within 12 hours of symptom onset received incremental doses of single-bolus tenecteplase (5–50 mg).

The rate of TIMI-3 flow was 59% for the 30-mg group and 64% for the 50-mg group. Combined TIMI-2 and TIMI-3 flows were similar for all doses tested (85%). Levels of coagulation parameters were affected only to a small extent when compared with levels after treatment with alteplase. In the TIMI-10B trial (6), 837 patients were randomized to single-bolus tenecteplase (30, 40, or 50 mg) or front-loaded alteplase (Fig. 1). TIMI-3 flow rates were identical after single-bolus administration of 40-mg tenecteplase compared with alteplase (63%). The 50-mg dose of tenecteplase had to be discontinued early because of an excess of intracranial hemorrhage. The incidence of serious bleeding complications, however, decreased in both groups after adjustment of heparin dosing during the study.

Subsequently, the safety of single-bolus administration of tenecteplase was evaluated in the ASSENT-1 study (44); 3325 patients received a single bolus of either 30- or 40-mg tenecteplase. An intracranial hemorrhage rate of 0.62% was observed in patients receiving 40-mg tenecteplase and a reduced dose of heparin. This rate compares favorably with previous rates observed with alteplase, possibly due to the increased fibrin specificity of tenecteplase.

In the double-blind ASSENT-2 trial (25), 16,949 patients were randomized to single-bolus tenecteplase or weight-adjusted front-loaded alteplase. Specifically designed as an equivalency trial, this study showed that tenecteplase and alteplase had equivalent 30-day mortality (6.18% vs. 6.15%, 90% CI 0.917–1.104) (Fig. 1). Mortality rates remained similar at one-year follow-up (45). The two treatments did not differ significantly in any subgroup analysis, except for a lower 30-day mortality with tenecteplase in patients treated after four hours of symptom onset. Although the rates of intracranial hemorrhage were similar for tenecteplase (0.93%) and alteplase (0.94%), female patients, elderly aged above 75 years, and patients weighing less than 67 kg tended to have lower rates of intracranial hemorrhage after treatment with tenecteplase (21). Noncerebral bleeding complications occurred less frequently in the tenecteplase group, and as a consequence there was less need for blood transfusion after tenecteplase. Differences were even more apparent in high-risk women. Thus, increased fibrin specificity of TNK may induce both a better outcome in late-treated patients and fewer bleeding complications especially in high-risk patients.

Different combinations of tenecteplase with abciximab or the low molecular weight heparin enoxaparin were studied in the ENTIRE study (46), in which 483 patients were randomized to (1) full-dose tenecteplase and unfractionated heparin, (2) full-dose tenecteplase and enoxaparin, (3) half-dose tenecteplase, abciximab, and unfractionated heparin, and (4) half-dose tenecteplase, abciximab, and enoxaparin. Enoxaparin achieved similar TIMI-3 flow rates compared with unfractionated heparin at 60 minutes but was associated with fewer ischemic events and major bleeding complications. The combination of half-dose tenecteplase, abciximab, and either enoxaparin or unfractionated heparin, however, did not further reduce the occurrence of postinfarct ischemic events when compared with full-dose tenecteplase and enoxaparin. The effect of half-dose tenecteplase plus abciximab or full-dose tenecteplase with either unfractionated heparin or enoxaparin on outcome was further studied in the ASSENT-3 study (47). Patients with STEMI received either full-dose weight-adjusted single-bolus tenecteplase with weight-adjusted enoxaparin (30 mg IV bolus followed by 1 mg/kg immediately and every 12 hours) or unfractionated heparin, or half-dose tenecteplase with weight-adjusted low-dose unfractionated heparin. Primary end points were the composites of 30-day mortality, in-hospital reinfarction, or refractory ischemia (primary efficacy end point), and the above plus in-hospital intracranial hemorrhage or major bleeding (primary efficacy plus safety end point). Both enoxaparin and abciximab significantly reduced the risk for ischemic complications after treatment with tenecteplase, although one-year mortality rates were similar across the three groups (48). More rapid and complete ST-segment resolution occurred in the abciximab group (49). Intracranial bleeding rates were very similar in the three treatment arms, but both major and minor bleeding complications were more frequent in the half-dose tenecteplase-abciximab arm. Because LMWH offers several advantages over conventional heparin, including easier administration and no need for coagulation monitoring, the combination of tenecteplase-enoxaparin has emerged as the most attractive treatment. In the recent ExTRACT study (50), enoxaparin was associated with a significantly lower incidence of the composite end point of death, nonfatal reinfarction, or nonfatal intracranial hemorrhage compared with unfractionated heparin in patients with STEMI receiving fibrinolytic therapy.

The combination of single-bolus tenecteplase plus enoxaparin has also been investigated in the prehospital setting in the ASSENT-3 PLUS trial; 1639 patients with STEMI received prehospital tenecteplase and were randomized to either enoxaparin or unfractionated heparin (51). A time gain of 47 minutes was observed, increasing the fraction of patients treated within two hours of symptom onset from 29% in ASSENT-3 to 52% in ASSENT-3 PLUS. Early treatment (<2 h) was associated with a lower 30-day mortality [4.4% vs. 6.2 (2–4 h) and 10.4% (4–6 h)], but no significant difference in outcome was observed between enoxaparin and heparin.

Staphylokinase

Staphylokinase, a bacterial profibrinolytic agent, is a 136-amino acid single-chain polypeptide with a unique structure and mechanism of action and of fibrin specificity (52). In contrast with streptokinase, staphylokinase is highly fibrin selective (53), but unlike alteplase and its mutants, staphylokinase is immunogenic (54). Staphylokinase variants with reduced immunogenicity and preserved lytic potency have been derivatized with PEG to reduce the plasma clearance by 2.5-fold (55). PEGylated variants detected only one-third of the antibodies generated by wild-type staphylokinase in patients with STEMI. In a pilot trial, PEG-staphylokinase was shown to be associated with promising patency rates (55). In an angiography-controlled dose-finding trial (CAPTORS II), patency rates for the highest doses of PEG-staphylokinase were lower than those in the pilot trial but remained comparable to those achieved with alteplase (56). Further clinical studies are currently being planned.

Lanoteplase

Lanoteplase is a deletion mutant of alteplase derived by deleting its fibronectin fingerlike and epidermal growth factor domains and mutating Asn (117) to Gln (117) (57), leading to decreased plasma clearance and improved resistance to PAI-1 (58). Unfortunately, these changes make lanoteplase less fibrin-specific compared with alteplase.

In the randomized double-blind IV nPA for the Treatment of Infarcting Myocardium Early (InTIME-I) trial (59), 602 patients within six hours of symptom onset received weight-adjusted single-bolus lanoteplase (15–120 kU/kg) or accelerated alteplase. Lanoteplase had a dose-dependent effect on coronary patency rates. The 60-kU/kg dose produced similar TIMI flow grade 3 rates compared with alteplase (44% vs. 37%) at 60 minutes. In the 120-kU/kg dose group, TIMI-3 flow rate was 47%. At 90 minutes, combined TIMI-2 and TIMI-3 flow was 72% and 83% for 60- and 120-kU/kg lanoteplase, respectively compared with 71% for alteplase. In the subsequent outcome trial (InTIME-II) (27), 15,078 patients were randomized in a 2:1 ratio to single-bolus lanoteplase (120 kU/kg) or accelerated alteplase. Thirty-day mortality was equivalent in both groups (6.75% vs. 6.61%; RR 1.02 one-sided 95% CI 1.137). At six months and one-year follow-up, mortality for both treatments remained similar, 8.7% vs. 8.9% and 10.0% vs 10.3%, respectively. Although the rate of combined hemorrhagic and ischemic strokes was not statis-tically different between the groups (1.87% for lanoteplase and 1.53% for alteplase), the rate of hemorrhagic strokes was significantly higher in patients treated with lanoteplase (1.12% vs. 0.64% for alteplase). Moreover, the incidence of mild bleeding was also significantly higher in the lanoteplase group (19.7% for lan-oteplase vs. 14.8% for alteplase). The increased risk for ICH and minor bleeding for lanoteplase are possibly related to its lower fibrin specificity when compared with alteplase and tenecteplase. Due to a decrease in heparin dose during the study, however, the rate of intracranial hemorrhage in the alteplase group was the lowest ever observed with this agent in a large trial (18). Nevertheless, further develop-ment has ceased because of its unfavorable risk profile compared with tenecteplase and reteplase.

Amediplase
Amediplase is a chimeric fusion protein consisting of the kringle 2 domain of t-PA and the catalytic domain of urokinase-type plasminogen activator (uPA). It is fibrin-specific and nonimmunogenic and can be given as a single bolus. In two angiographic studies (2k2 and 3k2), TIMI flow grade 3 was obtained in more than 50% of the patients in a dose of 0.8 to 1.2 mg/kg with a good safety profile (60,61). Currently, a phase-III trial investigating the safety and efficacy of this fibrinolytic agent is being prepared.

Monteplase
Monteplase, an alteplase mutant, has cysteine at position 84 replaced by serine. This single-amino acid deletion results in reduced plasma clearance and binding to PAI-1. Monteplase is given as a single bolus and is being developed in Japan. It has been tested mainly in the setting of facilitated PCI (62,63).

Pamiteplase
Another alteplase-derived fibrinolytic, pamiteplase, has arginine at position 275 replaced by glutaminic acid and the kringle 1 domain being deleted, which increases resistance to plasmin cleavage and further increases half-life (30–47 min) (64). Like monteplase, pamiteplase is given as a single bolus and has been exam-ined in the setting of facilitated PCI (65).

Saruplase
Saruplase is an unglycosylated single-chain recombinant uPA without immuno-genicity. Although not fibrin specific, it has a plasma half-life of nine minutes (66). Single- or double-bolus administration of saruplase was tested in the BASE trial (26); 192 patients received a 40-mg double bolus, a 60- or 80-mg single bolus, or a

standard regimen of a 20-mg bolus followed by a 60-mg continuous infusion. At 90 minutes, TIMI grade 3 flow rates were 73% with the 40-mg double bolus versus only 36% with the 60-mg single bolus and 72% with the continuous infusion. Unfortunately, the double-bolus regimen was associated with the highest rate of bleeding complications.

CONCLUSIONS

Fibrinolytic therapy significantly improves outcome after ST-segment elevation myocardial infarction. Over the last years, new bolus fibrinolytics with several other advantages over standard agents have been developed. Although they do not appear to have an impact on mortality, they are easier to administrate, are associated with a lower chance of dosing errors, and induce fewer side effects. Further improvements, however, will likely come from early detection of myocardial infarction in the community combined with prehospital bolus fibrinolysis. Also, new antithrombotic combinations with improved safety profile, especially in the elderly, need to be studied.

REFERENCES

1. de Vreede JJ, Gorgels AP, Verstraaten GM, et al. Did prognosis after acute myocardial infarction change during the past 30 years? A meta-analysis. J Am Coll Cardiol 1991; 18:698–706.
2. A comparison of continuous infusion of alteplase with double-bolus administration for acute myocardial infarction. The Continuous Infusion versus Double-Bolus Administration of Alteplase (COBALT) Investigators. N Engl J Med 1997; 337:1124–1130.
3. Cannon CP, McCabe CH, Diver DJ, et al. Comparison of front-loaded recombinant tissue-type plasminogen activator, anistreplase and combination thrombolytic therapy for acute myocardial infarction: results of the Thrombolysis in Myocardial Infarction (TIMI) 4 trial. J Am Coll Cardiol 1994; 24:1602–1610.
4. Gurwitz JH, Gore JM, Goldberg RJ, et al. Risk for intracranial hemorrhage after tissue plasminogen activator treatment for acute myocardial infarction. Participants in the National Registry of Myocardial Infarction 2. Ann Intern Med 1998; 129:597–604.
5. Comparison of invasive and conservative strategies after treatment with intravenous tissue plasminogen activator in acute myocardial infarction. Results of the thrombolysis in myocardial infarction (TIMI) phase II trial. The TIMI Study Group. N Engl J Med 1989; 320:618–627.
6. Cannon CP, Gibson CM, McCabe CH, et al. TNK-tissue plasminogen activator compared with front-loaded alteplase in acute myocardial infarction: results of the TIMI 10B trial. Thrombolysis in Myocardial Infarction (TIMI) 10B Investigators. Circulation 1998; 98:2805–2814.
7. Angeja BG, Alexander JH, Chin R, et al. Safety of the weight-adjusted dosing regimen of tenecteplase in the ASSENT-Trial. Am J Cardiol 2001; 88:1240–1245.
8. Leah V, Clark C, Doyle K, et al. Does a single bolus thrombolytic reduce door to needle time in a district general hospital? Emerg Med J 2004; 21(2):162–164.
9. Morrison LJ, Verbeek PR, McDonald AC, et al. Mortality and prehospital thrombolysis for acute myocardial infarction: a meta-analysis. JAMA 2000; 283:2686–2692.
10. Welsh RC, Goldstein P, Adgey J, et al. Variations in pre-hospital fibrinolysis process of care: insights from the Assessment of the Safety and Efficacy of a New Thrombolytic 3 Plus international acute myocardial infarction pre-hospital care survey. Eur J Emerg Med 2004; 11:134–140.
11. Fernandez-Aviles F, Alonso J, Castro-Beiras A, et al. Routine invasive strategy within 24 hours of thrombolysis versus ischaemia-guided conservative approach for acute myocardial infarction with ST-segment elevation. (GRACIA-1): a randomised controlled trial. Lancet 2004; 364:1045–1053.

12. Ross AM, Coyne KS, Reiner JS, et al. A randomized trial comparing primary angioplasty with a strategy of short-acting thrombolysis and immediate planned rescue angioplasty in acute myocardial infarction: the PACT trial. PACT investigators. Plasminogen-activator Angioplasty Compatibility Trial. J Am Coll Cardiol 1999; 34:1954–1962.

13. Fernandez-Aviles F, Alonso JJ, Castro-Beiras A, et al. Routine invasive strategy within 24 hours of thrombolysis versus ischaemia-guided conservative approach for acute myocardial infarction with ST-segment elevation (GRACIA-1): a randomised controlled trial. Lancet 2004; 364:1045–1053.

14. Primary versus tenecteplase-facilitated percutaneous coronary intervention in patients with ST-segment elevation acute myocardial infarction (ASSENT-4 PCI): randomised trial. Lancet 2006; 367:569–578.

15. Bottiger BW, Bode C, Kern S, et al. Efficacy and safety of thrombolytic therapy after initially unsuccessful cardiopulmonary resuscitation: a prospective clinical trial. Lancet 2001; 357:1583–1585.

16. Lederer W, Lichtenberger C, Pechlaner C, et al. Recombinant tissue plasminogen activator during cardiopulmonary resuscitation in 108 patients with out-of-hospital cardiac arrest. Resuscitation 2001; 50:71–76.

17. Spohr F, Arntz HR, Bluhmki E, et al. International multicentre trial protocol to assess the efficacy and safety of tenecteplase during cardiopulmonary resuscitation in patients with out-of-hospital cardiac arrest: the Thrombolysis in Cardiac Arrest (TROICA) Study. Eur J Clin Invest 2005; 35:315–323.

18. Giugliano RP, McCabe CH, Antman EM, et al. Lower-dose heparin with fibrinolysis is associated with lower rates of intracranial hemorrhage. Am Heart J 2001; 141:742–750.

19. Menon V, Berkowitz SD, Antman EM, et al. New heparin dosing recommendations for patients with acute coronary syndromes. Am J Med 2001; 110:641–650.

20. A comparison of reteplase with alteplase for acute myocardial infarction. The Global Use of Strategies to Open Occluded Coronary Arteries (GUSTO III) Investigators. N Engl J Med 1997; 337:1118–1123.

21. Van de Werf FJ, Barron HV, Armstrong PW, et al. Incidence and predictors of bleeding events after fibrinolytic therapy with fibrin-specific agents: a comparison of TNK-tPA and rt-PA. Eur Heart J 2001; 22:2253–2261.

22. Mehta SR, Eikelboom JW, Yusuf S. Risk of intracranial hemorrhage with bolus versus infusion thrombolytic therapy: a meta-analysis. Lancet 2000; 356:449–454.

23. ISIS-3: a randomised comparison of streptokinase vs tissue plasminogen activator vs anistreplase and of aspirin plus heparin vs aspirin alone among 41,299 cases of suspected acute myocardial infarction. ISIS-3 (Third International Study of Infarct Survival) Collaborative Group. Lancet 1992; 339:753–770.

24. Randomised, double-blind comparison of reteplase double-bolus administration with streptokinase in acute myocardial infarction (INJECT): trial to investigate equivalence. International Joint Efficacy Comparison of Thrombolytics. Lancet 1995; 346:329–336.

25. Single-bolus tenecteplase compared with front-loaded alteplase in acute myocardial infarction: the ASSENT-2 double-blind randomised trial. Assessment of the Safety and Efficacy of a New Thrombolytic Investigators. Lancet 1999; 354:716–722.

26. Bar FW, Meyer J, Boland J, et al. Bolus Administration of Saruplase in Europe (BASE), a Pilot Study in Patients with Acute Myocardial Infarction. J Thromb Thrombolysis 1998; 6:147–153.

27. Intravenous NPA for the treatment of infarcting myocardium early; InTIME-II, a double-blind comparison of single-bolus lanoteplase vs accelerated alteplase for the treatment of patients with acute myocardial infarction. Eur Heart J 2000; 21:2005–2013.

28. Eikelboom JW, Mehta SR, Pogue J, et al. Safety outcomes in meta-analyses of phase 2 vs phase 3 randomized trials: intracranial hemorrhage in trials of bolus thrombolytic therapy. JAMA 2001; 285:444–450.

29. Aylward P. Can we improve on front-loaded alteplase (r-TPA)? Aust N Z J Med 1998; 28:511–513.

30. Hoffmeister HM, Kastner C, Szabo S, et al. Fibrin specificity and procoagulant effect related to the kallikrein- contact phase system and to plasmin generation with double-bolus reteplase and front-loaded alteplase thrombolysis in acute myocardial infarction. Am J Cardiol 2000; 86:263–268.

31. Bode C, Smalling RW, Berg G, et al. Randomized comparison of coronary thrombolysis achieved with double-bolus reteplase (recombinant plasminogen activator) and front-loaded, accelerated alteplase (recombinant tissue plasminogen activator) in patients with acute myocardial infarction. The RAPID II Investigators. Circulation 1996; 94:891–898.
32. Smalling RW, Bode C, Kalbfleisch J, et al. More rapid, complete, and stable coronary thrombolysis with bolus administration of reteplase compared with alteplase infusion in acute myocardial infarction. RAPID Investigators. Circulation 1995; 91:2725–2732.
33. Topol EJ, Ohman EM, Armstrong PW, et al. Survival outcomes 1 year after reperfusion therapy with either alteplase or reteplase for acute myocardial infarction: results from the Global Utilization of Streptokinase and t-PA for Occluded Coronary Arteries (GUSTO) III Trial. Circulation 2000; 102:1761–1765.
34. Gurbel PA, Serebruany VL, Shustov AR, et al. Effects of reteplase and alteplase on platelet aggregation and major receptor expression during the first 24 hours of acute myocardial infarction treatment. GUSTO-III Investigators. Global Use of Strategies to Open Occluded Coronary Arteries. J Am Coll Cardiol 1998; 31:1466–1473.
35. Trial of abciximab with and without low-dose reteplase for acute myocardial infarction. Strategies for Patency Enhancement in the Emergency Department (SPEED) Group. Circulation 2000; 101:2788–2794.
36. Herrmann HC, Moliterno DJ, Ohman EM, et al. Facilitation of early percutaneous coronary intervention after reteplase with or without abciximab in acute myocardial infarction: results from the SPEED (GUSTO-4 Pilot) Trial. J Am Coll Cardiol 2000; 36:1489–1496.
37. Topol EJ. Reperfusion therapy for acute myocardial infarction with fibrinolytic therapy or combination reduced fibrinolytic therapy and platelet glycoprotein IIb/IIIa inhibition: the GUSTO V randomised trial. Lancet 2001; 357:1905–1914.
38. Merlini PA, Repetto A, Andreoli AM, et al. Effect of abciximab on prothrombin activation and thrombin generation in patients with acute myocardial infarction also receiving reteplase. Am J Cardiol 2004; 93:195–198.
39. Stewart RJ, Fredenburgh JC, Leslie BA, et al. Identification of the mechanism responsible for the increased fibrin specificity of TNK-tissue plasminogen activator relative to tissue plasminogen activator. J Biol Chem 2000; 275:10112–10120.
40. Collen D, Stassen JM, Yasuda T, et al. Comparative thrombolytic properties of tissue-type plasminogen activator and of a plasminogen activator inhibitor-1-resistant glycosylation variant, in a combined arterial and venous thrombosis model in the dog. Thromb Haemost 1994; 72:98–104.
41. Al Shwafi KA, de Meester A, Pirenne B, et al. Comparative fibrinolytic activity of front-loaded alteplase and the single-bolus mutants tenecteplase and lanoteplase during treatment of acute myocardial infarction. Am Heart J 2003; 145:217–225.
42. Binbrek AS, Rao NS, Neimane D, et al. Comparison of rapidity of coronary recanalization in men with tenecteplase versus alteplase in acute myocardial infarction. Am J Cardiol 2004; 93:1465–1468.
43. Cannon CP, McCabe CH, Gibson CM, et al. TNK-tissue plasminogen activator in acute myocardial infarction. Results of the Thrombolysis in Myocardial Infarction (TIMI) 10A dose-ranging trial. Circulation 1997; 95:351–356.
44. van de Werf FJ, Cannon CP, Luyten A, et al. Safety assessment of single-bolus administration of TNK tissue-plasminogen activator in acute myocardial infarction: the ASSENT-1 trial. The ASSENT-1 Investigators. Am Heart J 1999; 137:786–791.
45. Sinnaeve P, Alexander J, Belmans A, et al. One-year follow-up of the ASSENT-2 trial: a double-blind, randomized comparison of single-bolus tenecteplase and front-loaded alteplase in 16,949 patients with ST-elevation acute myocardial infarction. Am Heart J 2003; 146:27–32.
46. Antman EM, Louwerenburg HW, Baars HF, et al. Enoxaparin as adjunctive antithrombin therapy for ST-elevation myocardial infarction: results of the ENTIRE-Thrombolysis in Myocardial Infarction (TIMI) 23 Trial. Circulation 2002; 105:1642–1649.
47. Efficacy and safety of tenecteplase in combination with enoxaparin, abciximab, or unfractionated heparin: the ASSENT-3 randomised trial in acute myocardial infarction. Lancet 2001; 358:605–613.

48. Sinnaeve PR, Alexander JH, Bogaerts K, et al. Efficacy of tenecteplase in combination with enoxaparin, abciximab, or unfractionated heparin: one-year follow-up results of the Assessment of the Safety of a New Thrombolytic-3 (ASSENT-3) randomized trial in acute myocardial infarction. Am Heart J 2004; 147:993–998.
49. Armstrong W, Wagner G, Goodman SG, et al. ST segment resolution in ASSENT 3: insights into the role of three different treatment strategies for acute myocardial infarction. Eur Heart J 2003; 24:1515–1522.
50. Antman EM, Morrow DA, McCabe CH, et al. Enoxaparin versus Unfractionated Heparin with Fibrinolysis for ST-Elevation Myocardial Infarction. N Engl J Med 2006; 354:1477–1488.
51. Wallentin L, Goldstein P, Armstrong PW, et al. Efficacy and safety of tenecteplase in combination with the low-molecular-weight heparin enoxaparin or unfractionated heparin in the prehospital setting: the Assessment of the Safety and Efficacy of a New Thrombolytic Regimen (ASSENT)-3 PLUS randomized trial in acute myocardial infarction. Circulation 2003; 108:135–142.
52. Collen D, Vanderschueren S, van de Werf FJ. Fibrin-selective thrombolytic therapy with recombinant staphylokinase. Haemostasis 1996; 26(suppl):294–300.
53. Collen D, Moreau H, Stockx L, et al. Recombinant staphylokinase variants with altered immunoreactivity. II: Thrombolytic properties and antibody induction. Circulation 1996; 94:207–216.
54. Collen D, De Cock F, Demarsin E, et al. Recombinant staphylokinase variants with altered immunoreactivity. III: Species variability of antibody binding patterns. Circulation 1997; 95:455–462.
55. Collen D, Sinnaeve P, Demarsin E, et al. Polyethylene glycol-derivatized cysteine-substitution variants of recombinant staphylokinase for single-bolus treatment of acute myocardial infarction. Circulation 2000; 102:1766–1772.
56. Armstrong PW, Burton J, Pakola S, et al. Collaborative Angiographic Patency Trial Of Recombinant Staphylokinase (CAPTORS II). Am Heart J 2003; 146:484–488.
57. Nordt TK, Moser M, Kohler B, et al. Pharmacokinetics and pharmacodynamics of lanoteplase (n-PA). Thromb Haemost 1999; 82(Suppl 1):121–123.
58. Ogata N, Ogawa H, Ogata Y, et al. Comparison of thrombolytic therapies with mutant tPA (lanoteplase/SUN9216) and recombinant tPA (alteplase) for acute myocardial infarction. Jpn Circ J 1998; 62:801–806.
59. den Heijer P, Vermeer F, Ambrosioni E, et al. Evaluation of a weight-adjusted single-bolus plasminogen activator in patients with myocardial infarction: a double-blind, randomized angiographic trial of lanoteplase versus alteplase. Circulation 1998; 98:2117–2125.
60. Charbonnier B, Pluta W, De Ferrari G, et al. Evaluation of two weight-adjusted single bolus doses of Amediplase to patients with acute myocardial infarction: the 3k2 Trial. Circulation 2001; 107:I-538 (abstr).
61. Vermeer F, Oldrovd K, Pohl J, et al. Safety and angiography data of Amediplase, a new fibrin specific thrombolytic agent, given as a single bolus to patients with acute myocardial infarction: the 2K2 Dose Finding Trial. Circulation 2001; 104:I-538 (abstr).
62. Inoue T, Yaguchi I, Takayanagi K, et al. A new thrombolytic agent, monteplase, is independent of the plasminogen activator inhibitor in patients with acute myocardial infarction: initial results of the Combining Monteplase with Angioplasty (COMA) trial. Am Heart J 2002; 144:E5.
63. Inoue T, Nishiki R, Kageyama M, et al. Long-term benefits of monteplase before coronary angioplasty in acute myocardial infarction. Am J Cardiol 2005; 95:506–508.
64. Oikawa K, Kamimura H, Watanabe T, et al. Pharmacokinetic properties of a novel tissue-type plasminogen activator pamiteplase after single intravenous administration to rats, dogs, and monkeys. Thromb Res 2001; 101:493–500.
65. Watanabe K, Nagao K, Watanabe I, et al. Relationship between the door-to-TIMI-3 flow time and the infarct size in patients suffering from acute myocardial infarction: analysis based on the fibrinolysis and subsequent transluminal (FAST-3) trial. Circ J 2004; 68:280–285.
66. Bar FW, Vermeer F, Michels R, et al. Saruplase in Myocardial Infarction. J Thromb Thrombolysis 1995; 2:195–204.

6 Treatment Opportunities with Fibrinolytic Therapy

Robert C. Welsh and Paul W. Armstrong
Division of Cardiology, University of Alberta, Edmonton, Alberta, Canada

INTRODUCTION

Optimal patient outcomes in ST-elevation myocardial infarction (STEMI) are achieved with rapid, complete, and sustained coronary artery patency. The choice of reperfusion strategy [fibrinolysis or primary percutaneous coronary intervention (PCI)] is modulated by the time from symptom onset to first medical contact, the estimated baseline patient risk, and the predicted PCI-related delay, measured as the interval between initiation of fibrinolysis to first balloon inflation. Although debate persists relating to the acceptable limits of PCI-related delay, data from clinical trials and international registries support current American College of Cardiology/American Heart Association (ACC/AHA) STEMI guidelines that define a 60-minute interval as maximally acceptable.

Recent evidence has enhanced our knowledge regarding optimal pharmacological conjunctive therapy and appropriate mechanical cointervention in patients receiving fibrinolysis, thereby further improving pharmacological reperfusion strategies. Although primary PCI is considered the reperfusion strategy of choice if it can be delivered rapidly by an experienced interventionalist at a high-volume center, its applicability to the broad cross section of STEMI patients is logistically challenging. The key to addressing this challenge of optimizing therapy for all STEMI patients is to provide physicians and all health care providers with pragmatic and efficient approaches to treatment. In turn, these should be implemented through development of regional protocols and systematic approaches that facilitate prehospital cardiac care as well as overcoming both unnecessary delay and undertreatment of eligible patients.

THE IMPORTANCE OF REPERFUSION DELAY: IS IT ALL A MATTER OF TIME?

Experimental animal models of acute myocardial infarction (MI) demonstrate a continuous and progressive wave of myocardial necrosis dependent on the duration of ischemia induced by coronary artery ligation (1). The clinical impact of delay to reperfusion has been demonstrated in a meta-analysis of greater than 50,000 STEMI patients, where fibrinolysis within the first hour of symptom onset achieved twice the benefit of that observed within the second hour (65 vs. 37 lives saved/1000 patients treated) (2). Further support for this time-dependent concept arises from the In-TIME-2 study that demonstrated a 6% decrease in the likelihood of achieving myocardial reperfusion with each additional hour of delay in fibrinolytic treatment, as measured by complete (>70%) ST-segment resolution (3). These and other data focused attention on reducing time to reperfusion and spawned the familiar adages "golden hour" of reperfusion and "time is muscle."

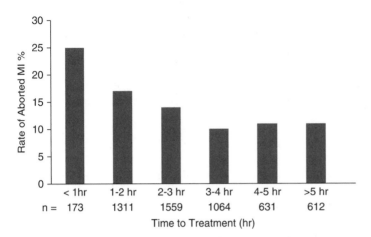

FIGURE 1 Aborted myocardial infarction: revisiting the "golden hour." In those patients receiving fibrinolysis within one hour of symptom onset, 25% "aborted" their myocardial infarction (4).

A newer concept supportive of early reperfusion therapy, entitled "aborted STEMI," has recently emerged. This entity refers to the circumstance where a patient with typical symptoms and an electrocardiographic diagnosis of STEMI exhibits prompt resolution of ST-elevation and minimal or no subsequent elevation of creatinine kinase after receiving reperfusion therapy. Within the ASSENT-3 trial (4), 25% of patients receiving fibrinolysis within the first hour of symptoms had their STEMI aborted compared with 13.3% in the entire study (Fig. 1). Overall, patients in this study had a median time to treatment of 2 hours and 42 minutes. Because aborted STEMI patients have an improved prognosis, it has been argued that this entity may serve as a useful proxy for reperfusion effectiveness in future trials (5).

Although the deleterious impact of temporal delay has been a well-accepted feature of fibrinolytic-treated patients, debate exists over whether the phenomenon is equally applicable to primary PCI. Resolution of this issue has been hampered by the limited number of patients enrolled in randomized clinical trials as well as the delay inherent in the performance of the PCI procedure. Specifically, only a few patients are able to receive primary PCI within the first two hours of symptom onset where the temporal window for myocardial salvage is maximal (6). The unfavorable impact of delay to first balloon inflation on mortality has been demonstrated in the two largest trials of primary PCI. Within DANAMI-2, there was a threefold increase in 30-day death, repeat MI, or stroke (4.7% vs. 12.2%) in patients with delay to randomization (Fig. 2A) (7). In GUSTO-2B, the in-hospital delay from randomization to first balloon inflation was associated with a sixfold increase in 30-day mortality when comparing patients treated within 60 minutes of randomization with those treated after 90 minutes of randomization (1% vs. 6.4%) (Fig. 2B) (8).

Analyses of large international registries have provided additional supportive evidence on the negative impact of delay to mechanical reperfusion. Within a cohort analysis of 29,222 STEMI patients treated with primary PCI within six hours of presentation at 395 National Registry of Myocardial Infarction (NRMI 3/4, 1999–2002) hospitals, longer door-to-balloon time was associated with increased in-hospital mortality rates of 3.0%, 4.2%, 5.7%, and 7.4% for door-to-balloon times of ≤90 minutes, 91 to 120 minutes, 121 to 150 minutes, and >150 minutes, respectively ($p < 0.01$ for trend) (9).

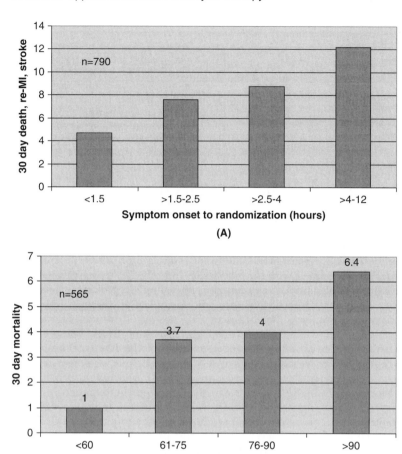

FIGURE 2   Temporal impact of delay to primary PCI on clinical events in STEMI. (**A**) The impact of delay from symptom onset to randomization on a composite clinical end point of 30-day death, repeat myocardial infarction, and stroke (DANAMI-2). Patients randomized within the first 90 minutes had a composite event rate of 4.7% compared with 12.2% in those randomized after four hours (67). (**B**) The impact of delay from randomization to PCI on 30-day mortality (GUSTO-2B). In those patients who received primary PCI within one hour of randomization, 30-day mortality was only 1% compared with 6.4% in those receiving primary PCI later than 90 minutes (8).

The increased mortality with increasing door-to-balloon times was seen regardless of either the symptom onset-to-door time or the patient's baseline clinical risk status.

REPERFUSION STRATEGY WHEN DELAY TO PRIMARY PCI IS UNAVOIDABLE

Although not observed in an individual trial, the Keely and Grines overview of 23 randomized studies comparing fibrinolysis with primary PCI demonstrated a mortality advantage with primary PCI (10). This publication accelerated the move

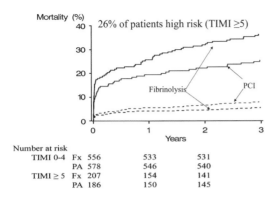

FIGURE 3   Impact of baseline risk, three-year mortality and choice of reperfusion therapy. In DANAMI-2, 26% of patients were found to have a baseline TIMI risk score greater than or equal to five, defining high risk. In these subjects, three-year mortality was significantly increased by greater than threefold and the benefit of primary PCI over fibrinolysis was evident. By contrast, there was no advantage of primary PCI over fibrinolytic therapy with TIMI scores of 0–4 (12).

to embracing mechanical reperfusion strategies despite a number of limitations in their analyses. Patients treated with fibrinolysis in these studies frequently received inferior pharmacological reperfusion strategies, including streptokinase, and non-state-of-the-art conjunctive antithrombotic and antiplatelet therapy. As well, mechanical cointervention, specifically rescue PCI, was used infrequently among fibrinolytic patients and was actually discouraged in some trials. These studies have also been criticized as not being representative of the real-world situation because the rapidity with which primary PCI was undertaken, represented by an average delay between fibrinolysis and primary PCI of only approximately 40 minutes. Moreover, the DANAMI-2 trial, which formed the largest component of the overview, enrolled patients with prior stroke and discouraged rescue PCI for fibrinolytic failure (11). This study was discontinued prior to planned enrollment because of perceived efficacy, thereby potentially overestimating the observed differences. Finally, and especially illuminating, the three-year follow-up of DANAMI-2 revealed that the benefit of PCI was limited to the one in four patients with advanced TIMI risk score, whereas no difference in outcome was evident among the large majority of STEMI patients (Fig. 3) (12).

On the basis of an analysis of these same randomized trials, the mortality benefit of PCI was shown to be time dependent. The 30-day mortality advantage of primary PCI decreased at an absolute rate of 0.94% with every 10-minute increase in PCI-related delay, defined as the temporal difference between door-to-balloon and door-to-needle time (13). With this rate of decline, the two reperfusion strategies became equivalent after 62 minutes from when fibrinolysis could have been administered prior to primary PCI. Although these time-dependent aspects have been debated with subsequent reanalyses (14–16), the results seem well aligned with registry data where the predicted advantage of primary PCI has not been consistently demonstrated (Fig. 4). Furthermore, this temporal target for reperfusion, and the notion of a 60-minute maximally accepted interval between strategies, has been incorporated in the ACC/AHA STEMI guidelines, as well as a Canadian perspective on these guidelines (17,18).

The relationship between reperfusion delay and outcomes appears non-linear and modulated by the total duration of symptoms. In the Myocardial Infarction and Triage Intervention (MITI) prehospital STEMI trial, patients treated with fibrinolysis within 70 minutes of symptom onset had a 30-day

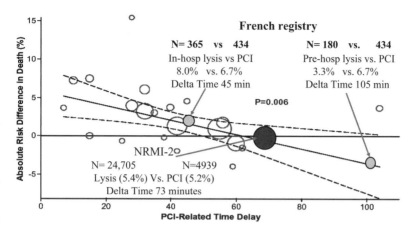

FIGURE 4 Mortality rates by mode of reperfusion and treatment delay. Randomized trials of fibrinolysis versus primary PCI demonstrate that with each 10 minutes of PCI-related delay, there is an associated 0.94% reduction in the benefit of primary PCI (13). PCI-related delay is defined as the time from first balloon inflation with primary PCI minus the time to administration of fibrinolysis. The size of the circles within this analysis represents the number of patients enrolled within the specific study. Overlying this analysis are data from the National Registry of Myocardial Infarction-2 (NRMI-2) in which 24,705 patients received fibrinolysis and 4939 patients received primary PCI with hospital mortality rates of 5.4% and 5.2%, respectively and a delta time between therapies of 73 minutes (74). The yellow circles represent French registry data (28). In those patients receiving in-hospital fibrinolysis compared with primary PCI, mortality rates of 8% and 6.7% were observed with a PCI-related delay of approximately 45 minutes. In contrast, those patients receiving prehospital fibrinolysis, compared with primary PCI, had mortality rates of 3.3% and 6.7%, respectively with a primary PCI-related delay of approximately 105 minutes.

mortality rate seven times lower than those treated later (1.2% vs. 8.7%, $p = 0.04$), demonstrating the impact of early fibrinolysis (19). The PRAGUE-2 study demonstrated that within three hours of symptom onset, 30-day mortality with primary PCI was similar to streptokinase (7.3% vs. 7.4%). The main advantage of primary PCI was in patients presenting after six hours of symptom onset (20). Although the CAPTIM trial was stopped prior to completing enrollment, the primary end point of death, repeat MI, and nonfatal disabling stroke was not different between prehospital fibrinolysis and prehospital triage for direct primary PCI. Interestingly, the mortality end point favored the prehospital fibrinolysis group at 30 days (3.8% vs. 4.8%) and one year (5.4% vs. 7.3%), although not statistically significant (21) (Table 1). Furthermore, when patients treated within two hours were analyzed, the 30-day mortality (2.2% vs. 5.7% $p = 0.058$) favored fibrinolysis with accelerated tissue plasminogen activator (rt-PA) with an associated reduction in the rate of cardiogenic shock (1.3% vs. 5.3%, $p = 0.032$) (22). These data support the notion that in patients that present early in the course of STEMI, excellent outcomes are achieved with fibrinolysis that are at least equivalent, if not superior, to primary PCI. As a consequence, a shorter time to equipoise between reperfusion therapies may be expected for patients who present early, when the thrombus is most amenable to fibrinolytic therapy.

TABLE 1   Clinical Trial and Registry Data—Mortality by Reperfusion Strategy

		Reperfusion therapy		
	Mortality	Prehospital fibrinolysis	In-hospital fibrinolysis	Primary PCI
Clinical trials				
CAPTIM	30-day mortality	3.8%		6.7%
	1-yr mortality	5.4%		7.3%
WEST	30-day mortality	2.4% (60%)		1%
Registry				
USIC	In-hospital mortality	3.3%	8.0%	6.7%
	1-yr mortality	6%	11%	11%
PURGE	In-hospital mortality	3.4%	8.0%	6.7%
SWEDISH	7-day mortality	5.9%	8.8%	3.5%
	30-day mortality	7.6%	11.4%	4.9%
	1-yr mortality	10.3%	15.9%	7.6%

REPERFUSION GUIDED BY PATIENT-SPECIFIC RISK PROFILE

Baseline patient risk varies substantially in STEMI patients with resultant mortality rates ranging from less than 3% to greater than 50% at 30 days (Fig. 5). Although the PRAGUE investigators demonstrated minimal risk of delay to reperfusion in a low-risk population, patients deemed to be at high risk suffered a substantial and progressive risk with delay to primary PCI, confirming the importance of rapid reperfusion in high-risk STEMI patients (23). Post hoc analysis of the DANAMI-2 trial, mentioned earlier, further added to this analysis with the long-term advantage of mechanical versus fibrinolysis reperfusion related to the 25% of patients with a high TIMI risk score (Fig. 3). In patients with cardiogenic shock, short- and long-term mortality is improved with urgent revascularization instead of medical stabilization (12). These data support the importance of patient risk stratification in determining optimal reperfusion strategy as well as the acceptable time delay.

The perceived benefit of primary PCI over fibrinolysis stratified by risk profiles has recently been addressed in the 22 clinical randomized trials of primary PCI versus fibrinolysis. Investigators, using baseline risk of the enrolled population, found that in patients with a mortality risk of less than 4.5%, benefit of primary PCI on 30-day mortality was unlikely (16). If this analysis was limited to those trials using fibrin-specific agents, equipoise was achieved at a predicted 30-day mortality of 4.8%. Furthermore, patient risk (regression coefficient 0.82, $p < 0.001$) and PCI-related delay (regression coefficiency 0.047, $p < 0.001$) were independently correlated with 30-day survival benefit of PCI or fibrinolytic therapy without interaction ($p = 0.5$).

Choice of reperfusion therapy is also affected by assessment of the patient risk of bleeding, especially intracranial hemorrhage, which occurs more frequently in the elderly, females, and patients with low body weight, prior stroke, and uncontrolled hypertension (24–27). Hence, the majority of incremental benefit of primary PCI compared with fibrinolytic therapy can be achieved by selecting patients presenting with high-risk clinical characteristics and/or contraindications to fibrinolysis. The majority of STEMI patients are likely best served by rapid reperfusion, regardless of mode of therapy.

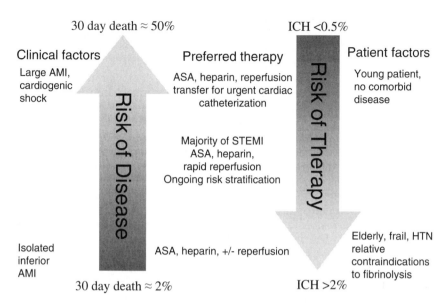

FIGURE 5 Risk and therapeutic choice in STEMI. Patient-specific risk factors assist in selection of appropriate reperfusion strategies. In patients suffering an isolated inferior STEMI, the mortality rate is low (approximately 2%). In contrast patients with a large anterior STEMI and cardiogenic shock have very high mortality rates (>50%). Similarly, complications of reperfusion therapy in young patients with no comorbid disease are low. In contrast, elderly frail patients, especially those with hypertension and female sex, have relative contraindications to reperfusion.

REAL WORLD INSIGHTS FROM REGISTRY DATA

Although randomized controlled trials provide the highest level of evidence evaluating novel therapies, they are frequently perceived to lack a "real world" relevance that allows generalizability of the results. This commonly relates to stringent patient and study site selection criteria. Although less rigorous in design, well-assembled and detailed registry data may be complementary by providing evaluation of the broader use and impact of such therapies.

Within the Service D'Aide Medicale D'urgence (SAMU) in France, physician-based triage at an emergency response center keys activation of mobile emergency care units manned with physicians responding to prehospital patients with suspected acute coronary syndromes. As a standard of care, this system provides expeditious decision making either to administer prehospital fibrinolysis or to transfer directly to a tertiary care PCI center. In a recent report of 1922 STEMI patients from 443 participating centers, the lowest in-hospital mortality was achieved in those receiving prehospital fibrinolysis compared with either in-hospital fibrinolysis or primary PCI (28). At one year, the benefit of prehospital fibrinolysis was maintained with 94% survival compared with 89% for both in-hospital fibrinolysis and primary PCI groups with a relative risk of death of 0.49 (95% CI 0.24–1.00; $p = 0.05$). Furthermore, in those patients treated early (prior to median time to hospital admission of 3.5 hours) with prehospital fibrinolysis, there was no in-hospital mortality and an excellent one-year survival of 99%. Compared with in-hospital fibrinolysis patients, the prehospital fibrinolysis group underwent more cardiac catheterization and PCI within the first day of admission, which may have contributed to the excellent outcomes (catheterization within 24 hours, 37% prehospital vs. 18% in-hospital fibrinolysis).

Relevant to the fact that only 25% of hospitals within the United States have primary PCI programs, NRMI (3/4, 1999–2002) has demonstrated substantial reperfusion delay in patients requiring transfer for primary PCI. Eighty-four percent of these patients transferred from a community hospital for primary PCI had greater than two hours reperfusion delay with a median door-to-balloon time of 180 minutes (29). Only 4.2% had a door-to-balloon time less than 90 minutes, revealing an important discrepancy between the performance of primary PCI in a real world setting and the strategy tested in randomized clinical trials.

A further analysis based on NRMI (2, 3, and 4, 1994–2003), with 192,509 patients from 645 hospitals who presented within 12 hours of symptom onset with STEMI, allows assessment of the relevance of the ACC/AHA STEMI guidelines suggesting that reperfusion strategy selection takes into account PCI-related reperfusion delay (30). The mean hospital-specific PCI reperfusion delay was of 78 minutes and increased to 148 minutes when restricted to patients requiring transfer, both results being substantially outside the 60-minute acceptable delay defined within guidelines (17). Although the door-to-needle time with fibrinolysis remained relatively constant across participating hospitals, the PCI delay varied significantly from 49 (±10.3) minutes in the lowest quartile to 141 (±19.2) minutes in the highest quartile, with low-volume PCI centers shown to have increased delay. After adjusting for patient-specific and hospital-specific characteristics, equipoise for mortality between mechanical and pharmacological reperfusion was achieved at 114 minutes [95% CI 96–132; $p < 0.001$] of PCI-related delay. Further analysis was undertaken addressing specific populations stratified by time from symptom onset to presentation, age, and STEMI location (Fig. 6). In patients less than 65 years of age presenting within two hours of symptom onset with an anterior wall or nonanterior wall STEMI, equipoise between reperfusion strategies was achieved after 40 and 58 minutes of PCI-related delay, respectively. Furthermore, in patients less than 65 years of age presenting after two hours of symptom onset with anterior wall STEMI, time to equipoise was only 43 minutes of PCI delay. Recognizing that 65% of patients presented within two hours of symptom onset, and that the mean age was 61 years within this registry, the vast majority of STEMI patients achieve equipoise between reperfusion strategies within a PCI-related delay of less than 60 minutes.

These "real world" analyses have resulted in major efforts to improve time to treatment with primary PCI including the current joint AHA/ACC door-to-balloon initiative (31–34). Proponents of a mechanical reperfusion strategy suggest that expansion of the benefits of primary PCI could be achieved by providing 24-hour-a-day service and increasing the number of interventional centers. Unfortunately, the efficacy of off-hour primary PCI service has been questioned based on 1702 consecutive STEMI patients within the Zwolle experience (35). Those treated during nonworking hours (18:00–8:00) were twice as likely to have failure of primary PCI (6.9% vs. 3.8%, $p < 0.01$) and experienced a greater than twofold increased 30-day mortality (4.2% vs. 1.9%, $p < 0.01$). The basis for this finding, which is supported by other analyses, is unclear but deserves further investigation regarding its implications for broader systems use of PCI (36,37). Furthermore, expanding the number of centers capable of performing primary PCI may prove problematic given the known inverse relationship between mortality and procedure volume in STEMI patients

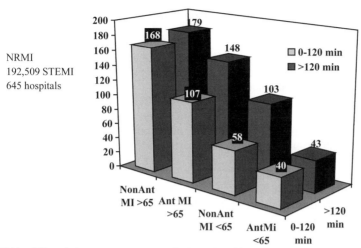

NRMI
192,509 STEMI
645 hospitals

Multi variable analysis –treatment type, age, gender, DM, HTN, Killip class, prior MI, infarct location, stroke, etc.
Also corrected for hospital covariates: STEMI volume, primary PCI volume, etc

FIGURE 6 Adjusted analysis of PCI-related delay in stratified STEMI populations. Impact of PCI-related delay in NRMI patients stratified by location of STEMI (anterior vs. non anterior), age (65 years of age), and time to presentation (120 minutes); adjusting for type of reperfusion, age, gender, diabetes mellitus, hypertension, Killip class, prior myocardial infarction, infarct location, past stroke, as well as hospital covariants including STEMI volume and primary PCI volume. Substantial variability of the time to equipoise between mechanical and pharmacological reperfusion therapy is evident as demonstrated by the PCI-related reperfusion delay across the stratified STEMI patient populations.

treated with primary PCI in low volume centers or by low volume interventionalists (38–42). The need to maintain adequate PCI center and operator volume to ensure high quality and competency requires a delicate balance and challenges the rational for widespread proliferation of primary PCI centers.

As stated in the 2004 ACC/AHA guidelines, "Given the current literature, it is not possible to say definitively that a particular reperfusion approach is superior for all patients, in all clinical settings, at all times of day" (17). The appropriate and timely use of some reperfusion therapy is likely more important than the choice of therapy, and timely reperfusion in as many eligible patients as possible is the most likely avenue to enhance the care of STEMI patients. Therefore, the wholesale abandonment of fibrinolysis in favor of mechanical reperfusion is unwise and impractical, given the desire to provide best patient care for the majority of patients with STEMI.

ENHANCING FIBRINOLYSIS: ADVANCES IN CONJUNCTIVE PHARMACOLOGICAL THERAPY

Over the past three decades, pharmacological reperfusion has evolved through multiple levels of investigation, including design and development of bolus fibrinolytic agents, and improved conjunctive pharmacological antithrombotic and antiplatelet therapies.

The GUSTO-1 trial established rt-PA as the gold standard fibrinolytic agent, achieving a 1% mortality advantage over streptokinase (43). Subsequent engineering of the rt-PA molecule led to new fibrinolytic agents, reteplase given as a double bolus over 30 minutes or single-bolus tenecteplase (44,45). Combined with ease of administration and efficacy, tenecteplase has decreased systemic bleeding compared with rt-PA (45).

Appropriate conjunctive therapy with antithrombotic agents is required with fibrinolysis to reduce thromboembolic complications and maintain coronary patency. Compared with unfractionated heparin, the low molecular weight heparin enoxaparin has enhanced sustained coronary patency and reduced reinfarction and recurrent ischemia rates. This benefit comes with an increased risk of bleeding in selected high-risk populations, specifically elderly low body weight females (25,46). The ExTRACT TIMI-25 trial compared enoxaparin and unfractionated heparin in fibrinolytic-treated STEMI patients ($n = 20,506$) and supported prior investigation demonstrating a 17% relative reduction in the dual end point of 30-day death and repeat MI [9.9% vs. 12%; RR 0.83 (77–90); $p = 0.001$] (47). This was achieved with an associated modest increased major bleeding risk [2.1% vs. 1.4%; RR 1.53 (1.23–1.89); $p < 0.001$] without increased risk of intracranial hemorrhage [0.8% vs. 0.7%; RR 1.7 (0.92–1.75); $p = 0.14$]. Importantly, in patients greater than 75 years, the intravenous dose of enoxaparin in ExTRACT was omitted and a subcutaneous dose reduction of 0.75 mg/kg was utilized, with an apparent maintenance of clinical efficacy without excess bleeding. Furthermore, secondary analysis has demonstrated consistent benefit in those patients within this trial undergoing cardiac catheterization and PCI while on enoxaparin. Investigation of other antithrombotic agents in conjunction with fibrinolysis has demonstrated no clear advantage in regards to reduced clinical end points with fondaparinux but reduced bleeding compared with placebo or unfractionated heparin (48). Importantly, there was an increased risk of thrombotic complications in conjunction with primary PCI, leading investigators to recommend additional unfractionated heparin use in this situation.

The importance of antiplatelet therapy in combination with fibrinolysis in STEMI patients has been known for several decades since ISIS-2 demonstrated the benefit of adding aspirin to streptokinase (49). Despite reasonable pathophysiological evidence predicting a benefit of more potent platelet inhibition, the combination of glycoprotein IIb/IIIa receptor blockers and fibrinolytic agents has failed to yield a net clinical benefit because of increased bleeding risk (50). Dual oral antiplatelet therapy with aspirin and clopidogrel has been shown to provide enhanced late coronary artery patency and improved clinical outcomes when combined with fibrinolysis (51,52). Further investigation into the impact of enhanced antiplatelet activity will be forthcoming with novel agents shown to have rapid onset of action and increased potency compared with aspirin or clopidogrel.

Although combinations of conjunctive therapy with fibrinolysis require further investigation, aspirin, clopidogrel, and enoxaparin were found to have 90.9% coronary patency rates two to three days following fibrinolysis and particularly low rates of cardiovascular death (3.2%), recurrent MI (3.0%), and major bleeding (1.8%) (53). Although direct comparison is not possible, the results achieved with modern pharmacological reperfusion are similar to those demonstrated with primary PCI.

ENHANCING FIBRINOLYSIS: ADVANCES
IN MECHANICAL COINTERVENTION

Attempts to improve patient outcomes following fibrinolysis through mechanical cointervention strategies continue to be an area of intense investigation, although the optimal interplay and appropriate timing remain unclear. Recognizing potential

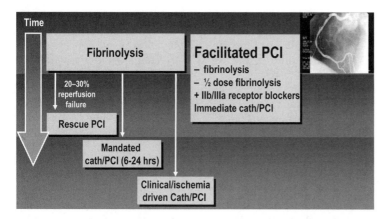

FIGURE 7 The role of mechanical intervention postfibrinolysis. After fibrinolysis, a host of options for mechanical cointervention strategies exists. In those patients with reperfusion failure, urgent rescue PCI is indicated. Debate exists regarding the need for coronary angiography (±PCI) in those patients subsequent to successful fibrinolysis. Modestly powered studies suggest potential benefit of mandated cardiac catheterization (±PCI) undertaken within the first 24 hours, although definitive investigations are required. In patients with evidence of recurrent or provoked myocardial ischemia or other high risk features, cardiac catheterization and PCI are recommended. Facilitated PCI, a strategy where all patients urgently proceed to cardiac catheterization (±PCI) following full-dose fibrinolysis or combination therapy is not supported by available research and remains investigational.

overlap between approaches, mechanical cointervention strategies currently include facilitated PCI, rescue PCI, mandated early cardiac catheterization with PCI as required, and cardiac catheterization based on clinical characteristics or evidence of residual myocardial ischemia (Fig. 7).

Recognizing the inherent delay for mechanical reperfusion and the suboptimal coronary patency achieved with pharmacological reperfusion, the concept of facilitated PCI has emerged over the last decade. This involves all patients receiving fibrinolysis, with the benefits of early reperfusion, and subsequently the patency advantage achieved in the cardiac catheterization laboratory through mechanical cointervention. This strategy was investigated in a host of small trials with varying results. The larger scale ASSENT-4 PCI trial designed to systematically assess the benefit of this strategy was stopped early after 1667 (planned $n = 4000$) patients were randomized, because of excess adverse events (facilitate PCI 19% vs. primary PCI 13%; death or congestive heart failure or shock within 90 days, $p = 0.0045$) (54). Given these results, as well as a systematic overview of facilitated PCI, there is no evidence to support mandated urgent cardiac catheterization and PCI following successful fibrinolysis, and this practice should be discouraged (55). The FINESSE trial further supports this conclusion with no benefit with facilitated PCI utilizing half-dose fibrinolysis (reteplase) in combination with abciximab or upstream abciximab alone in primary PCI (56).

Following fibrinolysis, failure of successful reperfusion as measured by lack of ST-segment resolution is known to be associated with adverse events. The strategy of rescue PCI, where mechanical cointervention is limited to this subset of patients or those experiencing high-risk electrical or hemodynamic features, strives to balance the potential risk of cardiac catheterization and PCI with the benefits of coronary patency and myocardial salvage. Although a logical approach, only limited data with mixed results have been available, and the concept has been challenging to investigate because of preconceived beliefs of practicing physicians. Utilizing a 90-minute ECG with less than 50% ST-elevation resolution after fibrinolysis denoting reperfusion failure, the REACT investigators demonstrated a reduction in adverse events with rescue PCI compared with conservative therapy or repeat fibrinolysis. The composite event rate (death, repeat MI, or cerebral vascular accident) was 15.3% for rescue PCI, 29.8% for conservative management, and 31.0% for repeat fibrinolysis ($p < 0.005$) (57). These data, combined with expert opinion, have led rescue angioplasty to be incorporated into major international STEMI guidelines.

Debate continues regarding the requirement for cardiac catheterization and its timing in STEMI patients that achieve successful reperfusion with fibrinolysis. The GRACIA-1 trial completed in Spain and Portugal assessed the benefit of cardiac catheterization following fibrinolysis with randomization to clinical ischemic driven versus mandated cardiac catheterization within 24 hours of fibrinolysis (58). With a median time to cardiac catheterization of 19.6 hours (SD 5.5) after symptom onset [16.7 hours (SD 5.6) following fibrinolysis], the mandated invasive catheterization group had a decreased one-year composite event rate of death, repeat MI, or revascularization (9% vs. 21%; $p = 0.008$) with a trend toward reduced death and repeat MI (7% vs. 12%; $p = 0.07$). This was achieved with 80% of patients in the invasive arm having PCI in the culprit artery and 26% having additional non-culprit PCI, compared with 21% of the standard therapy arm undergoing PCI for recurrent ischemia.

The Which Early ST-elevation myocardial infarction therapy study (WEST) was designed to assess differences between optimal pharmacological reperfusion without (group A) or with (groups B) protocol defined rescue PCI and cardiac catheterization and PCI as required within 24 hours of fibrinolysis, compared with primary PCI (group C) with a focus on expedited care (59). Within this modestly sized trial ($n = 306$), there was no difference in the primary composite clinical end points (30-day death, repeat MI, refractory ischemia, congestive heart failure, cardiogenic shock, and major ventricular arrhythmia) between the three reperfusion strategies. The rapid reperfusion achieved with symptom onset to fibrinolysis of two hours and first balloon inflation in less than three hours was associated with a 30-day mortality of only 2.0% (6/304). Post hoc analysis revealed that 30-day death and repeat MI was higher in the standard care fibrinolytic group (group A) compared with primary PCI (group C), whereas no difference was evident between primary PCI and the pharmacological reperfusion group with rescue and/or mandated cardiac catheterization within 24 hours (group B) [30-day death and re-MI, groups A = 13.0%, B = 6.7%, and C = 4.0%, p(log rank) = 0.02 A vs. C].

The optimal rate of rescue PCI following fibrinolysis remains unknown. The CAPTIM (21) and WEST (59) studies have demonstrated excellent clinical outcomes compared with primary PCI with the combination of early fibrinolysis and rescue PCI in 26% and 27% of patients, respectively, although CAPTIM did not have protocol recommendations. The WEST rescue substudy has shown that following fibrinolysis, 40.7% of patients had failure of ST-segment resolution greater than 50% at 90 minutes or clinical indications for rescue PCI, therefore further investigation into the optimal timing and appropriate rate of rescue referral are required (60). Because the WEST pharmacoinvasive strategy is attractive to many patient populations, including those presenting early to hospitals without the capability for experienced, timely PCI or activating the prehospital emergency medical system, plans are under way to further investigate this in a larger trial.

REGIONAL SYSTEMS APPROACH TO STEMI: FIRST POINT OF CARE STRATEGIES FOR DIAGNOSIS, TRIAGE, AND TREATMENT

Approximately half of STEMI patients activate the prehospital emergency medical system as the first contact for medical assistance (61,62). An analysis of randomized trials of prehospital versus in-hospital fibrinolysis has demonstrated a one-hour reduction in time to treatment with substantial improvement in patient mortality [1.7% absolute reduction, OR 0.83 (CI 0.70–0.98)] (63). In the two largest contemporary trials of prehospital fibrinolysis, median time to treatment of two hours was achieved in contrast to three hours in randomized trials of in-hospital fibrinolysis, with registry data documenting even further delays for in-hospital reperfusion (21,64–66). The fact that patients with STEMI who activate the prehospital emergency medical system can achieve rapid reperfusion and that this in turn portends excellent prognosis provides powerful impetus for health care systems to implement such programs.

Although international acceptance and implementation of prehospital reperfusion strategies have been variable, thought leaders in this arena have validated the concept from over two decades of research, clinical experience, and success. Contemporary trials have expanded our knowledge and addressed perceived limitations of past research and impediments to implementation of broad-scale prehospital reperfusion. In the 12 countries participating in the ASSENT-3+ prehospital fibrinolysis trial, substantial variability in population density, past experience with prehospital fibrinolysis (28% developed de novo programs), and prehospital emergency medical services resources was demonstrated (67). In 65% of study sites, a physician in the prehospital setting identified and treated patients. In other sites, paramedical personnel completed on-scene assessment, obtained and transmitted the 12-lead ECG for remote physician over-read, obtained informed consent, and administered fibrinolytic therapy (68). The presence of a physician in the prehospital setting was associated with greater adherence to protocol mandated therapies and procedures, but delay in time to treatment with no evidence of adverse events in those managed by paramedical personnel demonstrated. Although the clinical experience and enhanced training of a physician in the prehospital setting may represent the ideal situation, trials and the wealth of clinical experience worldwide have demonstrated efficacy, safety, and feasibility of paramedic based prehospital fibrinolysis programs (19,59,65,68–70). In the vast majority of health care systems worldwide, the presence of a prehospital physician is impractical and unrealistic. Therefore, empowering of adequately trained paramedical teams to administer lifesaving therapy, such as fibrinolysis prehospital, should be a high international priority. Recent calls for action in the United States have focused on shortening the delay to PCI and highlighting the value of prehospital ECG. Interestingly, the role of prehospital fibrinolysis is far less embraced possibly because of the complex sociopolitical, economic, and medical-legal environment (67,71,72).

Optimal therapy of STEMI patients in the current era requires a systematic, regionwide approach to early identification, diagnosis, triage, and treatment. Selecting the optimal reperfusion strategy for an individual patient requires assessing their presenting clinical and hemodynamic characteristics, including

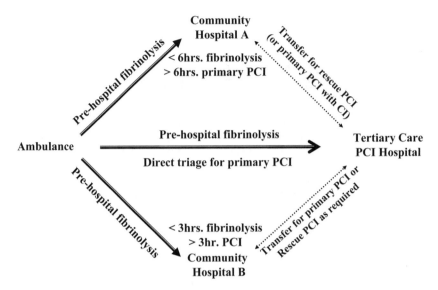

FIGURE 8 Regionalized system approach to STEMI. Reperfusion opportunities should be based on specific patient, hospital, and regional characteristics. Diagnosis and treatment at the point of first medical contact, including prehospital paramedical staff, should be facilitated to optimize time to reperfusion.

territory at risk on the ECG, as well as the risk of complications from reperfusion therapy. Additionally, modulating factors include time from symptom onset to presentation and potential PCI-related reperfusion delay (Fig. 5). Increasingly, debate about which reperfusion method is best is being supplanted by the afore-mentioned strategic approaches reflected in Figure 8.

For STEMI patients that activate the prehospital emergency medical system (approximately 50%), rapid EMS response, patient risk assessment, and stabilization with prehospital diagnosis, triage and treatment, as well as assessment of response to therapy allow seamless triage to the most appropriate hospital destination. In a substantial portion of these patients, treatment should include administration of prehospital fibrinolysis. In the presence of contraindications to fibrinolysis, and when patient characteristics justify primary PCI as the best reperfusion strategy, direct triage to an experienced interventional center with prehospital notification should minimize unnecessary delay to achieve first balloon inflation within 90 minutes. The knowledge and expertise required to safely triage and transport patients for primary PCI is entirely complementary to that required for administration of prehospital fibrinolysis.

For the patients presenting directly to hospital, specific patient, hospital, and regional characteristic should guide decision on the appropriate mode of reperfusion therapy. In patients who present to a community hospital (community hospital A, Fig. 8) and transfer to a tertiary care center for primary PCI and first balloon inflation cannot be consistently achieved within 60 minutes of when fibrinolysis could be administered, pharmacological reperfusion remains the strategy of choice. In patients presenting after six hours of symptom duration with indication for reperfusion, a longer, but not excessive, delay to primary PCI may be acceptable. Urgent transfer to a tertiary care hospital should occur in patients with

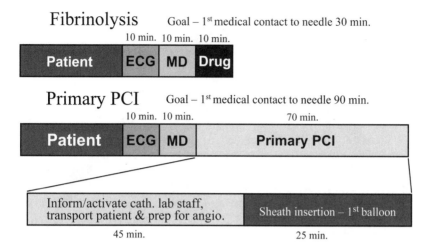

FIGURE 9 Understanding time to treatment: fibrinolysis and primary PCI. Guideline-derived time-to-treatment goals are based on the currently acceptable delay between fibrinolysis and primary PCI (60 minutes). Time from first medical contact with physician assessment and ECG-assisted diagnosis are denoted as two consecutive intervals of ≤10 minutes. Fibrinolysis should be administered within 10 minutes after confirmed diagnosis. With primary PCI, first balloon inflation should occur within 60 minutes of the time fibrinolysis could have been initiated. Since first balloon inflation occurs approximately 20 to 25 minutes after sheath insertion, the entire period to inform and activate the catheterization laboratory staff, transport, and prepare and drape the patient for diagnostic angiography must occur within 45 minutes.

contraindications to fibrinolysis, following fibrinolysis if rescue PCI is indicated, or if high-risk clinical characteristics exist. In patients who present to a community hospital (community hospital B, Fig. 8) where rapid triage to primary PCI can be consistently achieved, both pharmacological and mechanical reperfusion strategies should be employed with fibrinolysis preferred in early presenting patients (less than three hours) and rapid transfer for primary PCI in those presenting after three hours. Finally, in tertiary care PCI hospitals, primary PCI should be the reperfusion strategy of choice. This must occur in conjunction with experienced operators available 24 hours a day, 7 days per week and capable of achieving first balloon inflation within 60 minutes of diagnosis. If this cannot be achieved, a dual reperfusion strategy should be employed. Realistic assessment of time to reperfusion based on hospital and site-specific quality assurance data is mandatory with regular feedback to ensure treatment goals are being achieved (Fig. 9).

Although this chapter has focused on the management of STEMI patients, enhanced prehospital care establishes a platform from which to improve outcomes in a broad range of cardiovascular diseases (Fig. 10). Cardiac arrest is associated with a very poor prognosis that can be substantially improved with early CPR, automated external defibrillators, rapid EMS response, and initiation of definitive therapy including appropriate reperfusion (73). Moreover, enhancing prehospital treatment platforms could facilitate incorporation of novel evidence-based therapies, such as patient "cooling" following cardiac arrest early in the course of treatment. High-risk non-ST-elevation acute coronary syndrome patients would also benefit from early administration of effective antiplatelet and anticoagulant

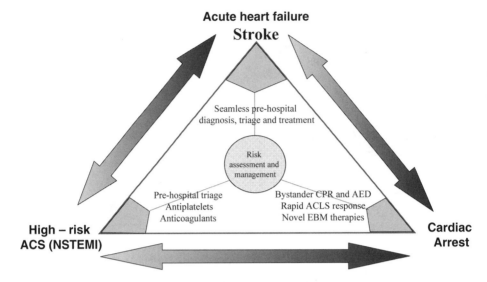

FIGURE 10 Opportunities for advancing prehospital cardiovascular care. Maximizing outcome in STEMI patients through prehospital management establishes an ideal platform from which to launch enhanced care for other high-risk, time-dependant cardiovascular problems.

therapy with triage to a center capable of invasive investigation and management. Moving forward to optimize prehospital cardiac care resources will require the engagement of information technologies, optimal pharmacological and mechanical therapies, and the cooperative work of a spectrum of health care professionals (Fig. 11). The clear recognition that the point of first medical contact has been relocated to the prehospital setting is key not only to encouraging patients to augment this mode of access but also ensuring they receive the best care at the right time and in the right place.

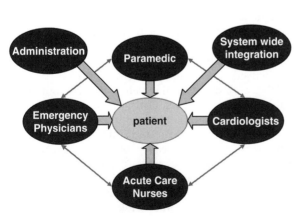

FIGURE 11 Reflections on STEMI care: success through cooperation. Optimizing the care of STEMI patients require all stakeholder, medical, and paramedical groups to collaborate seamlessly. Cardiologists, emergency physicians, and acute care nurses in conjunction with prehospital paramedical staff all provide direct patient care, ideally in a collaborative systematic fashion. This requires support from hospital and health regional administration to facilitate the process as well as reporting and promoting the positive outcomes.

REFERENCES

1. Reimer KA, Lowe JE, Rasmussen MM, et al. The wavefront phenomenon of ischemic cell death. 1. Myocardial infarct size vs duration of coronary occlusion in dogs. Circulation 1977; 56:786–794.
2. Boersma E, Maas AC, Deckers JW, et al. Early thrombolytic treatment in acute myocardial infarction: reappraisal of the golden hour. Lancet 1996; 348:771–775.
3. Antman EM, Cooper HA, Gibson CM, et al. Determinants of improvement in epicardial flow and myocardial perfusion for ST elevation myocardial infarction; insights from TIMI 14 and InTIME-II. Eur Heart J 2002; 23:928–933.
4. Taher T, Fu Y, Wagner GS, et al. Aborted myocardial infarction in patients with ST-segment elevation: insights from the Assessment of the Safety and Efficacy of a New Thrombolytic Regimen-3 Trial Electrocardiographic Substudy. J Am Coll Cardiol 2004; 44:38–43.
5. Verheugt FW, Gersh BJ, Armstrong PW. Aborted myocardial infarction: a new target for reperfusion therapy. Eur Heart J 2006; 27:901–904.
6. Gersh BJ, Stone GW, White HD, et al. Pharmacological facilitation of primary percutaneous coronary intervention for acute myocardial infarction: is the slope of the curve the shape of the future? JAMA 2005; 293:979–986.
7. Welsh RC, Ornato J, Armstrong PW. Prehospital management of acute ST-elevation myocardial infarction: a time for reappraisal in North America. Am Heart J 2003; 145:1–8.
8. Berger PB, Ellis SG, Holmes DR Jr., et al. Relationship between delay in performing direct coronary angioplasty and early clinical outcome in patients with acute myocardial infarction: results from the global use of strategies to open occluded arteries in Acute Coronary Syndromes (GUSTO-IIb) trial. Circulation 1999; 100:14–20.
9. McNamara RL, Wang Y, Herrin J, et al. Effect of door-to-balloon time on mortality in patients with ST-segment elevation myocardial infarction. J Am Coll Cardiol 2006; 47:2180–2186.
10. Keeley EC, Boura JA, Grines CL. Primary angioplasty versus intravenous thrombolytic therapy for acute myocardial infarction: a quantitative review of 23 randomised trials. Lancet 2003; 361:13–20.
11. Andersen HR, Nielsen TT, Rasmussen K, et al. A comparison of coronary angioplasty with fibrinolytic therapy in acute myocardial infarction. N Engl J Med 2003; 349:733–742.
12. Thune JJ, Hoefsten DE, Lindholm MG, et al. Simple risk stratification at admission to identify patients with reduced mortality from primary angioplasty. Circulation 2005; 112:2017–2021.
13. Nallamothu BK, Bates ER. Percutaneous coronary intervention versus fibrinolytic therapy in acute myocardial infarction: is timing (almost) everything? Am J Cardiol 2003; 92:824–826.
14. Betriu A, Masotti M. Comparison of mortality rates in acute myocardial infarction treated by percutaneous coronary intervention versus fibrinolysis. Am J Cardiol 2005; 95:100–101.
15. Boersma E. Does time matter? A pooled analysis of randomized clinical trials comparing primary percutaneous coronary intervention and in-hospital fibrinolysis in acute myocardial infarction patients. Eur Heart J 2006; 27:779–788.
16. Tarantini G, Razzolini R, Ramondo A, et al. Explanation for the survival benefit of primary angioplasty over thrombolytic therapy in patients with ST-elevation acute myocardial infarction. Am J Cardiol 2005; 96:1503–1505.
17. Antman EM, Anbe DT, Armstrong PW, et al. ACC/AHA guidelines for the management of patients with ST-elevation myocardial infarction; A report of the American College of Cardiology/American Heart Association Task Force on Practice Guidelines (Committee to Revise the 1999 Guidelines for the Management of patients with acute myocardial infarction). J Am Coll Cardiol 2004; 44:e1–e211.
18. Bogaty P, Buller CE, Dorian P, et al. Applying the new STEMI guidelines: 1. Reperfusion in acute ST-segment elevation myocardial infarction. CMAJ 2004; 171:1039–1041.
19. Weaver WD, Cerqueira M, Hallstrom AP, et al. Prehospital-initiated vs hospital-initiated thrombolytic therapy. The Myocardial Infarction Triage and Intervention Trial. JAMA 1993; 270:1211–1216.

20. Widimsky P, Budesinsky T, Vorac D, et al. Long distance transport for primary angioplasty vs immediate thrombolysis in acute myocardial infarction. Final results of the randomized national multicentre trial–PRAGUE-2. Eur Heart J 2003; 24:94–104.
21. Bonnefoy E, Lapostolle F, Leizorovicz A, et al. Primary angioplasty versus prehospital fibrinolysis in acute myocardial infarction: a randomised study. Lancet 2002; 360:825–829.
22. Steg PG, Bonnefoy E, Chabaud S. Impact of time to treatment on mortality after prehospital fibrinolysis or primary angioplasty: data from the CAPTIM randomized clinical trial. Circulation 2003; 108:2851–2856.
23. Henriques JP, Zijlstra F, van 't Hof AW, et al. Primary percutaneous coronary intervention versus thrombolytic treatment: long term follow up according to infarct location. Heart 2006; 92:75–79.
24. Angeja BG, Alexander JH, Chin R, et al. Safety of the weight-adjusted dosing regimen of tenecteplase in the ASSENT-Trial. Am J Cardiol 2001; 88:1240–1245.
25. Armstrong PW, Chang WC, Wallentin L, et al. Efficacy and safety of unfractionated heparin versus enoxaparin: a pooled analysis of ASSENT-3 and -3 PLUS data. CMAJ 2006; 174:1421–1426.
26. Sinnaeve PR, Huang Y, Bogaerts K, et al. Age, outcomes, and treatment effects of fibrinolytic and antithrombotic combinations: findings from Assessment of the Safety and Efficacy of a New Thrombolytic (ASSENT)-3 and ASSENT-3 PLUS. Am Heart J 2006; 152:684–689.
27. Van de WF, Barron HV, Armstrong PW, et al. Incidence and predictors of bleeding events after fibrinolytic therapy with fibrin-specific agents: a comparison of TNK-tPA and rt-PA. Eur Heart J 2001; 22:2253–2261.
28. Danchin N, Blanchard D, Steg PG, et al. Impact of prehospital thrombolysis for acute myocardial infarction on 1-year outcome: results from the French Nationwide USIC 2000 Registry. Circulation 2004; 110:1909–1915.
29. Nallamothu BK, Bates ER, Herrin J, et al. Times to treatment in transfer patients undergoing primary percutaneous coronary intervention in the United States: National Registry of Myocardial Infarction (NRMI)-3/4 analysis. Circulation 2005; 111:761–767.
30. Pinto DS, Kirtane AJ, Nallamothu BK, et al. Hospital delays in reperfusion for ST-elevation myocardial infarction: implications when selecting a reperfusion strategy. Circulation 2006; 114:2019–2025.
31. Bradley EH, Roumanis SA, Radford MJ, et al. Achieving door-to-balloon times that meet quality guidelines: how do successful hospitals do it? J Am Coll Cardiol 2005; 46:1236–1241.
32. Bradley EH, Herrin J, Wang Y, et al. Strategies for reducing the door-to-balloon time in acute myocardial infarction. N Engl J Med 2006; 355:2308–2320.
33. Bradley EH, Herrin J, Wang Y, et al. Door-to-drug and door-to-balloon times: where can we improve? Time to reperfusion therapy in patients with ST-segment elevation myocardial infarction (STEMI). Am Heart J 2006; 151:1281–1287.
34. Bradley EH, Curry LA, Webster TR, et al. Achieving rapid door-to-balloon times: how top hospitals improve complex clinical systems. Circulation 2006; 113:1079–1085.
35. Henriques JP, Haasdijk AP, Zijlstra F. Outcome of primary angioplasty for acute myocardial infarction during routine duty hours versus during off-hours. J Am Coll Cardiol 2003; 41:2138–2142.
36. De Luca G, Suryapranata H, Ottervanger JP, et al. Circadian variation in myocardial perfusion and mortality in patients with ST-segment elevation myocardial infarction treated by primary angioplasty. Am Heart J 2005; 150:1185–1189.
37. Magid DJ, Wang Y, Herrin J, et al. Relationship between time of day, day of week, timeliness of reperfusion, and in-hospital mortality for patients with acute ST-segment elevation myocardial infarction. JAMA 2005; 294:803–812.
38. Magid DJ, Calonge BN, Rumsfeld JS, et al. Relation between hospital primary angioplasty volume and mortality for patients with acute MI treated with primary angioplasty vs thrombolytic therapy. JAMA 2000; 284:3131–3138.
39. Malenka DJ, McGrath PD, Wennberg DE, et al. The relationship between operator volume and outcomes after percutaneous coronary interventions in high volume

hospitals in 1994–1996: the northern New England experience. Northern New England Cardiovascular Disease Study Group. J Am Coll Cardiol 1999; 34:1471–1480.

40. McGrath PD, Wennberg DE, Malenka DJ, et al. Operator volume and outcomes in 12,998 percutaneous coronary interventions. Northern New England Cardiovascular Disease Study Group. J Am Coll Cardiol 1998; 31:570–576.

41. McGrath PD, Wennberg DE, Dickens JD Jr., et al. Relation between operator and hospital volume and outcomes following percutaneous coronary interventions in the era of the coronary stent. JAMA 2000; 284:3139–3144.

42. Moscucci M, Share D, Smith D, et al. Relationship between operator volume and adverse outcome in contemporary percutaneous coronary intervention practice: an analysis of a quality-controlled multicenter percutaneous coronary intervention clinical database. J Am Coll Cardiol 2005; 46:625–632.

43. An international randomized trial comparing four thrombolytic strategies for acute myocardial infarction. The GUSTO investigators. N Engl J Med 1993; 329:673–682.

44. A comparison of reteplase with alteplase for acute myocardial infarction. The Global Use of Strategies to Open Occluded Coronary Arteries (GUSTO III) Investigators. N Engl J Med 1997; 337:1118–1123.

45. Van de WF, Adgey J, Ardissino D, et al. Single-bolus tenecteplase compared with front-loaded alteplase in acute myocardial infarction: the ASSENT-2 double-blind randomised trial. Lancet 1999; 354:716–722.

46. Theroux P, Welsh RC. Meta-analysis of randomized trials comparing enoxaparin versus unfractionated heparin as adjunctive therapy to fibrinolysis in ST-elevation acute myocardial infarction. Am J Cardiol 2003; 91:860–864.

47. Antman EM, Morrow DA, McCabe CH, et al. Enoxaparin versus unfractionated heparin with fibrinolysis for ST-elevation myocardial infarction. N Engl J Med 2006; 354: 1477–1488.

48. Yusuf S, Mehta SR, Chrolavicius S, et al. Effects of fondaparinux on mortality and reinfarction in patients with acute ST-segment elevation myocardial infarction: the OASIS-6 randomized trial. JAMA 2006; 295:1519–1530.

49. Randomised trial of intravenous streptokinase, oral aspirin, both, or neither among 17,187 cases of suspected acute myocardial infarction: ISIS-2. ISIS-2 (Second International Study of Infarct Survival) Collaborative Group. Lancet 1988; 2:349–360.

50. De Luca G, Suryapranata H, Stone GW, et al. Abciximab as adjunctive therapy to reperfusion in acute ST-segment elevation myocardial infarction: a meta-analysis of randomized trials. JAMA 2005; 293:1759–1765.

51. Chen ZM, Jiang LX, Chen YP, et al. Addition of clopidogrel to aspirin in 45,852 patients with acute myocardial infarction: randomised placebo-controlled trial. Lancet 2005; 366: 1607–1621.

52. Sabatine MS, Cannon CP, Gibson CM, et al. Addition of clopidogrel to aspirin and fibrinolytic therapy for myocardial infarction with ST-segment elevation. N Engl J Med 2005; 352:1179–1189.

53. Sabatine MS, Morrow DA, Montalescot G, et al. Angiographic and clinical outcomes in patients receiving low-molecular-weight heparin versus unfractionated heparin in ST-elevation myocardial infarction treated with fibrinolytics in the CLARITY-TIMI 28 Trial. Circulation 2005; 112:3846–3854.

54. Primary versus tenecteplase-facilitated percutaneous coronary intervention in patients with ST-segment elevation acute myocardial infarction (ASSENT-4 PCI): randomised trial. Lancet 2006; 367:569–578.

55. Collet JP, Montalescot G, Le May M, et al. Percutaneous coronary intervention after fibrinolysis: a multiple meta-analyses approach according to the type of strategy. J Am Coll Cardiol 2006; 48:1326–1335.

56. Ellis SG, Armstrong P, Betriu A, et al. Facilitated percutaneous coronary intervention versus primary percutaneous coronary intervention: design and rationale of the Facilitated Intervention with Enhanced Reperfusion Speed to Stop Events (FINESSE) trial. Am Heart J 2004; 147:E16.

57. Gershlick AH, Stephens-Lloyd A, Hughes S, et al. Rescue angioplasty after failed thrombolytic therapy for acute myocardial infarction. N Engl J Med 2005; 353:2758–2768.

58. Fernandez-Aviles F, Alonso JJ, Castro-Beiras A, et al. Routine invasive strategy within 24 hours of thrombolysis versus ischaemia-guided conservative approach for acute myocardial infarction with ST-segment elevation (GRACIA-1): a randomised controlled trial. Lancet 2004; 364:1045–1053.
59. Armstrong PW. A comparison of pharmacologic therapy with/without timely coronary intervention vs. primary percutaneous intervention early after ST-elevation myocardial infarction: the WEST (Which Early ST-elevation myocardial infarction Therapy) study. Eur Heart J 2006; 27:1530–1538.
60. Buller CE, Welsh RC, Westerhout CM, Webb JG, O'Neill B, Gallo R, Armstrong PW. Guideline adjudicated fibrinolytic failure: incidence, findings, and management in a contemporary clinical trial. Am Heart J. 2008; 155:121–127.
61. Hirvonen TP, Halinen MO, Kala RA, et al. Delays in thrombolytic therapy for acute myocardial infarction in Finland. Results of a national thrombolytic therapy delay study. Finnish Hospitals' Thrombolysis Survey Group. Eur Heart J 1998; 19:885–892.
62. Lambrew CT, Bowlby LJ, Rogers WJ, et al. Factors influencing the time to thrombolysis in acute myocardial infarction. Time to Thrombolysis Substudy of the National Registry of Myocardial Infarction-1. Arch Intern Med 1997; 157:2577–2582.
63. Morrison LJ, Verbeek PR, McDonald AC, et al. Mortality and prehospital thrombolysis for acute myocardial infarction: a meta-analysis. JAMA 2000; 283:2686–2692.
64. Goldberg RJ, Steg PG, Sadiq I, et al. Extent of, and factors associated with, delay to hospital presentation in patients with acute coronary disease (the GRACE registry). Am J Cardiol 2002; 89:791–796.
65. Wallentin L, Goldstein P, Armstrong PW, et al. Efficacy and safety of tenecteplase in combination with the low-molecular-weight heparin enoxaparin or unfractionated heparin in the prehospital setting: the Assessment of the Safety and Efficacy of a New Thrombolytic Regimen (ASSENT)-3 PLUS randomized trial in acute myocardial infarction. Circulation 2003; 108:135–142.
66. Welsh RC, Ornato J, Armstrong PW. Prehospital management of acute ST-elevation myocardial infarction: a time for reappraisal in North America. Am Heart J 2003; 145:1–8.
67. Welsh RC, Goldstein P, Adgey J, et al. Variations in pre-hospital fibrinolysis process of care: insights from the Assessment of the Safety and Efficacy of a New Thrombolytic 3 Plus international acute myocardial infarction pre-hospital care survey. Eur J Emerg Med 2004; 11:134–140.
68. Welsh RC, Chang W, Goldstein P, et al. Time to treatment and the impact of a physician on prehospital management of acute ST elevation myocardial infarction: insights from the ASSENT-3 PLUS trial. Heart 2005; 91:1400–1406.
69. Rosenberg DG, Levin E, Lausell A, et al. Feasibility and timing of prehospital administration of reteplase in patients with acute myocardial infarction. J Thromb Thrombolysis 2002; 13:147–153.
70. Morrow DA, Antman EM, Sayah A, et al. Evaluation of the time saved by prehospital initiation of reteplase for ST-elevation myocardial infarction: results of The Early Retavase-Thrombolysis in Myocardial Infarction (ER-TIMI) 19 trial. J Am Coll Cardiol 2002; 40:71–77.
71. Henry TD, Unger BT, Sharkey SW, et al. Design of a standardized system for transfer of patients with ST-elevation myocardial infarction for percutaneous coronary intervention. Am Heart J 2005; 150:373–384.
72. Menssen K, Henry T, Unger B, et al. Use of emergency medical services by patients with ST-elevation myocardial infarction in a regional network. Acad Emerg Med 2007; 14(5 suppl 1):S23.
73. Vaillancourt C, Stiell IG. Cardiac arrest care and emergency medical services in Canada. Can J Cardiol 2004; 20:1081–1090.
74. Tiefenbrunn AJ, Chandra NC, French WJ, et al. Clinical experience with primary percutaneous transluminal coronary angioplasty compared with alteplase (recombinant tissue-type plasminogen activator) in patients with acute myocardial infarction: a report from the Second National Registry of Myocardial Infarction (NRMI-2). J Am Coll Cardiol 1998; 31:1240–1245.

7 Primary Percutaneous Coronary Intervention

Nestor Mercado
Division of Cardiovascular Diseases, Scripps Clinic, La Jolla, California, U.S.A.

Simon R. Dixon
Division of Cardiology, William Beaumont Hospital, Royal Oak, Michigan, U.S.A.

William W. O'Neill
Division of Cardiology, Department of Internal Medicine, University of Miami, Miller School of Medicine, Miami, Florida, U.S.A.

INTRODUCTION

Primary percutaneous coronary intervention (PCI) for ST-segment elevation myocardial infarction (STEMI) is defined as a strategy of emergent angiography followed by mechanical revascularization of the infarct-related artery (IRA) with a balloon catheter (with or without the subsequent placement of a coronary stent), without prior administration of fibrinolytic therapy (FT). This approach has emerged as the preferred reperfusion strategy for STEMI patients when performed by an experienced team in a timely fashion.

In this chapter, we review the key steps in the evolution of primary PCI as well as discuss its clinical impact, provide some practical recommendations regarding the catheterization procedure and pre- and postprocedural patient care, and finally describe the limitations and future directions of primary PCI.

HISTORICAL BACKGROUND

STEMI usually occurs as a result of atherosclerotic plaque rupture of a coronary artery that previously was not severely narrowed (1), creating a potent stimulus for platelet aggregation, thrombus formation, and total arterial occlusion. In the early 1970s, the only method known to normalize myocardial blood supply was coronary artery bypass graft surgery (CABG). Berg and colleagues (2) performed coronary angiography prior to emergency CABG in a small number of patients and reported a 77% incidence of total occlusion of the IRA. These observations were in remarkable agreement with the findings of DeWood et al. (3). In his landmark study, 322 patients with acute myocardial infarction (AMI) underwent coronary angiography. A total coronary occlusion was present in 87% of patients studied within four hours of the onset of symptoms; this proportion decreased to 65%, when patients were evaluated 12 to 24 hours after the onset of symptoms. These two studies provided the first in vivo evidence that most cases of transmural AMI were indeed due to total coronary occlusion. Subsequently, Rentrop et al. (4) demonstrated in a small series of patients that the IRA could be recanalized by the intracoronary infusion of streptokinase. In 1983, Khaja et al. (5) carried out a randomized trial that confirmed the effectiveness of intracoronary FT to restore coronary patency. Reestablishment of coronary flow occurred in 80% of patients treated with streptokinase compared with 10% treated with placebo within six hours of the onset of AMI symptoms. In the same year, Kennedy et al. reported the results of the Western Washington Intracoronary Streptokinase (WWIC) trial (6). This trial randomized patients to receive intracoronary streptokinase versus standard therapy. The remarkable finding of this study was a threefold reduction in 30-day mortality for patients receiving streptokinase (3.7%) compared with the placebo group (11.2%).

THE BEGINNING OF MECHANICAL REPERFUSION

Gruntzig introduced percutaneous transluminal coronary balloon angioplasty (PTCA) in 1977 to treat patients with chronic stable angina (7). At that time, the prototype balloon catheters had a short, stiff wire mounted at the tip of the balloon that was not steerable. These devices were much more prone to cause arterial injury than were later, over-the-wire balloons, and the risk was increased in patients with AMI because there was no angiographic road map for advancing the balloon beyond the site of total occlusion (8). This prompted the initial use of guidewires and non–balloon catheters in patients with AMI. The first case series (9) included 13 patients in which recanalization of a totally occluded artery was attempted. The intervention was performed within 7.8 ± 8.3 hours of the onset of AMI symptoms, and restoration of antegrade flow after pullback of the recanalization device was achieved in 54% of patients.

As technology evolved, device safety also increased and several groups recognized the potential role for angioplasty to mechanically restore flow in the IRA during AMI. In the early 1980s, a number of observational studies confirmed the feasibility of balloon angioplasty in this setting. The first 41 patients reported by Hartzler et al. (10) were treated with PTCA either following intracoronary FT (29 patients with total occlusions) or directly (12 patients with subtotal occlusions) with a clinical success rate of 98% (one death occurred in a patient presenting with cardiogenic shock). Because of the necessity of coronary angiography prior to this treatment, it became apparent that a severe residual stenosis persisted in most patients after successful thrombolysis. The University of Michigan group demonstrated that balloon angioplasty could more effectively relieve the residual stenosis than FT, and this resulted in less recurrent ischemia and greater recovery of ventricular function (11). However, a number of logistic constraints, including lack of trained operators and catheterization facilities, hindered further development and widespread application of this technique in the mid-1980s.

ROUTINE PCI AFTER FIBRINOLYTIC THERAPY

The Gruppo Italiano per lo Studio della Sopravvivenza nell' Infarto Miocardico (GISSI) (12) and International Study of Infarct Survival-2 (ISIS-2) (13) trials, published in the mid-1980s, provided definitive evidence that intravenous FT improved survival in AMI patients. Intravenous streptokinase and aspirin became the standard of care as reperfusion therapy for AMI. However, concern remained regarding the severe residual stenosis seen in most patients after successful FT and the potential increased risk for reoclussion of the IRA. Three randomized clinical trials, the Thrombolysis and Angioplasty in Myocardial Infarction (TAMI-1) (14), the European Cooperative Study Group for Recombinant Tissue-Type Plasminogen Activator (ESCG) (15), and the Thrombolysis in Myocardial Infarction (TIMI)-2A (16), were performed in the late 1980s to determine the potential role of routine PCI in decreasing the incidence of reoclusion or reinfarction, or improving ventricular function after FT. The results of these studies were disappointing. PCI appeared to be harmful with higher transfusion rates, need for emergency CABG, as well as a trend for increased mortality. On the basis of these data, the strategy of routine PCI after FT was abandoned in the early 1990s. However, a number of important limitations with these studies preclude extrapolation of these data to the current era of mechanical reperfusion. Most notably, the lack of preprocedural treatment with aspirin or adequate doses of unfractionated heparin in some of these studies increased risk of abrupt vessel closure. There was also a failure to systematically monitor activated clotting time (ACTs), and in some cases the treatment of non-signifcant coronary lesions was allowed.

PRIMARY PCI WITH BALLOON

The results of the TAMI-1 (14), ESCG (15), and TIMI-2A(16) trials suggested that PCI after FT was harmful. A few years later, the Global Utilization of Streptokinase and Tissue Plasminogen Activator for Occluded Coronary Arteries (GUSTO-I) trial (17) and its angiographic substudy (18) demonstrated that new and aggressive FT strategies were associated with more complete angiographic reperfusion and improved clinical outcomes compared with standard FT regimens in AMI patients. As a result, the paths of mechanical and pharmacological reperfusion started to diverge and were viewed as competing, rather than complementary, strategies. However, interest still persisted in the use of PCI without antecedent FT (primary PCI), and large credit should be given to Hartzler and colleagues (19), who reported a series of primary PCI in 500 consecutive AMI patients with high success rates in reestablishing IRA patency and salvaging ischemic myocardium, resulting in low in-hospital and long-term mortality. At the same time, Brodie et al. (20) and O'Neill et al. (21) concluded that primary PCI had been inadequately tested as a reperfusion strategy. This prompted the development of randomized controlled trials to define the clinical efficacy and safety of primary PCI compared with FT.

In 1993, the Primary Angioplasty in Myocardial Infarction (PAMI) study group (22), the Zwolle group (23), and the Mayo Clinic (24) published the results of the first three large randomized trials comparing primary PCI with FT. Although there was marked heterogeneity between these trials in terms of study design and fibrinolytic agent used, these studies demonstrated the benefit of primary PCI over FT and established primary PCI as a legitimate and competing reperfusion strategy for AMI. Despite these early encouraging results, controversy persisted regarding the relative benefits of primary PCI versus FT for AMI. Primary PCI was regarded as reasonable alternative to FT but was not widely used due to logistical problems and limited data to support its clinical benefit.

RANDOMIZED CLINICAL TRIALS OF PRIMARY PCI
WITH BALLOON COMPARED WITH FIBRINOLYTIC THERAPY

In the early 1990s, 10 randomized trials of primary PCI with balloon compared with FT were performed (22–31). The largest of these were the PAMI-1 (22), Zwolle (23), and GUSTO-IIb (28) trials.

The PAMI-1 trial (22) randomized 395 patients to primary PCI with balloon or tissue plasminogen activator (t-PA) within 12 hours of the onset of AMI symptoms. Compared with the t-PA group, patients assigned to primary PCI with balloon had a significantly lower incidence of in-hospital death or nonfatal reinfarction (5.1% vs. 12%; $p = 0.02$), less recurrent ischemia (10.3% vs. 28%; $p < 0.001$), and a lower risk of intracranial hemorrhage (0% vs. 2%; $p = 0.05$). Similar early results were also seen in the larger GUSTO-IIb trial (28), which randomized 1138 patients to primary PCI with balloon or accelerated t-PA. In this study, primary PCI with balloon was associated with a 33% reduction in the primary end point of death, reinfarction, or disabling stroke at 30 days (9.6% vs. 13.7%; $p = 0.03$). However, the late results were less impressive, and in contrast to the PAMI-1 and Zwolle trials no clear clinical advantage was seen with primary PCI with balloon at six months. These discordant results may have been related to the fact that primary PCI with balloon was performed less often in patients randomized to the procedure in GUSTO-IIb than PAMI-1 and was also associated with a lower rate of final TIMI-3 flow in the IRA.

Although most of these trials demonstrated a clinical advantage with primary PCI with balloon, none were large enough to detect a difference in mortality rates between these reperfusion strategies. In 1997, Weaver et al. performed a quantitative analysis of 10 randomized trials comparing primary PCI with balloon with FT (32). Primary PCI with balloon was associated with a lower 30-day mortality rate (4.4% vs. 6.5%; $p = 0.02$), lower incidence of reinfarction (2.9% vs. 5.3%; $p = 0.002$), and lower incidence of death or reinfarction (7.2% vs. 11.9%; $p = 0.001$). Primary PCI with balloon was also associated with a significant reduction in the risk of stroke (0.7% vs. 2%; $p = 0.02$) and hemorrhagic stroke (0.1% vs. 1.1%; $p < 0.001$). Moreover, the initial results of improved clinical outcomes with primary PCI with balloon were maintained at two- (33) and five-year follow-up (34).

MECHANISM OF CLINICAL BENEFIT OF PRIMARY PCI

Several mechanisms appear to contribute to the clinical superiority of primary PCI over FT. Probably the most important of these factors is that significantly higher TIMI-3 flow rates can be achieved with primary PCI compared with FT. In most of the primary PCI trials, normal epicardial flow was achieved in >90% of patients, whereas only 29% to 54% of patients achieve TIMI-3 flow with FT. Data from the GUSTO-I angiographic substudy clearly established the importance of restoring normal antegrade flow in the IRA after reperfusion (18). Patients with TIMI-3 grade flow 90 minutes after FT had significantly better left ventricular function and survival at follow-up, compared with patients with incomplete reperfusion (<TIMI-3 flow). In addition, patients with TIMI-2 grade flow had a prognosis similar to patients with TIMI-0 to TIMI-1 flow. These data indicate that only TIMI-3 flow should be regarded as a satisfactory angiographic end point after reperfusion therapy. The importance of achieving TIMI-3 flow after reperfusion is further highlighted by the fact that there appears to be an inverse relationship between the rate of TIMI-3 flow after primary PCI or FT and 30-day survival (Fig. 1). Although newer pharmacological regimens have achieved higher rates of TIMI-3 flow at 90 minutes compared with FT alone, these rates are still lower than those achieved with primary PCI (35).

Unlike FT, primary PCI creates a widely patent lumen, so that most patients have no significant residual stenosis at the site of IRA occlusion. This reduction in residual stenosis accounts for the lower incidence of recurrent ischemia and IRA reocclusion observed after primary PCI compared with FT. Two studies have demonstrated that 25% to 30% of patients with an initially patent IRA after FT have reocclusion at follow-up catheterization (36–38). In contrast, only 9% to 16% of patients have reocclusion of the IRA after primary PCI, and this rate has been

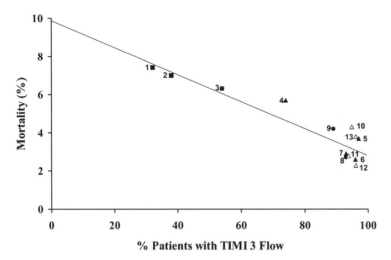

FIGURE 1 Relationship between in-hospital or 30-day death and rate of TIMI-3 flow in IRA after FT or primary PCI for AMI. *Source*: From Ref. 147.

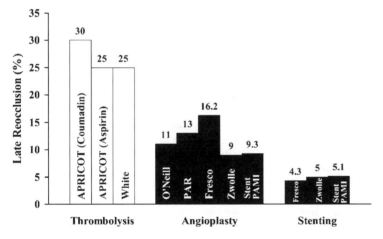

FIGURE 2 Late reocclusion of IRA after FT or primary PCI with balloon or stenting for AMI. *Source*: From Ref. 147.

reduced to about 5% with the advent of coronary stents (Fig. 2) (21,39,40). Several studies have confirmed the importance of IRA patency after AMI for both recovery of left ventricular function and long-term survival (41,42).

PRIMARY PCI WITH BARE METAL STENTS

The main factors limiting the clinical efficacy of primary PCI with balloon are restenosis and reocclusion of the IRA. Data from the PAMI-2 trial demonstrated that a suboptimal angiographic result after balloon angioplasty (residual stenosis >30% or coronary artery dissection) was associated with adverse clinical outcomes (43). Because coronary stents can effectively seal dissection planes and achieve a larger postprocedural lumen diameter than PCI with balloon alone, adjunctive stenting emerged as a promising means of improving early and late outcomes after mechanical reperfusion. However, stenting was initially avoided in AMI because of concern about the risk of stent thrombosis (ST), and it was not until the importance of optimal stent deployment and effective platelet inhibition was recognized that primary PCI with bare metal stents (BMS) became feasible. Initial pilot studies confirmed the safety of stenting in AMI and paved the way for prospective randomized clinical trials (44–47).

RANDOMIZED CLINICAL TRIALS OF PRIMARY PCI WITH BARE METAL STENT COMPARED WITH BALLOON ANGIOPLASTY

Eleven randomized clinical trials of primary PCI with BMS compared with balloon angioplasty in AMI were reported between 1998 and 2002 (48–58). It is important to recognize that these trials differ markedly with respect to sample size, stent design, crossover rates, and use of adjunctive GP IIb/IIIa inhibitors. The results of nine of these trials were summarized in two meta-analyses (59,60). In the first systematic overview (59), primary PCI with BMS was not associated with a lower 6- to 12-month mortality rate (3.7% vs. 3.6%; $p = 0.90$) or a lower incidence of reinfarction (2.1% vs. 2.9%; $p = 0.13$). However, primary PCI with BMS was associated with a significant reduction in target vessel revascularization (TVR) (9.2% vs. 18.7%; $p < 0.0001$) and the composite end point of major adverse cardiac events (MACE) (13.3 vs. 22.5; $p < 0.001$) when compared with primary PCI with balloon. Similarly, in the meta-analysis by Nordmann et al. (60), primary PCI with BMS was not associated with a lower mortality rate but was associated with a significant reduction in TVR when compared with primary PCI with balloon at 30 days, six months, and one year. Contrary to the meta-analysis by Zhu et al. (59), this study found a substantial reduction in reinfarction rates in patients treated with primary PCI with BMS, owing to a difference in the inclusion of eligible trials.

The largest of these trials, the stent-PAMI (54) and Controlled Abciximab and Device Investigation to Lower Late Angioplasty Complications (CADILLAC) (58) trials, deserve further consideration. In the stent-PAMI trial (54), 900 patients with infarct arteries suitable for stenting were randomized to primary PCI with balloon or PCI with BMS implantation. Stenting resulted in a larger minimal lumen diameter, less residual stenosis, and fewer dissections than angioplasty alone. At six months, stenting was associated with a lower incidence of the combined end point of death, reinfarction, disabling stroke, or TVR (12.6% vs. 20.1%; $p < 0.01$). This was primarily due to a lower rate of TVR in the stent group (7.7% vs. 17%; $p < 0.001$). Furthermore, primary PCI with BMS was associated with a lower incidence of restenosis compared with primary PCI with balloon alone (20.3% vs. 33.5%; $p < 0.001$). Despite these encouraging data, enthusiasm for routine BMS implantation was tempered by the fact that stenting was associated with a lower rate of final TIMI-3 flow (89% vs. 93%; $p = 0.006$) and a higher 12-month mortality rate than primary PCI with balloon (5.8% vs. 3.1%; $p = 0.07$). Concern was raised that stenting might increase the risk of distal embolization as a result of the bulky stent-delivery system or high-pressure postdilatation. For these reasons, it was recommended that stenting should be reserved for patients with a suboptimal angiographic result or dissection following primary PCI with balloon.

Fortunately, these concerns were alleviated after the results of the larger CADILLAC trial were reported (58). In contrast to previous trials, this was the only study to use a second-generation stent design and include adjunctive therapy with a GP IIb/IIIa inhibitor.

In this trial, 2082 patients with an IRA stenosis of >70% and a reference vessel diameter of 2.5 to 3.75 mm were randomized to one of four treatment arms: primary PCI with BMS (with or without abciximab) or balloon (with or without abciximab). Angiographic exclusion criteria included unprotected left main disease (>60% stenosis), culprit lesion in a saphenous vein or internal mammary graft, presence of a major side branch, or need for multivessel PCI during the acute phase. At six months, there was a significant improvement in event-free survival with stent implantation compared with balloon angioplasty with bailout stenting (primary end point of MACE 10.9% vs. 19.3%; $p = 0.001$). This benefit was primarily due to a reduction in the incidence of TVR. Importantly, stenting was not associated with a reduction in TIMI-3 flow as seen in the stent-PAMI trial, and no difference in late mortality was observed between any of the treatment arms.

On the basis of these results, routine primary PCI with BMS is recommended in patients undergoing mechanical reperfusion for AMI. Primary PCI with balloon alone remains an excellent strategy when either an optimal angiographic result can be achieved or the patient has coronary anatomy that is unfavorable for stent implantation.

OVERVIEW OF RANDOMIZED CLINICAL TRIALS OF PRIMARY PCI WITH BALLOON OR BARE METAL STENT COMPARED WITH FIBRINOLYTIC THERAPY

In 2003, Keeley et al. performed a quantitative analysis of 23 randomized trials comparing primary PCI with balloon or BMS compared with FT for STEMI patients (61). In this overview, primary PCI was associated with a lower short-term mortality (5% vs. 7%; $p = 0.0002$), lower incidence of nonfatal reinfarction (3% vs. 7%; $p < 0.0001$), and lower incidence of stroke (1% vs. 2%; $p = 0.0004$) (Fig. 3). Compared with FT, primary PCI showed a 27% reduction in short-term mortality, an estimated survival benefit of 21 lives saved per 1000 patients treated. The reduction in risk was less pronounced in fibrin-specific lytic trials (20% risk reduction) than in streptokinase trials (47% risk reduction), with statistical evidence of heterogeneity between these two groups of trials. Primary PCI was also associated with a dramatically lower incidence of intracranial hemorrhage than FT (0.05% vs. 1.1%; $p < 0.0001$), but the overall risk of major bleeding (mostly access site bleeding) was higher with PCI (7% vs. 5%; $p = 0.032$). A lower risk of bleeding was noted in the 13 most recent trials, attributable to lower doses of intravenous heparin, smaller sheath sizes, and improved operator technique. The relative treatment effect appeared to be similar across all subgroups of patients.

PRIMARY PCI WITH DIRECT BARE METAL STENTING

Direct stenting refers to stent positioning and deployment without prior balloon dilatation of the stenosis. Potential advantages of direct stenting include decrease in procedural duration, flouroscopic exposure time, and radiographic contrast use (62).

In STEMI patients, primary PCI with direct BMS may also reduce embolization of plaque material, lowering the incidence of the no-reflow phenomenon, thereby increasing myocardial perfusion and salvage. At least four observational studies carried out in the late 1990s support the concept that direct stenting is both feasible and safe with success rates between 80% and 100% with appropriate case selection (no major calcification, no significant angulation proximal to the lesion,

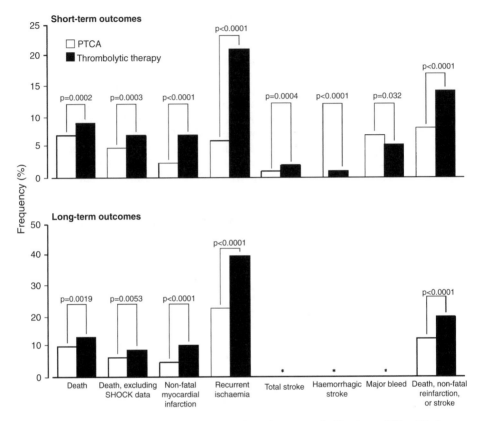

FIGURE 3 Short and long-term clinical outcomes in patients treated with primary PCI or FT. *Source*: From Ref. 61.

vessel size >2.5–3.0 mm, and lesion length <25 mm) (63–66). The proportion of STEMI patients included in these studies ranged from 6.5% (63) to 37.5% (66). The efficacy of primary PCI with direct BMS in STEMI patients was evaluated by Loubeyre and colleagues (67). In this study, 206 patients with infarct arteries suitable for direct stenting were randomized to direct stent implantation or stent implantation after balloon predilatation. Although the incidence of TIMI-3 flow and the corrected TIMI frame count were the same with both approaches, the incidence of the composite angiographic end point (slow and no-reflow or distal embolization) was significantly lower with direct stenting (11.7% vs. 26.9%; $p = 0.01$), and ST-segment resolution was more frequent with direct stenting as well (79.8% vs. 61.9%; $p = 0.01$). There were no significant differences in terms of in-hospital clinical outcomes between the two treatment strategies.

PRIMARY PCI WITH DRUG-ELUTING STENTS

Drug-eluting stents (DES), both sirolimus-eluting stent (SES) (68) and paclitaxel-eluting stent (PES) (69), have been proven to be very effective in reducing the rates of restenosis and TVR after elective PCI compared with BMS, but their role in treating STEMI patients undergoing primary PCI is less clear.

The first case-control study that evaluated the clinical efficacy of SES in STEMI patients was published in 2004 (70). Primary PCI with SES was performed in 186 STEMI patients who were compared with 183 patients treated with BMS as part of the Rapamycin-Eluting Stent Evaluated At Rotterdam Cardiology Hospital (RESEARCH) registry. At 10 months of follow-up, primary PCI with SES was not associated with a reduction in mortality (8.3% vs. 8.2%; $p = 0.8$) or the composite end point of mortality and nonfatal reinfarction (8.8% vs. 10.4%; $p = 0.5$). However, primary PCI with SES was associated with a significant reduction in TVR (1.1% vs. 8.2%; $p < 0.01$). Furthermore, the risk of subacute ST (24 hours to 30 days after stent implantation) did not appear higher compared with BMS (0% vs. 1.6%; $p = 0.1$). Despite this encouraging data, there was still concern that the incidence of ST with DES could be higher in the setting of STEMI. Moreover, the benefits of DES may not be as great as with elective PCI, since the incidence of TVR is relatively low with the use of BMS in patients with STEMI (7.7% in the BMS group of stent-PAMI and 5.2% in the BMS plus abciximab group of CADILLAC). This prompted the design of several trials comparing DES with BMS in STEMI.

RANDOMIZED CLINICAL TRIALS OF PRIMARY PCI WITH DRUG-ELUTING STENT COMPARED WITH BARE METAL STENT

In 2006, two randomized trials found conflicting results with the use of DES versus BMS in STEMI patients. The Trial to Assess the Use of Cypher Stent in Acute Myocardial Infarction Treated with Balloon Angioplasty (TYPHOON) trial randomized 712 STEMI patients to primary PCI with SES or any commercially available BMS (71). The primary end point, a composite of target vessel–related death, reinfarction, or TVR at one year, was significantly lower in SES group than in the BMS group (7.3% vs. 14.3%; $p = 0.004$). This reduction was driven by a decrease in the rate of TVR (5.6% vs. 13.4%; $p < 0.001$). There were no differences between the two groups in the rate of death (2.3% vs. 2.2%; $p = 1.00$), reinfarction (1.1% vs. 1.4%; $p = 1.00$), or ST (3.4% vs. 3.6%; $p = 1.00$).

The Paclitaxel-Eluting Stent versus Conventional Stent in Myocardial Infarction with ST-Segment Elevation (PASSION) trial randomized 619 STEMI patients to primary PCI with PES or BMS (either Express 2 or Liberte) (72). The primary end point was a composite of death from cardiac causes, reinfarction, or target-lesion revascularization at one year. A statistically nonsignificant trend in favor of PES as compared with BMS was observed for the primary end point (8.8% vs. 12.8%; $p = 0.09$) and each of the components of the primary end point, including death from cardiac causes (3.9% vs. 6.2%; $p = 0.20$), reinfarction (1.7% vs. 2.0%; $p = 0.74$), and target-lesion revascularization (5.3% vs. 7.8%; $p = 0.23$). There were no differences between the two groups in the rate of ST (1% vs. 1%; $p = 0.99$). A number of explanations can account for the differences in TVR between TYPHOON and PASSION. The TVR rates for both DES were very similar (5.6% for SES and 5.3% for PES), and the main difference was in the TVR rates in the BMS groups (13.4% in TYPHOON vs. 7.8% in PASSION). A subset of 174 patients underwent systematic angiographic follow-up at six months in the TYPHOON trial. This may have potentially triggered additional revascularization procedures. Moreover, in the TYPHOON trial any BMS was allowed, whereas in the PASSION trial only two specific BMS were used. This discrepancy may also explain why the TVR rates were higher in the TYPHOON trial than in the PASSION trial.

The safety of DES has been recently scrutinized. A meta-analysis of all randomized studies showed an increase in total mortality and Q-wave myocardial infarction with SES compared with BMS (6.3% vs. 3.9%; $p = 0.03$). No significant difference was found when PES was compared with BMS (2.3% vs. 2.6%; $p = 0.68$) (73). This analysis was hampered by incomplete data in publications, abstracts, and Internet sources and not considered completely correct from a methodological standpoint. However, it raised significant concern and prompted a patient-level meta-analysis of the four pivotal randomized SES trials (RAVEL, SIRIUS, E-SIRIUS, and C-SIRIUS) (74) and the five pivotal randomized PES trials (TAXUS I, II, IV, V, and VI) (75). This analysis demonstrated an increased rate of ST with both SES (5 events for SES vs. 0 for BMS; $p = 0.025$) and PES (9 events for PES vs. 2 events for BMS; $p = 0.028$) between one and four years of follow-up. The overall incidence of death and Q-wave myocardial infarction did not differ significantly between the groups with SES and BMS (8.2% vs. 6.3%; $p = 0.12$), and PES and BMS (7.5% vs. 7.3%; $p = 0.95$).

It is important to note that at the present time, DES for STEMI patients is still considered an off-label indication, and as such STEMI patients undergoing primary PCI with DES are at an increased risk for DES thrombosis, as recently suggested by data from a large two-institutional cohort study. In this analysis, 8146 consecutive patients underwent DES implantation. ST occurred in 152 patients; of whom acute and subacute ST developed in 91 patients (60%) and late ST in 61 patients (40%). The risk of ST between 30 days and 3 years was 0.6% per year. More importantly, acute coronary syndrome (ACS) at presentation was associated with a hazard ratio of 2.28 (1.29–4.03) for ST (76).

There are a number of ongoing and planned studies that will help to clarify the safety issues of DES. The HORIZONS-AMI trial is randomizing 3400 patients with AMI to DES versus BMS. The hypothesis tested is that the PES will safely reduce the one-year rate of ischemia-driven TVR. The e-SELECT Registry and INSIGHT randomized trial will be a 30,000 patient global registry incorporating a U.S. randomized trial of standard versus long duration clopidogrel. The PROTECT randomized trial will be an 8000 patient global randomized trial of the Endeavor versus the Cypher stent with a primary end point of ST. The ST study will enroll at least 10,000 consecutive patients receiving DES in whom aspirin and clopidogrel responsiveness will be assessed at baseline and throughout a two- to five-year follow-up for ST.

PRIMARY PCI WHEN FIBRINOLYTIC THERAPY IS CONTRAINDICATED

Observational studies have demonstrated that patients with contraindications to FT have an estimated baseline short-term mortality risk of 15% to 25% (77,78). In such patients, primary PCI appears to improve clinical outcomes in association with substantial salvage of ischemic myocardium (79). Data from the National Registry of Myocardial Infarction (NRMI) 2, 3, and 4 indicate that the mortality benefit of mechanical revascularization also extends to this high-risk group (80). In this propensity analysis, patients who were selected to receive immediate revascularization had a 46% relative reduction in the risk of hospital mortality compared with patients who did not undergo revascularization (10.9% vs. 20.1%; OR 0.48; 95% CI 0.43–0.55). More importantly, the study also provided insight into the alarmingly low utilization of mechanical reperfusion in FT ineligible patients. Of the 19,917 patients in the study, only 4707 (24%) underwent revascularization.

A similar clinical benefit was suggested in a meta-analysis that derived treatment estimates from trials of primary PCI versus FT and FT versus placebo. The absolute reduction in mortality with primary PCI in patients with contraindications to FT was 9.3% (95% CI 5.3–13.2%) (81). Overall, these findings strongly support routine adoption of mechanical reperfusion for FT ineligible patients as well as the need to improve access to centers with invasive facilities.

IMPACT OF TIME TO REPERFUSION

In experimental studies, the relationship between the duration of coronary artery occlusion and extent of myocardial necrosis is unequivocal (82). Accordingly, the primary goal of reperfusion therapy is to restore blood flow in the IRA as early as possible to salvage jeopardized myocardium, limit infarct size, and preserve ventricular function. Data from a number of randomized trials of FT have confirmed this notion (83,84). In aggregate, these studies suggest that the mortality benefit of FT is strongly time dependent, with the greatest response observed in those patients presenting early after symptom onset (85).

In contrast, the relationship between time-to-treatment and clinical outcomes has been the subject of intense debate for patients undergoing primary PCI. This controversy has been fueled, in part, by the discordant results of clinical studies. Some reports have identified an association between time to reperfusion and survival (86–90), while others have found no clear relationship (91–94). Difficulty in interpretation of these data is further compounded by our inability to account for the dynamic nature of coronary occlusion in humans, failure to examine the importance of collateral circulation, differences in study design and analysis, and marked patient heterogeneity depending on time to presentation.

Notwithstanding these limitations, the available data do suggest that efforts should be made to minimize the time to reperfusion during primary PCI, although the impact of presentation and treatment delay is less important than for patients treated with FT, as shown by Boersma and colleagues (95). In this patient-level meta-analysis of 22 studies, 6763 patients were randomized to primary PCI ($n = 3380$) or FT ($n = 3383$). Time to treatment was categorized into presentation delay (time from symptom onset to randomization) as 0–1, >1–2, >2–3, >3–6, and >6 hours. At 30 days, primary PCI was associated with a lower mortality compared with FT (5.3% vs. 7.9%; $p < 0.001$). Primary PCI was also superior to FT irrespective of the presentation delay. Mortality reduction by primary PCI widened from 1.3% in patients randomized in the first hour after symptom onset to 4.2% for those randomized for more than six hours but the absolute mortality rates for primary PCI increased with increasing presentation delay and PCI-related delay (Fig. 4). This effect may be explained, in part, by the findings of a pooled analysis of four recent trials of primary or rescue PCI in which the primary end point was infarct size (96). In this analysis of 1234 patients, a longer duration from symptom onset to first balloon inflation was strongly predictive of a greater infarct size, with both presentation delay and PCI-related delay contributing to a larger infarct size. Infarct size was smaller when reperfusion was accomplished within two hours of symptom onset, intermediate with reperfusion between two and three hours, and larger when first balloon inflation was performed for more than three hours of symptom onset, with little impact of further delays beyond three hours. These data affirm current recommendations for patient transport to tertiary centers after symptom onset as soon as possible,

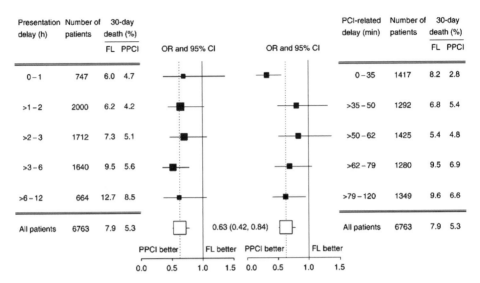

FIGURE 4 OR and 95% CI for 30-day death in patients randomized to primary PCI when compared with FT according to presentation delay (left panel) and PCI-related delay (right panel). *Source*: From Ref. 95.

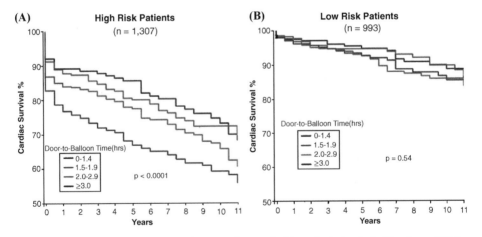

FIGURE 5 Kaplan-Meier estimates of late cardiac survival in patients treated with primary PCI for STEMI according to door-to-balloon times. (**A**) High-risk patients. (**B**) Low-risk patients. *Source*: From Ref. 99.

and to try to minimize door-to-balloon times, with 90 minutes as a suitable benchmark (97). Finally, the impact of time to reperfusion during primary PCI appears to be closely related to the baseline risk profile (Fig. 5) (98,99), most notably for patients with cardiogenic shock or those stratified as "high-risk" (Killip class 3–4, age >70 years, or anterior STEMI).

PRACTICAL CONSIDERATIONS IN PRIMARY PCI: PREPROCEDURAL CARE, CATHETERIZATION PROCEDURE, AND MANAGEMENT OF COMPLICATIONS AND POSTPROCEDURAL CARE

Preprocedural Care

The initial history and physical examination should be abbreviated, focusing on pertinent aspects of the cardiovascular system to avoid treatment delays. Once the diagnosis of STEMI is established in the emergency department, the patient should be transferred as quickly as possible to the cardiac catheterization laboratory. Adequate pain relief and supplemental oxygen are mandatory, as the patient will have to endure angiography and likely PCI.

All patients should receive aspirin (325 mg nonenteric coated for more rapid delivery of the drug) and intravenous heparin [5000–10,000 International Units (IU) or weight adjusted (70 IU/Kg) if a GP IIb/IIIa inhibitor is used] in an attempt to increase initial patency rates of the IRA (100). Intravenous β-blockade should be attempted to lower oxygen consumption and alleviate myocardial ischemia, unless contraindicated (contraindications: HR <60 beats/min, SBP <100 mmHg, moderate or severe left ventricular failure, signs of peripheral hypoperfusion, PR interval >0.24 sec, second- or third-degree atrioventricular (AV) block, severe COPD or history of asthma requiring home oxygen or oral steroids). Intravenous β-blockade may improve myocardial recovery and reduce mortality at 30 days in patients untreated with oral β-blockers before admission (101).

Abciximab as pretreatment and adjuvant therapy can be recommend for most patients (58,102). Clopidogrel is used in almost all patients with an ACS and should be started with a loading dose of at least 300 mg (103). The preoperative use of clopidogrel in patients undergoing CABG has been associated with a significant increased risk of bleeding and blood transfusions (104) but in our experience, only a minority of STEMI patients (<5%) will undergo CABG in the first few days.

Catheterization Procedure

Vascular access is generally performed from the femoral approach, but some centers prefer brachial or radial access. Venous access is generally avoided unless hemodynamic instability or bradycardia necessitates placement of a pulmonary artery catheter or temporary pacemaker. The activated clotting time should be checked after arterial access is achieved, and supplemental heparin titrated to prolong the activated clotting time >300 seconds (or 250 seconds if a GP IIb/IIIa inhibitor is used). A low osmolar ionic contrast agent is preferable to minimize hemodynamic complications and prothrombotic effects associated with other contrast agents (105).

Angiography of the non-IRA is usually undertaken to allow identification of multivessel disease and collateral flow into the infarct zone. We generally defer left ventriculography until after PCI to avoid delays in reperfusion. However, it may be useful to perform left ventriculography before intervention to assess the severity of left ventricular and valvular dysfunction or to help determine the IRA if this uncertain. In rare cases, papillary muscle rupture, ventricular septal defect, or even free wall rupture will be demonstrated when not previously suspected. On the other hand, demonstration of normal left ventricular function may raise concern about a nonischemic diagnosis such as acute pericarditis or aortic dissection.

Primary PCI is usually feasible in >90% of patients with STEMI. Angiographic exclusions to PCI include unprotected left main disease (>60%), IRA stenosis <70% with TIMI-3 flow, IRA that supplies a small area of myocardium (risks outweigh benefits), or an IRA with TIMI-3 flow and lesion morphology that is high risk for no-reflow or other complications. Emergency surgery may be considered for patients with left main disease, severe coronary anatomy unsuitable for percutaneous revascularization, multivessel disease with cardiogenic shock, mechanical complications, or failed angioplasty if there is ongoing myocardial ischemia.

Coronary intervention is generally performed with 6F or 7F guide catheters, although larger catheters may be required if non-balloon or stent devices are considered. The 7F guiding catheter system gives better support and torque control, as well as better visualization, during contrast injection around the balloon and stent delivery systems. Often some flow will be reestablished in the artery once the lesion is crossed with a soft or floppy-tipped 0.014-inch steerable guidewire. The soft tip usually crosses the fresh thrombus and is less traumatic than stiffer wires. The guidewire is then advanced down the IRA to ensure that it is located in the true lumen and not in a small side branch or under an intimal dissection. If the IRA is initially totally occluded, reperfusion will often be achieved after crossing with the guidewire, but it may be preferable to cross the occlusion with a balloon and then withdraw the balloon without inflating it to establish reperfusion. The more gradual reperfusion provided with the wire or balloon may result in less reperfusion arrhythmias than rapidly inflating the balloon immediately after crossing the lesion. After this, it is often possible to have a first impression of the distal vessel, and boluses of intracoronary nitrates are useful in avoiding underestimation of the true arterial size. PCI is performed by use of conventional techniques with an appropriately sized balloon using an approximately 1 or 1.1 to 1 balloon-to-artery ratio, followed by stenting if there is a significant residual stenosis or coronary artery dissection. Optimal angiographic visualization of the lesion and the distal artery in multiple projections are often necessary to assess the result and define the need for further balloon inflations and stenting. The operator should strive for an optimal result with <20% postprocedural residual stenosis, TIMI-3 flow, and evidence of myocardial reperfusion (106).

Usually, only the IRA is treated in the acute setting (107), except in rare circumstances such as cardiogenic shock, because this places additional myocardium at jeopardy if there is a complication. Recently, with the increased safety of PCI with stents and the recognition that there may be rupture of multiple unstable plaques in STEMI patients (108), primary PCI of more than one artery is sometimes performed, but this should be done with sound judgment and only when the risk of recurrent ischemia or infarction from a second ruptured plaque outweighs the risk of a non-IRA PCI.

Management of Complications

With increasing operator experience, improved equipment and patient selection, and the availability of stents, major catheterization laboratory complications with primary PCI have become infrequent. Acute catheterization laboratory complications from the stent-PAMI trial in nonshock patients are shown in Table 1. Laboratory death and emergency CABG for failed PCI are rare. Ventricular tachycardia or fibrillation, asystole and bradycardia (including second- and third-degree AV block), and hypotension are the most common complications and often occur

TABLE 1 Acute Cardiac Catheterization Laboratory Complications With Primary PCI with Balloon and Bare Metal Stents from the Stent-PAMI Trial

Complication	Balloon, $n = 448$ (%)	Stent, $n = 451$ (%)	Combined, $n = 899$ (%)
Laboratory death	0	0.2	0.1
Emergency CABG	0.2	0.2	0.2
Ventricular tachycardia/fibrillation requiring electric cardioversion	4.7	3.1	3.9
Cardiopulmonary resuscitation requiring chest compressions	0.4	0.9	0.7
Endotracheal intubation	0.7	0.2	0.4
Asystole/bradycardia requiring atropine or temporary pacing	8.5	9.3	8.9
Sustained hypotension requiring vasopressors or intra-aortic balloon counterpulsation	8.3	7.8	8.0

immediately after reperfusion. These complications can usually be managed effectively and often prevented with anticipation.

The non-reflow phenomenon (TIMI-0 to TIMI-1 flow) or slow reflow (TIMI-2 flow) may occur transiently or may persist after primary PCI for STEMI in 10% to 25% of patients. This is generally due to microvascular dysfunction from coronary spasm, distal embolization, or endothelial injury and is associated with poorer recovery of left ventricular function and a higher incidence of postprocedural complications (109,110). When slow reflow or non-reflow occurs, TIMI-3 flow usually can be reestablished with the use of intracoronary adenosine (6 mg of adenosine in 100 cc normal saline = 60 μg/cc, 1 cc every 1 minute until 1200–2400 μg have been given), nitroprusside (6.25 mg of nitroprusside in 250 cc D5W = 25 μg/cc, 2 cc up to 200 μg total dose, watch for hypotension), or verapamil (2.5 mg of verapamil in 10 cc normal saline = 250 μg/cc, 100–200 μg boluses, watch for bradycardia) (111) given through the guiding catheter (for slow reflow) or through an infusion catheter or the distal lumen of the balloon catheter (for non-reflow). Repeated boluses of intracoronary adenosine is our preferred approach for managing non-reflow phenomenon in STEMI patients because it can have the additional benefit of limiting infarct size. Heart block is frequent but resolves in seconds. The no-reflow phenomenon may sometimes be prevented by early administration of GP IIb/IIIa inhibitors or by preadministration of adenosine or verapamil (112). Intracoronary epinephrine can be used if the no-reflow phenomenon occurs with hypotension (1:10.000 dilution, 1 cc in 10 cc = 10 μg/cc; incremental doses of 1 cc, watch for hypertension and ventricular arrhythmias).

Caution should be used in stenting lesions with no-reflow, because poor run-off may increase the likelihood of ST, and placement of an intra-aortic balloon pump should be considered if the blood pressure low or if multivessel disease is present with severe left ventricular dysfunction.

Postprocedural Care

In regard to vascular access management, early sheath removal is strongly recommended. Vascular sheaths should be removed when the ACT <190 to 170 seconds in order to minimize the risk of vascular complications. Anticoagulation may be resumed after four to six hours from sheath removal for other indications (atrial fibrillation, prosthetic valves, large AMI, poor left ventricular function, residual thrombus). If the GP IIb/IIIa inhibitors are being used, heparin should not be restarted after the procedure. Patients at low risk can be transferred from the catheterization laboratory directly to a step-down unit (rather than the coronary care unit) and targeted for early discharge.

Postprocedure care has been standardized in the stent-PAMI and CADILLAC trials (54,58). Following the interventional procedure, heparin should be held until the ACT is less than 190 to 170 seconds, at which time the sheath should be removed in order to minimize the risk of vascular complications. Minidose heparin may be given subcutaneously while patients are in bed rest for prophylaxis against deep venous thrombosis. Low-risk patients can be transferred from the catheterization laboratory directly to the subacute unit and can be targeted for discharge on day 2 or 3 (day 0 = day of admission) (113). Patients should be treated with clopidogrel 75 mg and aspirin 325 mg for one month after BMS implantation, three months after SES implantation, and six months after PES implantation, and ideally, up to 12 months if they are not at high risk for bleeding (114). β-Blockers, angiotensin-converting enzyme (ACE) inhibitors, and statins should be given according to current standards. Patients who develop symptoms or electro-cardiographic changes of recurrent ischemia or reinfarction should undergo emergency repeat catheterization and intervention when indicated.

COST VS. CLINICAL BENEFIT OF PRIMARY PCI

Critics of primary PCI often voice concerns about cost issues as a major drawback of this reperfusion strategy compared with FT, in particular, the high up-front cost of cardiac catheterization and primary PCI in an era in which healthcare costs are steadily climbing. Contrary to this perception, data from several of the randomized trials comparing primary PCI and FT have shown that primary PCI can be performed with similar or reduced costs (113,115,116). In the Mayo Clinic (115) and PAMI-1 (116) trials, total hospital charges were significantly lower per patient with primary PCI compared with FT. Although primary PCI is initially more expensive because of catheterization charges, this is later offset by a reduction in adverse events such as recurrent ischemia and reinfarction during hospitalization and a reduced length of hospital stay. Another major advantage is that cardiac catheterization also provides important prognostic information for risk stratification and triage of patients at low risk for early hospital discharge. The safety and cost savings of this early discharge strategy were confirmed in the PAMI-2 trial (113).

However, since these earlier trials were performed, primary PCI techniques have evolved considerably, particularly with the introduction of stents and GP IIb/IIIa inhibitors. Data from the stent-PAMI trial suggest that although primary PCI with BMS may increase the cost of the initial procedure, this incremental cost is partially offset by the long-term reduction in need for rehospitalization and repeat TVR with primary PCI with BMS compared with balloon alone (117). The CADILLAC investigators found that primary PCI with BMS and adjunctive GP IIb/IIIa inhibitors increased aggregate costs at one year by about $1200 compared with standard therapy (118). Abciximab was not cost-effective unless non-significant differences in one-year mortality were incorporated into the analysis.

LIMITATIONS OF PRIMARY PCI

Beyond TIMI-3 Flow and the Importance of Microvascular Reperfusion

Although primary PCI restores normal epicardial coronary artery flow in >90% of patients with STEMI, there is evidence that deleterious effects to the myocardium, independent of distal embolization, may occur at the time of reperfusion resulting in suboptimal myocardial perfusion (119). The mechanisms of this reperfusion injury are not well understood but are thought to be related to a complement-dependent inflammatory response, formation of oxygen-free radicals, or ischemia-induced microvascular damage. Studies utilizing sensitive measures of myocardial perfusion, such as ST-segment resolution, angiographic blush scores, contrast echocardiography, and cardiac magnetic resonance imaging, have shown worse clinical outcomes in patients with poor tissue level flow (120–124).

In this context, there is a growing interest to develop and test potential novel adjunctive therapies for primary PCI. Unfortunately, trials evaluating several pharmacological and mechanical approaches designed to enhance myocardial perfusion, reduce reperfusion injury, and improve myocardial salvage have been largely disappointing, but some studies have shown promise.

Adenosine could potentially reduce reperfusion injury by suppressing free-radical formation and by preventing neutrophil activation. The Acute Myocardial Infarction STudy of ADenosine (AMISTAD) 1 trial found a 33% relative reduction in infarct size in STEMI patients treated with adenosine as an adjunct to FT compared with placebo. This benefit was limited to patients with anterior STEMI (15% vs. 45.5%; $p = 0.014$), and the trial was underpowered to evaluate clinical outcomes (125). In the larger AMISTAD 2 trial, adenosine was tested as an adjunct to either primary PCI or FT in anterior STEMI patients. There was a nonsignificant trend toward reduction in infarct size (17% vs. 27%; $p = 0.074$) and clinical events at six months (16% vs. 18%; $p = 0.43$) compared with placebo (126). The greatest clinical benefit of adenosine appeared to be in patients who had early reperfusion therapy (<3 hours of symptom onset) with significant reduction in one- (5.2% vs. 9.2%; $p = 0.014$) and six-month mortality (7.3% vs. 11.2%; $p = 0.033$) (127).

The COMplement inhibition in Myocardial infarction treated with Angio-plasty (COMMA) trial evaluated the effect of pexelizumab, a novel C5 complement inhibitor, in reducing reperfusion injury. Although there was no difference in infarct size between study groups, there was a surprising 90-day mortality benefit in STEMI patients treated with primary PCI and pexelizumab bolus plus infusion compared with placebo (1.8% vs. 5.9%; $p = 0.014$) (128). This finding raised questions regarding the potential mechanisms of this mortality benefit and launched the Assessment of Pexelizumab in Acute Myocardial Infarction (APEX MI) trial, which was designed to evaluate the effect of pexelizumab on survival in patients with STEMI undergoing primary PCI (129). The trial was stopped early due to lower than expected mortality rates at the time of the first interim analysis and the negative results of a parallel phase-3 trial of pexelizumab in CABG patients (Pexelizumab for the Reduction In Myocardial infarction and MOrtality in CABG II) that was released at the same time (130). Notwithstanding the above, 30-day mortality was unaffected by pexelizumab (4.06% vs. 3.92%; $p = 0.78$).

Mechanical approaches to improve myocardial perfusion include systemic hypothermia, hyperoxemic reperfusion, and devices to limit the effects of distal embolization. Experimental studies have demonstrated that mild hypothermia reduces metabolic demand in the risk region and limits infarct size (131,132). Moreover, systemic hypothermia initiated prior to reperfusion may potentially reduce reperfusion injury (133). New cooling systems have been developed using catheters placed in the inferior vena cava via the femoral vein through which cold saline is circulated. These systems can provide rapid cooling and have been evaluated in the hypothermia as an adjunctive therapy to PCI in patients with acute myocardial infarction (COOL-MI) (134) and Intravascular Cooling adjunctivE to Percutaneous Coronary InTervention (ICE-IT) (135) trials. Neither trial met its primary end point (reduction in infarct size), but both trials suggested that hypothermia reduced infarct size in patients with anterior STEMI who are cooled to target temperature prior to reperfusion. Currently, the COOL-MI 2 trial is evaluating the effect of systemic hypothermia in patients with anterior STEMI who are cooled to target temperatures prior to reperfusion.

Hyperoxemic reperfusion, utilizing intracoronary infusion of blood supersaturated with oxygen, also appears to be a promising adjunctive therapy. In experimental models of AMI, administration of hyperbaric oxygen during ischemia or early after reperfusion was associated with a reduction in infarct size (136). This served as the rationale for testing this concept in STEMI patients. A pilot study of hyperoxemic reperfusion employing aqueous oxygen after primary PCI demonstrated that the technique was safe and feasible (137). The Acute Myocardial Infarction with HyperOxemic Therapy (AMI-HOT) trial was designed to determine whether hyperoxemic reperfusion with aqueous oxygen would improve ventricular function or limit infarct size after primary PCI. The trial was negative as there were no differences in the three coprimary end points (ST-segment resolution, infarct size, and change in the regional wall motion score index) or 30-day MACE rate. In post hoc analysis, anterior STEMI patients reperfused less than six hours from symptom onset who were treated with aqueous oxygen had greater improvement in regional wall motion (0.75 vs. 0.54; $p = 0.03$), smaller infarct size (9% vs. 23%; $p = 0.04$), and improved ST-segment resolution compared with normoxemic controls (138). The AMI-HOT 2 trial is currently in progress and will evaluate the efficacy of aqueous oxygen therapy in patients with anterior STEMI reperfused within six hours of symptom onset.

Finally, techniques to limit the effects of distal embolization include the use of thrombectomy devices or distal protection systems. A recent meta-analysis of 14 trials included 2630 STEMI patients treated with primary PCI with or without antiembolic devices (139). There were no differences in surrogate end points (postprocedural myocardial blush grade <3 and ST-segment resolution) or clinical events in patients treated with antiembolic devices prior to PCI compared with standard PCI.

Improving the Availability of Primary PCI

Although the use of mechanical reperfusion has increased over the last decade, most patients with STEMI are admitted to hospitals without facilities or trained personnel to perform primary PCI (140–142). Traditionally, FT has been the preferred first-line reperfusion strategy in these patients, although nearly 50% of patients are subsequently transferred to a PCI facility (142). Given the overwhelming advantages of primary PCI, particularly in high-risk patients, three major strategies including patient transfer for primary PCI (143), primary PCI

TABLE 2 Strategies for Reducing the Door-To-Balloon Time in STEMI Patients

Strategy	Mean reduction in door-to-balloon time (min)
Having ED physician activate the catheterization laboratory	8.2
Having a single call to a central page operator to activate laboratory	13.8
Having the ED department to activate the catheterization laboratory while the patient is en route to the hospital	15.4
Expecting staff to arrive in the catheterization laboratory within 20 min after being paged (vs. > 30 min)	19.3
Having an attending cardiologist always on site	14.6
Having staff in the ED and the catheterization laboratory use real-time data feedback	8.6

Source: From Ref. 146.

without on-site surgery (144), and regionalization of STEMI care (the heart attack center) (145) have evolved to optimize management of patients presenting to noninvasive centers. Of these new approaches, the patient transfer for primary PCI strategy has had the greatest impact on clinical practice patterns.

CONCLUSIONS

Mechanical reperfusion therapy has become the preferred reperfusion strategy for patients with STEMI when it can be performed by skilled operators in a timely fashion. Outcomes have improved with the use of coronary stents, GP IIb/IIIa inhibitors, and with increased experience, and there is a promise that outcomes can become even better with new methods to enhance myocardial reperfusion and reduce reperfusion injury and with new anticoagulants and DES. Recent trends from the NRMI have shown that the frequency of use of primary PCI has increased and has surpassed FT, but primary PCI is still used to treat a minority of patients with STEMI (142). A major challenge for clinicians for the next decade will be to find new ways to reduce door-to-balloon times (Table 2) (146) with the goal of making primary PCI more available to patients with STEMI, especially for high-risk patients presenting at noninterventional hospitals.

REFERENCES

1. Ambrose JA, Tannenbaum MA, Alexopoulos D, et al. Angiographic progression of coronary artery disease and the development of myocardial infarction. J Am Coll Cardiol 1988; 12:56–62.
2. Berg R, Jr., Everhart FJ, Duvoisin G, et al. Operation for acute coronary occlusion. Am Surg 1976; 42:517–521.
3. DeWood MA, Spores J, Notske R, et al. Prevalence of total coronary occlusion during the early hours of transmural myocardial infarction. N Engl J Med 1980; 303:897–902.
4. Rentrop KP, Blanke H, Karsch KR, et al. Acute myocardial infarction: intracoronary application of nitroglycerin and streptokinase. Clin Cardiol 1979; 2:354–363.
5. Khaja F, Walton JA, Jr., Brymer JF, et al. Intracoronary fibrinolytic therapy in acute myocardial infarction. Report of a prospective randomized trial. N Engl J Med 1983; 308:1305–1311.
6. Kennedy JW, Ritchie JL, Davis KB, et al. Western Washington randomized trial of intracoronary streptokinase in acute myocardial infarction. N Engl J Med 1983; 309:1477–1482.

7. Gruntzig A. Transluminal dilatation of coronary-artery stenosis. Lancet 1978; 1:263.
8. Rentrop KP. Development and pathophysiological basis of thrombolytic therapy in acute myocardial infarction: Part II. 1977–1980 The pathogenetic role of thrombus is established by the Goettingen pilot studies of mechanical interventions and intracoronary thrombolysis in acute myocardial infarction. In: Timmis GC, ed. Thrombolytic Therapy. Armonk: Futura Publishing Company, 1999:13–36.
9. Rentrop KP, Blanke H, Karsch KR, et al. Initial experience with transluminal recanalization of the recently occluded infarct-related coronary artery in acute myocardial infarction—comparison with conventionally treated patients. Clin Cardiol 1979; 2:92–105.
10. Hartzler GO, Rutherford BD, McConahay DR, et al. Percutaneous transluminal coronary angioplasty with and without thrombolytic therapy for treatment of acute myocardial infarction. Am Heart J 1983; 106:965–973.
11. O'Neill W, Timmis GC, Bourdillon PD, et al. A prospective randomized clinical trial of intracoronary streptokinase versus coronary angioplasty for acute myocardial infarction. N Engl J Med 1986; 314:812–818.
12. Effectiveness of intravenous thrombolytic treatment in acute myocardial infarction. Gruppo Italiano per lo Studio della Streptochinasi nell'Infarto Miocardico (GISSI). Lancet 1986; 1:397–402.
13. Randomised trial of intravenous streptokinase, oral aspirin, both, or neither among 17,187 cases of suspected acute myocardial infarction: ISIS-2. ISIS-2 (Second International Study of Infarct Survival) Collaborative Group. Lancet 1988; 2:349–360.
14. Topol EJ, Califf RM, George BS, et al. A randomized trial of immediate versus delayed elective angioplasty after intravenous tissue plasminogen activator in acute myocardial infarction. N Engl J Med 1987; 317:581–588.
15. Simoons ML, Arnold AE, Betriu A, et al. Thrombolysis with tissue plasminogen activator in acute myocardial infarction: no additional benefit from immediate percutaneous coronary angioplasty. Lancet 1988; 1:197–203.
16. Immediate vs delayed catheterization and angioplasty following thrombolytic therapy for acute myocardial infarction. TIMI II A results. The TIMI Research Group. JAMA 1988; 260:2849–2858.
17. An international randomized trial comparing four thrombolytic strategies for acute myocardial infarction. The GUSTO investigators. N Engl J Med 1993; 329:673–682.
18. The effects of tissue plasminogen activator, streptokinase, or both on coronary-artery patency, ventricular function, and survival after acute myocardial infarction. The GUSTO Angiographic Investigators. N Engl J Med 1993; 329:1615–1622.
19. O'Keefe JH, Jr., Rutherford BD, McConahay DR, et al. Early and late results of coronary angioplasty without antecedent thrombolytic therapy for acute myocardial infarction. Am J Cardiol 1989; 64:1221–1230.
20. Brodie BR, Weintraub RA, Stuckey TD, et al. Outcomes of direct coronary angioplasty for acute myocardial infarction in candidates and non-candidates for thrombolytic therapy. Am J Cardiol 1991; 67:7–12.
21. O'Neill WW, Weintraub R, Grines CL, et al. A prospective, placebo-controlled, randomized trial of intravenous streptokinase and angioplasty versus lone angioplasty therapy of acute myocardial infarction. Circulation 1992; 86:1710–1717.
22. Grines CL, Browne KF, Marco J, et al. A comparison of immediate angioplasty with thrombolytic therapy for acute myocardial infarction. The Primary Angioplasty in Myocardial Infarction Study Group. N Engl J Med 1993; 328:673–679.
23. Zijlstra F, de Boer MJ, Hoorntje JC, et al. A comparison of immediate coronary angioplasty with intravenous streptokinase in acute myocardial infarction. N Engl J Med 1993; 328:680–684.
24. Gibbons RJ, Holmes DR, Reeder GS, et al. Immediate angioplasty compared with the administration of a thrombolytic agent followed by conservative treatment for myocardial infarction. The Mayo Coronary Care Unit and Catheterization Laboratory Groups. N Engl J Med 1993; 328:685–691.
25. De Wood MA. Direct PTCA vs. intravenous t-PA in acute myocardial infarction: results from a prospective randomized trial. Proceedings from the Thrombolysis and Interventional

Therapy in Acute Myocardial Infarction Symposium VI. Washington D.C.: George Washington University Press; 1990:28–29.

26. Ribeiro EE, Silva LA, Carneiro R, et al. Randomized trial of direct coronary angioplasty versus intravenous streptokinase in acute myocardial infarction. J Am Coll Cardiol 1993; 22:376–380.

27. Grinfeld LB, Berrocal D, Belardi J. Fibrinolytics vs. primary angioplasty in acute myocardial infarction (FAP): a randomized trial in a community hospital in Argentina. J Am Coll Cardiol 1996; 29(suppl A):222A.

28. A clinical trial comparing primary coronary angioplasty with tissue plasminogen activator for acute myocardial infarction. The Global Use of Strategies to Open Occluded Coronary Arteries in Acute Coronary Syndromes (GUSTO IIb) Angioplasty Substudy Investigators. N Engl J Med 1997; 336:1621–1628.

29. Zijlstra F, Beukema WP, van't Hof AW, et al. Randomized comparison of primary coronary angioplasty with thrombolytic therapy in low risk patients with acute myocardial infarction. J Am Coll Cardiol 1997; 29:908–912.

30. Ribichini F, Steffenino G, Dellavalle A, et al. Comparison of thrombolytic therapy and primary coronary angioplasty with liberal stenting for inferior myocardial infarction with precordial ST-segment depression: immediate and long-term results of a randomized study. J Am Coll Cardiol 1998; 32:1687–1694.

31. Garcia E, Elizaga J, Perez-Castellano N, et al. Primary angioplasty versus systemic thrombolysis in anterior myocardial infarction. J Am Coll Cardiol 1999; 33:605–611.

32. Weaver WD, Simes RJ, Betriu A, et al. Comparison of primary coronary angioplasty and intravenous thrombolytic therapy for acute myocardial infarction: a quantitative review. JAMA 1997; 278:2093–2098.

33. Nunn CM, O'Neill WW, Rothbaum D, et al. Long-term outcome after primary angioplasty: report from the primary angioplasty in myocardial infarction (PAMI-I) trial. J Am Coll Cardiol 1999; 33:640–646.

34. Zijlstra F, Hoorntje JC, de Boer MJ, et al. Long-term benefit of primary angioplasty as compared with thrombolytic therapy for acute myocardial infarction. N Engl J Med 1999; 341:1413–1419.

35. Antman EM, Giugliano RP, Gibson CM, et al. Abciximab facilitates the rate and extent of thrombolysis: results of the thrombolysis in myocardial infarction (TIMI) 14 trial. The TIMI 14 Investigators. Circulation 1999; 99:2720–2732.

36. Meijer A, Verheugt FW, Werter CJ, et al. Aspirin versus coumadin in the prevention of reocclusion and recurrent ischemia after successful thrombolysis: a prospective placebo-controlled angiographic study. Results of the APRICOT Study. Circulation 1993; 87:1524–1530.

37. Veen G, de Boer MJ, Zijlstra F, et al. Improvement in three-month angiographic outcome suggested after primary angioplasty for acute myocardial infarction (Zwolle trial) compared with successful thrombolysis (APRICOT trial). Antithrombotics in the Prevention of Reocclusion In COronary Thrombolysis. Am J Cardiol 1999; 84:763–767.

38. White HD, French JK, Hamer AW, et al. Frequent reocclusion of patent infarct-related arteries between 4 weeks and 1 year: effects of antiplatelet therapy. J Am Coll Cardiol 1995; 25:218–223.

39. Brodie BR, Grines CL, Ivanhoe R, et al. Six-month clinical and angiographic follow-up after direct angioplasty for acute myocardial infarction. Final results from the Primary Angioplasty Registry. Circulation 1994; 90:156–162.

40. Nakagawa Y, Iwasaki Y, Kimura T, et al. Serial angiographic follow-up after successful direct angioplasty for acute myocardial infarction. Am J Cardiol 1996; 78:980–984.

41. Brodie BR, Stuckey TD, Kissling G, et al. Importance of infarct-related artery patency for recovery of left ventricular function and late survival after primary angioplasty for acute myocardial infarction. J Am Coll Cardiol 1996; 28:319–325.

42. White HD, Cross DB, Elliott JM, et al. Long-term prognostic importance of patency of the infarct-related coronary artery after thrombolytic therapy for acute myocardial infarction. Circulation 1994; 89:61–67.

43. Stone GW, Marsalese D, Brodie BR, et al. A prospective, randomized evaluation of prophylactic intraaortic balloon counterpulsation in high risk patients with acute

myocardial infarction treated with primary angioplasty. Second Primary Angioplasty in Myocardial Infarction (PAMI-II) Trial Investigators. J Am Coll Cardiol 1997; 29:1459–1467.

44. Ahmad T, Webb JG, Carere RR, et al. Coronary stenting for acute myocardial infarction. Am J Cardiol 1995; 76:77–80.

45. Rodriguez AE, Fernandez M, Santaera O, et al. Coronary stenting in patients undergoing percutaneous transluminal coronary angioplasty during acute myocardial infarction. Am J Cardiol 1996; 77:685–689.

46. Berland G, Block P, DeLoughery T, et al. Clinical one-year outcomes after stenting in acute myocardial infarction. Cathet Cardiovasc Diagn 1997; 40:337–341.

47. Stone GW, Brodie BR, Griffin JJ, et al. Prospective, multicenter study of the safety and feasibility of primary stenting in acute myocardial infarction: in-hospital and 30-day results of the PAMI stent pilot trial. Primary Angioplasty in Myocardial Infarction Stent Pilot Trial Investigators. J Am Coll Cardiol 1998; 31:23–30.

48. Suryapranata H, van't Hof AW, Hoorntje JC, et al. Randomized comparison of coronary stenting with balloon angioplasty in selected patients with acute myocardial infarction. Circulation 1998; 97:2502–2505.

49. Antoniucci D, Santoro GM, Bolognese L, et al. A clinical trial comparing primary stenting of the infarct-related artery with optimal primary angioplasty for acute myocardial infarction: results from the Florence Randomized Elective Stenting in Acute Coronary Occlusions (FRESCO) trial. J Am Coll Cardiol 1998; 31:1234–1239.

50. Rodriguez A, Bernardi V, Fernandez M, et al. In-hospital and late results of coronary stents versus conventional balloon angioplasty in acute myocardial infarction (GRAMI trial). Gianturco-Roubin in Acute Myocardial Infarction. Am J Cardiol 1998; 81:1286–1291.

51. Jacksch R, Niehues R, Knobloch W, et al. PTCA versus stenting in acute myocardial infarction (AMI). Circulation 1998; 98(suppl I):I–307 (abstr).

52. Saito S, Hosokawa G, Tanaka S, et al. Primary stent implantation is superior to balloon angioplasty in acute myocardial infarction: final results of the primary angioplasty versus stent implantation in acute myocardial infarction (PASTA) trial. PASTA Trial Investigators. Catheter Cardiovasc Interv 1999; 48:262–268.

53. Kawashima A, Ueda K, Nishida Y, et al. Quantitative angiographic analysis of restenosis of primary stenting using wiktor stent for acute myocardial infarction: results from a multicenter randomized PRISAM study. Circulation 1999; 100(suppl 1):1–856 (abstr).

54. Grines CL, Cox DA, Stone GW, et al. Coronary angioplasty with or without stent implantation for acute myocardial infarction. Stent Primary Angioplasty in Myocardial Infarction Study Group. N Engl J Med 1999; 341:1949–1956.

55. Maillard L, Hamon M, Khalife K, et al. A comparison of systematic stenting and conventional balloon angioplasty during primary percutaneous transluminal coronary angioplasty for acute myocardial infarction. STENTIM-2 Investigators. J Am Coll Cardiol 2000; 35:1729–1736.

56. Schwimmbeck PL, Spencker S, Hohmann C, et al. Results from the Berlin Stent Study in Acute Myocardial Infarction. Circulation 2000; 102(suppl II):II–813 (abstr).

57. Scheller B, Hennen B, Severin-Kneib S, et al. Long-term follow-up of a randomized study of primary stenting versus angioplasty in acute myocardial infarction. Am J Med 2001; 110:1–6.

58. Stone GW, Grines CL, Cox DA, et al. Comparison of angioplasty with stenting, with or without abciximab, in acute myocardial infarction. N Engl J Med 2002; 346:957–966.

59. Zhu MM, Feit A, Chadow H, et al. Primary stent implantation compared with primary balloon angioplasty for acute myocardial infarction: a meta-analysis of randomized clinical trials. Am J Cardiol 2001; 88:297–301.

60. Nordmann AJ, Hengstler P, Harr T, et al. Clinical outcomes of primary stenting versus balloon angioplasty in patients with myocardial infarction: a meta-analysis of randomized controlled trials. Am J Med 2004; 116:253–262.

61. Keeley EC, Boura JA, Grines CL. Primary angioplasty versus intravenous thrombolytic therapy for acute myocardial infarction: a quantitative review of 23 randomised trials. Lancet 2003; 361:13–20.

62. Barbato E, Marco J, Wijns W. Direct stenting. Eur Heart J 2003; 24:394–403.

63. Figulla HR, Mudra H, Reifart N, et al. Direct coronary stenting without predilatation: a new therapeutic approach with a special balloon catheter design. Cathet Cardiovasc Diagn 1998; 43:245–252.
64. Pentousis D, Guerin Y, Funck F, et al. Direct stent implantation without predilatation using the MultiLink stent. Am J Cardiol 1998; 82:1437–1440.
65. Hamon M, Richardeau Y, Lecluse E, et al. Direct coronary stenting without balloon predilation in acute coronary syndromes. Am Heart J 1999; 138:55–59.
66. de la Torre Hernandez JM, Gomez I, Rodriguez-Entem F, et al. Evaluation of direct stent implantation without predilatation by intravascular ultrasound. Am J Cardiol 2000; 85:1028–1030.
67. Loubeyre C, Morice MC, Lefevre T, et al. A randomized comparison of direct stenting with conventional stent implantation in selected patients with acute myocardial infarction. J Am Coll Cardiol 2002; 39:15–21.
68. Morice MC, Serruys PW, Sousa JE, et al. A randomized comparison of a sirolimus-eluting stent with a standard stent for coronary revascularization. N Engl J Med 2002; 346:1773–1780.
69. Stone GW, Ellis SG, Cox DA, et al. A polymer-based, paclitaxel-eluting stent in patients with coronary artery disease. N Engl J Med 2004; 350:221–231.
70. Lemos PA, Saia F, Hofma SH, et al. Short- and long-term clinical benefit of sirolimus-eluting stents compared to conventional bare stents for patients with acute myocardial infarction. J Am Coll Cardiol 2004; 43:704–708.
71. Spaulding C, Henry P, Teiger E, et al. Sirolimus-eluting versus uncoated stents in acute myocardial infarction. N Engl J Med 2006; 355:1093–1104.
72. Laarman GJ, Suttorp MJ, Dirksen MT, et al. Paclitaxel-eluting versus uncoated stents in primary percutaneous coronary intervention. N Engl J Med 2006; 355:1105–1113.
73. Camenzid E, Steg PG, Wijns W. A meta-analysis of first generation drug eluting stent programs. World Congress of Cardiology, Barcelona, Spain, September 2–5, 2006.
74. Stone GW. Independent physician-led patient-level analysis: CYPHER randomized trials. Presented at Transcatheter Cardiovascular Therapeutics, Washington D.C., USA, October 22–27, 2006.
75. Leon MB. Independent physician-led patient-level analysis: TAXUS randomized trials. Presented at Transcatheter Cardiovascular Therapeutics. Washington D.C., USA, October 22–27, 2006.
76. Daemen J, Wenaweser P, Tsuchida K, et al. Early and late coronary stent thrombosis of sirolimus-eluting and paclitaxel-eluting stents in routine clinical practice: data from a large two-institutional cohort study. Lancet 2007; 369:667–678.
77. Behar S, Gottlieb S, Hod H, et al. The outcome of patients with acute myocardial infarction ineligible for thrombolytic therapy. Israeli Thrombolytic Survey Group. Am J Med 1996; 101:184–191.
78. Zahn R, Schuster S, Schiele R, et al. Comparison of primary angioplasty with conservative therapy in patients with acute myocardial infarction and contraindications for thrombolytic therapy. Maximal Individual Therapy in Acute Myocardial Infarction (MITRA) Study Group. Catheter Cardiovasc Interv 1999; 46:127–133.
79. Kastrati A, Mehilli J, Nekolla S, et al. A randomized trial comparing myocardial salvage achieved by coronary stenting versus balloon angioplasty in patients with acute myocardial infarction considered ineligible for reperfusion therapy. J Am Coll Cardiol 2004; 43:734–741.
80. Grzybowski M, Clements EA, Parsons L, et al. Mortality benefit of immediate revascularization of acute ST-segment elevation myocardial infarction in patients with contraindications to thrombolytic therapy: a propensity analysis. JAMA 2003; 290:1891–1898.
81. Massel D. Primary angioplasty in acute myocardial infarction: hypothetical estimate of superiority over aspirin or untreated controls. Am J Med 2005; 118:113–122.
82. Reimer KA, Lowe JE, Rasmussen MM, et al. The wavefront phenomenon of ischemic cell death. 1. Myocardial infarct size vs duration of coronary occlusion in dogs. Circulation 1977; 56:786–794.

83. Newby LK, Rutsch WR, Califf RM, et al. Time from symptom onset to treatment and outcomes after thrombolytic therapy. GUSTO-1 Investigators. J Am Coll Cardiol 1996; 27:1646–1655.
84. Goldberg RJ, Mooradd M, Gurwitz JH, et al. Impact of time to treatment with tissue plasminogen activator on morbidity and mortality following acute myocardial infarction (The second National Registry of Myocardial Infarction). Am J Cardiol 1998; 82:259–264.
85. Boersma E, Maas AC, Deckers JW, et al. Early thrombolytic treatment in acute myocardial infarction: reappraisal of the golden hour. Lancet 1996; 348:771–775.
86. Brodie BR, Stuckey TD, Wall TC, et al. Importance of time to reperfusion for 30-day and late survival and recovery of left ventricular function after primary angioplasty for acute myocardial infarction. J Am Coll Cardiol 1998; 32:1312–1319.
87. Berger PB, Ellis SG, Holmes DR Jr., et al. Relationship between delay in performing direct coronary angioplasty and early clinical outcome in patients with acute myocardial infarction: results from the global use of strategies to open occluded arteries in Acute Coronary Syndromes (GUSTO-IIb) trial. Circulation 1999; 100:14–20.
88. Kent DM, Lau J, Selker HP. Balancing the benefits of primary angioplasty against the benefits of thrombolytic therapy for acute myocardial infarction: the importance of timing. Eff Clin Pract 2001; 4:214–220.
89. Nallamothu BK, Bates ER. Percutaneous coronary intervention versus fibrinolytic therapy in acute myocardial infarction: is timing (almost) everything? Am J Cardiol 2003; 92:824–826.
90. De Luca G, Suryapranata H, Ottervanger JP, et al. Time delay to treatment and mortality in primary angioplasty for acute myocardial infarction: every minute of delay counts. Circulation 2004; 109:1223–1225.
91. Cannon CP, Gibson CM, Lambrew CT, et al. Relationship of symptom-onset-to-balloon time and door-to-balloon time with mortality in patients undergoing angioplasty for acute myocardial infarction. JAMA 2000; 283:2941–2947.
92. Brodie BR, Stone GW, Morice MC, et al. Importance of time to reperfusion on outcomes with primary coronary angioplasty for acute myocardial infarction (results from the Stent Primary Angioplasty in Myocardial Infarction Trial). Am J Cardiol 2001; 88:1085–1090.
93. Brodie BR, Stuckey TD, Hansen CJ, et al. Effect of treatment delay on outcomes in patients with acute myocardial infarction transferred from community hospitals for primary percutaneous coronary intervention. Am J Cardiol 2002; 89:1243–1247.
94. Zijlstra F, Patel A, Jones M, et al. Clinical characteristics and outcome of patients with early (<2 h), intermediate (2–4 h) and late (>4 h) presentation treated by primary coronary angioplasty or thrombolytic therapy for acute myocardial infarction. Eur Heart J 2002; 23:550–557.
95. Boersma E. Does time matter? A pooled analysis of randomized clinical trials comparing primary percutaneous coronary intervention and in-hospital fibrinolysis in acute myocardial infarction patients. Eur Heart J 2006; 27:779–788.
96. Stone GW, Dixon SR, Grines CL, et al. Predictors of infarct size after primary angioplasty: pooled patient level analysis from four contemporary randomized trials. Am J Cardiol 2007; 100:1370–1375.
97. Antman EM, Anbe DT, Armstrong PW, et al. ACC/AHA guidelines for the management of patients with ST-elevation myocardial infarction: a report of the American College of Cardiology/American Heart Association Task Force on Practice Guidelines (Committee to Revise the 1999 Guidelines for the Management of Patients with Acute Myocardial Infarction). Circulation 2004; 110:e82–e292.
98. De Luca G, Suryapranata H, Zijlstra F, et al. Symptom-onset-to-balloon time and mortality in patients with acute myocardial infarction treated by primary angioplasty. J Am Coll Cardiol 2003; 42:991–997.
99. Brodie BR, Hansen C, Stuckey TD, et al. Door-to-Balloon time with primary percutaneous coronary intervention for acute myocardial infarction impacts late cardiac mortality in high-risk patients and patients presenting early after the onset of symptoms. J Am Coll Cardiol 2006; 47:289–295.

100. Zijlstra F, Ernst N, de Boer MJ, et al. Influence of prehospital administration of aspirin and heparin on initial patency of the infarct-related artery in patients with acute ST elevation myocardial infarction. J Am Coll Cardiol 2002; 39:1733–1737.
101. Halkin A, Grines CL, Cox DA, et al. Impact of intravenous beta-blockade before primary angioplasty on survival in patients undergoing mechanical reperfusion therapy for acute myocardial infarction. J Am Coll Cardiol 2004; 43:1780–1787.
102. Montalescot G, Barragan P, Wittenberg O, et al. Platelet glycoprotein IIb/IIIa inhibition with coronary stenting for acute myocardial infarction. N Engl J Med 2001; 344:1895–1803.
103. Mehta SR, Yusuf S, Peters RJ, et al. Effects of pretreatment with clopidogrel and aspirin followed by long-term therapy in patients undergoing percutaneous coronary intervention: the PCI-CURE study. Lancet 2001; 358:527–533.
104. Leong JY, Baker RA, Shah PJ, et al. Clopidogrel and bleeding after coronary artery bypass graft surgery. Ann Thorac Surg 2005; 80:928–933.
105. Grines CL, Schreiber TL, Savas V, et al. A randomized trial of low osmolar ionic versus nonionic contrast media in patients with myocardial infarction or unstable angina undergoing percutaneous transluminal coronary angioplasty. J Am Coll Cardiol 1996; 27:1381–1386.
106. Henriques JP, Zijlstra F, van't Hof AW, et al. Angiographic assessment of reperfusion in acute myocardial infarction by myocardial blush grade. Circulation 2003; 107:2115–2119.
107. Roe MT, Cura FA, Joski PS, et al. Initial experience with multivessel percutaneous coronary intervention during mechanical reperfusion for acute myocardial infarction. Am J Cardiol 2001; 88:170–173.
108. Goldstein JA, Demetriou D, Grines CL, et al. Multiple complex coronary plaques in patients with acute myocardial infarction. N Engl J Med 2000; 343:915–922.
109. Morishima I, Sone T, Okumura K, et al. Angiographic no-reflow phenomenon as a predictor of adverse long-term outcome in patients treated with percutaneous transluminal coronary angioplasty for first acute myocardial infarction. J Am Coll Cardiol 2000; 36:1202–1209.
110. Mehta RH, Harjai KJ, Boura J, et al. Prognostic significance of transient no-reflow during primary percutaneous coronary intervention for ST-elevation acute myocardial infarction. Am J Cardiol 2003; 92:1445–1447.
111. Taniyama Y, Ito H, Iwakura K, et al. Beneficial effect of intracoronary verapamil on microvascular and myocardial salvage in patients with acute myocardial infarction. J Am Coll Cardiol 1997; 30:1193–1199.
112. Marzilli M, Orsini E, Marraccini P, et al. Beneficial effects of intracoronary adenosine as an adjunct to primary angioplasty in acute myocardial infarction. Circulation 2000; 101:2154–2159.
113. Grines CL, Marsalese DL, Brodie B, et al. Safety and cost-effectiveness of early discharge after primary angioplasty in low risk patients with acute myocardial infarction. PAMI-II Investigators. Primary Angioplasty in Myocardial Infarction. J Am Coll Cardiol 1998; 31:967–972.
114. Smith SC Jr., Feldman TE, Hirshfeld JW Jr., et al. ACC/AHA/SCAI 2005 Guideline Update for Percutaneous Coronary Intervention–summary article: a report of the American College of Cardiology/American Heart Association Task Force on Practice Guidelines (ACC/AHA/SCAI Writing Committee to Update the 2001 Guidelines for Percutaneous Coronary Intervention). Circulation 2006; 113:156–175.
115. Reeder GS, Bailey KR, Gersh BJ, et al. Cost comparison of immediate angioplasty versus thrombolysis followed by conservative therapy for acute myocardial infarction: a randomized prospective trial. Mayo Coronary Care Unit and Catheterization Laboratory Groups. Mayo Clin Proc 1994; 69:5–12.
116. Stone GW, Grines CL, Rothbaum D, et al. Analysis of the relative costs and effectiveness of primary angioplasty versus tissue-type plasminogen activator: the Primary Angioplasty in Myocardial Infarction (PAMI) trial. The PAMI Trial Investigators. J Am Coll Cardiol 1997; 29:901–907.

117. Cohen DJ, Taira DA, Berezin R, et al. Cost-effectiveness of coronary stenting in acute myocardial infarction: results from the stent primary angioplasty in myocardial infarction (stent-PAMI) trial. Circulation 2001; 104:3039–3045.
118. Bakhai A, Stone GW, Grines CL, et al. Cost-effectiveness of coronary stenting and abciximab for patients with acute myocardial infarction: results from the CADILLAC (Controlled Abciximab and Device Investigation to Lower Late Angioplasty Complications) trial. Circulation 2003; 108:2857–2863.
119. Ito H, Tomooka T, Sakai N, et al. Lack of myocardial perfusion immediately after successful thrombolysis. A predictor of poor recovery of left ventricular function in anterior myocardial infarction. Circulation 1992; 85:1699–1705.
120. van't Hof AW, Liem A, de Boer MJ, et al. Clinical value of 12-lead electrocardiogram after successful reperfusion therapy for acute myocardial infarction. Zwolle Myocardial infarction Study Group. Lancet 1997; 350:615–619.
121. Wu KC, Zerhouni EA, Judd RM, et al. Prognostic significance of microvascular obstruction by magnetic resonance imaging in patients with acute myocardial infarction. Circulation 1998; 97:765–772.
122. van't Hof AW, Liem A, Suryapranata H, et al. Angiographic assessment of myocardial reperfusion in patients treated with primary angioplasty for acute myocardial infarction: myocardial blush grade. Zwolle Myocardial Infarction Study Group. Circulation 1998; 97:2302–2306.
123. Claeys MJ, Bosmans J, Veenstra L, et al. Determinants and prognostic implications of persistent ST-segment elevation after primary angioplasty for acute myocardial infarction: importance of microvascular reperfusion injury on clinical outcome. Circulation 1999; 99:1972–1977.
124. Gibson CM, Cannon CP, Murphy SA, et al. Relationship of TIMI myocardial perfusion grade to mortality after administration of thrombolytic drugs. Circulation 2000; 101:125–130.
125. Mahaffey KW, Puma JA, Barbagelata NA, et al. Adenosine as an adjunct to thrombolytic therapy for acute myocardial infarction: results of a multicenter, randomized, placebo-controlled trial: the Acute Myocardial Infarction STudy of ADenosine (AMISTAD) trial. J Am Coll Cardiol 1999; 34:1711–1720.
126. Ross AM, Gibbons RJ, Stone GW, et al. A randomized, double-blinded, placebo-controlled multicenter trial of adenosine as an adjunct to reperfusion in the treatment of acute myocardial infarction (AMISTAD-II). J Am Coll Cardiol 2005; 45:1775–1780.
127. Kloner RA, Forman MB, Gibbons RJ, et al. Impact of time to therapy and reperfusion modality on the efficacy of adenosine in acute myocardial infarction: the AMISTAD-2 trial. Eur Heart J 2006; 27:2400–2405.
128. Granger CB, Mahaffey KW, Weaver WD, et al. Pexelizumab, an anti-C5 complement antibody, as adjunctive therapy to primary percutaneous coronary intervention in acute myocardial infarction: the COMplement inhibition in Myocardial infarction treated with Angioplasty (COMMA) trial. Circulation 2003; 108:1184–1190.
129. Armstrong PW, Granger CB, Adams PX, et al. Pexelizumab for acute ST-elevation myocardial infarction in patients undergoing primary percutaneous coronary intervention: a randomized controlled trial. JAMA 2007; 297:43–51.
130. Smith PK, Levy JH, Shernan SK. Pexelizumab, a terminal complement inhibitor in coronary artery bypass graft surgery: results from the Pexelizumab for the Reduction in Myocardial Infarction and Mortality in CABG II trial. 55th Annual American College of Cardiology Scientific Session. Atlanta, GA, USA, March 11–14, 2006.
131. Chien GL, Wolff RA, Davis RF, et al. "Normothermic range" temperature affects myocardial infarct size. Cardiovasc Res 1994; 28:1014–1017.
132. Duncker DJ, Klassen CL, Ishibashi Y, et al. Effect of temperature on myocardial infarction in swine. Am J Physiol 1996; 270:H1189–H1199.
133. Hale SL, Dave RH, Kloner RA. Regional hypothermia reduces myocardial necrosis even when instituted after the onset of ischemia. Basic Res Cardiol 1997; 92:351–357.
134. Dixon SR, Kuntz RE, Griffin JJ, et al. Mild hypothermia during primary percutaneous coronary intervention for acute myocardial infarction: a randomized trial. (Submitted for publication.)

135. Grines CL. Intravascular Cooling adjunctive to percutaneous coronary intervention. Presented at Transcatheter Cardiovascular Interventions 2004. Washington D.C., USA, September 27–October 1, 2004.
136. Buras J. Basic mechanisms of hyperbaric oxygen in the treatment of ischemia-reperfusion injury. Int Anesthesiol Clin 2000; 38:91–109.
137. Dixon SR, Bartorelli AL, Marcovitz PA, et al. Initial experience with hyperoxemic reperfusion after primary angioplasty for acute myocardial infarction: results of a pilot study utilizing intracoronary aqueous oxygen therapy. J Am Coll Cardiol 2002; 39:387–392.
138. O'Neill WW, Martin JL, Dixon SR, et al. Acute myocardial infarction with hyperoxemic therapy (AMIHOT): a prospective, randomized trial of intracoronary hyperoxemic reperfusion after percutaneous coronary intervention. J Am Coll Cardiol 2007; 50:397–405.
139. Kunadian B, Dunning J, Vijayalakshmi K, et al. Meta-analysis of randomized trials comparing anti-embolic devices with standard PCI for improving myocardial reperfusion in patients with acute myocardial infarction. Catheter Cardiovasc Interv 2007; 69:488–496.
140. Every NR, Parsons LS, Fihn SD, et al. Long-term outcome in acute myocardial infarction patients admitted to hospitals with and without on-site cardiac catheterization facilities. MITI Investigators. Myocardial Infarction Triage and Intervention. Circulation 1997; 96:1770–1775.
141. Rogers WJ, Canto JG, Lambrew CT, et al. Temporal trends in the treatment of over 1.5 million patients with myocardial infarction in the US from 1990 through 1999: the National Registry of Myocardial Infarction 1, 2 and 3. J Am Coll Cardiol 2000; 36: 2056–2063.
142. Rogers WJ, Canto JG, Barron HV, et al. Treatment and outcome of myocardial infarction in hospitals with and without invasive capability. Investigators in the National Registry of Myocardial Infarction. J Am Coll Cardiol 2000; 35:371–379.
143. Nallamothu BK, Bates ER, Wang Y, et al. Driving times and distances to hospitals with percutaneous coronary intervention in the United States: implications for pre-hospital triage of patients with ST-elevation myocardial infarction. Circulation 2006; 113:1189–1195.
144. Dehmer GJ, Blankenship J, Wharton TP Jr., et al. The current status and future direction of percutaneous coronary intervention without on-site surgical backup: an expert consensus document from the Society for Cardiovascular Angiography and Interventions. Catheter Cardiovasc Interv 2007; 69:471–478.
145. Topol EJ, Kereiakes DJ. Regionalization of care for acute ischemic heart disease: a call for specialized centers. Circulation 2003; 107:1463–1466.
146. Bradley EH, Herrin J, Wang Y, et al. Strategies for reducing the door-to-balloon time in acute myocardial infarction. N Engl J Med 2006; 355:2308–2320.
147. Dixon SR, O'Neill WW. Interventions in acute myocardial infarction. Curr Probl Cardiol 2001; 26:613–672.

8 Rescue PCI

Damian J. Kelly and Anthony H. Gershlick
Department of Cardiology, University Hospitals of Leicester, Glenfield Hospital, Leicester, United Kingdom

INTRODUCTION

Each year in the United States, an estimated 500,000 patients develop an acute ST-segment elevation myocardial infarction (STEMI) (1). Despite advances in reperfusion therapy, 30-day mortality following reperfusion treatment for STEMI in Europe and the United States remains relatively high at 6% to 7% (2,3). STEMI treatment aims to provide rapid, complete, and sustained restoration of infarct-related artery (IRA) patency. Mechanical reperfusion by "primary" percutaneous coronary intervention (P-PCI) has been shown to deliver superior clinical outcomes compared with fibrinolysis. A meta-analysis of randomized clinical trials demonstrated a reduction in recurrent myocardial infarction or stroke at 30 days from 14% with fibrinolysis to 8% with PPCI (OR 0.53; 95% CI, 0.45–0.53; number needed to treat = 14; $p < 0.001$), irrespective of whether transfer to a PCI center was required (4). A linear relationship exists between long-term mortality and time delay before P-PCI, making prompt delivery of PPCI vital (5,6). Guidelines emphasize that P-PCI should be preferred to fibrinolysis if it can be delivered by an experienced team within 90 minutes of first medical contact (1,7).

Real-world data suggest widespread delivery of P-PCI is challenging, requiring reorganization of paramedic activities and heavy investment in training and facilities (1,7). The most recent published data of over 150,000 patients developing STEMI from 1998 through 2002 from the U.S. National Registry of Myocardial Infarction (NRMI) suggest that 53% received early reperfusion therapy, with 52% receiving intravenous fibrinolytic therapy; the remainder were treated by P-PCI (8,9). Fibrinolysis is supported by a large body of evidence. Trials recruiting over 45,000 patients with STEMI or left bundle branch block demonstrate 20 to 30 lives saved per 1000 patients treated within 12 hours of symptom onset (10). By virtue of its ease of use and widespread availability, fibrinolysis will continue to be first-line treatment for patients with STEMI in geographically isolated areas or in the areas that lack an established network for referral for P-PCI. In other hospitals, it may be considered a better option than investing in personnel and facilities that need to be maintained 24 hours per day, seven days per week. It is likely that reperfusion therapy using fibrinolysis as the first-line option will remain important for the foreseeable future. However, there are drawbacks to using fibrinolytic therapy, including reduced patency rates.

Successful reperfusion, defined by Thrombolysis in Myocardial Infarction (TIMI) grade 3 flow at angiography, correlates strongly with improved left ventricular function and better long-term clinical outcome (11). P-PCI produces TIMI grade 2 or 3 IRA flow in over 90% of patients, whereas patency rates after fibrinolysis are only 30% to 60% and are associated with higher residual diameter stenoses (11–13).

Failed fibrinolysis is estimated to affect up to 75,000 patients in the United States per year (2). How we define lytic failure will be discussed later in this chapter. The resultant burden of morbidity and mortality is significant, with estimates of relative risk for in-hospital mortality ranging from 1.56 (95% CI, 1.0–2.44; $p = 0.048$) when data from the conservative arms of rescue PCI (R-PCI) trials are used to 2.8 when data from available registry data are used as the source (2). Evidence of lytic failure on clinical grounds has been reported in up to 40% of patients in the fibrinolytic trials and is associated with reductions of up to 30% in short- and long-term survival rates (10).

Until recently, there was no consensus on how to best treat patients with failed reperfusion following lytic therapy. Wide variations exist in clinical practice utilizing R-PCI or conservative care or repeated attempts at fibrinolysis (14). R-PCI is defined as mechanical reperfusion for failed fibrinolysis with the goal of restoration of coronary flow, limitation of infarct size, and improved survival. While R-PCI may appear intuitive, the patients involved are inherently different from those eligible for P-PCI. They present later, have already received systemic fibrinolytic therapy, and have higher risk profiles. Randomized trial data are now available, however, to guide the management of patients who fail fibrinolysis.

THE PATHOPHYSIOLOGY OF FAILED FIBRINOLYSIS

Many theoretical reasons exist to suggest that fibrinolysis has the potential to fail. Susceptibility to fibrinolytic therapy varies between individuals, being mediated by comorbid and anatomical factors that tend to be immutable. Therefore, further attempts at lytic therapy are likely to be unsuccessful since the system is already lytic saturated anyway. Thrombosis involves a balance between local thrombosis and endogenous fibrinolysis. Following rupture of a coronary atherosclerotic plaque, exposed subendothelial lipid and inflammatory cells provoke intense platelet activation and aggregation. Coronary occlusion occurs because of rapid formation of a dense "white thrombus" composed of activated platelets enmeshed in cross-linked fibrin, while downstream from this occlusion, an erythrocyte-rich "red" thrombus predominates. Platelets play a central role in mediating lytic resistance. Levels of platelet-derived inhibitors of fibrinolysis such as platelet activator inhibitor-1 and thrombin activatable fibrinolysis inhibitor vary among individuals. In vitro studies suggest that a dominant platelet-mediated lytic inhibitory effect may develop within older thrombus, or when levels of lytic within the thrombus are suboptimal (15). Following lytic failure, residual "white" platelet-rich thrombus predominates. Whereas "red" thrombus is easily lysed, white thrombi are relatively resistant to lysis with tissue plasminogen activator (t-PA) (16).

In some patients, arterial occlusions are inherently lytic resistant. Interindividual variability in local thrombin levels may promote resistant fibrin architecture (17). A "stump" coronary occlusion may impair access of fibrinolytic agent if there are no patent side branches to allow distal perfusion of the drug. Coronary hypoperfusion, as occurs in the setting of cardiogenic shock, greatly reduces fibrinolytic efficacy. Late administration of lytic (>4 hours after symptom onset) substantially reduces the likelihood of reperfusion (18). With increasing duration of occlusion, the effect of fibrinolytic therapy is attenuated as fibrin cross-links mature and the thrombus becomes organized, with reduced rates of clinical reperfusion (19). Fibrinolytic agents have been shown to induce a transient procoagulant effect mediated through increased thrombin activity (20). Further administration of fibrinolytic therapy may be paradoxically self-defeating by releasing trapped thrombin and enhancing platelet activation, while depleting endogenous fibrinogen stores and reducing the likelihood of further attempts at pharmacological fibrinolysis being successful (12,21).

DIAGNOSING FAILED FIBRINOLYSIS

Rapid, accurate assessment of the adequacy of reperfusion following fibrinolytic therapy is difficult, but vital in determining whether there is likely to be a satisfactory outcome. Nine landmark fibrinolysis trials show a linear relationship between delayed reperfusion and survival, with each additional hour of delay associated with a reduction in benefit of 1.6 (SD 0.6) lives saved per 1000 patients (10). Sophisticated techniques such as intracoronary Doppler-derived coronary flow and myocardial perfusion scores are available for sensitive detection of inadequate perfusion but are impractical when used as screening tests for failure of fibrinolysis.

Angiographic studies by the TIMI group confirm that even subtle reductions in myocardial perfusion following fibrinolysis impacted negatively on survival (22). Up to 40% of patients categorized as having TIMI grade 3 flow, and thus likely to have clinical evidence of satisfactory reperfusion, can be demonstrated to have impaired microvascular perfusion at angiography with delayed clearance of contrast from myocardium in the distribution of the IRA, a so-called abnormal "blush" or TIMI myocardial perfusion (TMP) score. Abnormal "blush" scores were an independent risk factor for 30-day mortality in the TIMI 10B trial, conferring a relative risk of 2.86 (95% CI, 0.98–9.33; $p = 0.054$). Failed reperfusion to a degree that would be manifest clinically (TIMI 0 or 1 flow) increased mortality 18-fold from 0.73% to 10.9% ($p < 0.001$) compared with optimal reperfusion.

Clinical markers of failed reperfusion taken in isolation are largely unhelpful (23). Relief of pain is an insensitive indicator of reperfusion, affected by large variations in individual pain threshold and response to analgesics. In the Middlesborough Early Revascularization to Limit Infarction (MERLIN) trial (24) of R-PCI, chest pain was neither a reliable predictor of persistent arterial occlusion when present nor a good indicator of arterial patency when absent: 43% of patients in the R-PCI group had TIMI grade flow less than 3 but were pain-free at the time of randomization based on electrocardiographic criteria of failed reperfusion. A substudy of the TAMI-5 trial (25) showed that clinical variables failed to predict recurrent myocardial ischemia or the need for urgent intervention in the days following fibrinolysis. Of 16 variables analyzed, only age and presence of anterior myocardial infarction were predictive of high risk. Neither did the indication for urgent angiography predict IRA patency. The IRA was patent (TIMI 2 or 3 flow) in 60% of patients with recurrent chest pain, in 45% with recurrent ST-segment elevation, and in 23% with systolic hypotension.

However, noninvasive markers of failed reperfusion are crucial to allow triage of patients for R-PCI and to facilitate clinical protocols. There is evidence that altered ratios of biochemical markers from pre- to postlysis may indicate arterial patency. Of these, myoglobin has shown promise because of its rapid release into and degradation from the circulation. A 60 minute to baseline ratio of myoglobin levels of less than 4 has been proposed as a biochemical marker to be combined with clinical and electrocardiographic indices to detect lytic failure. Biochemical markers are limited by poor specificity despite high sensitivity and a tendency to overdiagnose failed reperfusion (using myoglobin; sensitivity 92%, specificity 59%) (26).

Electrocardiographic assessment of fibrinolytic efficacy has the advantage of objectivity and ease of use. Several classification systems for detection of lytic failure have been proposed on the basis of angiographic substudies of lytic trials. Schröder et al. (27) defined a three-component definition based on the sum of ST-segment resolution after fibrinolysis: complete (>70%), partial (30–70%), or absent (<30%) reperfusion. A strong stepwise correlation exists across a series of lytic trials between the degree of ST-segment resolution and clinical outcome (28,29). More recently, analysis of resolution of maximal ST-segment elevation in a single lead has been shown to be able discriminate for death and development of heart failure. Adoption of a 50% cutoff for ST-segment resolution appears to confer similar sensitivity (around 90%) to that of less than 70% maximal ST-segment resolution threshold, with fewer false-positive results (specificity around 60% at the 50% threshold) (30).

We advocate adoption of a single criterion of less than 50% ST-segment resolution (measured from the isoelectric baseline to 80 milliseconds beyond the J point) in the lead with previous maximal ST elevation. This measure lends ease-of-use and clarity to the postfibrinolytic assessment of STEMI patients for trial purposes. Furthermore, a 50% ST-segment resolution cutoff equips physicians and nursing staff with a simple bedside tool to diagnose lytic failure, without resort to complex calculations or measuring tools. There is little evidence to suggest that combined noninvasive approaches offer significantly better discrimination in clinical practice (31,32).

TRIALS OF REPEATED FIBRINOLYSIS

Some have advocated repeat lytic therapy as a way of managing lytic failure. Only three RCTs, including the Rescue Angioplasty versus Conservative Treatment or Repeat Thrombolysis (REACT) trial, have involved randomization to repeat fibrinolysis or to conservative management (33–35). The lytic agent in all three trials was recombinant tissue plasminogen activator (rt-PA), with 100% follow-up at six months. Meta-analysis of these trials was featured in a recent paper by Wijeysundra et al. (36). They report that repeated fibrinolytic therapy in 410 patients failed to reduce the rates of all-cause mortality (RR 0.68; 95% CI, 0.41–1.14; $p = 0.14$) or reinfarction (RR 1.79; 95% CI, 0.92–3.48; $p = 0.09$). The incidence of heart failure in 283 patients from the REACT trial did not differ between the fibrinolytic and conservative arms (7% vs. 7.8%). Across the trials, minor bleeding was significantly increased with repeat fibrinolytic therapy versus conservative therapy (RR 1.84; 95% CI, 1.06–3.18; $p = 0.03$), but no significant increase was observed in major bleeding. Data were insufficient to comment on repeat fibrinolytic therapy and the risk of stroke. However, there were more major bleeds in the REACT trial in the repeat lytic arm, although these numbers as stated did not reach statistical significance. They included one case of hemopericardium and two cases of intracranial hemorrhage. On the basis of these intuitive and trial data, repeat fibrinolytic therapy cannot be advocated for the treatment of lytic-resistant STEMI.

EARLY CLINICAL TRIALS OF R-PCI

Determining the best treatment for failed fibrinolysis has been challenging. Enrollment of patients in RCTs has always been difficult, perhaps biased in early trials by using angiographic recruitment criteria. Conclusions from meta-analyses should be interpreted in light of heterogeneity between trials in definition of lytic failure, timing of PCI, and choice of angiographic and clinical end points (Table 1).

Six RCTs were conducted between 1992 and 2004 and recruited over 900 patients with suspected failed fibrinolysis randomized to R-PCI or conservative therapy (24,33,37–40) (Table 2). These six trials have formed the basis for contemporary meta-analyses (36,41,42). In addition, the Limburg Myocardial Infarction

TABLE 1 Trial Design of Rescue PCI Trials

Trial	Year	Randomized to R-PCI or control (n)	Inclusion criteria	Follow-up	Anterior wall (%)	Mean age (yrs)	Men (%)	Time from symptom onset to		1° E-P
								Lytic (min)	PCI (min)	
REACT (33)	2005	285*	<50% STR at 90 min with TIMI < 3	6-month	43	61	78	140 (95–220)†	414 (350–505)†	Death, non-fatal MI, stroke, heart failure at 30d & 6m
MERLIN (24)	2004	307	<50% STR at 60 min	30-day	44	63	72	180 ± 120	327 ± 121	All-cause mortality at 30d and 1 yr
RESCUE II (40)	2000	29	TIMI 2	30-day	59	63	93	210 ± 156	294 ± 252	LVEF at 30d
RESCUE (38)	1994	151	TIMI 0 or 1	30-day	100	59	82	N/A	270 ± 110	LVEF at 30d
TAMI (44)	1994	108	TIMI 2	In-hospital	41	57	81	176 ± 62	268 ± 71	LVEF at 7–10d
Belenkie et al. (37)	1992	28	TIMI 0	In-hospital	56	58	44	<180	257 ± 57	In-hospital mortality

*REACT randomized a further 142 patients to repeat lysis.
†Inter-Quartile range.
Abbreviations: 1° E-P, primary end-point definition; STR, reduction in maximal ST-segment elevation; TIMI, Thrombolysis In Myocardial Infarction angiographic perfusion grade; LVEF, left ventricular ejection fraction.

TABLE 2 Mortality and Outcome Data

Trial	No. of patients	Mortality	RR (95% CI)	Heart failure	RR (95% CI)	Stroke	RR (95% CI)
REACT (33) R-PCI (conservative)	144 (141)	5% (10.6%)	0.46 (0.19–1.09)	4% (7%)	0.59 (0.22–1.57)	1.4% (0.7%)	1.96 (0.18–21.36)
MERLIN (24) R-PCI (conservative)	153 (154)	9.8% (11%)	0.89 (0.46–1.71)	24% (30%)	0.81 (0.56–1.17)	4% (0.6%)	7.05 (0.88–56.58)*
RESCUE II (40) R-PCI (conservative)	14 (15)	7% (0)	3.20 (0.14–72.62)	–	–	–	–
RESCUE (38) R-PCI (conservative)	78 (73)	5% (9.6%)	0.53 (0.16–1.75)	1.3% (7%)	0.19 (0.02–1.56)	–	–
TAMI (44) R-PCI (conservative)	49 (59)	8.2% (3.4%)	NS	18.4% (23.7%)	NS	–	–
Belenkie et al. (37) R-PCI (conservative)	16 (12)	6% (33%)	0.19 (0.02–1.47)	–	–	6% (0%)	2.29 (0.10–51.85)*

*Wide confidence intervals (CI) for stroke are indicative of low absolute event rates.

Abbreviations: RR, relative risk of adverse outcome; NS, no significant difference between groups, where RR not quoted in original paper.

Source: Adapted from Patel TN, et al. *Am J Cardiol.* 2006;97:1685–1690, with permission.

(LIMI) trial recorded data on 75 patients undergoing R-PCI (43). This was a pilot study of primary (balloon-only) PCI rather than R-PCI; however, its results are included in one meta-analysis (42). The first prospective R-PCI trial was the Thrombolysis and Angioplasty in Myocardial Infarction (TAMI)-5 trial (44), in which 575 patients were enrolled between 1988 and 1989 in a 3×2 factorial design. TAMI-5 investigated combination thrombolytic regimens and whether immediate coronary angiography with mandated R-PCI in the event of lytic failure, defined as TIMI 0 or 1 flow in the IRA, was superior to delayed angiography with or without PCI after 5 to 10 days. Patients treated with immediate angiography showed a trend toward improved predischarge IRA patency (94% vs. 90%; $p = 0.065$) with a modest reduction in in-hospital adverse outcomes (55% vs. 67%; $p = 0.004$) and improved left ventricular function and less recurrent ischemia compared with a strategy of delayed or ischemia-driven intervention. Subsequently, a reanalysis of the earlier TAMI-1 trial, investigating immediate angioplasty in all patients following fibrinolysis versus continued medical therapy, showed marginal improvements in left ventricular ejection fraction at 7 to 10 days with the invasive approach (39). The TAMI trials were important, as they rekindled interest in the concept of R-PCI and in the development of noninvasive methods for detection of lytic failure.

Following publication by Belenkie et al. of a pilot 28 patient study (37) showing a trend toward improved in-hospital survival in the R-PCI group (RR 0.19; 95% CI, 0.02–1.47; $p = 0.13$), the first major R-PCI trial was RESCUE-1, which ran from 1990 to 1993 (38). This trial enrolled 151 patients with anterior myocardial infarction and persistent TIMI grade 0 or 1 flow following fibrinolysis and randomized them to conservative therapy with aspirin, heparin, and nitrates or R-PCI by balloon angioplasty. There was moderate improvement in left ventricular ejection fraction after exercise at 30 days in those treated by R-PCI compared with conservative therapy (43% vs. 38%; $p = 0.04$) and reduction in a composite of mortality and heart failure of borderline significance (6.4% vs. 16.6%, $p = 0.05$), although this was not a prespecified end point.

The hypothesis of the RESCUE-2 trial (40) was that R-PCI for patients with moderate to large infarcts and TIMI 2 flow would improve outcome compared with conservative therapy. The study suffered from slow recruitment and difficulties with study-site indemnity and was published only as part of a pooled analysis of nine RCTs (including PCI in patent IRAs), although its results are included in contemporary meta-analyses. A pooled analysis of 1456 patients from these early pre-stent studies reported a reduction in the occurrence of severe heart failure following R-PCI (3.8% vs. 11.7%; $p = 0.04$) and improved survival at one year in patients with moderate to large infarcts (92% vs. 87%; $p = 0.001$) (39). R-PCI conferred no significant benefit for any single clinical end point.

CONTEMPORARY CLINICAL TRIALS OF R-PCI

MERLIN Trial

Rapid improvement in PCI techniques occurred during the 1990s. Coronary stents, improved antiplatelet therapy, and activated clotting time monitoring with reduced heparin dosing increased procedural success rates and reduced complications. The first R-PCI trial to report in the post-stent era was the MERLIN trial (24). This was commenced after the initiation of the REACT trial but its recruitment, being a single-centre trial, was faster. Conducted in the northeast of the United Kingdom, MERLIN randomized 307 patients with persistent 50% ST elevation at 60 minutes postfibrinolysis (almost exclusively streptokinase) to R-PCI or conservative management with heparin use at the discretion of the treating physician. Stent use (50.3%) and glycoprotein IIb/IIIa inhibitor (GPI) administration rates (3.3%) in the intervention arm were much lower than in contemporary practice. There was no significant difference in the primary end point of all-cause mortality at 30 days between the groups (9.8% vs. 11%; $p = 0.7$), although these event rates were higher than seen in similar trials. There was a reduction in a composite secondary end point of death, reinfarction, stroke, unplanned revascularization, or heart failure at 30 days in the R-PCI group (27.3% vs. 50%; $p = 0.02$). The only significant risk reduction seen with R-PCI was in the requirement for revascularization procedures, a soft end point and potentially subject to bias in an unblinded study.

The MERLIN authors noted an increase in (predominantly ischemic) stroke (4.6% vs. 0.6%; $p = 0.03$) and need for transfusion (11.1% vs. 1.3%; $p = 0.01$) following PCI. The reasons for the unexpectedly high rate of ischemic stroke is a matter of conjecture but may be related to trial design and the procoagulant potential of streptokinase, which may increase plasmin-mediated thrombin activity in the setting of catheter intervention (45). The absolute numbers contributing to this excess are small (7 strokes in 153 patients from the R-PCI group). Of these seven patients, one did not proceed to angiography, while four patients suffered their stroke later than 24 hours postprocedure, inviting some doubt as to whether PCI itself was the culprit.

Blood transfusions were needed more commonly in the R-PCI group (11.1% vs. 1.3%; $p < 0.001$), mainly due to femoral access site–related bleeding with no excess of gastrointestinal or cerebrovascular hemorrhage. One-year follow-up data have subsequently been published showing persistence of reduction in the composite secondary end point with R-PCI versus conservative treatment (43.1% vs. 57.8%; OR 0.85; 95% CI, 0.74–0.96; $p = 0.01$) driven largely by a reduction in unplanned revascularization but no difference in all-cause mortality (14.4% vs. 13.0%; $p = 0.7$) (45).

Recently published three-year results again indicate no significant difference in the rate of reinfarction (0.7% vs. 0.7%) or heart failure (2.7% vs. 1.3%) between one and three years in the R-PCI and conservative arms (46). However, the need for unplanned revascularization at three years was greater in the conservative arm (33.8% vs. 14.4%; risk difference 19.4%; 95% CI, 10–28.7; $p < 0.01$), with most events occurring within one year. The MERLIN group concluded that the first year carries the highest risk of clinical events in patients with failed reperfusion, beyond which the rate of clinical events is low.

Several factors may explain the apparent lack of mortality benefit of R-PCI in the MERLIN trial. The authors themselves report that the trial was underpowered for differences in mortality between the groups because of an overestimate in the potential benefit of R-PCI, which required a 67% relative reduction (from 18% to 6%) in the risk of death at 30 days to satisfy the power calculation (45). The observed 9.2% 30-day mortality following R-PCI was higher than 6%. The trial did not mandate PCI for all patients in the R-PCI arm and therefore was in reality a trial of conservative therapy versus angiographically directed urgent PCI rather than R-PCI. Of those randomized to R-PCI ($n = 153$), only 66% underwent PCI. The remaining patients were included in the R-PCI intention-to-treat analysis, accruing an 18.1% incidence of unplanned revascularization within one year.

The low rates of stent and GPI use in the MERLIN trial may also have contributed to a higher than expected rate of adverse events in the R-PCI group. There is now evidence of benefit for both these therapies, stenting during R-PCI being independently associated with improved myocardial salvage compared with balloon angioplasty alone (47) and small-scale studies, suggesting fewer ischemic complications and improved left ventricular function at the expense of higher rates of minor bleeding following abciximab administration during R-PCI (48). Other factors may have contributed to a low observed mortality (11% at 30 days) in the conservative treatment group. The choice of an early 60-minute time point at which to declare lytic failure may have biased the results by enrolling patients destined to reperfuse successfully beyond one hour. This supposition is supported by the fact that 40% of patient in the R-PCI arm had TIMI grade 3 flow in the IRA upon initial angiography. In addition, rigorous risk stratification in the conservative treatment group led to a 20% incidence of unplanned revascularization by PCI within 30 days, further diluting the treatment effect of R-PCI.

REACT Trial

The UK multicenter Rescue Angioplasty versus Conservative Treatment or Repeat Thrombolysis (REACT) trial was conducted between 1999 and 2004 and is the largest trial of R-PCI (33). Patients were considered for the REACT trial if they failed to resolve ST-segment elevation to <50% on the 90-minute ECG. Consenting patients ($n = 427$) were randomized to one of three trial groups: repeat (fibrin specific) lysis, standard management (heparin for 24 hours with routine care), or R-PCI. Median time from randomization to repeat lytic administration was 190 minutes (3.2 hours) and to R-PCI 274 minutes (4.6 hours). The times from pain to these respective randomized treatments were 330 and 414 minutes. Recruitment and funding difficulties necessitated early termination of the trial. In contrast to MERLIN, the rate of use of stents (68.5% vs. 50.3%) and GPIs (43.4% vs. 3.3%) was higher and more representative of modern interventional practice.

The primary end point (a composite of death, reinfarction, stroke, or severe heart failure within six months) occurred in 15.3% of patients treated by R-PCI compared with 29.8% of conservative care patients and 31% of those given repeat fibrinolysis. Event-free survival at six months was significantly improved in patients randomized to R-PCI [84.6%, compared with 68.7% for repeated fibrinolysis and 70.1% for conservative therapy ($p = 0.004$)]. The adjusted hazard ratios (HR) for R-PCI versus conservative therapy was 0.47 (95% CI, 0.28–0.79; $p = 0.004$), for R-PCI versus repeated fibrinolysis 0.43 (95% CI, 0.26–0.72; $p = 0.001$), and for repeated fibrinolysis versus conservative treatment 1.09 (95% CI, 0.71–1.67; $p = 0.67$ (Fig. 1). The observed benefit of R-PCI was largely driven by a reduction in recurrent myocardial infarction (2.1% vs. 8.5%; $p < 0.01$). Although not powered to detect a difference in survival, there was a trend toward lower six-month mortality in the R-PCI arm versus conservative care (6.2% vs. 12.8%, $p = 0.12$). Increased nonfatal bleeding, mostly sheath-related, was seen in 22.9% of the R-PCI patients versus 5.7% managed conservatively, but with no increase in major bleeding or bleeding-related deaths in the R-PCI group. An important and major contribution of REACT was to conclusively demonstrate that repeat fibrinolysis confers no benefit over conservative management.

Twelve-month follow-up data for the REACT trial data has recently become available (49). These data confirm persistence of the clear survival benefit following R-PCI. At one year, the rate of event-free survival in those patients randomized to R-PCI was 81.5% compared with 67.5% in those with conservative therapy and 64.1% in those with repeated fibrinolysis ($p = 0.004$). The important hard end point of late mortality has recently been demonstrated in follow-up out to 5 years

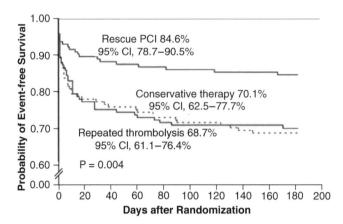

No. of Event-free Patients

Repeated thrombolysis 110 106 105 101   99   99   96   95   93
Conservative therapy   109 104 102   99   98   97   96   95   93
Rescue PCI   129 127 124 122 120 118 117 116 115

FIGURE 1 Kaplan-Meier estimates of the cumulative rate of the composite primary end point (death, recurrent myocardial infarction, severe heart failure, or cerebrovascular event) within six months. *Abbreviations*: PCI, percutaneous coronary intervention; CI, confidence interval. *Source*: From Ref. 33.

(submitted for publication). Mortality was dramatically reduced by R-PCI versus repeated fibrinolysis (HR 0.41; 95% CI, 0.22–0.75; $p = 0.004$) or conservative therapy (HR 0.43; 95% CI, 0.23–0.79; $p = 0.006$) with no alteration after sensitivity analysis. Similarly, the adjusted HR for freedom from unplanned revascularization by PCI or CABG were clearly in favor of R-PCI in comparison with conservative treatment (HR 0.50; 95% CI, 0.30–0.83, $p = 0.007$) or repeated fibrinolysis. In those patients who did not survive, time to death after a median follow-up period of 4.4 years was 14 days (range 0–1470) for repeated fibrinolysis, 33.5 days (range 0–1854) for conservative therapy, but 142.5 days (range 0–2215) for R-PCI ($p = 0.10$).

The probability of procedural success was high in the MERLIN and REACT trials (94% and 92.8%, respectively), although previous studies have reported in-hospital mortality rates of up to 30% in the small number of patients in whom R-PCI does not restore coronary patency (24,38). Adequate data are not available to delineate risk reduction by infarct territory, although most patients in the MERLIN and REACT trials (55.7% and 57.5%, respectively) had nonanterior STEMI (as per real world presentation).

The reasons for the fundamental differences between the results of MERLIN and REACT, particularly the mortality benefit with R-PCI, despite debate remain unclear. One pertinent difference was in the definition of heart failure. In MERLIN, heart failure was defined by requirement for diuretics and by clinical and chest X ray characteristics, whereas the REACT definition encompassed only severe heart failure (New York Heart Association functional class III or IV). Perhaps R-PCI prevents the development of severe heart failure symptoms, although this would not totally explain the differences in late mortality.

The clear reductions in late mortality seen in REACT following R-PCI are compelling, since the mortality data were obtained independently and in a blinded fashion through a national government registry. Ultimately, the difference between the trials are likely to relate to differences in sample size, stent and GPI use, time to ECG assessment, higher rates of stroke in the MERLIN R-PCI cohort, and the higher mortality rates in the MERLIN R-PCI arm.

META-ANALYSES OF THE R-PCI TRIALS

Three systematic reviews have been published since 2006 supporting the use of R-PCI following lytic failure (36,41,42). When two major trials such as MERLIN and REACT show disparity of results, meta-analyses should be viewed with caution, as the benefits of one are likely to be attenuated by the negativity of the other. Wijeysundra et al. (36) analyzed data from six trials (24,33,37–40) enrolling 908 patients randomized to R-PCI or conservative care and concluded that R-PCI was associated with improved clinical outcomes for STEMI patients after failed fibrinolysis. There were significant reductions in the risk of reinfarction (RR 0.58; 95% CI, 0.35–0.97; $p = 0.04$) and development of heart failure (RR 0.73; 95% CI, 0.54–1.00; $p = 0.05$). There was a trend toward reduced all-cause mortality (RR 0.69; 95% CI, 0.46–1.05; $p = 0.09$), although the authors comment that even the pooled estimates were underpowered with a calculated power of 0.48 to detect a 30% relative risk reduction in mortality. R-PCI did confer an increased risk of stroke (RR 4.98; 95% CI, 1.10–22.5; $p = 0.04$) and minor bleeding (RR 4.58; 95% CI, 2.46–8.55; $p = 0.001$). The increased risk of stroke was driven almost entirely by seven embolic events (4.6%) in the intervention arm of MERLIN.

Patel et al. (41) confined their analysis to five randomized controlled trials (24,33,37,38,40) specifically addressing R-PCI and demonstrated a significant reduction in the risk of death (RR 0.64; 95% CI, 0.41–1.00; $p = 0.048$) in the rescue arm, with a trend toward reduced risk of heart failure (RR 0.72; 95% CI, 0.51–1.01; $p = 0.06$) and increased risk of thromboembolic stroke in the R-PCI groups (RR 3.61; 95% CI, 0.91–14.27; $p = 0.07$).

Finally, Collet et al. (42) performed a meta-analysis comparing R-PCI with conservative therapy along with a pooled analysis of trials comparing systematic and early PCI (within 24 hours of fibrinolysis) with delayed, ischemia-driven PCI. Their findings in support of R-PCI were broadly in agreement with the other published meta-analyses, with a borderline-significant reduction in mortality (RR 0.63; 95% CI, 0.39–0.99; $p = 0.055$) and a significant reduction in the risk of death or reinfarction (RR 0.60; 95% CI, 0.41–0.89; $p = 0.012$). With longer follow-up (up to one year), there was a trend toward reduced mortality in the R-PCI group compared with conservative treatment (8.9% vs. 12.0%; OR 0.69; 95% CI, 0.41–1.57; $p = 0.16$) (Fig. 2). Overall, their conclusions were strongly in favor of R-PCI for failed fibrinolysis and more cautiously in favor of a strategy of systematic early PCI following *successful* fibrinolysis. This later strategy remains controversial, although interestingly there was a clear disparity of benefit between the trials conducted in the pre- and post-stent eras.

R-PCI trials have differed in their definition of bleeding complications, the consistent theme being that R-PCI for failed fibrinolysis conferred an increased risk of minor (mostly sheath related) nonfatal bleeding, but no increase in major gastrointestinal or intracranial bleeding compared with conservative management. These findings are compatible with the PRAGUE trial (50) and the trial by Vermeer et al. (43) examining STEMI management strategies at community hospitals which reported similar rates of major bleeding between conservative and R-PCI arms, but increased minor bleeding in the latter.

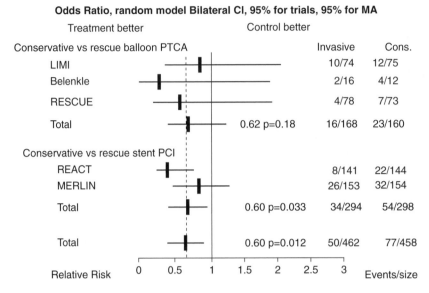

FIGURE 2 Meta-analysis showing lower rates of death or reinfarction within 30 days of lytic failure among 920 patients treated with rescue PCI versus conservative care. Overall OR 0.60; 95% CI, 0.41–0.89; $p = 0.012$. *Abbreviation*: LIMI, Limburg Myocardial Infarction trial. *Source*: From Ref. 42.

In summary, the results of the REACT trial showing significant reduction in mortality at one-year following R-PCI for failed fibrinolysis are confirmed by subsequent meta-analyses. There is a clear reduction in recurrent ischemia following R-PCI compared with conservative care at the expense of an approximate fourfold increase in nonfatal minor (mostly access site) bleeding and a possible increase in the rate of thromboembolic stroke. It should be emphasized that the absolute number of strokes involved was small and the effect largely driven by the excess incidence in the MERLIN R-PCI cohort. There is <u>no role</u> for repeat administration of fibrinolytic therapy following initial lytic failure.

ANTIPLATELET THERAPY IN R-PCI

Platelet inhibition encourages endogenous fibrinolysis and maintenance of IRA patency following R-PCI. Sustained platelet activation is required to maintain thrombus integrity. Thrombus stability appears to be dependant on continuous activation of the platelet GP IIb/IIIa receptor mediated by constant stimulation of the platelet P_2Y_1 and P_2Y_{12} [adenosine diphosphate (ADP)] receptors (51). Clopidogrel inhibits the platelet ADP receptor and acts additively with aspirin. Laboratory tests of platelet aggregation suggest that maximal clopidogrel–induced platelet inhibition occurs around two hours following a 600-mg loading dose (52). There are no safety data on the use of a 600-mg loading dose with full-dose fibrinolytic therapy.

The "final common pathway" of platelet aggregation involves bridging of adjacent platelets by fibrinogen via the platelet GP IIb/IIIa receptor. Concern has been raised regarding the safety of administering GPIs with full-dose thrombolytic agents. Most patients treated with GPI during R-PCI currently receive periprocedural abciximab. Current data, pending the results of the FINESSE randomized trial, do not support the use of combination reperfusion therapy with fibrinolytic and GPI (so called "facilitated" PCI) (53).

GP IIb/IIIa receptor inhibition may usefully negate the antifibrinolytic effects of platelet activation and thus facilitate endogenous fibrinolysis (54). Abciximab has been shown to attenuate capillary plugging by interfering with integrin receptors that mediate adherence of granulocytes to the injured vessel wall (55). Both stent thrombosis and embolization of platelet aggregates to the distal microcirculation are relatively common events following R-PCI that might theoretically be mitigated by abciximab use. Efforts to protect the microcirculation may be clinically relevant when a large thrombus burden is visible at angiography (56). Unfortunately, definitive data is lacking on GPI use during R-PCI.

RECOMMENDATIONS FOR ADJUNCTIVE PHARMACOLOGICAL AGENTS

We recommend GPI use during R-PCI in selected patients after careful assessment of each patient's bleeding risk. Rates of intracranial hemorrhage appear unacceptably high when GPIs are used following streptokinase, so we advise against the use of GPI with this lytic agent or when the patient is older than 75 years (57). A loading dose of clopidogrel may be justified in patients at low risk of bleeding if clopidogrel was not given at the time of fibrinolysis. In the absence of data specific to R-PCI, clopidogrel either 300 mg or 600 mg should be given as early as possible prior to transfer to the PCI center.

Reassuringly, most periprocedural bleeds appear to be related to the femoral artery sheath, with no fatalities due to bleeding in any of the R-PCI trials. There are scant safety data regarding use with the intra-aortic balloon pump or with radial artery access. The radial artery route can be expected to produce fewer access site bleeding complications.

Overall, bleeding complications have fallen with widespread use of controlled, weight-adjusted periprocedural intravenous heparin. Regular ACT monitoring should be performed targeting an activated clotting time of 200 to 250 seconds. Coronary stents should be implanted routinely as per normal practice. There are no data to support the use of low molecular-weight heparin during R-PCI.

LIMITATIONS OF THE APPLICABILITY OF AVAILABLE DATA

R-PCI has been less extensively studied than P-PCI for STEMI, and data are lacking in patients over the age of 85 years or presenting later than seven hours after symptom onset (33). Further attempts to elucidate the mechanisms of benefit in R-PCI are warranted, along with studies to determine the time window for intervention following lytic failure. It is striking to note that a sustained mortality benefit was achieved in the REACT trial, despite the 6.9-hour mean time from symptom onset to R-PCI. These areas may be addressed by future research trials. In the absence of specific data, we advise that clinicians continue to weigh the individual risks and potential benefits of intervention for each patient, performing angiography with or without PCI, unless contraindications or patient preference for conservative therapy exist.

CONCLUSIONS

R-PCI is effective in reducing adverse outcomes in patients with STEMI following failure of fibrinolytic therapy. Repeat lytic therapy administration increases bleeding risk and confers no clinical benefit. Clinicians should not consider administration of fibrinolytic therapy as the final act in acute STEMI management but must be vigilant in order to detect failed reperfusion. The REACT trial and subsequent meta-analyses have focused attention on the importance of routine electrocardiographic assessment of reperfusion success following fibrinolysis. Emergency room or coronary care ward staff should habitually record an electrocardiogram 90 minutes after completion of administration of lytic therapy, checking for the presence of $\geq 50\%$ resolution of maximal ST-segment resolution. If this is not present, an urgent referral should be made for consideration of R-PCI in appropriate candidates.

In the REACT trial, the mean time for transfer from referring district hospitals was 85 minutes. If transfer to a PCI center is required, every effort should be made to reduce transfer delays. An explanation of treatment options and administration of clopidogrel should occur prior to transfer with informed consent reconfirmed by the operator at the PCI center. If the patient reperfuses en route, subsequent planned investigation may be performed at the PCI center. An integrated approach including key stakeholders such as paramedics and the cath lab team is critical, building upon established networks for P-PCI. Continuing staff training and audit of patient outcomes are important for success.

R-PCI is the only treatment that has been shown to benefit patients who fail to reperfuse following fibrinolytic therapy. Robust clinical systems are required to allow rapid detection of failed fibrinolysis and rapid referral via clear logistical pathways to a PCI center. A high index of suspicion for failed fibrinolysis is the crucial first step to improve outcomes for the many thousands of STEMI patients who fail to reperfuse each year. R-PCI should be part of mandated AMI management strategies.

REFERENCES

1. Antman EM, Anbe DT, Armstrong PW, et al. ACC/AHA guidelines for the management of patients with ST-elevation myocardial infarction—executive summary. Report of the American College of Cardiology/American Heart Association task force on practice guidelines (writing committee to revise the 1999 guidelines for the management of patients with myocardial infarction). Circulation 2004; 110:588–636.
2. Wiviott SD, Morrow DA, Frederick PD, et al. Performance of the thrombolysis in myocardial infarction risk index in the National Registry of Myocardial Infarction-3 and —4. A simple index that predicts mortality in ST-segment elevation myocardial infarction. J Am Coll Cardiol 2004; 44:783–789.
3. Mandelzweig L, Battler A, Boyko V, et al., and Euro Heart Survey Investigators. The second Euro Heart Survey on acute coronary syndromes: characteristics, treatment, and outcome of patients with ACS in Europe and the Mediterranean Basin in 2004. Eur Heart J 2006; 27:2285–2293.
4. Keeley EC, Boura JA, Grines CL. Primary angioplasty versus intravenous thrombolytic therapy for acute myocardial infarction: a quantitative review of 23 randomised trials. Lancet 2003; 361:13–20.
5. De Luca G, Suryapranata H, Ottervanger JP, et al. Time delay to treatment and mortality in primary angioplasty for acute myocardial infarction: every minute of delay counts. Circulation 2004; 109:1223–1225.
6. Williams DO. Treatment delayed is treatment denied. Circulation 2004; 109:1806–1808.
7. Van de Werf F, Ardissino D, Betriu A, et al. Management of acute myocardial infarction in patients presenting with ST-segment elevation. The task force on the management of acute myocardial infarction of the European Society of Cardiology. Eur Heart J 2003; 24:28–66.
8. Rogers WJ, Canto JG, Lambrew CT, et al. Temporal trends in the treatment of over 1.5 million patients with myocardial infarction in the U.S. from 1990 through 1999. The National Registry of Myocardial Infarction 1, 2 and 3. J Am Coll Cardiol 2000; 36:2056–2063.

9. Wiviott SD, Morrow DA, Guigliano RP, et al. Performance of the thrombolysis in myocardial infarction risk index for early acute coronary syndrome in the National Registry of Myocardial Infarction: a simple risk index predicts mortality in both ST and non-ST elevation myocardial infarction. J Am Coll Cardiol 2003; 41:365A–366A (abstr).

10. Indications for fibrinolytic therapy in suspected acute myocardial infarction: collaborative overview of early mortality and major morbidity results from all randomised trials of more than 1000 patients. Fibrinolytic Therapy Trialists' (FTT) Collaborative Group. Lancet 1994; 343:311–322.

11. Anderson JL, Karagounis LA, Califf RA, et al. Meta-analysis of five reported studies on the relation of early coronary patency grades with mortality and outcomes after acute myocardial infarction. Am J Cardiol 1996; 78:1–8.

12. Prasad A, Gersh BJ. Management of microvascular dysfunction and reperfusion injury. Heart 2005; 91:1530–1532.

13. Nunn CM, O'Neill WW, Rothbaum D, et al. Long-term outcome after Primary Angioplasty in Myocardial Infarction (PAMI-1) trial. J Am Coll Cardiol 1999; 33:640–646.

14. Prendergast BD, Shandall A, Buchalter MB. What do we do when thrombolysis fails? A United Kingdom survey. Int J Cardiol 1997; 61:39–42.

15. Guimaraes AH, Barrett-Bergshoeff MM, Criscuoli M, et al. Fibrinolytic efficacy of amediplase, tenecteplase and scu-PA in different external plasma clot lysis models: sensitivity to the inhibitory action of thrombin activatable fibrinolysis inhibitor (TAFI). Thromb Haemost 2006; 96:325–330.

16. Jang IK, Gold HK, Ziskind AA, et al. Differential sensitivity of erythrocyte-rich and platelet-rich arterial thrombi to lysis with recombinant tissue-type plasminogen activator. A possible explanation for resistance to coronary thrombolysis. Circulation 1989; 79:920–928.

17. Collet JP, Allali Y, Lesty C, et al. Altered fibrin architecture is associated with hypofibrinolysis and premature coronary atherothrombosis. Arterioscler Thromb Vasc Biol 2006; 26:2567–2573.

18. Anderson JL. Why does lysis fail? Am J Cardiol 1997; 80:1588–1590.

19. Newby LK, Rutsch WR, Califf RM, et al. Time from symptom onset to treatment and outcomes after thrombolytic therapy. GUSTO-1 Investigators. J Am Coll Cardiol 1996; 27:1646–1655.

20. Owen J, Friedman KD, Grossman BA, et al. Thrombolytic therapy with tissue plasminogen activator or streptokinase induces transient thrombin activity. Blood 1998; 72:616–620.

21. Topol EJ. Early myocardial reperfusion: an assessment of current strategies in acute myocardial infarction. Eur Heart J 1996; 17(suppl E):42–48.

22. Gibson CM, Cannon CP, Murphy SA, et al. Relationship of TIMI myocardial perfusion grade to mortality after administration of thrombolytic drugs. Circulation 2000; 101:125–130.

23. Califf RM, O'Neill W, Stack RS, et al. Failure of simple clinical methods to predict perfusion status after intravenous thrombolysis. Ann Intern Med 1998; 108:658–662.

24. Sutton AGC, Campbell PG, Graham R, et al. A randomized trial of rescue angioplasty versus a conservative approach for failed fibrinolysis in ST-segment elevation myocardial infarction: the Middlesbrough Early Revascularization to Limit Infarction (MERLIN) trial. J Am Coll Cardiol 2004; 44:287–296.

25. Muller DWM, Topol EJ, Ellis SG, et al., and The TAMI-5 study group. Determinants of the need for early acute intervention in patients treated conservatively after thrombolytic therapy for acute myocardial infarction. J Am Coll Cardiol 1991; 18:1594–1601.

26. Stewart JT, French JK, Theroux P, et al. Early non-invasive identification of failed reperfusion after intravenous thrombolytic therapy in acute myocardial infarction. J Am Coll Cardiol 1998; 31:1499–1505.

27. Schröder R, Dissmann R, Bruggemann T, et al. Extent of early ST-segment elevation resolution: a simple but strong predictor of outcome in patients with acute myocardial infarction. J Am Coll Cardiol 1994; 24:384–391.

28. Schröder R, Wegscheider K, Scröder K, et al. Extent of early ST-segment resolution: a substudy of the International Joint Efficacy Comparison of Thrombolytics (INJECT) trial. J Am Coll Cardiol 1995; 26:1657–1664.

29. Schröder R, Zeymer U, Wegscheider K, et al. Comparison of the predictive value of ST-segment elevation resolution in patients with thrombolysis for myocardial infarction: results from the angiographic sub-study of the Hirudin for Improvement of Thrombolysis (HIT)-4 trial. Eur Heart J 2001; 22:769–775.
30. de Lemos JA, Antman EM, Guigliano RP, et al. Comparison of a 60- versus 90-minute determination of ST-segment resolution after thrombolytic therapy for acute myocardial infarction. Am J Cardiol 2000; 86:1235–1237.
31. de Lemos JA, Gibson CM, Antman EM, et al. Correlation between the TIMI myocardial perfusion grade and ST-segment resolution after fibrinolytic therapy. Circulation 2000; 102(suppl II):775 (abstr).
32. Eeckhout E. Rescue percutaneous coronary intervention: does the concept make sense? Heart 2007; 93:632–638.
33. Gershlick AH, Stevens-Lloyd A, Hughes A, et al. Rescue angioplasty after failed thrombolytic therapy for acute myocardial infarction. N Engl J Med 2005; 353:2758–2768.
34. Mounsey JP, Skinner JS, Hawkins T, et al. Rescue thrombolyis: alteplase as adjuvant treatment after streptokinase in acute myocardial infarction. Br Heart J 1995; 74:348–353.
35. Sarullo FM, Americo L, Di Pasquale P, et al. Efficacy of rescue thrombolysis in patients with acute myocardial infarction: preliminary findings. Cardiovasc Drugs Ther 2000; 14:83–89.
36. Wijeysundra HC, Vijayaraghavan R, Nallamothu BK, et al. Rescue angioplasty or repeat fibrinolysis after failed fibrinolytic therapy for ST-segment myocardial infarction: a meta-analysis of randomized trials. J Am Coll Cardiol 2007; 49:422–430.
37. Belenkie I, Traboulsi M, Hall CA, et al. Rescue angioplasty during myocardial infarction has a beneficial effect on mortality: a tenable hypothesis. Can J Cardiol 1992; 8:357–362.
38. Ellis SG, Ribeiro da Silva E, Heyndrickx G, et al. Randomized comparison of rescue angioplasty with conservative management of patients with early failure of thrombolysis for acute anterior myocardial infarction. Circulation 1994; 90:2280–2284.
39. Ellis SG, Lincoff AM, George BS, et al. Randomized evaluation of coronary angioplasty for early TIMI 2 flow after thrombolytic therapy for the treatment of acute myocardial infarction: a new look at an old study. The Thrombolysis and Angioplasty in Myocardial Infarction (TAMI) study group. Coron Artery Dis 1994; 5:611–615.
40. Ellis SG, Ribiero da Silva E, Spaulding C, et al. Review of immediate angioplasty after fibrinolytic therapy for acute myocardial infarction: insights from the RESCUE I, RESCUE II, and other contemporary clinical experiences. Am Heart J 2000; 139:1046–1053.
41. Patel TN, Bavry AA, Kumbhani DJ, et al. A meta-analysis of randomized trials of rescue percutaneous coronary intervention after failed fibrinolysis. Am J Cardiol 2006; 97:1685–1690.
42. Collet JP, Montalescot G, Le May M, et al. Percutaneous coronary intervention after fibrinolysis: a multiple meta-analyses approach according to the type of strategy. J Am Coll Cardiol 2006; 48:1326–1335.
43. Vermeer F, Oude Ophuis AJ, vd Berg EJ, et al. Prospective randomised comparison between thrombolysis, rescue PTCA and primary PTCA in patients with extensive myocardial infarction admitted to a hospital without PTCA facilities: a safety and feasibility study. Heart 1999; 82:426–431.
44. Califf RM, Topol EJ, Stack RS et al. Evaluation of combination thrombolytic therapy and timing of cardiac catheterization in acute myocardial infarction. Results of Thrombolysis and Angioplasty in Myocardial Infarction (TAMI)-phase 5 randomized trial. TAMI Study Group. Circulation 1991; 83:1543–1556.
45. Sutton AGC, Campbell PG, Graham R, et al. One year results of the Middlesbrough early revascularisation to limit infarction (MERLIN) trial. Heart 2005; 91:1330–1337.
46. Kunadian B, Sutton AG, Vijayalakshmi K, et al. Early invasive versus conservative treatment in patients with failed fibrinolysis—no late survival benefit: the final analysis of the Middlesborough Early Revascularisation to Limit Infarction (MERLIN) randomized trial. Am Heart J 2007; 153:763–771.
47. Schomig A, Ndrepepa G, Mehilli J, et al. A randomized trial of coronary stenting versus balloon angioplasty as a rescue intervention after failed thrombolysis in patients with acute myocardial infarction. J Am Coll Cardiol 2004; 44:2073–2079.

48. Petronio AS, Musumeci G, Limbruno U, et al. Abciximab improves 6-month clinical outcome after rescue coronary angioplasty. Am Heart J 2002; 143:334–341.
49. Gershlick AH, Fairbrother K, Carver A, et al. The REACT (Rescue Angioplasty versus Conservative treatment or repeat thrombolysis) trial: longer term follow-up. Heart 2007; 93(suppl 1):A5.
50. Widimsky P, Groch L, Zelizko M, et al. Multi-centre randomized trial comparing transport to primary angioplasty vs immediate thrombolysis vs combined strategy for patients with acute myocardial infarction presenting to a community hospital without a catheterization laboratory. The PRAGUE study. Eur Heart J 2000; 21:823–831.
51. Goto S, Tamura N, Ishida H, et al. Dependence of platelet thrombus stability on sustained glycoprotein IIb/IIIa activation through adenosine 5'-diphosphate receptor stimulation and cyclic calcium signaling. J Am Coll Cardiol 2006; 47:155–162.
52. Von Beckerath N, Taubert D, Pogatsa-Murray G, et al. Absorption, metabolization, and antiplatelet effects of 300-, 600-, and 900-mg loading doses of clopidogrel: results of the ISAR-CHOICE Trial. Circulation 2005; 112:2946–2950.
53. Keeley EC, Boura JC, Grines CL. Comparison of primary and facilitated percutaneous coronary intervention for ST-elevation myocardial infarction: qualitative review of randomized trials. Lancet 2006; 367:579–588.
54. Collet JP, Montalescot G, Lesty C, et al. Effects of abciximab on the architecture of platelet-rich clots in patients with acute myocardial infarction undergoing primary coronary intervention. Circulation 2001; 103:2328–2331.
55. Neumann FJ, Zohlnhofer D, Fakhoury L, et al. Effect of glycoprotein IIb/IIIa receptor blockade on platelet-leukocyte interaction and surface expression of the leukocyte integrin Mac-1 in acute myocardial infarction. J Am Coll Cardiol 1999; 34:1420–1426.
56. Kirtane AJ, Vafai JJ, Murphy SA, et al. Angiographically evident thrombus following fibrinolytic therapy is associated with impaired myocardial perfusion in STEMI: a CLARITY-TIMI 28 substudy. Eur Heart 2006; 27:2040–2045.
57. Antman EM, Giugliano RP, Gibson CM, et al. Abciximab facilitates the rate and extent of thrombolysis: results of the thrombolysis in myocardial infarction (TIMI) 14 trial. Circulation 1999; 99:2720–2732.

Facilitated Percutaneous Coronary Intervention in Acute Myocardial Infarction

E. Magnus Ohman
Division of Cardiovascular Medicine, Duke University Medical Center,
Duke Clinical Research Institute, Durham, North Carolina, U.S.A.

Mauricio G. Cohen
Division of Cardiology, Department of Medicine, The University of
North Carolina at Chapel Hill, Chapel Hill, North Carolina, U.S.A.

INTRODUCTION

The management of acute myocardial infarction (AMI) has undergone a dramatic change over the last several decades. Although the majority of patients receive fibrinolysis worldwide, many patients are now receiving percutaneous coronary interventions (PCI) in AMI. In fact, PCI has become the standard therapy in the United States, and many strategies have been developed to increase the efficiency of bringing patients to the cardiac catheterization laboratory as quickly as possible. Fibrinolytic therapy (FT) is the simplest method of reperfusion therapy and can almost always be given within 30 minutes in any prehospital or hospital setting. However, complete reperfusion is only achieved in about 60% to 75% of cases and there is a small, but catastrophic, risk of life-threatening bleeding associated with this therapy (1). Thus, strategies have been developed to optimize reperfusion therapy by combining pharmacological and mechanical approaches. This chapter will focus on facilitated PCI and review current data for the rationale and results with this therapy.

WHAT IS FACILITATED PCI?

Facilitated PCI is defined as a combination of a pharmacological strategy that uses one or a combination of medical therapies to restore reperfusion as quickly as possible, followed by acute cardiac catheterization to define the coronary anatomy, and a mechanical approach such as PCI with or without stenting to complete reperfusion and treat the underlying lesion. The term facilitated PCI was first coined by a group of investigators who were working on different combinations of pharmacological strategies evaluated by acute cardiac catheterization, usually within 60 minutes of administering the medical therapy (2). They observed good clinical outcomes in patients initially treated with a combination of low-dose FT and a glycoprotein IIb/IIIa inhibitor (GPI), who were immediately taken to the cardiac catheterization laboratory for PCI. Facilitated PCI differs from "rescue PCI" in that it is a planned mechanical strategy regardless of whether or not reperfusion is successful. It also differs from "primary PCI," as a pharmacological strategy is given as soon as possible during the first medical contact (prehospital or emergency department) to enhance early reperfusion before PCI.

The concept of facilitated PCI came from two studies exploring the role of medical therapy for AMI with PCI. In the Strategies for Patency Enhancement in the Emergency Department (SPEED) trial (2), different dosing schemes of reteplase (r-PA) in combination with abciximab were tested with 88% of patients having coronary angiography at a median of 63 minutes after initiating drug therapy. Facilitated PCI was attempted in 323 (61%) patients, with stents used in 78%, and the PCI success rate [Thrombolysis in Myocardial Infarction (TIMI) grade 3 flow rate and residual stenosis <50% in the infarct-related artery (IRA)] was 88%. Facilitated PCI was associated with a reduction of the composite end point of death, reinfarction, and recurrent ischemia leading to urgent revascularization compared with a conservative strategy (5.6% vs. 16%, $p < 0.001$). In addition, it was noted that the procedural success rate was higher among those patients who had a patent IRA before PCI, suggesting that an open artery was a better target for PCI. Similar findings were observed in the Plasminogen-Activator Angioplasty Compatibility Trial (PACT) (3), where 606 patients were randomized to low-dose tissue-type plasminogen activator (t-PA) (50-mg bolus only) or placebo. There was no difference between the two groups, but two important observations were made. First, patients with TIMI grade 3 flow prior to PCI had an ejection fraction of 62.4% compared with 57.9% among those with TIMI grade flow 0 to 2 on arrival, and successful PCI with postprocedure TIMI grade 3 flow ($p < 0.004$), and 54.7% among those in whom normal flow was never restored before or after the PCI. Second, in a group of 32 patients with TIMI grade 3 flow before PCI, the composite end point of death, reinfarction, emergency target vessel revascularization (TVR), and recurrent ischemia occurred in 0%, while it occurred in 43% of the 109 patients with TIMI grade 3 flow not treated with PCI ($p < 0.01$) (4). Thus, both studies suggested that facilitated PCI conceptually could offer a new strategy for treating patients with AMI.

IMPORTANCE OF TIME TO REPERFUSION

It has now been accepted beyond doubt that the sooner normal reperfusion is established, the lower the morbidity and mortality in AMI (5–7). However, while primary PCI is a very attractive method to establish reperfusion, it is complicated to operationally organize so that the majority of patients have reperfusion established within 90 minutes of arrival to the hospital. It has also been established that there is a 7.5% relative increase in mortality with every 30-minute delay for primary PCI (Fig. 1) (6). In a meta-regression analysis of trials that compared primary PCI with FT (8), it was observed that the beneficial effect of PCI on mortality was lost when the time to primary PCI exceeded the time to fibrinolytic administration by more than 62 minutes (Fig. 2). Thus, in many clinical settings, such as local community hospitals without PCI capability, it makes sense to explore strategies that combine an early pharmacological strategy with an obligatory mechanical approach. Facilitated PCI provides an opportunity to build on the superior aspects of primary PCI and to extend it with administration of early medical reperfusion therapy. This could be of particular value in settings where excessive delays in transferring patients for PCI could be expected, such as in non-urban community hospitals (9).

FACILITATING PCI: IMPORTANCE OF ESTABLISHING NORMAL REPERFUSION (TIMI GRADE 3 FLOW) BEFORE PCI IN AMI

Establishing and sustaining normal reperfusion in the IRA is important for lowering morbidity and mortality in AMI, irrespective of reperfusion strategy used (medical or mechanical). In the Global Utilization of Streptokinase and Tissue Plasminogen Activator for Occluded Coronary Arteries (GUSTO) trial (10,11), the

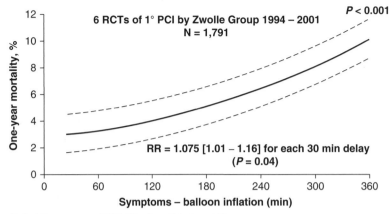

Dotted lines represent 95% CIs of predicted mortality.

FIGURE 1 Relationship between symptom onset to balloon time and mortality in primary PCI for STEMI. *Abbreviations*: PCI, percutaneous coronary interventions; STEMI, ST segment elevation myocardial infarction. *Source*: Adapted from Ref. 62.

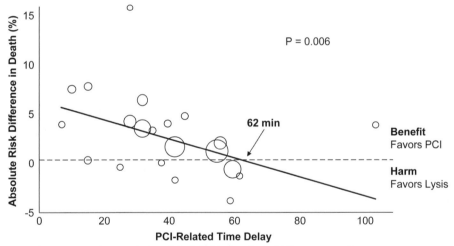

Circle sizes represent the sample size of the individual study. Solid line represent the weighted meta-regression.

FIGURE 2 Relationship between symptom onset to balloon time and mortality in primary PCI for STEMI. *Abbreviations*: PCI, percutaneous coronary interventions; STEMI, ST segment elevation myocardial infarction. *Source*: Adapted from Ref. 8.

benefit with accelerated t-PA over streptokinase (SK) was ascribed to higher 90-minute TIMI grade 3 flow rate with t-PA. Normal reperfusion is also important for prevention of reinfarction and other morbidities such as heart failure (12,13). In a pooled analysis of four Primary Angioplasty in Myocardial Infarction (PAMI) studies involving 2327 patients within 12 hours of AMI, the importance of normal

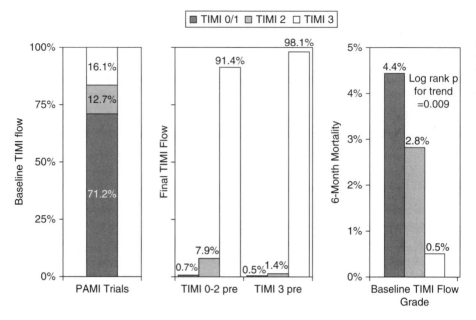

FIGURE 3 Relationship of TIMI grade 3 flow before PCI to six month survival. *Abbreviations*: TIMI, Thrombolysis in Myocardial Infarction; PCI, percutaneous coronary interventions. *Source*: Adapted from Ref. 14.

reperfusion before and after primary PCI was explored (14). This study was one of the first to demonstrate an association between pre-PCI TIMI grade flow and six-month mortality. Upon arrival to the catheterization laboratory, normal flow (TIMI grade 3) in the IRA was only observed in 15.7% of patients, with suboptimal reperfusion (TIMI grade 2) in 12.6% and no reperfusion (TIMI grade 0 or 1) in 71.2% (Fig. 3). Patients with spontaneous TIMI grade 3 flow were more likely to arrive at hospital without heart failure (Killip class 1) and to have a more benign hospital course with less heart failure and hypotension and less need for mechanical ventilation compared with patients with TIMI grade 0–2 flow. Lower grades of preprocedure reperfusion (TIMI grade 0–2) were associated with higher six-month mortality (TIMI grade 0–1, 4.4%; TIMI grade 2, 2.8%, and TIMI grade 3, 0.5%; $p = 0.009$). Factors independently associated with higher six-month mortality by multivariable analysis were advanced age, female gender, anterior MI location, and preprocedural TIMI grade 0–2 flow. In addition, the mortality at six months was 22.2% among patients with post-PCI TIMI grade 0–1 flow, 6.1% among patients with TIMI grade 2 flow, and 2.6% among patients with TIMI grade 3 flow ($p < 0.0001$).

Similar observations have been made by the Zwolle Group that has had a dedicated approach to primary PCI in their community over the last several decades (15). They found among 1791 primary PCI patients that pre-PCI TIMI grade 3 flow was an independent predictor of one-year mortality compared with pre-PCI TIMI grade 0–1 flow (3.8% vs. 17%; $p = 0.005$). The same group of investigators also explored the effect of early administration of aspirin (500 mg) and heparin (5000 U) on reperfusion rates (TIMI grade 2–3 flow). A group of 860 patients transferred from community hospitals received these therapies almost 1 hour earlier than

842 patients initially presenting to the emergency department in a PCI hospital. Pre-PCI reperfusion rates were 17% in the patients transferred for PCI versus 10% in patients treated at the PCI hospital. Patients who had TIMI grade 2–3 flow prior to PCI had smaller infarct size (as measured by cardiac biomarkers), better left ventricular function, and lower 30-day mortality (1.6% vs. 3.4%, $p = 0.04$) compared with patients who had TIMI grade 0–1 flow. These findings in aggregate suggest that among patients receiving primary PCI, outcomes will be better if normal flow is present at baseline angiography before primary PCI.

A pooled analysis from several angiographic trials in AMI showed that the observations on coronary flow can be extended to tissue level reperfusion using TIMI frame count and myocardial blush scores (13,16). Higher TIMI frame count in the IRA 90 minutes after FT, indicating less tissue perfusion, was an independent predictor of 30-day mortality. When examined in relationship to PCI in the IRA, preprocedural higher TIMI grade flow (hazard ratio 0.41, $p < 0.001$), lower TIMI frame count (hazard ratio 0.92, $p = 0.02$), and higher myocardial blush score (hazard ratio 0.51, $p = 0.038$) were all independently associated with a lower two-year mortality using multivariate analysis adjusting for important variable predicting mortality (age, gender, heart rate, anterior MI location) (17). Thus, the importance of pre-PCI flow can also be extended from epicardial coronary flow to tissue level reperfusion explaining the better outcomes on a myocardial salvage level.

THERAPEUTIC OPTIONS FOR FACILITATED PCI

Three different pharmacological options for establishing early reperfusion for facilitated PCI have been studied. These options include FT alone, GPI alone, or the combination of low-dose FT and GPI. The majority have been studied in addition to standard AMI therapy including aspirin and heparin. The results of these various options will be discussed in detail.

Full-Dose Fibrinolytic Therapy with PCI
Fibrin-Specific Fibrinolytic Agents
Early studies. Nearly two decades ago, a number of studies explored the possibility of combining full-dose FT and PCI. These were carried out before the use of stents in AMI and the use of aspirin was variable. The primary end point in these trials was typically ejection fraction at discharge. The TIMI IIa trial (18) randomized 389 patients to immediate PCI versus delayed PCI, 18 to 48 hours after standard dose t-PA. There was no difference in ejection fraction at discharge between the two groups, but there was significantly more bleeding and need for coronary artery bypass grafting (CABG) among patients randomized to early PCI. In the Thrombolysis and Angioplasty in Myocardial Infarction (TAMI)-1 trial (19), 386 patients were treated with t-PA achieving a patency rate (TIMI grade 2–3 flow) of 75% in the IRA at 90 minutes after administration. The 197 patients with an open IRA and suitable anatomy were randomized to immediate PCI versus delayed PCI (7–10 days later). There was no difference in ejection fraction or left ventricular recovery at 7 to 10 days between the groups. Early PCI was associated with more bleeding, while delayed PCI was associated with more recurrent ischemia. The European Cooperative Study Group (ECSG) trial (20) included 367 patients who were randomized to immediate PCI versus conservative management after t-PA. Ejection fraction was evaluated 10 to 22 days later and was found to be similar in both groups. There was a

significant lower rate of the composite end point of death, recurrent ischemia, and bleeding among patients randomized to the conservative arm.

In a meta-analysis of these three trials (21), there was a significantly higher mortality rate among the patients randomized to early PCI (6.5% vs. 3.4%, $p = 0.04$). In addition, bleeding rates were consistently higher in the immediate PCI-treated patients. While these trials were all disappointing, the concept of rescue PCI came out of the early experience of these studies.

Recent studies. Since the early PCI trials, major improvement in PCI results has occurred with the advent of new technologies such as stents, and intravenous antiplatelet agents and more careful attention to aspirin and heparin dosing. This led to a revisiting of the concept of immediate PCI after FT. However, the majority of these trials included only a few hundred patients. Nevertheless, they added important observations that rekindled interest in the field.

The Dutch Limburg Myocardial Infarction (LIMI) trial (22) included 224 patients that were randomized to t-PA alone, t-PA with transfer for possible rescue PCI, or transfer for primary PCI. The composite end point of death and MI at 42 days was 16% in the t-PA group alone, 14% in the t-PA with transfer for rescue PCI group, and 8% in the primary PCI group. The majority of this difference was driven by lower rates of reinfarction among patients having PCI (7% with t-PA, 4% with t-PA and rescue PCI, 1% with primary PCI; $p = 0.14$). Among patients who underwent cardiac catheterization, initial patency (TIMI grade 2–3 flow) in the IRA was higher in patients receiving t-PA compared with primary PCI (71% vs. 23%). The promising aspect of this small trial was the low reinfarction rates after primary or rescue PCI.

The Southwest German Interventional Study in AMI (SIAM) III trial (23) enrolled 163 patients who were randomized to transfer for immediate primary PCI (with stenting), or immediate t-PA followed by transfer and later PCI. Although the immediate PCI group had a lower combined rate of death, MI, and need for TVR (25.6% vs. 50.6%, $p = 0.001$), patients randomized to facilitated PCI had better six-month left ventricular function (61.5% vs. 56.4%, $p = 0.018$). The clinical outcomes were mostly driven by the difference in recurrent ischemia that favored the primary PCI group (4.9% vs. 28.4%). This trial was the first to show that the facilitated PCI may be a viable alternative to transfer for primary PCI.

In the Grupo de Analisis de la Cardiopatia Isquernica Aguda (GRACIA)-1 trial (24), 500 patients received t-PA and then were randomized to early ("next day") angiography followed by PCI if indicated versus ischemia-driven conservative management. Patients with early angiography had significantly lower rates of death, reinfarction, and revascularization at one year (primary end point) compared with patients managed conservatively (9% vs. 21%, $p = 0.0008$). Although this is not technically a trial of facilitated PCI, as many patients received PCI more than 12 hours after FT, the study suggested that an early invasive strategy offered some benefits over a more conservative strategy in AMI. This was followed by the GRACIA-2 trial (25), where 205 patients were randomized to full-dose tenecteplase and enoxaparin followed by PCI within 3 to 12 hours versus primary PCI with abciximab within 3 hours of randomization. The facilitated PCI group had better TIMI grade 3 flow rates at baseline angiography compared with the primary PCI group (67% vs. 14%). Interestingly, post-PCI myocardial blush grade 3 rates were significantly higher in patients treated with facilitated PCI (50%) compared with patients treated with primary PCI (25%). The composite end point (death, nonfatal MI, and ischemia driven TVR at 6 months) favored the facilitated PCI group, but was not statistically different (9.6% vs. 12.0%). The major bleeding rates were also similar in both groups (2% vs. 3%), indicating a good safety profile with facilitated PCI.

The Combined Angioplasty and Pharmacological Intervention Versus Thrombolysis Alone in Acute Myocardial Infarction (CAPITAL-AMI) trial (26) randomized 170 high-risk AMI patients within six hours of symptom onset to two strategies. Facilitated PCI patients received Tenecteplase (TNK) followed by PCI, whereas patients randomized to TNK alone could have rescue PCI for clinically failed reperfusion. Only 9.5% had rescue PCI in the TNK alone arm. The facilitated PCI group had a significantly lower rate of the composite end point of death, reinfarction, recurrent unstable ischemia, or stroke during hospitalization compared with the TNK alone group (8.1% vs. 21.4%, $p = 0.02$). The most pronounced effect was the reduction in reinfarction (3.5% vs. 13.1%, $p = 0.03$) among the facilitated PCI patients. There were similar outcomes with both strategies on left ventricular function and clinical events such as new heart failure and cardiogenic shock. There was a nonsignificant trend to more bleeding with the facilitated PCI strategy (23.3% vs. 13.1%; $p = 0.11$), but hospital stay was shorter (5 days vs. 6 days, $p = 0.009$). The composite end point at 30 days similarly favored facilitated PCI (9.3% vs. 21.7%, $p = 0.03$). While there was no difference in mortality (2.3% vs. 3.6%), the facilitated PCI group had a lower reinfarction rate at 30 days (4.7% vs. 13.3%). Although the outcomes favor the facilitated PCI arm in this trial, the ischemic event rate in the TNK alone arm was higher than expected, which makes it hard to interpret this trial compared with other trials of facilitated PCI.

The Canadian Which Early ST elevation myocardial infarction Therapy (WEST) trial (27) randomized 304 patients into three different strategies: TNK alone and conservative management, TNK with transfer to a PCI center within 24 hours for cardiac catheterization and PCI, or immediate transfer for primary PCI. Although the composite primary end point (30-day death, reinfarction, refractory ischemia, congestive heart failure, cardiogenic shock, and major ventricular arrhythmia) was similar in the three groups (25%, 24%, and 23%, respectively), the rate of death or reinfarction favored the more aggressively treated patients with early invasive management with PCI or primary PCI (13.0%, 6.7%, 4.0%, $p = 0.02$). The bleeding rates were also low (1.0%, 1.9%, 1.0%, respectively) and no patient had an intracranial hemorrhage. This study therefore did not include facilitated PCI, but similar to GRACIA-1, showed that an early invasive strategy appeared superior to a more conservative strategy of FT alone with or without rescue PCI.

The largest trial to date to test the hypothesis of facilitated PCI with TNK alone was the Assessment of the Safety and Efficacy of a New Treatment Strategy with Percutaneous Coronary Intervention (ASSENT-4 PCI) trial (28). In this trial, patients were randomized to either primary PCI or facilitated PCI after full-dose TNK. This trial had a planned enrollment of 4000 patients, but was terminated early by the Data and Safety Committee after 1665 patients had been enrolled because of a higher in-hospital mortality in the facilitated PCI arm (6% vs. 3%, $p = 0.01$). The primary end point of death, heart failure, or shock at 90 days was significantly lower among patients randomized to primary PCI compared with facilitated PCI (13.4% vs. 18.6%, $p = 0.0045$). The 30-day mortality individual end point also favored the primary PCI arm (3.8% vs. 6.0%; $p = 0.04$), but this difference was no longer statistically significant at 90 days (4.9% vs. 6.7% ; $p = 0.14$). Although major bleeding rates were similar between the two groups (4.4% vs. 5.6%, $p = 0.31$), there was a significantly higher rate of in-hospital intracranial hemorrhage among patients receiving TNK in the facilitated PCI arm (1.8% vs. 0%, $p < 0.0001$). Of note, the time from randomization to balloon inflation was short (115 and 107 minutes in the facilitated PCI and primary PCI arms, respectively) limiting the extrapolation of these results to a real-world scenario where delays can be longer than three hours, especially if transport to a tertiary care center is involved. In addition, the study protocol did not allow clopidogrel loading, maintenance IV heparin infusion, or GPI administration in the TNK arm, except in bailout situations, which may have compromised IRA patency during the follow-up period. This trial provides an interesting perspective as it mimics the older trials of PCI and full-dose t-PA (18–20). Similar to those trials, mortality was higher with PCI after t-PA, raising the question whether a fibrin-specific agent plus PCI causes a prothrombotic state. While this is difficult to prove, there have been observations that suggest that rescue PCI performed with less fibrin-specific agents such as r-PA may be associated with better outcomes compared with those after t-PA (29).

Although the full-dose FT trials with facilitated PCI are not encouraging, the Canadian Trial of Routine Angioplasty and Stenting after Fibrinolysis to Enhance Reperfusion in Acute Myocardial Infarction (TRANSFER-AMI) trial has completed enrollment in 2007 with a total of 1060 patients (30). The design of TRANSFER-AMI differs significantly from the ASSENT-4 PCI design in that all patients received standard dose TNK and then were randomized to PCI with or without GPI within six hours of fibrinolysis (pharmacoinvasive strategy) versus standard care, which could involve rescue PCI (on the basis of persistent ST-segment elevation, or continued symptoms). Because patients were only randomized in community hospitals without PCI capability, the "cross-over" is likely to be minimal. The primary end point is the 30-day composite of death, reinfarction, recurrent ischemia, new or worsening heart failure, and cardiogenic shock. Secondary end points include bleeding events, infarct size, and six-month and one-year death and reinfarction rates. The results of this study will be presented at the meeting of the American College of Cardiology in March 2008.

Trials with Streptokinase
The use of SK to facilitate reperfusion prior to PCI is associated with several challenges. First, SK TIMI grade 3 flow rates are only around 30% to 40% (11). Second, standard dose SK induces a fibrinolytic state to which adding intravenous heparin typically increases the risk of bleeding and intracranial hemorrhage (10). In general, the trials using SK have not been successful for facilitated PCI.

Early studies. The first trial to randomize patients to SK and PCI versus primary PCI was the Streptokinase and Angioplasty in Myocardial Infarction (SAMI) trial (31). Patients were randomized to full-dose SK followed by PCI versus primary PCI. A total of 122 patients were enrolled and the primary end point was left ventricular function at six months. There was no difference in the primary end point between primary PCI and facilitated PCI using SK (51% in both arms). At 24 hours, the left ventricular ejection fraction was numerically higher in the primary PCI arm (52% vs. 50%), but this difference was not statistically different. However, the transfusion rates were significantly higher in the SK and PCI arm compared with primary PCI (39% vs. 8%, $p = 0.0001$). In addition, there was significantly more CABG in the SK plus PCI arm (10.5% vs. 1.6%, $p = 0.03$), indicating a more complicated PCI procedure. This trial was performed before stents were available and patients with dissection in the IRA had to be sent to CABG unless prolonged balloon inflation could stabilize the patient.

Recent studies. The most widely used TT outside North America is SK. Thus, all the recent trials that have examined SK have been from outside the United States. The Primary Angioplasty in Patients Transferred from General Community Hospitals to Specialized PTCA Units with or without Emergency Thrombolysis (PRAGUE)-1 study (32) enrolled 300 AMI patients in Eastern Europe. Patients were randomized into three strategies: on-site SK, transfer for primary PCI, or SK during transfer for primary PCI. Patency rates (TIMI grade 2 or 3 flow) in patients pretreated with SK were higher than in patient transferred for primary PCI (47% vs. 27%), and stents were used in 79%. The composite clinical end point (death, reinfarction, or stroke at 30 days) was significantly lower in the primary PCI group compared with facilitated PCI, or SK alone (8%, 15%, 23% respectively, $p = 0.02$). Bleeding rates were significantly higher in the facilitated PCI group compared with the other two groups ($p < 0.001$), highlighting the challenges in managing peri-PCI anticoagulation and GPI use. Another study using SK in combination with GPI has also found higher bleeding rates (33). Therefore SK is not an appropriate FT for facilitated PCI strategies.

GPIs Only as a Facilitated PCI Strategy

GPI have been studied extensively for PCI in both stable and emergency clinical settings. A meta-analysis of all interventional trials evaluating abciximab in AMI has shown a 46% significant reduction in the combination of death, reinfarction, and ischemic TVR, and a nonsignificant trend toward a reduction in the combination of death or reinfarction (odds ratio 72; 95% CI, 0.49–1.05) (34). In aggregate, these studies suggest that GPI is an important adjunctive therapy for primary PCI. In some of these trials, GPI were given prior to the patient's arrival to the cardiac catheterization laboratory and therefore experience was gained with GPI in addition to aspirin and heparin as a reperfusion strategy and facilitation strategy. As a matter of fact, a meta-analysis that included six trials (931 patients) comparing early (before transfer to the cardiac catheterization laboratory) versus late (in the catheterization laboratory) administration of GPI in the setting of acute MI showed better rates of TIMI grade 3 flow at baseline angiography (20% vs. 12%, $p < 0.001$) and a nonsignificant trend toward decreased mortality in patients treated early with GPI (3.4 vs. 4.7%) (35).

GPI as a Sole Reperfusion Strategy

Abciximab has been shown to disaggregate platelets in the setting of acute IRA occlusion. The mechanism in man may involve the ability of abciximab to reduce the size of platelet aggregates and to increase fibrin exposure in platelet-rich thrombus, thereby improving endogenous fibrinolysis causing clot lysis (36,37). Although the effect is modest, several studies have now shown this effect to be time dependent; it has also been documented with small molecule GPI as shown in Figure 4 (38–43).

Abciximab. Several studies have reported the TIMI grade 3 flow rate prior to PCI in AMI. The first study by Gold et al. (38) showed an 8% TIMI grade 3 flow rate 10 minutes after abciximab administration. A subsequent study from The Netherlands

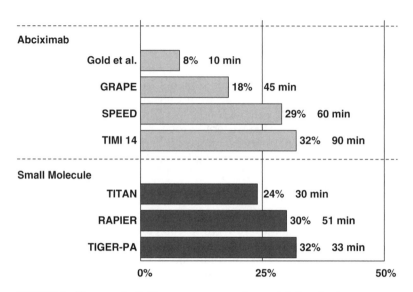

FIGURE 4 Glycoprotein IIb/IIIa receptor antagonists and dethrombosis.

showed the rate to be 18% at 45 minutes (39). TIMI 14 (40) and SPEED (41) were phase II angiographic trials that examined IRA patency with different combinations of reduced-dose FT with abciximab and also included arms with abciximab monotherapy. In these two trials, the TIMI grade 3 flow rate was 27% at 60 minutes and 32% at 90 minutes, a rate that was similar to SK alone in the angiographic substudy of the GUSTO trial (11), suggesting that GPI therapy alone would not be effective enough as reperfusion therapy, but may be considered as adjunctive to facilitated PCI. This concept was explored in the Abciximab before Direct Angioplasty and Stenting in Myocardial Infarction Regarding Acute and Long-term Follow-up (ADMIRAL) trial (42), where over 25% of patients received abciximab in the emergency department (ED) or in the ambulance compared with just prior to PCI. While this was not a prespecified end point, the ED-treated patients had a significant reduction in the 30-day composite end point of death, reinfarction and urgent TVR (2.5% vs. 21.1%, $p = 0.005$) compared with placebo-treated patients. Similar findings were observed at one year (2.5% vs. 23.7%, $p = 0.004$) as shown in Figure 5. A small randomized clinical trial with 112 patients showed similar results in terms of IRA patency rates with early administration of abciximab (44). TIMI grade 3 flow rates at baseline angiography were 16% in the early administration group (38 minutes before angiography) versus 2% in the late administration group (immediately before angiography). In addition, early abciximab administration was associated with more complete ST segment resolution post-PCI despite similar rates of post-PCI TIMI 3 flow. Another small study including 55 patients showed better TIMI 3 flow rates with early abciximab administration (29% vs. 7%, $p = 0.042$) (45).

Small molecule GPI. Three relatively small trials randomized patients to tirofiban in the ED compared with just prior to PCI in AMI. The Tirofiban Given in the Emergency Room Before Primary Angioplasty (TIGER-PA) trial (46) showed a TIMI grade 3 flow rate of 32%, with significant improvement in corrected TIMI frame count ($p = 0.05$) and myocardial tissue perfusion grade ($p = 0.001$) favoring ED administration of

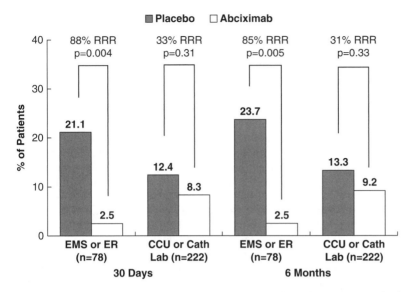

FIGURE 5 Differences in outcomes according to location of abciximab administration in the ADMIRAL trial. *Abbreviations*: ADMIRAL, Abciximab Before Direct Angioplasty and Stenting in Myocardial Infarction Regarding Acute and Long-term Follow-up; RRR, relative risk reduction; EMS, emergency medical services; ER, emergency room; CCU, coronary care unit. *Source*: Adapted from Ref. 42.

GPI. On the other hand, the Ongoing Tirofiban in Myocardial Infarction Evaluation (ON-TIME) trial (47) showed a nonsignificant difference in baseline TIMI 3 flow in patients treated with tirofiban before transfer for primary PCI compared with patients who received tirofiban at the time of PCI (19% vs. 15%, $p = 0.22$). A strategy of early tirofiban was associated with a reduction in TIMI 0 flow rates (44% vs. 59%, $p = 0.0013$) and a reduction in the presence of coronary thrombus (25% vs. 32%, $p = 0.06$), compared with the delayed tirofiban strategy. It is unclear why there is such a discrepancy between these two tirofiban trials. A third study by Cutlip et al. (48) with 58 patients showed a nonsignificant trend toward better patency with early administration (63 minutes before angiography) of tirofiban (32% vs. 20%, $p > 0.20$).

Eptifibatide has also been evaluated in two studies in AMI. The first was an observational study in 30 patients that showed a patency rate (TIMI flow grade 2–3) of 57% after double bolus eptifibatide (180 µg/kg × 2) given 51 minutes before angiography (43). This was followed by the Time to Integrilin Therapy in Acute Myocardial Infarction (TITAN) trial (49) that compared administration of eptifibatide in the ED versus in the catheterization laboratory prior to PCI in 343 patients. The primary end point was corrected TIMI frame count prior to PCI, which was found to be marginally improved among those who received eptifibatide in the ED (77 vs. 84, $p = 0.049$). Early administration was also associated with better rates of myocardial blush grade 3 (24.3% vs. 14.2%, $p = 0.026$). However, baseline TIMI 3 flow rates were not statistically significant between groups (24% vs. 19%, $p =$ NS). There was no difference in in-hospital mortality (2.3% vs. 2.1%), while there was a trend toward less congestive heart failure favoring the ED eptifibatide arm (2.9% vs. 7.1%, $p = 0.08$). Thus, the data appears to be more robust with abciximab as opposed to the small molecule GPI in establishing reperfusion in AMI prior to PCI.

Combination Therapy with Reduced FT Plus GPI
as a Facilitation Strategy

The combination of reduced dose FT with full-dose GPI has undergone extensive evaluation as a reperfusion strategy in AMI. A number of dose-ranging trials were followed by the large GUSTO-V trial (50) that examined 30-day mortality in over 16,000 patients in AMI. Patients were randomized to half-dose r-PA with standard dose abciximab or standard r-PA alone. At 30 days, the mortality was 5.6% in the combination arm versus 5.9% in the r-PA alone arm ($p = 0.43$). By one year, this difference had narrowed to become identical in both arms (8.4%) (51). In the elderly (age > 75), there was an absolute 1% increase in intracranial hemorrhage in the combination arm compared with the r-PA alone arm. While the results with combination therapy were disappointing, a few trials have explored the combination therapy as a facilitation strategy.

The Bavarian Reperfusion Alternatives Evaluation (BRAVE) trial (52) randomized 253 patients within 12 hours of symptom onset. Patients were randomized to combination therapy (abciximab + r-PA) versus abciximab both given in the ED. The combination therapy patients had better TIMI grade 3 flow prior to PCI (40% vs. 18%, $p = 0.001$) compared with the abciximab alone arm. There was also a trend toward more major bleeding in the combination arm (5.6% vs. 1.6%, $p = 0.16$). The primary end point was SPECT infarct size measured at 5 to 10 days after admission to hospital. There was no difference in left ventricular infarct size between the two groups (13.0% vs. 11.5%, $p = 0.81$). The composite of death, reinfarction, or stroke was also similar (3.2% vs. 1.6%).

The Addressing the Value of Facilitated Angioplasty After Combination Therapy or Eptifibatide Monotherapy in Acute Myocardial Infarction (ADVANCE-MI) trial (53), using a similar trial design with TNK and eptifibatide, was stopped after 146 out of 5640 patients were enrolled because of slow enrollment rates. The primary end point was death or new or worsening heart failure. The patients randomized to the combination arm (double bolus eptifibatide and half-dose TNK) had significantly higher patency rates (TIMI grade 2 or 3 flow) at pre-PCI angiogram compared with eptifibatide alone (67% vs. 33%, $p < 0.001$). However, there was a trend toward higher event rates (10% vs. 3%, $p = 0.09$) and major bleeding rates (20% vs. 10%, $p = 0.09$).

Prehospital combination therapy prior to PCI has also been explored in two trials. A trial from Germany administered combination therapy (r-PA and abciximab) in the prehospital setting with subsequent randomization to PCI versus conservative care (54). The primary end point was cardiac MRI measurement of infarct size, which was lower in the facilitated PCI arm (5.3% of the left ventricle vs. 10.5%, $p = 0.001$) compared with the combination therapy alone arm. The clinical outcomes also favored facilitated PCI treated patients with a composite outcome of 15% vs. 25% ($p = 0.1$), while bleeding surprisingly was in a similar direction (11.3% vs. 20.5%, $p = 0.1$). In aggregate, these trials have shown promising reperfusion rates with combination therapy for facilitated PCI, but the clinical event rates have trended to more harm.

Because of the plethora of data, mostly from small underpowered trials, a couple of meta-analyses have tried to provide a more conclusive answer about the role of facilitated PCI in clinical practice. A large meta-analysis (55) including 17 trials with different facilitation strategies showed higher rates of baseline TIMI 3 flow with the facilitated approach (37% vs. 15%, $p = 0.0001$), but an increase in the rates of death (5% vs. 3%, $p = 0.04$), nonfatal reinfarction (3% vs. 2%, $p = 0.006$), and TVR (4% vs. 1%, $p = 0.01$). Safety was also a concern with facilitated

PCI with higher rates of major bleeding (7% vs. 5%, $p = 0.01$) and hemorrhagic stroke (0.7% vs. 0.1%, $p = 0.0014$). Of note, this meta-analysis included studies that used fibrin- and non-fibrin-specific FT, some studies with obsolete interventional technologies, including a study performed almost two decades ago when the safety of antithrombotic therapies were not clearly understood. Moreover, the majority of the studies included approximately 100 patients per arm or less, therefore the results were driven by the ASSENT-4 PCI trial that had limitations in its design and conduct as mentioned above. In fact, the detrimental effect of facilitated PCI is most noticeable in the trials that included FT in its initial pharmacological approach. A second meta-analysis (56) with a more stringent selection of trials was designed to specifically examine combined FT and GPI versus GPI alone as facilitation strategy. Only four trials with a total of 725 patients were pooled. These trials were more homogeneous, using fibrin-specific FT with contemporary interventional technology. Major bleeding was more frequent with strategies that included FT (9.5% vs. 4.7%, $p = 0.007$), but there were no significant differences in 30-day mortality and reinfarction rates.

Two larger trials have recently been reported and provide more insight on the role of facilitated PCI in the management of myocardial infarction.

The Combined Abciximab Reteplase Stent Study in Acute Myocardial Infarction (CARESS in AMI) trial (57) randomized 600 high-risk MI patients in European hospitals without PCI capability to routine transfer for facilitated PCI versus transfer only for rescue PCI (36% of patients) for persistent ST segment elevation 90 minutes after initial treatment with abciximab and half-dose r-PA. The primary end point of 30-day death, reinfarction, and refractory ischemia occurred in 4.1% of the immediate PCI group versus 11.1% of the rescue PCI group [OR 0.34 (0.17–0.68); $p = 0.001$]. The main difference was in refractory ischemia (0.7% vs. 5.0%), but not in death (3.1% vs. 4.4%) or reinfarction (0.3% vs. 1.7%). In terms of safety, the facilitated PCI group had a higher incidence of bleeding (12.2% vs. 7.4%; $p = 0.3$), including trends toward more stroke (1.4% vs. 0.7%), intracerebral bleeding (4.0% vs. 1.0%), and transfusions (3.7% vs. 2.0%).

The Facilitated Intervention with Enhanced Reperfusion Speed to Stop Events (FINESSE) trial (58) was a placebo-controlled double-blind study designed to recruit 3000 patients, but was terminated after enrollment of 2452 patients with AMI because of slow recruitment. Patients were randomized 1:1:1 to primary PCI with abciximab administration in the catheterization laboratory, early abciximab administration alone followed by PCI, and combination therapy (half-dose r-PA plus abciximab). The rates of TIMI 3 flow at baseline angiography were 13%, 15%, and 36%, respectively. Rates of post-PCI TIMI 3 flow were approximately 90% in the three treatment arms. The 90-day composite end point of death, cardiogenic shock, late ventricular fibrillation (>48 hours), and admission for heart failure occurred in 10.7%, 10.5%, 9.8%, respectively, a statistically insignificant difference. All cause mortality rates were 4.5%, 5.5%, and 5.2%, respectively. Bleeding rates were statistically increased in the combination group. TIMI minor or major bleeding occurred in 6.9%, 10.1%, and 14.5% of patients in each group respectively.

CONCLUSIONS

Facilitated PCI is a simple and attractive treatment strategy that has the potential to improve early reperfusion in many patients, particularly those patients seen and treated in community hospitals (59) (Fig. 6). Indeed, the angiographic outcomes

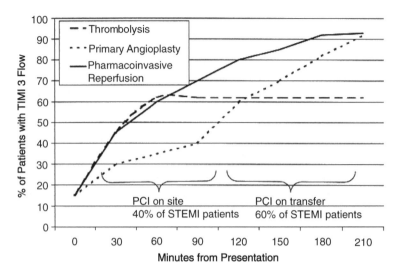

FIGURE 6   Combining optimal pharmacological reperfusion with PCI maximizes the ability to obtain normal flow in the IRA. *Abbreviation*: IRA, infarct-related artery. *Source*: From Ref. 59.

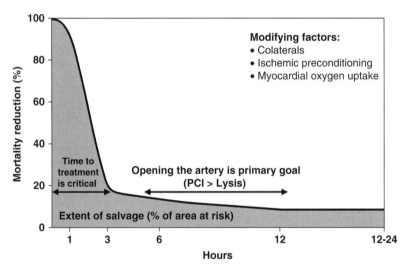

FIGURE 7   Relationship between mortality reduction and extent of salvage. *Source*: Adapted from Ref. 60.

have been improved in the majority of trials. Rather surprisingly, the clinical outcomes have not followed the path predicted by the reperfusion rates. This may be due to low event rates, indicating that the majority of trials were underpowered. Another explanation has been put forward by Gersh and colleagues (60), who suggested that the relationship between myocardial salvage and reduction in mortality is quite complex and is dependent on the duration of symptoms with maximal myocardial salvage only when reperfusion therapy can be administered within two to three hours of symptom onset (Fig. 7). Using this model, a cardiologist could now find exactly where each patient is on this curve and apply a tailored reperfusion therapy at each level to optimize salvage and reduce mortality. Thus, the benefit of facilitated PCI has been difficult to prove in the setting of AMI.

Results to date suggest that the only current viable facilitation strategy is to use early GPI therapy either in the ED or at first medical contact with the patient. At least this strategy appears safe and may be associated with some clinical benefits (35). There is increasing evidence indicating that bleeding outcomes may be as important as ischemic outcomes in determining the prognosis of MI patients (61). Therefore, the individual bleeding risk has to be evaluated at the time of deciding on the use of a facilitated strategy. Another aspect to consider is the increased ability of our health systems to deliver rapid primary PCI that to some extent has negated the need for a strategy to combine early pharmacological therapy with PCI. Although rapid primary PCI will help thousands of patients each year, there are still a great majority of patients that could benefit from the combined approach, if only we could find the right tailored therapy for those individuals.

REFERENCES

1. The GUSTO Angiographic Investigators. The effects of tissue plasminogen activator, streptokinase, or both on coronary-artery patency, ventricular function, and survival after acute myocardial infarction. N Engl J Med 1993; 329:1615–1622.
2. Herrmann HC, Moliterno DJ, Ohman EM, et al. Facilitation of early percutaneous coronary intervention after reteplase with or without abciximab in acute myocardial infarction: results from the SPEED (GUSTO-4 Pilot) Trial. J Am Coll Cardiol 2000; 36:1489–1496.
3. Ross AM, Coyne KS, Reiner JS, et al. A randomized trial comparing primary angioplasty with a strategy of short-acting thrombolysis and immediate planned rescue angioplasty in acute myocardial infarction: the PACT trial. PACT investigators. Plasminogen-activator Angioplasty Compatibility Trial. J Am Coll Cardiol 1999; 34:1954–1962.
4. Ross AM, Coyne KS, Reiner JS, et al. Very early PTCA of infarct arteries with TIMI 3 flow is associated with improved clinical outcomes. J Am Coll Cardiol 2000; 35(2 suppl A):403 (abstr).
5. Indications for fibrinolytic therapy in suspected acute myocardial infarction: collaborative overview of early mortality and major morbidity results from all randomised trials of more than 1000 patients. Fibrinolytic Therapy Trialists' (FTT) Collaborative Group. Lancet 1994; 343:311–322.
6. De Luca G, Suryapranata H, Ottervanger JP, et al. Time delay to treatment and mortality in primary angioplasty for acute myocardial infarction: every minute of delay counts. Circulation 2004; 109:1223–1225.
7. Cannon CP, Gibson CM, Lambrew CT, et al. Relationship of symptom-onset-to-balloon time and door-to-balloon time with mortality in patients undergoing angioplasty for acute myocardial infarction. JAMA 2000; 283:2941–2947.
8. Nallamothu BK, Bates ER. Percutaneous coronary intervention versus fibrinolytic therapy in acute myocardial infarction: is timing (almost) everything? Am J Cardiol 2003; 92:824–826.
9. Angeja BG, Gibson CM, Chin R, et al. Predictors of door-to-balloon delay in primary angioplasty. Am J Cardiol 2002; 89:1156–1161.
10. An international randomized trial comparing four thrombolytic strategies for acute myocardial infarction. The GUSTO Investigators. N Engl J Med 1993; 329:673–682.
11. Ross AM, Coyne KS, Moreyra E, et al. Extended mortality benefit of early postinfarction reperfusion. GUSTO-I Angiographic Investigators. Global Utilization of Streptokinase and Tissue Plasminogen Activator for Occluded Coronary Arteries Trial. Circulation 1998; 97:1549–1556.
12. Ohman EM, Califf RM, Topol EJ, et al. Consequences of reocclusion after successful reperfusion therapy in acute myocardial infarction. TAMI Study Group. Circulation 1990; 82:781–791.

13. Gibson CM, Murphy SA, Rizzo MJ, et al. Relationship between TIMI frame count and clinical outcomes after thrombolytic administration. Thrombolysis in Myocardial Infarction (TIMI) Study Group. Circulation 1999; 99:1945–1950.
14. Stone GW, Cox D, Garcia E, et al. Normal flow (TIMI-3) before mechanical reperfusion therapy is an independent determinant of survival in acute myocardial infarction: analysis from the primary angioplasty in myocardial infarction trials. Circulation 2001; 104:636–641.
15. De Luca G, Ernst N, Zijlstra F, et al. Preprocedural TIMI flow and mortality in patients with acute myocardial infarction treated by primary angioplasty. J Am Coll Cardiol 2004; 43:1363–1367.
16. Gibson CM, Cannon CP, Murphy SA, et al. Relationship of TIMI myocardial perfusion grade to mortality after administration of thrombolytic drugs. Circulation 2000; 101:125–130.
17. Gibson CM, Cannon CP, Murphy SA, et al. Relationship of the TIMI myocardial perfusion grades, flow grades, frame count, and percutaneous coronary intervention to long-term outcomes after thrombolytic administration in acute myocardial infarction. Circulation 2002; 105:1909–1913.
18. Immediate vs delayed catheterization and angioplasty following thrombolytic therapy for acute myocardial infarction. TIMI II A results. The TIMI Research Group. JAMA 1988; 260:2849–2858.
19. Topol EJ, Califf RM, George BS, et al. A randomized trial of immediate versus delayed elective angioplasty after intravenous tissue plasminogen activator in acute myocardial infarction. N Engl J Med 1987; 317:581–588.
20. Simoons ML, Arnold AE, Betriu A, et al. Thrombolysis with tissue plasminogen activator in acute myocardial infarction: no additional benefit from immediate percutaneous coronary angioplasty. Lancet 1988; 1:197–203.
21. Gibson CM. Primary angioplasty, rescue angioplasty, and new devices. In: Hennekens CH, ed. Clinical Trials in Cardiovascular Disease: A Companion to Braunwald's Heart Disease. Philadelphia, PA: WB Saunders Co, 1999:185–197.
22. Vermeer F, Oude Ophuis AJ, vd Berg EJ, et al. Prospective randomised comparison between thrombolysis, rescue PTCA, and primary PTCA in patients with extensive myocardial infarction admitted to a hospital without PTCA facilities: a safety and feasibility study. Heart 1999; 82:426–431.
23. Scheller B, Hennen B, Hammer B, et al. Beneficial effects of immediate stenting after thrombolysis in acute myocardial infarction. J Am Coll Cardiol 2003; 42:634–641.
24. Fernandez-Aviles F, Alonso JJ, Castro-Beiras A, et al. Routine invasive strategy within 24 hours of thrombolysis versus ischaemia-guided conservative approach for acute myocardial infarction with ST-segment elevation (GRACIA-1): a randomised controlled trial. Lancet 2004; 364:1045–1053.
25. Fernandez-Aviles F, Alonso JJ, Pena G, et al. Primary angioplasty vs. early routine postfibrinolysis angioplasty for acute myocardial infarction with ST-segment elevation: the GRACIA-2 non-inferiority, randomized, controlled trial. Eur Heart J 2007; 28:949–960.
26. Le May MR, Wells GA, Labinaz M, et al. Combined angioplasty and pharmacological intervention versus thrombolysis alone in acute myocardial infarction (CAPITAL AMI study). J Am Coll Cardiol 2005; 46:417–424.
27. Armstrong PW. A comparison of pharmacologic therapy with/without timely coronary intervention vs. primary percutaneous intervention early after ST-elevation myocardial infarction: the WEST (Which Early ST-elevation myocardial infarction Therapy) study. Eur Heart J 2006; 27:1530–1538.
28. Primary versus tenecteplase-facilitated percutaneous coronary intervention in patients with ST-segment elevation acute myocardial infarction (ASSENT-4 PCI): randomised trial. Lancet 2006; 367:569–578.
29. Miller JM, Smalling R, Ohman EM, et al. Effectiveness of early coronary angioplasty and abciximab for failed thrombolysis (reteplase or alteplase) during acute myocardial infarction (results from the GUSTO-III trial). Global Use of Strategies To Open occluded coronary arteries. Am J Cardiol 1999; 84:779–784.
30. Cantor WJ, Fitchett D, Borgundvaag B, et al. Rationale and design of the Trial of Routine ANgioplasty and Stenting After Fibrinolysis to Enhance Reperfusion in Acute Myocardial Infarction (TRANSFER-AMI). Am Heart J 2008; 155:19–25.

31. O'Neill WW, Weintraub R, Grines CL, et al. A prospective, placebo-controlled, randomized trial of intravenous streptokinase and angioplasty versus lone angioplasty therapy of acute myocardial infarction. Circulation 1992; 86:1710–1717.
32. Widimsky P, Groch L, Zelizko M, et al. Multicentre randomized trial comparing transport to primary angioplasty vs immediate thrombolysis vs combined strategy for patients with acute myocardial infarction presenting to a community hospital without a catheterization laboratory. The PRAGUE study. Eur Heart J 2000; 21:823–831.
33. Ronner E, van Kesteren HA, Zijnen P, et al. Safety and efficacy of eptifibatide vs placebo in patients receiving thrombolytic therapy with streptokinase for acute myocardial infarction. A phase II dose escalation, randomized, double-blind study. Eur Heart J 2000; 21:1530–1536.
34. Kandzari DE, Hasselblad V, Tcheng JE, et al. Improved clinical outcomes with abciximab therapy in acute myocardial infarction: a systematic overview of randomized clinical trials. Am Heart J 2004; 147:457–462.
35. Montalescot G, Borentain M, Payot L, et al. Early vs late administration of glycoprotein IIb/IIIa inhibitors in primary percutaneous coronary intervention of acute ST-segment elevation myocardial infarction: a meta-analysis. JAMA 2004; 292:362–366.
36. Collet JP, Montalescot G, Lesty C, et al. Disaggregation of in vitro preformed platelet-rich clots by abciximab increases fibrin exposure and promotes fibrinolysis. Arterioscler Thromb Vasc Biol 2001; 21:142–148.
37. Collet JP, Montalescot G, Lesty C, et al. Effects of abciximab on the architecture of platelet-rich clots in patients with acute myocardial infarction undergoing primary coronary intervention. Circulation 2001; 103:2328–2331.
38. Gold HK, Garabedian HD, Dinsmore RE, et al. Restoration of coronary flow in myocardial infarction by intravenous chimeric 7E3 antibody without exogenous plasminogen activators. Observations in animals and humans. Circulation 1997; 95:1755–1759.
39. van den Merkhof LF, Zijlstra F, Olsson H, et al. Abciximab in the treatment of acute myocardial infarction eligible for primary percutaneous transluminal coronary angioplasty. Results of the Glycoprotein Receptor Antagonist Patency Evaluation (GRAPE) pilot study. J Am Coll Cardiol 1999; 33:1528–1532.
40. Trial of abciximab with and without low-dose reteplase for acute myocardial infarction. Strategies for Patency Enhancement in the Emergency Department (SPEED) Group. Circulation 2000; 101:2788–2794.
41. de Lemos JA, Antman EM, Gibson CM, et al. Abciximab improves both epicardial flow and myocardial reperfusion in ST-elevation myocardial infarction. Observations from the TIMI 14 trial. Circulation 2000; 101:239–243.
42. Montalescot G, Barragan P, Wittenberg O, et al. Platelet glycoprotein IIb/IIIa inhibition with coronary stenting for acute myocardial infarction. N Engl J Med 2001; 344:1895–1903.
43. Cutlip DE, Cove CJ, Irons D, et al. Emergency room administration of eptifibatide before primary angioplasty for ST elevation acute myocardial infarction and its effect on baseline coronary flow and procedure outcomes. Am J Cardiol 2001; 88:A6, 62–64.
44. Zorman S, Zorman D, Noc M. Effects of abciximab pretreatment in patients with acute myocardial infarction undergoing primary angioplasty. Am J Cardiol 2002; 90:533–536.
45. Gyongyosi M, Domanovits H, Benzer W, et al. Use of abciximab prior to primary angioplasty in STEMI results in early recanalization of the infarct-related artery and improved myocardial tissue reperfusion - results of the Austrian multi-centre randomized ReoPro-BRIDGING Study. Eur Heart J 2004; 25:2125–2133.
46. Lee DP, Herity NA, Hiatt BL, et al. Adjunctive platelet glycoprotein IIb/IIIa receptor inhibition with tirofiban before primary angioplasty improves angiographic outcomes: results of the TIrofiban Given in the Emergency Room before Primary Angioplasty (TIGER-PA) pilot trial. Circulation 2003; 107:1497–1501.
47. van't Hof AW, Ernst N, de Boer MJ, et al. Facilitation of primary coronary angioplasty by early start of a glycoprotein 2b/3a inhibitor: results of the ongoing tirofiban in myocardial infarction evaluation (On-TIME) trial. Eur Heart J 2004; 25:837–846.
48. Cutlip DE, Ricciardi MJ, Ling FS, et al. Effect of tirofiban before primary angioplasty on initial coronary flow and early ST-segment resolution in patients with acute myocardial infarction. Am J Cardiol 2003; 92:977–980.

49. Gibson CM, Kirtane AJ, Murphy SA, et al. Early initiation of eptifibatide in the emergency department before primary percutaneous coronary intervention for ST-segment elevation myocardial infarction: results of the Time to Integrilin Therapy in Acute Myocardial Infarction (TITAN)-TIMI 34 trial. Am Heart J 2006; 152:668–675.
50. Topol EJ. Reperfusion therapy for acute myocardial infarction with fibrinolytic therapy or combination reduced fibrinolytic therapy and platelet glycoprotein IIb/IIIa inhibition: the GUSTO V randomised trial. Lancet 2001; 357:1905–1914.
51. Lincoff AM, Califf RM, Van de Werf F, et al. Mortality at 1 year with combination platelet glycoprotein IIb/IIIa inhibition and reduced-dose fibrinolytic therapy vs conventional fibrinolytic therapy for acute myocardial infarction: GUSTO V randomized trial. JAMA 2002; 288:2130–2135.
52. Kastrati A, Mehilli J, Schlotterbeck K, et al. Early administration of reteplase plus abciximab vs abciximab alone in patients with acute myocardial infarction referred for percutaneous coronary intervention: a randomized controlled trial. JAMA 2004; 291: 947–954.
53. Facilitated percutaneous coronary intervention for acute ST-segment elevation myocardial infarction: results from the prematurely terminated ADdressing the Value of facilitated ANgioplasty after Combination therapy or Eptifibatide monotherapy in acute Myocardial Infarction (ADVANCE MI) trial. Am Heart J 2005; 150:116–122.
54. Thiele H, Engelmann L, Elsner K, et al. Comparison of pre-hospital combination-fibrinolysis plus conventional care with pre-hospital combination-fibrinolysis plus facilitated percutaneous coronary intervention in acute myocardial infarction. Eur Heart J 2005; 26:1956–1963.
55. Keeley EC, Boura JA, Grines CL. Comparison of primary and facilitated percutaneous coronary interventions for ST-elevation myocardial infarction: quantitative review of randomised trials. Lancet 2006; 367:579–588.
56. Sinno MC, Khanal S, Al-Mallah MH, et al. The efficacy and safety of combination glycoprotein IIbIIIa inhibitors and reduced-dose thrombolytic therapy-facilitated percutaneous coronary intervention for ST-elevation myocardial infarction: a meta-analysis of randomized clinical trials. Am Heart J 2007; 153:579–586.
57. Di Mario C, on behalf of the CARESS in MI Investigators. Combined abciximab reteplase stent study in acute myocardial infarction. Presented at: European Congress of Cardiology, 2007; Vienna.
58. Ellis SG, on behalf of the FINESS Investigators. Facilitated intervention with enhanced reperfusion speed to stop events. Presented at: European Congress of Cardiology, 2007; Vienna.
59. Dauerman HL, Sobel BE. Synergistic treatment of ST-segment elevation myocardial infarction with pharmacoinvasive recanalization. J Am Coll Cardiol 2003; 42:646–651.
60. Gersh BJ, Stone GW, White HD, et al. Pharmacological facilitation of primary percutaneous coronary intervention for acute myocardial infarction: is the slope of the curve the shape of the future? JAMA 2005; 293:979–986.
61. Rao SV, Jollis JG, Harrington RA, et al. Relationship of blood transfusion and clinical outcomes in patients with acute coronary syndromes. JAMA 2004; 292:1555–1562.
62. DeLuca G, Suryapranata H, Ottervanger JP, et al. Time delay to treatment and mortality in primary angioplasty for acute myocardial infarction. Circulation 2004; 109:1223–1225.

10 Primary PCI with Off-Site Cardiac Surgery Backup

Thomas P. Wharton
Section of Cardiology and Cardiac Catheterization Laboratory,
Exeter Hospital, Exeter, New Hampshire, U.S.A.

INTRODUCTION

Primary percutaneous coronary intervention (PCI) has become the standard of care for reperfusion therapy in patients with ST-elevation myocardial infarction (STEMI) when delivered rapidly and expertly. However, this standard is not being met for a majority of the population in the United States. Data from the National Registries of Myocardial Infarction (NRMI) indicate that only 20% of patients with STEMI are treated with primary PCI (1,2). Over one-third of patients with STEMI still do not receive any type of reperfusion therapy. The lack of widespread and rapid delivery of primary PCI into the community represents an urgent public health problem.

REPERFUSION OPTIONS FOR PATIENTS WITH STEMI PRESENTING TO COMMUNITY HOSPITALS

Most patients with STEMI present to community hospitals that do not have cardiac surgery programs (3) and seldom provide primary PCI. Many states still have regulations that restrict PCI to surgical centers, including emergent procedures for STEMI. Patients that present to hospitals without PCI have two reperfusion options: (1) fibrinolytic therapy, now demonstrated to be suboptimal even when administered before hospital arrival, when transfer for immediate and expert PCI is available (4,5), or (2) rapid transfer or prehospital ambulance triage to a primary PCI center for emergent intervention.

Randomized trials from Denmark (6) and Prague (7) compared local fibrinolytic therapy to rapid transfer for primary PCI for patients with acute STEMI. (It is notable that two of the seven PCI centers in the Prague study did not have cardiac surgery capability.) These trials, and a recent meta-analysis that included these and similar trials (8), demonstrated superior outcomes in patients that were transferred compared with those treated locally with fibrinolytic therapy.

Early rapid transfer and pre-hospital ambulance triage to PCI centers have been appropriately advocated to meet the need to increase access to primary PCI (9), but there are many limitations inherent in these strategies. Their usefulness is generally limited to urban areas, since the transport time must be short. Air transport is not always a reliable option due to weather. Pre-hospital ambulance triage to PCI centers is also not an option in the 50% of STEMI patients that do not arrive by ambulance (10). Liability issues associated with interhospital transport or triage of unstable patients with AMI can be a deterrent, as can extraneous pressures such as institutional pride and fear of loss of reimbursement.

More importantly, even when effective rapid transport is available, some STEMI patients are too unstable to be sent from one hospital to another. In the Denmark and

Prague trials, 4% and 1% of patients, respectively, were too unstable to travel and some of these patients died; deaths during transfer also occurred (6,7). Patients too unstable to travel are the ones at highest risk and thus might be among those expected to benefit the most if primary PCI were available at the point of first presentation. Patients with cardiogenic shock are at particular risk during interhospital transfer; rapid primary PCI can be lifesaving in this group. The Should We Emergently Revascularize Occluded Coronaries for Cardiogenic Shock (SHOCK) study (11) demonstrated that the group randomized to mechanical revascularization within the first six hours of infarction had the greatest survival advantage of all subgroups.

The most important limitation of interhospital transfer for PCI is that of delay in time to reperfusion. Although pilot studies of the strategies of rapid transfer for PCI in Boston, Durham, and Minneapolis have shown promising initial results (12–14), and although nearly 80% of the U.S. population lives within 60 minutes of a PCI hospital (15), recent data from NRMI unfortunately show that door-to-balloon times in the United States are still 71 minutes longer for patients transferred for primary PCI than for those receiving PCI at the point of first presentation (16). Since the transfer delay in NRMI was approximately one hour greater than that in the Denmark and Prague studies, the data from these randomized trials that show superiority of transfer for PCI over local fibrinolytic therapy may not be applicable to most hospitals in the United States (17).

Door-to-balloon times of 2.5 to 3 hours, often seen in patients transferred for PCI in the United States, are associated with a 60% increase in mortality compared to times of less than two hours (18). Only 15% of patients transferred for primary PCI in the NRMI registries received it even within 120 minutes (19). In striking contrast, eight studies of primary PCI at hospitals with off-site surgery backup, which include over 5000 patients, indicate that primary PCI at such centers can be performed within 80 to 110 minutes of first presentation (20–28); no study of primary PCI with off-site backup has door-to-balloon times of longer than 110 minutes.

One other potential limitation should also be considered—the currently active primary PCI centers, which also perform a heavy caseload of nonemergent procedures, might have difficulty in accommodating the extra caseload if primary PCI were to be delivered to 80% to 90% instead of 20%, of patients with acute STEMI. The load will continue to increase, since the volume of patients with STEMI can be expected to increase progressively due to the aging of population and the currently accelerating epidemics of obesity and diabetes.

THE EMERGING ROLE OF LOCAL PCI CENTERS WITH OFF-SITE SURGERY BACKUP

To increase access to primary PCI for more of the population, there is an urgent need for more centers that can provide expert primary PCI in broader geographical regions. For reasons already discussed, the options of interhospital transfer and pre-hospital ambulance triage for primary PCI are not sufficient solutions for the problem of providing rapid and universal access. Increasing the number of STEMI centers that are capable of providing primary PCI can reduce the risk and delay, and even the barrier, of transport for PCI. This does not imply a need for more cardiac surgery centers; indeed the volume of cardiac surgery procedures has plateaued and may be declining. Uncoupling PCI programs from the requirement for on-site cardiac surgery should reduce the demand for opening new low-volume cardiac surgery programs merely to support PCI programs.

Approximately 600 hospitals have diagnostic cardiac catheterization without cardiac surgery (29); of these, only relatively few provide primary PCI. But many of the rest may have the potential to launch primary PCI programs if they can meet rigorous requirements, which include experienced interventionalists and support personnel, equipment and supplies, and off-site backup support from a surgery center.

REQUIREMENTS FOR PRIMARY PCI PROGRAMS WITH OFF-SITE SURGERY BACKUP

The American College of Cardiology (ACC)/American Heart Association (AHA)/ Society for Cardiovascular Angiography and Interventions (SCAI) PCI and ACC/ AHA STEMI Guidelines (30,31) have affirmed rigorous criteria for operators and institutions that seek to establish primary PCI programs with off-site surgery backup (based on criteria originally published from our institution (21)). Tables 1 and 2 show our latest adaptation of these criteria. Basic requirements include experienced high-volume interventionalists on staff who routinely also perform nonemergent PCI, a cath lab staff experienced in coronary intervention, an on-call system to provide 24/7/365 coverage, a full array of equipment including aspiration thrombectomy and distal protection devices, covered stents, an intra-aortic balloon pump, strict adherence to rigorous clinical and angiographic selection criteria for the performance of primary PCI and for emergency transfer to a tertiary surgery center (Table 2), and established protocols and agreements to accomplish emergency transfers expeditiously (Table 3).

A critical hospital-wide pathway for primary PCI from pre-hospital contact through to hospital discharge (32), such as the one shown in Figure 1, can help assure rapid door-to-balloon times, appropriate in-hospital management, and optimal outcomes. It is equally important to monitor outcomes rigorously and initiate continuous quality improvement measures (33–35). We strongly advocate that all hospitals providing PCI participate in the ACC National Cardiovascular Data Registry (ACC-NCDR) and enlist a dedicated data and quality coordinator.

TABLE 1 Operator and Institutional Criteria for Primary PCI Programs at Hospitals With Off-Site Cardiac Surgery Backup

1. Experienced high-volume interventionalists
2. Experienced nursing and technical CCL staff with training in interventional laboratories
3. Well-equipped and well-stocked CCL, with IABP support on site
4. Experienced CCU nursing staff, comfortable with invasive hemodynamic monitoring and IABP management
5. Formalized written protocols and agreements for emergency transfer of patients to the nearest cardiac surgical facility (Table 3)
6. Full support from hospital administration in fulfilling the above institutional requirements
7. Rigorous clinical and angiographic selection criteria for PCI and for emergency transfer (Table 2)
8. Performance of primary PCI as the treatment of first choice for STEMI to ensure streamlined care paths and increased case volumes
9. Primary PCI coverage on a 24-hour, 7-day per week basis
10. Performance of at least 3 to 4 primary PCI procedures per month
11. Ongoing outcomes analysis and formalized periodic case review

Abbreviations: CABG, coronary artery bypass graft; CCL, cardiac catheterization laboratory; CCU, cardiac care unit; IABP, intra-aortic balloon pump; PCI, percutaneous coronary intervention; STEMI, ST-segment acute myocardial infarction.
Source: Adapted from Ref. 21.

TABLE 2 Selection for Primary PCI and Emergency Aortocoronary Bypass Surgery at Hospitals With Off-Site Cardiac Surgery Backup

Avoid intervention in

- Patients with severe left main disease proximal to infarct-related lesion
- Extremely long or angulated target lesions with TIMI grade 3 flow at high-risk for PCI failure
- Lesions in other than the infarct artery (unless they appeared to be flow limiting in patients with hemodynamic instability or ongoing symptoms)
- Lesions with TIMI grade 3 flow that are not amenable to stenting in patients with left-main or three-vessel disease who will require coronary bypass surgery

Transfer emergently for coronary bypass surgery

- Patients with high-grade residual left main or three-vessel coronary disease and clinical or hemodynamic instability after angioplasty of occluded vessels when appropriate and preferably with intra-aortic balloon pump support
- Patients with failed or unstable PCI result and ongoing ischemia, with intra-aortic balloon pump support during transfer

Abbreviations: PCI, percutaneous coronary intervention; TIMI, thrombolysis in myocardial infarction.
Source: Adapted from Ref. 21.

TABLE 3 Elements of a Cardiac Transfer Agreement and Protocol for Primary Angioplasty Programs at Hospitals With Off-Site Cardiac Surgery Backup: A Proven Plan for Rapid Access to Cardiac Surgery

1. Cardiologist will establish a good working relationship with cardiac surgeons at receiving facility[a].
2. Cardiac surgeons from referral cardiac surgery hospital will formally agree to provide cardiac surgery back up for urgent and emergent cases at all hours.
3. Surgeon will assure that the patient will be accepted for services based on factors such as medical condition, capacity of surgeons to provide services at the time of request, and availability of facility and staff resources.
4. Cardiologist will review with surgeon the potential needs and risks of the patient being transferred for emergency care.
5. Referring facility will establish a rigorous medical protocol for the safe and rapid transfer of patients to receiving cardiac surgery hospital.
6. EMS ambulance supplier will be formally contracted to be available on-site within 15–20 minutes of a call on a 24-hour, 7-day per week basis.
7. The hospital's transport team will include critical care nurses, paramedics and CCL personnel with IABP expertise. All members of the team should be ACLS certified.
8. EMS ambulance provider will have available and/or be able to accommodate the following: portable cardiac ECG and pressure monitoring, sufficient O_2 supply, suction, multiple drips, ACLS drugs, resuscitation equipment, defibrillator, and IABP.
9. Transferring physician will obtain consent from patient or appropriate consenting party.
10. Review of transferred patients will be ongoing and include feedback from referring facility regarding problems in transfer process, teaching opportunities through catheterization conferences, and periodic review of the outcomes of the surgical program with special emphasis on outcomes of transferred patients.
11. Cardiac surgeon will be credentialed to visit patients and families at referring hospital to review medical options if time allows.
12. Hospital administrations from both referring and accepting facilities will endorse the transfer agreement.

[a]Cardiologists must collaborate with their cardiac surgeons to ensure a seamless transition of care from the primary hospital to the surgical center. Measures to foster a good working relationship include the surgeon's attendance at cardiac catheterization conferences and becoming credentialed at the referring hospital. This will enable bedside consultation on nonemergent inpatients with review of treatment options with cardiologists, patients and families, and encourage frequent personal interaction between the surgeon and the cardiologist. A very important element of this relationship will also include outcomes feedback from the surgeon to the referring cardiologist.
Abbreviations: ACLS, advanced cardiac life support; CCL, cardiac catheterization laboratory; ECG, electrocardiogram; EMS, emergency medical services; IABP, intra-aortic balloon pump.
Source: From Exeter Hospital. Developed by Wharton TP, Sinclair N, Hiett D, and Cresta D, Exeter Hospital, Exeter, NH.

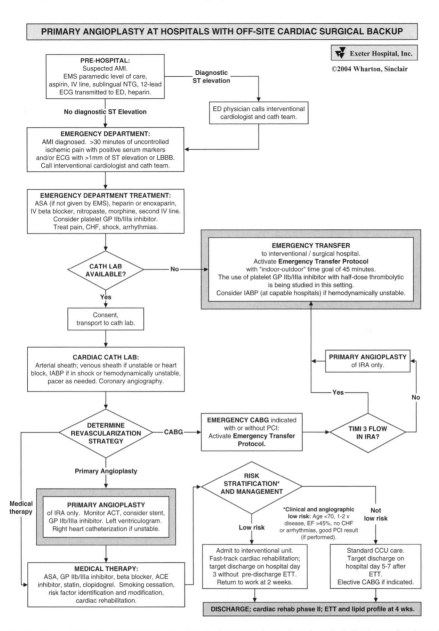

FIGURE 1 Critical pathway from pre-hospital contact through to hospital discharge for the primary angioplasty program at Exeter Hospital, Exeter, New Hampshire, which is a community hospital with off-site cardiac surgery backup. *Abbreviations*: ACE, angiotensin converting enzyme; ACT, activated clotting time; AMI, acute myocardial infarction; ASA, aspirin; BP, blood pressure; CABG, coronary artery bypass graft; CCU, cardiac care unit; CHF, congestive heart failure; ED, emergency department; EF, ejection fraction; ECG, electrocardiogram; EMS, emergency medical services; ETT, exercise tolerance test; GP, glycoprotein; IABP, intra-aortic balloon pump; IRA, infarct-related artery; IV, intravenous; LBBB, left bundle branch block; NTG, nitroglycerin; PCI, percutaneous coronary intervention; TIMI, thrombolysis in myocardial infarction. *Source*: From Ref. 32. Wharton TP and Sinclair N.

It is imperative to provide primary PCI around the clock at any PCI center, with or without on-site cardiac surgery, as routine standard of care for all patients with acute STEMI (36). Emergency medical services providers should be equipped with diagnostic 12-lead electrocardiography and the ability to transmit the electrocardiogram (ECG) to the hospital's emergency department (ED). The ED physicians should be empowered to call in the interventionalist and cath team directly for all patients with ST-segment elevation, even before patient arrival when ST-segment elevation is seen on pre-hospital ECG, eliminating the "door-to-decision" time. These practices alone can significantly reduce door-to-balloon times (37–41) and thus should be expected to improve patient outcomes.

The resulting streamlined, well-practiced critical pathways will set a single high standard of care rather than a double standard that depends on the hour of the day or the interposition and preference of a non-interventional physician. Such standards will also increase institutional volumes of primary PCI, and this volume increase should also improve outcomes; higher institutional volumes of primary PCI produce more rapid reperfusion times and improved mortality rates. NRMI-2 demonstrated that the mortality rate of primary PCI was 33% lower at institutions that performed more than 33 primary PCI procedures per year than at institutions that performed fewer than 12 per year, and that door-to-balloon times were shorter (42). Thus, the current ACC PCI and STEMI Guidelines (30,31) recommend a minimum volume of 36 primary PCI procedures per year for hospitals that perform primary PCI without onsite cardiac surgery. Cardiac surgery centers should also meet this guideline.

CURRENT ACC/AHA GUIDELINES FOR PRIMARY PCI AT HOSPITALS WITHOUT ONSITE CARDIAC SURGERY

The 2001 ACC/AHA PCI Guidelines (43) designated primary PCI at hospitals without on-site cardiac surgery with a "Class IIb" indication, which is used to describe therapeutic options whose "usefulness/efficacy [is] less well established by evidence/opinion." Unfortunately, the recent revision of the ACC/AHA Guidelines for STEMI (31) and the current revision of the ACC/AHA/SCAI Guidelines for PCI (30) maintain this Class IIb indication. We believe that there is now enough evidence to support an upgrade to a Class IIa indication, which means that the "weight of evidence/opinion is in favor of [the] usefulness/efficacy" of this therapeutic option at qualified hospitals with off-site surgery backup.

There are at least 15 registries and studies of primary PCI at hospitals without cardiac surgery programs (20–28,44–53). The 2001 ACC/AHA PCI Guidelines (43) cites five of these studies (20,21,44,47,49), which report a total of 1026 procedures at nine hospitals. On the basis of the excellent outcomes in these five studies, the 2001 PCI Guidelines Committee concluded that primary PCI at hospitals with off-site surgery backup was indicated at the Class IIb level.

There are at least 10 additional studies and registries of primary PCI at hospitals without cardiac surgery (22–28,45,46,48,50–53), all but one of which (48) were published after the 2001 ACC/AHA PCI guidelines. One of these new studies (24) is the first (and likely the only) randomized trial of primary PCI versus fibrinolytic therapy at hospitals with off-site surgery backup. These newer studies and the randomized trial include over 7000 more patients at 180 sites, or seven times as many patients reported from 20 times as many sites as recognized in the 2001 PCI Guidelines. In these more recent studies, the outcomes remained excellent; the rate of PCI success was 95% in those six studies reporting this outcome; the mortality rate over all studies was only 5.8%, including cardiogenic shock in five of the studies. The rate of emergency coronary bypass surgery for PCI failure was very low at 0.53% in 2055 patients in the four studies that reported this outcome.

Most remarkably, the door-to-balloon times, reported in 8 of the 15 studies (including over 5000 patients), ranged from 80 to 110 minutes, as noted above. These reperfusion times were 1 to 1.5 hours faster than in patients transferred for PCI in U.S. hospitals in the NRMI registry for 2003 (16). Recent data from a cohort of over 33,000 patients treated with primary PCI from 1999 through 2002 showed faster door-to-balloon times at hospitals that did not have on-site cardiac surgery compared with tertiary surgical centers (54).

These fifteen studies demonstrate that qualified community hospitals can deliver primary PCI safely, effectively, and rapidly, with outcomes that are similar to those reported from tertiary centers. The benefits that community PCI centers can provide in increasing the access to rapid and expert primary PCI at the point of first patient contact should far outweigh any theoretical risk of having cardiac surgery backup off-site rather than on-site.

In view of this mounting evidence, we feel that there is quite sufficient justification, at a "Level of Evidence B" (data derived from a single randomized trial or nonrandomized) to advance the Class IIb indication to a Class IIa for primary PCI at hospitals with off-site cardiac surgery backup, provided such hospitals can meet rigorous standards.

It is unlikely that there will be any more randomized trials of primary PCI with off-site backup. In lieu of a randomized trial, we advocate that all hospitals that perform PCI with off-site cardiac surgery backup should be required to submit their data to the ACC-NCDR. As the amount of data increases, the likelihood of future Guidelines modifications should also increase—not only for primary PCI, but also for non-emergent PCI at hospitals with off-site surgery backup.

SOME OF THE EXPERT OPINIONS IN THE LITERATURE DIFFER FROM THE GUIDELINES

Many cardiology thought-leaders have recently encouraged primary PCI at qualified hospitals with off-site surgery backup or have directly advocated an advance to a IIa classification. Ryan states, "... for rural America, it is important to nurture and further develop existing institutions without nearby surgical capability that can demonstrate their ability to undertake lifesaving techniques, such as primary PCI, safely and effectively to make that technology more available to the patient in need" (55).

Cannon writes, "... if a community hospital makes a strong institutional commitment to establishing a comprehensive program, performance of primary PCI will be beneficial to patients" (56).

Weaver calls for more qualified nonsurgical hospitals to establish primary PCI programs to meet the growing need (57). Regarding the fact that some states require on-site cardiac surgery for hospitals performing PCI, he states, "In my mind, these restrictive regulations must be changed." Weaver continues, "Geography should not determine the type of treatment we receive for life-threatening conditions such as STEMI." He adds, "Too often in cardiology, we generate evidence to support a new treatment [primary PCI] but fail to effectively implement it. This cannot be another such example!"

Brodie directly advocates this advance to Class IIa, "... I believe the data presented by Wharton et al. provide sufficient evidence to revise these guidelines to provide a class IIa indication ... for primary PCI at hospitals with catheterization laboratories but without on-site surgery" (2). He continues, "We, as a cardiology community, should vigorously promote making mechanical reperfusion more available. The performance of primary PCI at facilities with interventional capabilities but without on-site cardiac surgery will help us toward this goal."

Bahr emphasizes, "The morbidity and mortality for the heart attack problem remains the number one public health problem facing our nation. We are at a point in cardiology where we can exert a major impact on these horrendous statistics... the time is ripe for the nation to move ahead and set up quality PCI centers in properly trained community hospitals to serve as "centers of excellence" in this new strategy" (58).

Moscucci and Eagle note, "it is likely that the next decade will be characterized by further expansion of primary PCI for acute STEMI in hospitals with cardiac catheterization laboratories" (59).

CONCLUSIONS

One of the most urgent public health problems in the Unites States is to increase the access to primary PCI, to make primary PCI rapidly available to most patients with STEMI—not merely to a small minority. Encouraging the wider availability of primary PCI in broader geographic locations by uncoupling PCI from the requirement from on-site bypass surgery is a key step toward this goal. Community hospitals that can meet rigorous standards can provide primary PCI just as safely and effectively, and often more rapidly, than cardiac surgery centers. To encourage more hospitals to establish primary PCI programs, we advocate advancing the indication for primary PCI at hospitals with off-site surgery backup to Class IIa in the STEMI and PCI Guidelines.

There is a strong and steadily growing grass roots movement to offer primary PCI at community hospitals. These hospitals are motivated by the commitment to provide this "best" therapy for STEMI to their patients, despite the controversies that invariably accompany such efforts and the extraordinary and costly efforts required. Unfortunately, this movement has little support from the ACC/AHA Guidelines, and has no one with direct experience on the Guidelines Committees. This movement deserves the encouragement that a Class IIa Guidelines indication would provide.

Many hospitals have successfully challenged and changed state regulations that formerly prohibited any PCI without on-site surgery, but restrictive regulations still prevail in many states. An upgrade to a Class IIa indication would help greatly to facilitate changes in inappropriately restrictive regulations.

The ACC/AHA Guidelines for AMI and PCI have evolved considerably over the 19 years since the first 1988 ACC/AHA PTCA Guidelines (60), which strongly opposed all PTCA at all hospitals without onsite surgery. Despite this initial and firm position, many community hospitals without on-site cardiac surgery (including ourselves) stepped out "ahead of the curve" and began offering primary PCI in the early 1990s, when the advantages of primary PCI became recognized. We hope for and look forward to the further evolution of the Guidelines, which will be a crucial step in increasing the number of AMI centers in the United States capable of offering primary PCI, and thus in increasing access to PCI for a broader segment of our population.

REFERENCES

1. Rogers WJ, Canto JG, Lambrew CT, et al. Temporal trends in the treatment of over 1.5 million patients with myocardial infarctions in the U.S. from 1990–1999. J Am Coll Cardiol 2000; 36:2056–2063.
2. Brodie BR. Primary percutaneous intervention at hospitals without onsite cardiac surgery. J Am Coll Cardiol 2004; 43:1951–1953.
3. Mehta RH, Stalhandske EJ, McCargar PA, et al. Elderly patients at highest risk with acute myocardial infarction are more frequently transferred from community hospitals to tertiary centers: reality or myth? Am Heart J 1999; 138:688–695.
4. Boersma E, and the Primary Coronary angioplasty vs. Thrombolysis Group. Does time matter? A pooled analysis of randomized clinical trials comparing primary percutaneous coronary intervention and in-hospital fibrinolysis in acute myocardial infarction patients. Eur Heart J 2006; 27:779–788.
5. Stenestrand U, Lindback J, Wallentin L. Long-term outcome of primary percutaneous coronary intervention vs prehospital and in-hospital thrombolysis for patients with ST-elevation myocardial infarction. JAMA 2006; 296:1749–1756.
6. Andersen HR, Nielsen TT, Rasmussen K, et al. A comparison of coronary angioplasty with fibrinolytic therapy in acute myocardial infarction. N Engl J Med 2003; 349:733–742.
7. Widimsky P, Budesinsky T, Vorac D, et al. Long distance transport for primary angioplasty vs immediate thrombolysis in acute myocardial infarction. Eur Heart J 2003; 24:94–104.
8. Dalby M, Bouzamondo A, Lechat P, et al. Transfer for primary angioplasty versus immediate thrombolysis in acute myocardial infarction: a meta-analysis. Circulation 2003; 108:1809–1814.
9. Henry TD, Atkins JM, Cunningham MS, et al. ST-segment elevation myocardial infarction: recommendations on triage of patients to heart attack centers. Is it time for a national policy for the treatment of ST-segment elevation myocardial infarction? J Am Coll Cardiol 2006; 47:1339–1345.
10. Canto JG, Zalenski RJ, Ornato JP, et al. Use of emergency medical services in acute myocardial infarction and subsequent quality of care. Observations from the National Registry of Myocardial Infarction 2. Circulation 2002; 106:3018–3023.
11. Hochman JS, Sleeper LA, Webb JG, et al. Early revascularization in acute myocardial infarction complicated by cardiogenic shock. SHOCK Investigators. Should we emergently revascularize occluded coronaries for cardiogenic shock. N Engl J Med 1999; 341:625–634.
12. Moyer P, Feldman J, Levine J, et al. Implications of the mechanical (PCI) vs thrombolytic controversy for ST segment elevation myocardial infarction on the organization of emergency medical services. The Boston EMS experience. Crit Pathw Cardiol 2004; 3:53–61.
13. Waters RE II, Singh KP, Roe MT, et al. Rationale and strategies for implementing community-based transfer protocols for primary percutaneous coronary intervention for acute ST-segment elevation myocardial infarction. J Am Coll Cardiol 2004; 43:2153–2159.
14. Larson DM, Sharkey SW, Unger BT, et al. Is rapid transfer of ST-elevation myocardial infarction patients for primary angioplasty feasible in the United States? Am J Cardiol 2003; 92(suppl 6A):152L–153L (abstr).
15. Nallamothu BK, Bates ER, Wang Y, et al. Driving times and distances to hospitals with percutaneous coronary intervention in the United States: implications for prehospital triage of patients with ST-elevation myocardial infarction. Circulation 2006; 113:1189–1195.
16. Gibson CM. NRMI and current treatment patterns for ST-elevation myocardial infarction. Am Heart J 2004; 148:S29–S33.
17. Hermann HC. Transfer for primary angioplasty: the importance of time. Circulation 2005; 111:718–720.
18. Cannon CP, Gibson CM, Lambrew CT, et al. Relationship of symptom-onset-to-balloon time and door-to-balloon time with mortality in patients undergoing angioplasty for acute myocardial infarction. JAMA 2000; 283:2941–2947.
19. Nallamothu BK, Bates ER, Herrin J, et al. Times to treatment in transfer patients undergoing primary percutaneous coronary intervention in the United States. National Registry of Myocardial Infarction (NRMI)-3/4 analysis. Circulation 2005; 111:761–767.

20. Weaver WD, Litwin PE, Martin JS. Use of direct angioplasty for treatment of patients with acute myocardial infarction in hospitals with and without on-site cardiac surgery. Circulation 1993; 88:2067–2075.
21. Wharton TP, McNamara NS, Fedele FA, et al. Primary angioplasty for the treatment of acute myocardial infarction: experience at two community hospitals without cardiac surgery. J Am Coll Cardiol 1999; 33:1257–1265.
22. Ribichini F. Experiences with primary angioplasty without on site-cardiac surgery. Semin Interv Cardiol 1999; 4:47–53.
23. Ribichini F, Steffenino G, Dellavalle A. Primary angioplasty without surgical back-up at all. Results of a five years experience in a community hospital in Europe (abstract). J Am Coll Cardiol 2000; 35:364A.
24. Aversano T, Aversano LT, Passamani E, et al. Thrombolytic therapy vs primary percutaneous coronary intervention for myocardial infarction in patients presenting to hospitals without on-site cardiac surgery: a randomized controlled trial. JAMA 2002; 287:1943–1951.
25. Aversano T. Primary angioplasty at hospitals without cardiac surgery: C-PORT Registry outcomes (abstract). Circulation 2003; 108:IV-613 (abstr).
26. Politi A, Zerboni S, Galli M, et al. Primary angioplasty in acute myocardial infarction: experience and results in the first 1,000 consecutive patients. Ital Heart J Suppl 2003; 4:755–763.
27. Sanborn TA, Jacobs AK, Frederick PD, et al. Comparability of quality-of-care indicators for emergency coronary angioplasty in patients with acute myocardial infarction regardless of on-site cardiac surgery (Report from the National Registry of Myocardial Infarction). Am J Cardiol 2004; 93:1335–1339.
28. Wharton TP Jr., Grines LL, Turco MA, et al. Primary Angioplasty in Acute Myocardial Infarction at Hospitals With No Surgery On-Site (the PAMI-No SOS study) versus transfer to surgical centers for primary angioplasty. J Am Coll Cardiol 2004; 43:1943–1950.
29. Sheldon WC. Trends in cardiac catheterization laboratories in the United States. Catheter Cardiovasc Interv 2001; 53:40–45.
30. Smith SC Jr., Feldman TE, Hirshfeld JW Jr., et al. ACC/AHA/SCAI 2005 guideline update for percutaneous coronary intervention: a report of the American College of Cardiology/American Heart Association Task Force on Practice Guidelines (ACC/AHA/SCAI Writing Committee to Update the 2001 © 2005 by the American College of Cardiology Foundation and the American Heart Association, Inc. Guidelines for Percutaneous Coronary Intervention). Available at: http://www.acc.org/qualityandscience/clinical/guidelines/percutaneous/update/index.pdf.
31. Antman EM, Anbe DT, Armstrong PW, et al. ACC/AHA guidelines for the management of patients with ST-elevation myocardial infarction: a report of the American College of Cardiology/American Heart Association Task Force on Practice Guidelines (Committee to Revise the 1999 Guidelines for the Management of Patients With Acute Myocardial Infarction). 2004. Available at: http://www.acc.org/clinical/guidelines/stemi/index.pdf.
32. Sinclair N, Wharton TP Jr. Critical pathways for primary angioplasty in acute myocardial infarction at community hospitals without cardiac surgery. In: Cannon C, O'Gara P, eds. Critical Pathways in Cardiology, 2nd ed. Philadelphia, PA: Lippincott Williams & Wilkins, 2006:108–128.
33. Moscucci M, Rogers EK, Montoye C, et al. Association of a continuous quality improvement initiative with practice and outcome variations of contemporary percutaneous coronary interventions. Circulation 2006; 113:814–822.
34. Brindis RG, Dehmer GJ. Continuous quality improvement in the cardiac catheterization laboratory: are the benefits worth the cost and effort? Circulation 2006; 113:767–770.
35. Caputo RP, Kosinski R, Walford G, et al. Effect of continuous quality improvement analysis on the delivery of primary percutaneous revascularization for acute myocardial infarction: a community hospital experience. Catheter Cardiovasc Interv 2005; 64:428–433.
36. Nallamothu BK, Wang Y, Magid DJ, et al. Relation between hospital specialization with primary percutaneous coronary intervention and clinical outcomes in ST-segment

elevation myocardial infarction. National Registry of Myocardial Infarction-4 analysis. Circulation 2006; 113:222–229.

37. Curtis JP, Portnay EL, Wang Y, et al. The pre-hospital electrocardiogram and time to reperfusion in patients with acute myocardial infarction, 2000–2002: findings from the National Registry of Myocardial Infarction-4. J Am Coll Cardiol 2006; 47:1544–1552.

38. Garvey JL, MacLeod BA, Sopko G, et al. Pre-hospital 12-lead electrocardiography programs: a call for implementation by emergency medical services systems providing advanced life support. J Am Coll Cardiol 2006; 47:485–491.

39. Bradley EB, Roumanis SA, Radford MJ, et al. Achieving door-to-balloon times that meet quality guidelines: how do successful hospitals do it? J Am Coll Cardiol 2005; 46:1236–1241.

40. Bradley EH, Herrin J, Wang Y, et al. Strategies for reducing the door-to-balloon time in acute myocardial infarction. N Engl J Med 2006; 355:2308–2320.

41. Moscucci M, Eagle KA. Reducing the door-to-balloon time for myocardial infarction with ST-segment elevation. N Engl J Med 2006; 355:2364–2365.

42. Canto JG, Every NR, Magid DJ, et al. The volume of primary angioplasty procedures and survival after acute myocardial infarction. N Engl J Med 2000; 342:1573–1580.

43. Smith SC. Jr., Dove JT, Jacobs AK, et al. ACC/AHA guidelines for percutaneous coronary intervention: executive summary and recommendations. A report of the American College of Cardiology/American Heart Association Task Force on Practice Guidelines (Committee to Revise the 1993 Guidelines for Percutaneous Transluminal Coronary Angioplasty). J Am Coll Cardiol 2001; 37:2215–2238.

44. Iannone LA, Anderson SM, Phillips SJ. Coronary angioplasty for acute myocardial infarction in a hospital without cardiac surgery. Tex Heart Inst J 1993; 20:99–104.

45. Weaver WD, Parsons L, Every N, et al. Primary coronary angioplasty in hospitals with and without surgery backup. J Invasive Cardiol 1995; 7:34F–39F.

46. Weaver WD, for the MITI project investigators. PTCA in centers without surgical backup—outcome, logistics and technical aspects. J Invasive Cardiol 1997; 9:20B–23B.

47. Brush JE, Thompson S, Ciuffo AA, et al. Retrospective comparison of a strategy of primary coronary angioplasty versus intravenous thrombolytic therapy for acute myocardial infarction in a community hospital without cardiac surgical backup. J Invasive Cardiol 1996; 8:91–98.

48. Moquet B, Huguet RG, Cami G, et al. Primary angioplasty in acute myocardial infarction: a one-year experience in a small urban community. Arch Mal Coeur Vaiss 1997; 90:11–15.

49. Smyth DW, Richards AM, Elliott JM. Direct angioplasty for myocardial infarction: one-year experience in a center with surgical back-up 220 miles away. J Invasive Cardiol 1997; 9:324–332.

50. Kutcher MA, Klein LW, Wharton TP, et al. Clinical outcomes in coronary angioplasty centers with off-site versus on-site cardiac surgery capabilities: a preliminary report from the American College of Cardiology-National Cardiovascular Data Registry. J Am Coll Cardiol 2004; 43:96a (abstr).

51. Foster JK, Klein LW, Veledar E, et al. On-site surgical backup as a predictor of mortality among PCI patients with STEMI, NSTEMI, or no AMI. Circulation 2005; 112(suppl II):II–737.

52. Singh M, Ting HH, Berger PB, et al. Rationale for on-site cardiac surgery for primary angioplasty: a time for reappraisal. J Am Coll Cardiol 2002; 39:1881–1889.

53. Wennberg DE, Lucas FL, Siewers AE, et al. Outcomes of percutaneous coronary interventions performed at centers without and with onsite coronary artery bypass graft surgery. JAMA 2004; 292:1961–1968.

54. Magid DJ, Wang Y, Herrin J, et al. Relationship between time of day, day of week, timeliness of reperfusion, and in-hospital mortality for patients with acute ST-segment elevation myocardial infarction. JAMA 2005; 294:803–812.

55. Ryan TJ. Primary percutaneous coronary intervention without nearby surgical capability: a reassuring response from rural America. Mayo Clin Proc 2004; 79:731–732.

56. Cannon CP. Primary percutaneous coronary intervention for all? JAMA 2002; 287:1987–1989.

57. Weaver WD. All hospitals are not equal for treatment of patients with acute myocardial infarction. Circulation 2003; 108:1768–1771.
58. Bahr RD. Comment on "Increasing the speed and delivery of primary percutaneous coronary intervention in the community: should the ACC/AHA guidelines be revisited?" Crit Pathw Cardiol 2006; 5:44–45.
59. Moscucci M, Eagle K. Door-to-balloon time in primary percutaneous coronary intervention: is the 90-minute gold standard an unreachable chimera? Circulation 2006; 113:1048–1050.
60. Guidelines for percutaneous transluminal coronary angioplasty. A report of the American College of Cardiology/American Heart Association Task Force on Assessment of Diagnostic and Therapeutic Cardiovascular Procedures (Subcommittee on Percutaneous Transluminal Coronary Angioplasty). J Am Coll Cardiol 1988; 12:529–545.

11 Interhospital Transfer for Primary PCI

Brahmajee K. Nallamothu
*Department of Internal Medicine, Division of Cardiovascular Medicine,
University of Michigan, Ann Arbor, Michigan, U.S.A.*

INTRODUCTION

Primary percutaneous coronary intervention (PCI) is superior to fibrinolytic therapy as a reperfusion strategy in ST-elevation myocardial infarction (STEMI) when performed rapidly and by experienced operators. Compared with fibrinolytic therapy, primary PCI results in higher infarct artery patency rates and lower rates of reinfarction, stroke, and death (1). However, PCI programs are available in just 25% of acute-care hospitals in the United States and even fewer hospitals worldwide (2,3). As a result, only a minority of STEMI patients present directly to PCI hospitals and many receive care initially at local hospitals without cardiac catheterization laboratories. Clinicians at hospitals without PCI capability are left with two treatment options: immediate on-site fibrinolytic therapy or emergent interhospital transfer for primary PCI.

In recent years, the precise role of interhospital transfer for primary PCI versus immediate fibrinolytic therapy has been debated vigorously in the literature. Although recent clinical trials have supported the use of interhospital transfer for primary PCI, there is still a limited understanding of its applicability in the "real-world" setting given the markedly long delays to reperfusion that are frequently associated with this strategy. Because of the strong relationship between time to reperfusion and clinical outcomes in primary PCI (4,5), the benefits of interhospital transfer may not be reproducible in clinical practice, particularly in the United States, where long transport times are common. This chapter reviews evidence from recent clinical trials on interhospital transfer for PCI and practical limitations with its implementation as a routine strategy.

CLINICAL TRIALS

Early reports from the late 1980s suggested that interhospital transfer of patients with STEMI was a safe and feasible approach under select circumstances (6–8). However, this strategy was largely reserved for patients with uncertain diagnoses, clear contraindications to fibrinolytic therapy, high-risk features like anterior location or delayed presentation after symptom onset, or cardiogenic shock.

Recently, six randomized clinical trials have specifically tested whether a strategy of interhospital transfer for primary PCI was superior to immediate on-site fibrinolytic therapy in a broader population of patients with STEMI (9–14). A quantitative review of these six trials suggested that interhospital transfer for primary PCI significantly reduced the incidence of a 30-day composite end point of death, reinfarction, and stroke by 42% ($p < 0.001$) (Table 1) (15). The overall number needed to treat (NNT) to prevent one of these major adverse events was 19 on the basis of these findings. When the end points were examined individually in the quantitative review, reinfarction and stroke were significantly reduced by 68% and 56%, respectively, while there was a strong trend in mortality with a 19% reduction ($p = 0.08$).

TABLE 1 Six Trials Comparing the Incidence of a Combined End Point of Death, Reinfarction, or Stroke in Patients Undergoing Interhospital Transfer for Primary PCI with Immediate On-Site Fibrinolytic Therapy

| | Death/reinfarction/stroke | | |
| | Number of events/number of patients | | |
	PCI	Lysis	Risk ratio
Maastricht	8/75	14/75	0.57
PRAGUE	8/101	23/99	0.34
Air-Pami	6/71	9/66	0.62
CAPTIM	26/421	34/419	0.76
DANAMI-2	63/790	107/782	0.58
PRAGUE-2	36/429	64/421	0.55
Total	147/1887	251/1863	0.58[a]

[a] $p < 0.001$ for summary RR.
Source: Adapted from Ref. 15.

Although statistical tests of heterogeneity were nonsignificant across these studies, it is important to note key differences in the designs of these trials. Two trials, PRAGUE-2 and DANAMI-2, were large multicenter trials and their results substantially influenced the quantitative review given their large number of patients (13,14). The PRAGUE-2 trial (13) randomized 850 patients with STEMI from the Czech Republic to either immediate on-site fibrinolytic therapy with streptokinase or emergent interhospital transfer for primary PCI up to a maximum distance of 120 km. Despite these distances, the median time from randomization to balloon inflation was 97 minutes and there was a nonsignificant trend toward lower mortality among patients who underwent primary PCI (6.8% vs. 10.0%; $p = 0.12$). An important additional finding from the PRAGUE-2 trial was an apparent interaction between time from symptom onset to presentation and the clinical benefits of primary PCI. Of the 551 patients treated within three hours of symptom onset, there was no difference between reperfusion strategies in 30-day mortality (7.3% for primary PCI vs. 7.4% for streptokinase; $p = $ NS). In contrast, the 299 patients randomized more than three hours after symptom onset had significantly lower 30-day mortality rates with primary PCI (6% vs. 15.3%; $p < 0.02$).

In the DANAMI-2 trial (14), 1129 patients with STEMI were randomized in Denmark at non-PCI hospitals to transfer for primary PCI or on-site fibrinolytic therapy with accelerated t-PA. (An additional 443 patients presenting directly to PCI hospital also were randomized to the two reperfusion strategies but are not discussed here.) Patients were transferred up to 150 km, and the median time from randomization to balloon inflation was 90 minutes. A primary 30-day composite end point of death, reinfarction, or disabling stroke occurred in 14.2% of patients receiving fibrinolytic therapy compared with 8.5% of patients who underwent primary PCI. There was no significant difference in 30-day mortality, with the majority of difference in the composity endpoint driven by reductions in reinfarction with primary PCI (1.9% vs. 6.2%; $p < 0.001$). Interestingly, these investigators have gone on to report an important interaction between risk status and the effectiveness of primary PCI (16). In 1134 patients identified as low-risk on the basis of a Thrombolysis in Myocardial Infarction (TIMI) risk score of four or less, there was a nonsignificant trend toward lower mortality with fibrinolytic therapy (5.6% vs. 8.0%; $p = 0.11$). In contrast, fibrinolytic therapy was associated with higher mortality when compared with primary PCI in 438 patients with TIMI risk scores greater than 4 (36.2% vs. 25.3%; $p = 0.02$).

Another critical trial that was included in the quantitative review was the French CAPTIM trial (11), which compared "optimal" pharmacological reperfusion with interhospital transfer for primary PCI. The use of the term "optimal" specification referred to prehospital fibrinolytic therapy in this study, because randomization in the CAPTIM trial occurred in the prehospital setting. Overall, this trial showed no significant differences between the two reperfusion strategies in a 30-day composite end point that included death, reinfarction, and stroke. In addition, some potential for harm was noted as interhospital transfer for primary PCI was associated with a higher rate of developing cardiogenic shock (2.1% vs. 0%; $p = 0.004$), presumably because of longer delays to reperfusion. An additional difference was that the CAPTIM trial required that all patients be transferred to tertiary care centers for subsequent care even after successful fibrinolytic therapy. The protocol for mandatory transfer allowed for greater use of rescue PCI and early invasive risk stratification in contrast to other trials, such as DANAMI-2, which rarely permitted crossover in their protocols.

OBSERVATIONAL STUDIES

It is important to note that for many of the trials that evaluated interhospital transfer for primary PCI, the average time from randomization at the initial hospital to first balloon inflation at the PCI hospital was relatively short. In trials performed in European countries with highly organized national emergency medical systems, the overall median door-to-balloon time was approximately 95 minutes. In the only trial to include PCI hospitals in the United States, the time from randomization to first balloon inflation was much longer, at 120 minutes (12).

For many years, data on time after interhospital transfer were unknown in the United States. In 2005, Nallamothu and colleagues reported that overall times to reperfusion may be substantially delayed in this population, potentially placing them at risk and diminishing the benefits of primary PCI (17). Using data from 1999 to 2002 in the National Registry of Myocardial Infarction (NRMI), these investigators found that the median "total" door-to-balloon time from arrival at the referral hospital to balloon inflation at the PCI hospital was 180 minutes in 4278 patients with STEMI who were transferred for primary PCI. Of these patients, only 4.2% had door-to-balloon inflation times of less than 90 minutes. More contemporary data from the American College of Cardiology National Cardiovascular Data Registry suggest that time delays have not changed dramatically during recent years (18).

No study to date has reported the extent to which interhospital transfer is being used in the United States. Anecdotally, there appears to have been an increase in recent years with the publication of several studies that have demonstrated favorable outcomes with interhospital transfer. In addition, a number of investigators have begun to publish reports from single-center experiences that suggest health care systems may be able to overcome some of the challenges associated with interhospital transfer. In Minnesota, Henry and colleagues have published data on reductions in total door-to-balloon time from 192 to 98 minutes at a large tertiary care hospital (19). The network that these investigators established now incorporates 30 community hospitals in the area and combines the use of fibrinolytic therapy with mechanical reperfusion based on the patient's clinical characteristics, location, and anticipated time to reperfusion. Similar programs have been developed in other states to help hospitals overcome the formidable barriers to rapid transfer of patients between hospitals often encountered in the United States (20). However, the overall applicability of these types of protocols to the broader population of patients with STEMI across the United States has been challenged (21).

CURRENT RECOMMENDATIONS

Guidelines from the ACC, AHA, and the European Society of Cardiology have recommended a treatment goal of 90 minutes or less for door-to-balloon times (or the time from initial medical contact to treatment) (22,23). This treatment goal also has been incorporated into national, publicly reported quality indicators for hospital performance in the United States (24), although patients who undergo primary PCI after interhospital transfer are routinely excluded from data collection.

The ultimate decision about whether to transfer patients for primary PCI should be made only after balancing the potential benefits of primary PCI against the potential dangers of delaying reperfusion in patients who are otherwise eligible for fibrinolytic therapy. When both reperfusion strategies can be rapidly performed, there is little question that the preponderance of evidence strongly supports the use of primary PCI. PCI also is the best option in patients with cardiogenic shock and the only option in those with contraindications to fibrinolytic therapy (25,26). When primary PCI is not available, however, fibrinolytic therapy remains a practical option for many patients. With regard to mortality, the advantages of primary PCI over fibrinolytic therapy are modest (~1% to 2% absolute mortality risk reduction at 30 days) even in clinical trials where it is optimally performed (27).

Thus, the key question is, "How long a delay to primary PCI would make fibrinolytic therapy the preferred strategy for reperfusion?" Several meta-regressions have attempted to answer this question by examining whether additional delays related to primary PCI (i.e., "PCI-related delay") correlated with mortality differences between primary PCI and fibrinolytic therapy reported by clinical trials (28–31). Results of these analyses varied substantially on the basis of which clinical trials were included. For example, an analysis that used only contemporary trials with fibrin-specific agents suggested that there was no mortality difference between reperfusion strategies when PCI-related delay exceeded 62 minutes (30). If fibrinolytic therapy can be delivered within 30 minutes of hospital arrival, this degree of PCI-related delay corresponds to a goal of 90 minutes or less for patients undergoing primary PCI. However, a recent pooled analysis by Boersma et al. of patient-level data on 6763 patients from several of the same clinical trials suggested that primary PCI was preferred even when PCI-related delays exceeded 79 minutes, although absolute and relative mortality benefits were greatest with delays under 35 minutes (32) (chap. 7, Fig. 4).

These previous studies all used data from clinical trials where patients were highly selected and had rapid access to both reperfusion strategies. In the trials evaluated by Boersma et al., for example, the median times from randomization to fibrinolytic therapy and primary PCI were 19 and 76 minutes, respectively (32). Outside of clinical trials, patients often present more heterogeneously and with longer times to treatment. In a recent observational analysis of patients within NRMI, PCI-related delays associated with no mortality differences between the reperfusion strategies varied widely on the basis of patient age, location of infarct, and symptom duration (33) (chap. 6, Fig. 6). Younger patients with anterior

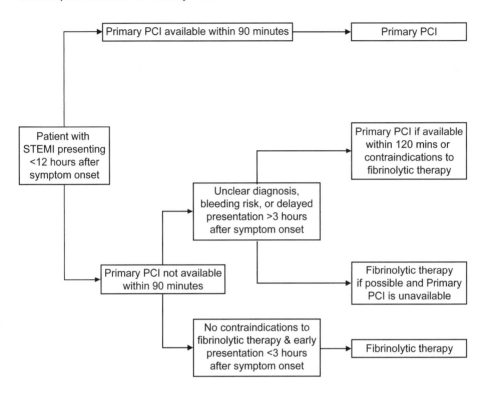

FIGURE 1 Example of triage protocol for patients with STEMI presenting to hospitals with and without the capability for primary PCI.

infarction and short symptom durations appeared most sensitive to longer PCI-related delays given the efficacy and safety of fibrinolytic therapy in this population and the critical importance of maximizing myocardial salvage during this time period. Rapid assessment of these factors and their incorporation into triage protocols may be needed to optimize the use of reperfusion strategies across patient populations (34,35).

An example of such a triage protocol is outlined in Figure 1. In this protocol, minimizing time to treatment is given greater priority than the particular type of reperfusion therapy utilized in patients presenting early after symptom onset (e.g., within 2–3 hours). After this early time period, however, the relative advantages and safety of primary PCI over fibrinolytic therapy increase and it becomes the preferred reperfusion therapy based on availability.

FUTURE DIRECTIONS

Combination Strategies

Given that there is a limit to how much door-to-balloon time may be shortened in patients undergoing interhospital transfer, ongoing studies are attempting to minimize the impact of delays on outcomes by combining both reperfusion strategies. In one strategy, commonly referred to as "facilitated PCI," pharmacological reperfusion with fibrinolytic therapy or glycoprotein IIb/IIIa receptor blockers is used to reestablish flow, immediately followed by emergent PCI to stabilize the infarct artery. When compared with primary PCI, clinical trials have failed to demonstrate that facilitated PCI improves outcomes and may actually result in higher mortality (36). However, many of these trials included patients at hospitals where primary PCI was already rapidly available. The approach has yet to be studied in a large number of transfer patients at high risk for prolonged delays to primary PCI.

Another widely discussed strategy is the "pharmacoinvasive approach," which is distinct from facilitated PCI. In this approach, immediate PCI is routinely performed for fibrinolytic therapy failure (i.e., rescue PCI). Routine, nonemergent cardiac catheterization is performed early after successful reperfusion. This strategy appears promising but has not been studied in any large populations of patients with STEMI (37). Although anecdotal reports indicate that clinicians are increasingly using facilitated PCI and the pharmacoinvasive approach, neither can be definitively recommended at this time.

STEMI Systems of Care

In recent years, there has been increasing motivation within the United States to coordinate prehospital emergency medical systems for triaging STEMI patients across regional health care systems and to expand primary PCI to more hospitals (38). The motivation for establishing these STEMI systems of care is to avoid delays associated with interhospital transfer by permitting more direct access to primary PCI. Yet many challenges will need to be overcome for these STEMI systems of care to succeed. Prehospital electrocardiography, which shortens the time from hospital arrival to PCI by permitting earlier activation of the cardiac catheterization laboratory and allows for direct transport protocols to nearby PCI hospitals, is limited to a few U.S. regions and used in less than 10% of patients (39,40). Challenges for implementing prehospital electrocardiography include device-related costs as well as training requirements for personnel. While the current distribution of patient populations and PCI hospitals supports the possibility of hospital bypass protocols in the future (2), these strategies will be difficult to implement in the competitive environment of the current U.S. health care system, where facilities may be reluctant to share revenue and responsibility for these patients (41).

Finally, the use of primary PCI at hospitals without on-site cardiac surgery is expanding in many states based on data from clinical trials, such as Cardiovascular Patient Outcomes Research Team (C-PORT) trial (42). In this trial, 11 community hospitals in Massachusetts and Maryland with cardiac catheterization laboratories but no on-site cardiac surgery randomized patients with STEMI to immediate on-site fibrinolytic therapy or primary PCI. All the hospitals underwent an intensive, formal PCI development program prior to the initiation of the trial. Overall, the six-month composite end point of death, reinfarction, and stroke was significantly lower in patients who underwent primary PCI (12.4% vs. 19.9%; $p = 0.03$). However, the expansion of routine PCI services to patients without STEMI at these hospitals and its potential to increase overall mortality related to PCI has been raised (43,44).

CONCLUSIONS

Recent clinical trials have supported the use of interhospital transfer for primary PCI. However, in the "real-world" setting, this strategy may lead to substantial delays to reperfusion and offset the advantages of primary PCI. For an individual patient, determining the role of interhospital transfer for primary PCI requires clinicians to balance its potential benefits against the risks of delaying reperfusion. Ideally, this decision should be influenced by the patients' clinical characteristics and their anticipated time to reperfusion with primary PCI.

REFERENCES

1. Keeley EC, Boura JA, Grines CL. Primary angioplasty versus intravenous thrombolytic therapy for acute myocardial infarction: a quantitative review of 23 randomised trials. Lancet 2003; 361:13–20.
2. Nallamothu BK, Bates ER, Wang Y, et al. Driving times and distances to hospitals with percutaneous coronary intervention in the United States: implications for prehospital triage of patients with ST-elevation myocardial infarction. Circulation 2006; 113:1189–1195.
3. Keeley EC, Grines CL. Should patients with acute myocardial infraction be transferred to a tertiary center for primary angioplasty or receive it at qualified hospitals in the community? The case for emergency transfer for primary percutaneous coronary intervention. Circulation 2005; 112:3520–3532.
4. De Luca G, Suryapranata H, Ottervanger JP, et al. Time delay to treatment and mortality in primary angioplasty for acute myocardial infarction: every minute of delay counts. Circulation 2004; 109:1223–1225.
5. McNamara RL, Wang Y, Herrin J, et al. Effect of door-to-balloon time on mortality in patients with ST-segment elevation myocardial infarction. J Am Coll Cardiol 2006; 47:2180–2186.
6. Bellinger RL, Califf RM, Mark DB, et al. Helicopter transport of patients during acute myocardial infarction. Am J Cardiol 1988; 61:718–722.
7. Gore JM, Corrao JM, Goldberg RJ, et al. Feasibility and safety of emergency interhospital transport of patients during early hours of acute myocardial infarction. Arch Intern Med 1989; 149:353–355.
8. Zijlstra F, van't Hof AW, Liem AL, et al. Transferring patients for primary angioplasty: a retrospective analysis of 104 selected high risk patients with acute myocardial infarction. Heart 1997; 78:333–336.
9. Vermeer F, Oude Ophuis AJ, vd Berg EJ, et al. Prospective randomised comparison between thrombolysis, rescue PTCA, and primary PTCA in patients with extensive myocardial infarction admitted to a hospital without PTCA facilities: a safety and feasibility study. Heart 1999; 82:426–431.
10. Widimsky P, Groch L, Zelizko M, et al. Multicentre randomized trial comparing transport to primary angioplasty vs immediate thrombolysis vs combined strategy for patients with acute myocardial infarction presenting to a community hospital without a catheterization laboratory. The PRAGUE study. Eur Heart J 2000; 21:823–831.
11. Bonnefoy E, Lapostolle F, Leizorovicz A, et al. Primary angioplasty versus prehospital fibrinolysis in acute myocardial infarction: a randomised study. Lancet 2002; 360:825–829.
12. Grines CL, Westerhausen DR. Jr., Grines LL, et al. A randomized trial of transfer for primary angioplasty versus on-site thrombolysis in patients with high-risk myocardial infarction: the Air Primary Angioplasty in Myocardial Infarction study. J Am Coll Cardiol 2002; 39:1713–1719.
13. Widimsky P, Budesinsky T, Vorac D, et al. Long distance transport for primary angioplasty vs immediate thrombolysis in acute myocardial infarction. Final results of the randomized national multicentre trial—PRAGUE-2. Eur Heart J 2003; 24:94–104.
14. Andersen HR, Nielsen TT, Rasmussen K, et al. A comparison of coronary angioplasty with fibrinolytic therapy in acute myocardial infarction. N Engl J Med. 2003; 349: 733–742.
15. Dalby M, Bouzamondo A, Lechat P, et al. Transfer for primary angioplasty versus immediate thrombolysis in acute myocardial infarction: a meta-analysis. Circulation 2003; 108:1809–1814.
16. Thune JJ, Hoefsten DE, Lindholm MG, et al. Simple risk stratification at admission to identify patients with reduced mortality from primary angioplasty. Circulation 2005; 112:2017–2021.

17. Nallamothu BK, Bates ER, Herrin J, et al. Times to treatment in transfer patients undergoing primary percutaneous coronary intervention in the United States: National Registry of Myocardial Infarction (NRMI)-3/4 analysis. Circulation 2005; 111:761–767.
18. Nallamothu BK, Wang Y, Rathore S, et al. Time-to-reperfusion in patients undergoing interhospital transfer for primary percutaneous coronary intervention in the United States: results from the National Cardiovascular Data Registry. Circulation 2006; 114:II-420 (abstr).
19. Henry TD, Unger BT, Sharkey SW, et al. Design of a standardized system for transfer of patients with ST-elevation myocardial infarction for percutaneous coronary intervention. Am Heart J 2005; 150:373–384.
20. Waters RE II, Singh KP, Roe MT, et al. Rationale and strategies for implementing community-based transfer protocols for primary percutaneous coronary intervention for acute ST-segment elevation myocardial infarction. J Am Coll Cardiol 2004; 43:2153–2159.
21. Rathore SS, Epstein AJ, Nallamothu BK, et al. Regionalization of ST-segment elevation acute coronary syndromes care: putting a national policy in proper perspective. J Am Coll Cardiol 2006; 47:1346–1349.
22. Antman EM, Anbe DT, Armstrong PW, et al. ACC/AHA guidelines for the management of patients with ST-elevation myocardial infarction: a report of the American College of Cardiology/American Heart Association Task Force on Practice Guidelines (Committee to Revise the 1999 Guidelines for the Management of Patients with Acute Myocardial Infarction). Circulation 2004; 110:e82–e292.
23. Van de Werf F, Ardissino D, Betriu A, et al. Management of acute myocardial infarction in patients presenting with ST-segment elevation. The Task Force on the Management of Acute Myocardial Infarction of the European Society of Cardiology. Eur Heart J 2003; 24:28–66.
24. Krumholz HM, Anderson JL, Brooks NH, et al. ACC/AHA clinical performance measures for adults with ST-elevation and non-ST-elevation myocardial infarction: a report of the American College of Cardiology/American Heart Association Task Force on Performance Measures (Writing Committee to Develop Performance Measures on ST-Elevation and Non-ST-Elevation Myocardial Infarction). Circulation 2006; 113:732–761.
25. Hochman JS, Sleeper LA, Webb JG, et al. Early revascularization in acute myocardial infarction complicated by cardiogenic shock. N Engl J Med 1999; 341:625–634.
26. Grzybowski M, Clements EA, Parsons L, et al. Mortality benefit of immediate revascularization of acute ST-segment elevation myocardial infarction in patients with contraindications to thrombolytic therapy: a propensity analysis. JAMA 2003; 290:1891–1898.
27. Melandri G. The obsession with primary angioplasty. Circulation 2003; 108:e162.
28. Kent DM, Lau J, Selker HP. Balancing the benefits of primary angioplasty against the benefits of thrombolytic therapy for acute myocardial infarction: the importance of timing. Eff Clin Pract 2001; 4:214–220.
29. Nallamothu BK, Bates ER. Percutaneous coronary intervention versus fibrinolytic therapy in acute myocardial infarction: is timing (almost) everything? Am J Cardiol 2003; 92:824–826.
30. Nallamothu BK, Antman EM, Bates ER. Primary percutaneous coronary intervention versus fibrinolytic therapy in acute myocardial infarction: does the choice of fibrinolytic agent impact on the importance of time-to-treatment? Am J Cardiol 2004; 94:772–774.
31. Betriu A, Masotti M. Comparison of mortality rates in acute myocardial infarction treated by percutaneous coronary intervention versus fibrinolysis. Am J Cardiol 2005; 95:100–101.
32. Boersma E. Does time matter? A pooled analysis of randomized clinical trials comparing primary percutaneous coronary intervention and in-hospital fibrinolysis in acute myocardial infarction patients. Eur Heart J 2006; 27:779–788.
33. Pinto DS, Kirtane AJ, Nallamothu BK, et al. Hospital delays in reperfusion for ST-elevation myocardial infarction: implications when selecting a reperfusion strategy. Circulation 2006; 114:2019–2025.
34. Kalla K, Christ G, Karnik R, et al. Implementation of guidelines improves the standard of care: the Viennese registry on reperfusion strategies in ST-elevation myocardial infarction (Vienna STEMI registry). Circulation 2006; 113:2398–2405.

35. Ting HH, Yang EH, Rihal CS. Narrative review: reperfusion strategies for ST-segment elevation myocardial infarction. Ann Intern Med 2006; 145:610–617.
36. Keeley EC, Boura JA, Grines CL. Comparison of primary and facilitated percutaneous coronary interventions for ST-elevation myocardial infarction: quantitative review of randomised trials. Lancet 2006; 367:579–588.
37. Armstrong PW. A comparison of pharmacologic therapy with/without timely coronary intervention vs. primary percutaneous intervention early after ST-elevation myocardial infarction: the WEST (Which Early ST-elevation myocardial infarction Therapy) study. Eur Heart J 2006; 27:1530–1538.
38. Jacobs AK, Antman EM, Ellrodt G, et al. Recommendation to develop strategies to increase the number of ST-segment-elevation myocardial infarction patients with timely access to primary percutaneous coronary intervention. Circulation 2006; 113:2152–2163.
39. Garvey JL, MacLeod BA, Sopko G, et al. Pre-hospital 12-lead electrocardiography programs: a call for implementation by emergency medical services systems providing advanced life support—National Heart Attack Alert Program (NHAAP) Coordinating Committee; National Heart, Lung, and Blood Institute (NHLBI); National Institutes of Health. J Am Coll Cardiol 2006; 47:485–491.
40. Curtis JP, Portnay EL, Wang Y, et al. The pre-hospital electrocardiogram and time to reperfusion in patients with acute myocardial infarction, 2000–2002: findings from the National Registry of Myocardial Infarction-4. J Am Coll Cardiol 2006; 47:1544–1552.
41. Nallamothu BK, Taheri PA, Barsan WG, et al. Broken bodies, broken hearts? Limitations of the trauma system as a model for regionalizing care for ST-elevation myocardial infarction in the United States. Am Heart J 2006; 152:613–618.
42. Aversano T, Aversano LT, Passamani E, et al. Thrombolytic therapy vs primary percutaneous coronary intervention for myocardial infarction in patients presenting to hospitals without on-site cardiac surgery: a randomized controlled trial. JAMA 2002; 287:1943–1951.
43. Wennberg DE, Lucas FL, Siewers AE, et al. Outcomes of percutaneous coronary interventions performed at centers without and with onsite coronary artery bypass graft surgery. JAMA 2004; 292:1961–1968.
44. Weaver WD. Is onsite surgery backup necessary for percutaneous coronary interventions? JAMA 2004; 292:2014–2016.

Farzin Beygui and Gilles Montalescot
Institut de Cardiologie, Pitié-Salpêtrière University Hospital, Paris, France

Reperfusion therapy is the major treatment for acute ST-elevation myocardial infarction (STEMI). Both mechanical and pharmacological reperfusion therapy are associated with reduced mortality rates in STEMI. (1–3) Antiplatelet therapy is also a pivotal therapy in reducing the rates of death and vascular events in STEMI where platelet activation and aggregation (consequences of coronary plaque rupture) represent the very first step in the chain reaction leading to occlusive coronary thrombosis (4). Furthermore, both percutaneous coronary intervention (PCI) and fibrinolysis lead to increased platelet activation and aggregation by different mechanisms. Hence, antiplatelet therapy as an adjunct to reperfusion therapy is recommended based on high levels of evidence by all expert guidelines (5–10).

ANTIPLATELET DRUGS (TABLE 1)

Aspirin

Aspirin partially inhibits platelet aggregation by irreversibly inactivating the cyclooxygenase activity (COX) of prostaglandin H synthase-1 and -2, through selective acetylation of a serine residue (Ser529 in COX-1 and Ser516 in COX-2). Acetylation blocks the platelet production of thromboxane A2. Thromboxane A2 is synthesized in platelets and released in response to various stimuli such as thrombin, adenosine diphosphate, collagen, and platelet activating factor; leading to vasoconstriction, amplification of the activation signal, and promotion of irreversible platelet aggregation. Aspirin inhibition of COX-1 is 170 times superior to its activity on COX-2, explaining its relatively poor anti-inflammatory effects.

After oral administration, aspirin is rapidly absorbed in the stomach and the upper intestine with a peak plasma level reached within 40 minutes of ingestion. Significant and long-lasting (up to seven days) inhibition of the platelet function occurs within an hour after a single oral dose of aspirin and within five minutes after an intravenous bolus. Chewed aspirin has a more rapid effect than oral aspirin.

Aspirin has been widely demonstrated to reduce the risk of vascular events (myocardial infarction [MI], stroke, and vascular death) in a broad spectrum of atherothrombotic diseases (4). These effects have been demonstrated for doses as low as 30 mg and as high as 1500 mg. There are no demonstrable therapeutic advantages for doses greater than 75–100 mg daily compared with higher doses, while higher doses are associated with more gastrointestinal side effects, especially in patients treated with combination antiplatelet therapy. The recommended daily doses are 75 to 325 mg in different settings of coronary artery disease.

Within 24 hours of STEMI, aspirin 160 mg daily was associated with a 23% five-week mortality reduction (95% CI, 15–30%, $2p < 0.00001$) in ISIS-2 trial (1). Antiplatelet therapy, essentially aspirin, in the subgroup of patients with MI in the Antithrombotic Trialists' Collaboration (15 controlled randomized trials pooling almost 20,000 patients), was associated with a 30% odds reduction for the composite vascular end point (MI, stroke, or vascular death), with significant risk reductions in each end point (4).

Thienopyridines

Thienopyridines irreversibly inhibit the platelet ADP $P2Y_{12}$ receptor, leading to an attenuated platelet aggregation response to ADP receptor stimulation. The mechanism of action of thienopyridines is complementary to the aspirin mechanism. The use of thienopyridines increased dramatically after ticlopidine, in combination with aspirin, was reported to reduce both the risks of subacute stent thrombosis and bleeding after stent placement compared with aspirin combined with warfarin (11). The use of ticlopidine was nevertheless restricted to the first 15 to 28 days after stent placement because of the potentially lethal risk of neutropenia (2.4%) (12). The general and long-term use of a thienopyridine derivative has become possible since clopidogrel became available.

Clopidogrel is a thienopyridine derivative structurally related to ticlopidine with fewer serious side effects (reported rates of neutropenia comparable to those of placebo) and both faster and longer duration of action. Clopidogrel is a prodrug, needing in vivo hepatic transformation for its antiplatelet effect. Significant platelet function inhibition is detected within two hours after a single oral dose of clopidogrel. With repeated daily doses of 75 mg, a steady state with 50% to 60% inhibition of platelet aggregation induced by ADP is reached in four to seven days. An initial standard loading dose of 300 mg is usually used to achieve the platelet inhibition effects more rapidly. Recent data show that more significant inhibitory effects can be achieved even faster with higher loading doses of 600 or 900 mg (13–15).

Clopidogrel in combination with aspirin has shown similar efficacy in reducing rates of subacute stent thrombosis compared with the combination of ticlopidine and aspirin (16,17). Moreover, pretreatment and prolonged therapy (9–12 months) by clopidogrel has been reported to be associated with a lower incidence of acute atherothrombotic events after PCI (18,19). The increase in the use of potentially more thrombogenic drug-eluting stents has also contributed to the recommendation of prolonged clopidogrel therapy (2–6 months) after placement of such stents (6,9).

GP IIb/IIIa Inhibitors

GP IIb/IIIa inhibitors block the binding of fibrinogen and von Willebrand factor to platelet GP IIb/IIIa receptors, consequently blocking the final common pathway of platelet aggregation. Unlike aspirin and thienopyridine derivatives, GP IIb/IIIa blockade results in platelet inhibition regardless of the initial aggregation stimuli.

Three IV inhibitors of platelet GP IIb/IIIa receptors—abciximab, eptifibatide and tirofiban—are commercially available (Table 1). All three agents provide significant antiplatelet action within minutes after an IV bolus. A 12- to 18-hour continuous infusion is needed to maintain the antiplatelet effect of the drugs after the procedure.

GP IIb/IIIa inhibitors have demonstrated variable degrees of efficacy in the setting of acute coronary syndromes and PCI. There is general consensus that a GP IIb/IIIa agent, particularly abciximab, is recommended in patients undergoing primary PCI for STEMI, NSTEMI, or planned PCI in high-risk patients such as diabetics. A meta-analysis of 20 studies, including 20,137 patients undergoing PCI, reported a significant and sustained reduction in the risk of death and acute MI after PCI by the use of GP IIb/IIIa inhibitors, with an increase in the risk of major

TABLE 1 Antiplatelet Drugs

Class	Drug	Antiplatelet action	Administration	Loading dose	First dose to effect time	Regimen after PCI	Dose adjustment in renal failure
Aspirin	Aspirin	Irreversible	Oral/IV[a]	162–325 mg PO 250–500 mg IV[a]	< 1 hr	75–100 mg daily	No
Thienopyridines	Ticlopidine	Irreversible	Oral	1000 mg	24–48 hr	250 mg twice daily	No
	Clopidogrel	Irreversible	Oral	300 600/900 mg[b]	6–24 hr 2–6 hr	75 mg daily	No
GP IIb/IIIa inhibitors	Abciximab	Irreversible	IV	0.25 mg/kg	minutes	0.125 µg/kg/min for 12 hr	No (not recommended if severe RF)
	Eptifibatide	Reversible	IV	180 µg/kg bolus × 2, 10 min apart	minutes	2 µg/kg/min for 18 hr	Yes (not recommended if severe RF)
	Tirofiban	Reversible	IV	0.4 µg/kg/min for 30 min (or 25 µg/kg)	minutes	0.1 µg/kg/min for 12 hr	Yes, half dose if CrCl < 30 mL/min

[a]In some countries.
[b]In untreated patients undergoing urgent PCI.
Abbreviation: RF, renal failure.

bleeding only in patients with continued postprocedure heparin therapy (20). The degree of evidence is best established for abciximab, especially in the setting of PCI for STEMI, less for eptifibatide, and least for tirofiban. Orally administered GP IIb/ IIIa inhibitors studied in a variety of coronary artery disease presentations were generally associated with poor outcomes and excess mortality (21,22).

Other Antiplatelet Agents

Other agents with some antiplatelet activity such as cilostazol, dipyridamole, and reversible COX-1 inhibitors (sulfinpyrazone, indobufen, triflusal) have been studied in clinical trials. There is no established evidence that these drugs have clinical benefit in any setting of coronary artery disease compared with aspirin or thieno-pyridines. Therefore, their use in the setting of primary PCI is not recommended.

ANTIPLATELET THERAPY IN THE SETTING OF CATHETER-BASED REPERFUSION THERAPY (TABLE 2)

Both mechanical reperfusion by primary PCI and pharmacologic reperfusion by fibrinolysis are efficient methods of restoring coronary flow in the infarct-related artery, reducing infarct size, and saving lives. While fibrinolysis is still used as the first-line reperfusion strategy in most countries, there is general consensus that when primary PCI is available, it is the best approach to reperfusion therapy, associated with more efficient reperfusion; lower rates of short- and long-term death, MI, recurrent ischemia, and stroke; but more major bleeding complications (3).

There are two major drawbacks to the benefit of primary PCI for acute STEMI. First, the successful recanalization of the infarct-related artery (IRA) does not always result in adequate myocardial perfusion because of potential distal embolization of thrombi during PCI. Second, the transfer delay may reduce the benefit of primary PCI (23–25). The early administration of powerful antiplatelet agents may be a solution to both drawbacks.

Aspirin

Although no specific data are available comparing aspirin with a placebo, or concerning the time of administration of aspirin in the setting of primary PCI, the general 30% and 50% vascular risk reductions associated with such medication in

TABLE 2   Use of Antiplatelet Drugs in the Setting of Primary PCI for STEMI

Antiplatelet agent	Initial administration	Therapy after PCI
Aspirin	As soon as possible 162–325 mg PO 250–500 mg IV[a]	75–100 mg PO indefinitely
Clopidogrel	As soon as possible 600/900 mg PO	75 mg daily for at least 1 month[b]
Abciximab	As soon as possible 0.25 mg/kg IV bolus 0.125 µg/kg/min IV infusion for 12 hours (max of 10 µg/min)	12 hr

[a]In some countries.
[b]In patients with sirolimus/paclitaxel eluting stents, at least 2/6 months, and in general 9 to 12 months' clopidogrel therapy is recommended.

the settings of acute MI and PCI justify the class I A recommendation of the ACC/ AHA and ESC experts. An initial 162 to 325 mg oral dose of aspirin should be administered as soon as possible, followed by an indefinite 75 to 162 mg daily maintenance dose in the setting of primary PCI in absence of contraindication to such therapy (4,5,26).

Clopidogrel

The antiplatelet action of clopidogrel is delayed after its oral administration. Nevertheless, with higher loading doses (600–900 mg) such delay can be significantly shortened (13,15). Similar to aspirin, there are no randomized data available comparing clopidogrel with placebo or concerning the time of administration or the dose of clopidogrel in the setting of primary PCI. Based on the higher risks of surgery-related bleeding among patients with NSTEMI treated with aspirin and clopidogrel in the CURE trial, the ACC/AHA guidelines recommend (class I B) the use of clopidogrel in all patients undergoing primary PCI, only after the initial angiography has excluded the need for surgical revascularization (5). This recommendation can be challenged, as the rates of primary surgical reperfusion for STEMI or urgent surgery after primary PCI are extremely low and the late administration of clopidogrel may delay reperfusion, favor distal embolization, and increase acute stent thrombosis. More recent ESC guidelines on PCI recommend (class I C) the administration of a 600 mg loading dose of clopidogrel in STEMI patients who are clinically eligible for primary PCI at the first medical contact (8). Such considerations need to be assessed by randomized trials but have already led to prehospital high-loading dose strategies in some countries. Clopidogrel is recommended for up to 12 months after primary PCI in association with aspirin.

Platelet GP IIb/IIIa Inhibitors (Table 3)

GP IIb/IIIa inhibitors are associated with reduced thrombotic events in a broad spectrum of PCI settings, including primary PCI. GP IIb/IIIa inhibitors decrease distal embolization and have been shown to reduce death and MI in acute coronary syndromes without increasing the risk of intracranial or severe hemorrhage (27).

GP IIb/IIIa inhibitors are powerful antiplatelet drugs, with rapid biological effects suited to primary PCI. The benefit of GPIIb/IIIa therapy in primary PCI has been widely demonstrated in terms of pre-PCI coronary flow, angiographic parameters, and the composite end point of death, MI, and urgent target vessel revascularization (28–31). The other GPIIb/IIIa inhibitors, eptifibatide and tirofiban, have been less extensively studied in this setting. Nevertheless, they have been reported to improve outcome in the general setting of PCI for acute coronary syndromes (20).

The ADMIRAL study (28) enrolled 300 patients with STEMI undergoing primary stenting. Patients were randomized to receive either a placebo or abciximab before catheterization. Patients treated by abciximab had higher IRA patency rates (TIMI 2/3 flow rates 25.9% vs. 10.8%) before revascularization and LVEF (61% vs. 57%) at six months follow-up. The rate of the primary composite end point of death, reinfarction, or need for subsequent target-vessel revascularization was significantly lower in patients treated by abciximab compared with the placebo at 30 days (6.0% vs. 14.6%, $p = 0.01$) and at six months (7.4% vs. 15.9%, $p = 0.02$).

The CADILLAC study (32) randomized 2082 acute MI patients (88% with STEMI) to primary PCI by balloon angioplasty alone versus stenting and to placebo versus abciximab in the catheterization laboratory after a qualifying angiogram.

The primary composite end point of death, reinfarction, revascularization, or disabling stroke was higher in the group assigned to balloon PCI alone (8.3%), compared with the other three groups (4.8% in balloon PCI plus abciximab, 5.7% in stenting alone, 4.4% in stenting plus abciximab groups). Nevertheless, abciximab-treated patients had significantly lower rates of death, recurrent MI, or urgent target vessel revascularization at 30 days compared with those treated by placebo (4.6% vs. 6.8%).

The ACE study randomized 400 patients to primary stenting alone or associated with abciximab immediately before the procedure. At 30 days, the incidence of the primary composite end point of death, reinfarction, target-vessel revascularization, or stroke was reduced in the stent plus abciximab group compared with the stent-alone group (4.5% vs. 10.5%; $p = 0.02$) (33).

The prior studies were all underpowered to demonstrate a mortality reduction with the use of abciximab. A recent meta-analysis of eight randomized trials comparing abciximab versus placebo as adjunctive therapy to primary PCI in STEMI demonstrated a significant mortality reduction at 30 days (2.4% vs. 3.4%, $p = 0.047$) and at 6 to 12 months (4.4% vs. 6.2%, $p = 0.01$). The authors estimated that the number of patients needed to be treated by abciximab to prevent one death was 100 at 30 days and 55.6 at 6 to 12 months, making this strategy cost-effective (34).

The level of evidence for a beneficial action of the two other GP IIb/IIIa inhibitors in the setting of primary PCI is extremely poor, limited to one feasibility angiographic study for eptifibatide (35) and one small randomized placebo controlled trial for tirofiban (36). In one recent randomized trial comparing standard dose abciximab with high dose tirofiban (0.25 μg/kg bolus followed by 0.15 μg/kg/min infusion) in patients undergoing primary PCI, the post-PCI TIMI flow grade, corrected TIMI frame count, and 30-day left ventricular function recovery were similar between the two groups (37) Randomized placebo-controlled trials of GPIIb/IIIa inhibitors in the setting of primary PCI are summarized in Table 3.

PRIMARY PCI WITH ABCIXIMAB OR FACILITATED PRIMARY PCI? (TABLE 4)

While the systematic use of abciximab as adjunctive therapy to primary PCI for STEMI is already recommended, the timing of the administration of GPIIb/IIIa inhibitors still remains a matter of debate.

Rationale for Facilitated Primary PCI

The rationale for the facilitation of primary PCI by a pharmacologic approach is based on three major considerations: (1) the progressive and irreversible nature of the ischemia-related myocardial necrosis (38,39); (2) the inverse relationship between time to reperfusion and both the extent of the salvaged myocardium and survival (23,25,40,41); and (3) the relationship between antegrade coronary flow prior to primary PCI and contractility recovery and survival after STEMI (42–44).

Hence, the facilitated PCI strategy providing an early restoration of a certain degree of flow prior to primary PCI appears to be a logical and attractive option in STEMI patients. Considering the unsuccessful or unresolved issues of fibrinolytic facilitation with or without GP IIb/IIIa inhibitors, the early administration of GP IIb/IIIa alone in STEMI patients prior to PCI remains the most realistic facilitation strategy.

TABLE 3 Randomized Trials Comparing Administration of GP IIb/IIIa Inhibitors Versus Placebo as Adjunctive Therapy to Primary PCI for STEMI

Study	Agent	No. of patients	Major findings
RAPPORT (31)	Abciximab	483	Abciximab-associated significant reduction of the composite of death, MI, urgent TVR at 30 days
ISAR-2 (76)	Abciximab	401	Abciximab-associated significant reduction of the composite of death, reinfarction and TLR at 30 days
ADMIRAL (28)	Abciximab	300	Abciximab-associated significant reduction of the composite of death, MI, urgent TVR at 30 days and 6 months
CADILLAC (32)	Abciximab	2082	No significant difference in the occurrence of the composite of death, MI, disabling stroke and ischemia driven TVR at 6 months between stent groups with or without abciximab
Petronio et al.[a] (77)	Abciximab	89	Abciximab-associated significant reduction of the composite of death, reinfarction, congestive heart failure, target lesion revascularization, or recurrent ischemia at 30-days and 6-months
Zorman et al. (47)	Abciximab	163	Lower rates of in-hospital and 6 month mortality in patients receiving abciximab (specially those receiving pre-angiography abciximab)
ACE (33)	Abciximab	400	Abciximab-associated significant reduction of the composite of death, MI, TVR and stroke at 1 month
Petronio et al (78)	Abciximab	31	Abciximab-associated better myocardial perfusion, preserved microvascular integrity and LV global and regional function recover assessed by cTFC, MCE and 99mTc-SPECT
Steen et al (36)	Tirofiban	53	In-hospital MRI-derived TFC, perfusion signal and regional wall motion significantly favored tirofiban

[a]Rescue PCI after failed thrombolysis.

GP IIb/IIIa Inhibitor Facilitated PCI

Early administration of abciximab in the emergency room or the mobile intensive care unit was tested for the first time in the ADMIRAL trial (28). Abciximab was associated with higher infarct-related artery patency rates and a trend towards higher risk reduction for the primary end point of the study (death/reinfarction/ urgent target vessel revascularization) in patients receiving the drug in the mobile intensive care units compared with those treated later at 30 days (OR = 0.12 vs. 0.67) and six months (OR = 0.11 vs. 0.69).

Several recent randomized trials have studied the effect of the early administration of GP IIb/IIIa inhibitors compared with their administration in the cardiac catheterization laboratory, prior or during primary PCI (Table 4). All these trials are underpowered to detect significant differences in hard clinical outcomes among the studied groups. Surrogate end points, such as pre-PCI TIMI flow grade and/or ST-segment elevation regression, were used to assess the efficacy of the early administration of GP IIb/IIIa inhibitors. While the results are quite heterogeneous between the trials, there is a general trend towards better myocardial perfusion, assessed by ST-segment resolution, and higher rates of infarct-related artery patency prior to PCI in patients with early GP IIb/IIIa therapy (45–52). A meta-analysis from

TABLE 4 Randomized Trials Comparing Early Versus Late Administration of GP IIb/IIIa Inhibitors as Adjunctive Therapy to Primary PCI for STEMI

Study	Agent	No. of patients		Pre-PCI TIMI 2/3		Pre-PCI TIMI 3	
		Early group	Late group	Early group	Late group	Early group	Late group
ON-TIME (49)	Tirofiban	251	256	43%[a]	34%	19%	15%
TIGER-PA (51)	Tirofiban	50	50	46%[a]	18%	32%[a]	10%
Cutlip et al. (45)	Tirofiban	28	30	39%	27%	32%	20%
TITAN[c]	Tirofiban	174	142	46%	37%	24%	19%
Zorman et al. (47)	Abciximab	56	56	32%[a]	13%	16%[a]	2%
REOMOBILE (50)	Abciximab	52	48	52%	48%	NA	NA
ERAMI (46)	Abciximab	36	38	31%	26%	11%	8%
REOPRO-BRIDGING (52)	Abciximab	28	27	61%[a]	33%	29%[a]	7%
INTAMI (48)	Eptifibatide	52	47[b]	42%	33%	34%[a]	10%

[a]Statistically significant ($p < 0.05$) differences between groups.
[b]Only 42 patients of the group had eptifibatide.
[c]Unpublished data, presented at the Texas Heart Institute, 2005.

our center in a pooled population of 931 STEMI patients studied the effect of early administration of GP IIb/IIIa inhibitors (tirofiban or abciximab) compared with administration during primary PCI. (53) The study showed a significant increase in rates of TIMI grade 2/3 flow (OR = 1.69, 95% CI = 1.28–2.22, $p < 0.001$] and TIMI grade 3 flow (OR = 1.85, 95% CI = 1.26–2.71, $p < 0.001$) by the early use of GP IIb/IIIa inhibitors. Odds ratios were similar between the two tested drugs. The analysis also showed a nonsignificant trend in favor of early GP IIb/IIIa therapy regarding mortality (OR = 0.72 95% CI = 0.37–1.4), reinfarction (OR = 0.73, 95% CI = 0.31–1.77), and the composite ischemic end point (OR = 0.78, 95% CI = 0.51–1.20).

A more recent meta-analysis including nine randomized trials enrolling 1074 patients undergoing primary PCI facilitated or not by GP IIb/IIIa inhibitors (5 trials with abciximab, 3 with tirofiban, and 1 with eptifibatide), has reported improved initial TIMI flow rates (26% vs. 15% $p = 0.0001$), but a similar incidence of early mortality (3% for both approaches), non fatal reinfarction (1% for both approaches), urgent target vessel revascularization (2% for both approaches), and a non significant trend towards a higher incidence of major bleeding (7% vs. 5%, $p = 0.3$) (54). The same meta-analysis showed deleterious effects of PCI facilitation by fibrinolytic therapy compared with placebo in terms of death, reinfarction, urgent target vessel revascularization and major bleeding.

The heterogeneity of the results concerning facilitation of primary PCI by GP IIb/IIIa inhibitors may have several explanations. First, despite a class effect, there might be differences between GP IIb/IIIa inhibitors in STEMI patients as has been reported in ACS or PCI settings (55,56). Moreover, abciximab is still the only GP IIb/IIIa inhibitor that has demonstrated its efficacy regarding hard clinical outcomes after primary PCI for STEMI. Indeed, a recent pooled analysis of six abciximab studies, comparing early to late administration, showed impressive results not only for admission patency rates but also for microvascular reperfusion as evaluated by ST-segment resolution. Furthermore, an absolute, but nonsignificant, 2% reduction in mortality was found with early abciximab administration (57). Second, there are differences between studies regarding the inclusion criteria (STEMI <6 or 12 hours) and the time from symptom to GP IIb/IIIa inhibitor administration, both in patients with early (average time from 38 to 259 minutes) and late (average time from 82 to 374 minutes) administration of the drug. The studies with very early administration of GP IIb/IIIa inhibitors (<2 hours after the symptom onset), appear to be those where the effect of the drug on the infarct-related pre-PCI flow and/or mortality is the most important (45,47,50,52). The longer time to presentation and to administration of the drug reduces the amount of myocardium to be salvaged and consequently may reduce the potential effect of the early administration of GP IIb/IIIa inhibitors. It may also change the architecture of the thrombus which becomes more resistant to the "dethrombotic" effect of the drugs.

There is strong evidence that abciximab reduces mortality by approximately 25% in the setting of primary PCI and its use is recommended (class IIa A or B) in absence of contraindications (5,6,8,26). Hence, the timing of its administration may no more be a true matter of debate. Considering the few downsides of the early GP IIb/IIIa facilitation strategy, its generalization may already be recommended in patients presenting with STEMI who are candidates for primary PCI.

Primary PCI Facilitated by Combination Fibrinolysis+GP IIb/IIIa Inhibitor Therapy

Based on high rates of infarct artery patency after low-dose lytic therapy combined with GP IIb/IIIa inhibitors and the potential synergistic effects of combination therapy in several phase II studies, two trials studied the benefit of this therapy compared with GP IIb/IIIa alone prior to primary PCI. The BRAVE trial (58) enrolled 253 STEMI patients who randomly received either half-dose reteplase and standard abciximab therapy or standard abciximab therapy alone. Despite significantly higher rates of initial TIMI grade 3 infarct artery flow, the study failed to show any difference in the post-PCI TIMI flow grades, infarct size, or clinical outcomes at one and six months. The ADVANCE MI trial comparing half-dose TNK plus eptifibatide versus eptifibatide alone prior to PCI was prematurely terminated because of slow recruitment. The underpowered analysis among the 148 patients showed significantly higher IRA patency before PCI, but higher rates of the composite rate of death or new/worsening severe heart failure at 30 days, and a two-fold increase in bleeding complications (59).

The GP IIb/IIIa inhibitor plus low-dose fibrinolytic combination prior to PCI cannot be recommended because of the lack of benefit and the potential bleeding risk. The results of the FINESSE trial support this conclusion.

ANTIPLATELET THERAPY IN THE SETTING OF FIBRINOLYTIC THERAPY

Fibrinolytic therapy remains the first line therapy for STEMI in many countries as it is universally available and can be initiated in primary centers, emergency rooms, and even prior to hospitalization in mobile intensive care units. Nevertheless, it is limited by low rates of infarct-related artery patency and high rates of recurrent ischemia, justifying antiplatelet adjunctive therapy and proximity of catheterization laboratories if rescue PCI is required. Fibrinolysis administered early (<3 hours) after the onset of STEMI is reported to be associated with similar rates of death but higher rates of urgent coronary revascularization compared with primary PCI (60,61). Whether facilitated primary PCI may provide better results compared with fibrinolysis needs to be assessed. The results of the recently published SWEDES study, showing higher rates of infarct artery patency and a trend towards better clinical outcomes in patients undergoing abciximab-facilitated PCI compared to those treated by fibrinolysis despite much shorter symptom to treatment time in the latter group (62), support such a hypothesis.

Aspirin
The ISIS-2 trial was a blinded, placebo-controlled study with a 2 × 2 factorial design testing aspirin alone (162.5 mg/d for 1 month), streptokinase alone, both, or neither in clinically suspected STEMI. The study enrolled 17,187 patients within 24 h of symptom onset (1). Streptokinase alone was associated with a 25% reduction in 35-day vascular mortality compared with placebo. Aspirin alone was associated with a 23% risk reduction for the same end point. The effects of aspirin and streptokinase were additive with a 42% reduction in vascular mortality in the dual therapy group. The addition of aspirin to streptokinase was also associated with reduced rates of reinfarction, cardiac arrest, cardiac rupture, and stroke. The ISIS-2 trial is the pivotal and only placebo-controlled trial leading to the class I A recommendation of the ACC/AHA and ESC experts suggesting an initial 162 to 325 mg oral dose of aspirin as soon as possible followed by an indefinite 75 to 162 mg daily maintenance dose in the setting of fibrinolysis for STEMI in absence of contraindication to such therapy (5,26).

Clopidogrel
The benefit of the association of clopidogrel with aspirin in the setting of fibrinolytic therapy was unknown until the publication of COMMIT and CLARITY trials. The COMMIT trial was a randomized, placebo-controlled study enrolling 45,852 patients within 24 hours of onset of STEMI, to receive clopidogrel 75 mg OD (without loading dose) or matching placebo until discharge or up to four weeks in-hospital (63). The 2 × 2 factorial design of the study allowed separate assessment of metoprolol versus placebo in the same population. The study demonstrated that the addition of clopidogrel to aspirin was associated with significant risk reductions for death (RRR 7%, $p = 0.03$), and the composite of death, reinfarction, or stroke (RRR 9%, $p = 0.002$), without significant excess risk of major bleeding. Among 55% of patients receiving fibrinolytic therapy, the risk of the composite primary end point was significantly lower in the clopidogrel group (8.8% vs. 9.9%, RRR 11%) with comparable major bleeding rates.

The CLARITY-TIMI 28 trial enrolled 3491 STEMI patients undergoing fibrinolytic therapy (64) who presented within 12 hours after symptom onset. They were randomly assigned to receive clopidogrel (300 mg loading dose, followed by 75 mg once daily) or placebo. All patients received aspirin and were scheduled to undergo angiography two to eight days after admission. The primary efficacy end point was a composite of angiographic IRA occlusion on day two to eight or death or recurrent MI before angiography. Clopidogrel was associated with a 36% ($p < 0.001$) reduction in the odds of the primary end point. Furthermore, clopidogrel was associated with a 31% reduction ($p = 0.02$) in the odds of recurrent MI, and a 20% reduction ($p = 0.03$) in the odds of the composite of death from cardiovascular causes, recurrent MI, or recurrent ischemia leading to urgent revascularization within 30 days after randomization.

The PCI-CLARITY trial was a prespecified substudy of the CLARITY trial, assessing the potential benefit of clopidogrel pretreatment in 1863 patients undergoing PCI after fibrinolytic therapy (65). Pretreatment with clopidogrel was associated with reductions in the incidence of MI or stroke prior to PCI (4.0% vs. 6.2%; $p = 0.03$); and cardiovascular death, MI, or stroke following PCI (3.6% vs 6.2%; $p = 0.008$). Overall, pretreatment with clopidogrel resulted in a reduction in cardiovascular death, MI, or stroke from randomization through 30 days (adjusted OR, 0.59; $p = 0.001$) with no significant excess in bleeding.

Clopidogrel (initial 300 mg loading dose followed by 75 mg daily) should be considered as adjunctive therapy to fibrinolytic therapy and aspirin.

GP IIb/IIIa Inhibitors

In vitro studies have demonstrated a synergic effect of GP IIb/IIIa inhibitors disaggregating the platelet rich clots and exposing fibrin to fibrinolytics, hence facilitating fibrinolysis and controlling the potential deleterious effects of lytic-induced thrombin generation (66–68).

Several trials assessing such associations were conducted, based on the hypotheses that (1) GP IIb/IIIa inhibitors alone or in association with fibrinolysis may lead to higher rates of infarct-related artery patency and (2) the association of GP IIb/IIIa inhibitors with half-dose fibrinolysis may reduce the risk of major bleeding in STEMI patients. Randomized trials comparing the administration of GP IIb/IIIa Inhibitors versus placebo as adjunctive therapy to thrombolysis in STEMI are summarized in Table 5.

The TIMI-14 trial randomized 888 patients with STEMI within 12 hours after symptom onset to receive either full-dose alteplase (100 mg), abciximab alone (bolus 0.25 mg/kg and a 12-hour infusion of 0.125 µg/kg/min) or abciximab in combination with reduced doses of alteplase (20 to 65 mg) or streptokinase (500,000 U to 1.5 MU) (69). Patients with abciximab regimens received low-dose heparin while those treated with full-dose alteplase received standard heparin doses. TIMI 3 flow rates were significantly higher in the 50 mg alteplase plus abciximab group compared with the full-dose alteplase group at both 60 minutes (72% vs. 43%; $p = 0.0009$) and 90 minutes (77% vs. 62%; $p = 0.02$).

The Intro AMI trial enrolled a total of 649 STEMI patients, who received either eptifibatide (4 different regimens) with low dose alteplase or full dose alteplase (70). The study showed significantly higher rates of TIMI 3 flow in the IRA at 60 minutes with eptifibatide (double 180/90 µg/Kg bolus + 2 µg/Kg/min infusion) compared with full-dose alteplase (56% vs. 40%, $p = 0.02$).

Three major clinical trials have studied the benefit of abciximab plus fibrinolytic combination therapy. The GUSTO V trial randomly assigned 16,588 patients presenting within six hours after STEMI to receive full-dose reteplase or half-dose reteplase plus abciximab (71). At 30 days, the rates of mortality (primary end point) were comparable between standard and combination therapy groups (5.9% vs. 5.6%). Compared with standard therapy, combination therapy was nevertheless associated with lower rates of reinfarction (2.3 vs. 3.5%; $p < 0.0001$), recurrent ischemia (11.3% vs. 12.8%; $p = 0.004$), and sustained ventricular tachycardia and ventricular fibrillation. Such findings were counterbalanced by higher rates of severe extracranial bleeding in the combination therapy group (1.1% vs. 0.5%, $p < 0.0001$). The one-year follow-up of patients enrolled in the GUSTO V trial did not show any difference in mortality rates between the two groups (72).

The ASSENT-III trial studied another fibrin-specific agent, tenecteplase (73). The study enrolled 6095 patients within six hours after STEMI and randomly assigned them to full-dose tenecteplase and enoxaparin, half-dose tenecteplase with low-dose unfractionated heparin and abciximab, or full-dose tenecteplase with standard-dose unfractionated heparin. The incidence of the primary composite end point (30-day mortality, in-hospital reinfarction, or in-hospital refractory ischemia) was lower in the enoxaparin and abciximab groups compared with the unfractionated heparin group

TABLE 5 Randomized Trials Comparing Administration of GP IIb/IIIa Inhibitors Versus Placebo as Adjunctive Therapy to Thrombolysis in STEMI

Study (Ref.)	GP IIb/IIIa inhibitor	Lytic	No. of patients	Major findings
TIMI 14 (69)	Abciximab	Reteplase	888	Higher rates of TIMI 3 flow at 60 and 90 min in the combination therapy group
SPEED (79)	Abciximab	Reteplase	198	Trend to higher rates of TIMI 3 flow at 60 to 90 min in the combination therapy group
ASSENT 3 (73)	Abciximab	Tenecteplase	6095	Lower rates of primary efficacy (30 days death/re-MI or refractory ischemia) and efficacy + safety (efficacy endpoint + intracranial or major bleeding) endpoints in the combination therapy group
ENTIRE-TIMI 23 (74)	Abciximab	Tenecteplase	483	Lower rates of 30 days death/re-MI in the combination therapy group
GUSTO V (71)	Abciximab	Reteplase	16588	Lower rates of 30 days death/re-MI in the combination therapy group
INTEGRITI (80)	Eptifibatide	Tenecteplase	140	Trend to higher rates of TIMI 3 flow at 60 min in the combination therapy group
INTRO MI (70)	Eptifibatide	Alteplase	305	Higher rates of TIMI 3 flow at 60 to 90 min in the combination therapy group
IMPACT-AMI (81)	Eptifibatide	Alteplase	48	Higher rates of TIMI 3 flow at 90 min in the combination therapy group
FASTER-TIMI 24 (82)	Tirofiban	Tenecteplase	409	Faster ST segment elevation resolution in combination therapy group

(11.4% and 11.1% vs. 15.4% $p < 0.0001$ and $p = 0.0002$, respectively). The efficacy plus safety end point (grouping the primary end point and intracranial or severe bleeding) also favored the enoxaparin and abciximab groups (13.7% and 14.2% vs. 17%, $p = 0.0037$ and $p = 0.014$, respectively).

Finally, the ENTIRE-TIMI 23 trial enrolled 483 patients with STEMI presenting less than six hours from symptom onset who were randomized to full-dose tenecteplase (with either unfractionated heparin or enoxaparin) or half-dose TNK plus abciximab (with either low dose unfractionated heparin or low dose enoxaparin) (74). The rates of TIMI 3 flow at 60 minutes were comparable among the four groups. The composit of death/recurrent MI with full-dose TNK occurred in 15.9% with UFH versus 4.4% with enoxaparin. Among patients receiving combination therapy, the rates of death/recurrent MI were 6.5% and 5.5%, with UFH and enoxaparin respectively. Thus, there was no difference in TIMI 3 flow rates or risk of major hemorrhage with enoxaparin, but there were fewer ischemic events.

The meta-analysis of the three previous trials failed to show a significant effect of abciximab use among fibrinolytic-treated patients in terms of 30-day or 6- to 12-month mortality, but the 30-day reinfarction rate was significantly reduced with combination therapy (2.3 vs. 3.6%; $p < 0.001$) (34). This finding was counterbalanced by higher rates of extracranial bleeding associated with the combination therapy (5.2% vs. 3.1%; $p < 0.001$). The fibrinolysis and GP IIb/IIIa inhibitor combination therapy appears to be associated with higher rates of bleeding and is not recommended by expert guidelines.

THE FUTURE OF ANTIPLATELET REGIMENS IN THE SETTING OF REPERFUSION THERAPY FOR STEMI

The benefit of low-dose fibrinolytic plus GP IIb/IIIa inhibitor combination therapy prior to PCI, the potential differences between different GP IIb/IIIa inhibitors, the identification of patient subgroups profiting most from different strategies, and the role of other antiplatelet regimens still remain unresolved issues. Specific and adequately sized trials are needed to answer these important questions.

The FINESSE trial (75) comparing an ADMIRAL strategy (preangiography abciximab alone) with a CADILLAC strategy (postangiography abciximab alone) and a combination facilitation strategy (half-dose reteplase with abciximab prior to angiography) recently presented at the American Heart Association 2007 scientific sessions did not support the facilitated PCI strategy.

Newer antiplatelet agents such as prasugrel, a thienopyridine derivative with potentially faster action and fewer nonresponders, other $P2Y_{12}$ receptor antagonists, and platelet thrombin receptor antagonists are being investigated and may improve antiplatelet therapy in the near future. Their place in the wide panel of antithrombotic regimens remains to be identified in the setting of reperfusion therapy for STEMI with higher clopidogrel loading doses and earlier timing of antiplatelet administration.

REFERENCES

1. Randomised trial of intravenous streptokinase, oral aspirin, both, or neither among 17,187 cases of suspected acute myocardial infarction: ISIS-2. ISIS-2 (Second International Study of Infarct Survival) Collaborative Group. Lancet 1988; 2:349–360.
2. Franzosi MG, Santoro E, De Vita C, et al. Ten-year follow-up of the first megatrial testing thrombolytic therapy in patients with acute myocardial infarction: results of the Gruppo Italiano per lo Studio della Sopravvivenza nell'Infarto-1 study. The GISSI Investigators. Circulation 1998; 98:2659–2665.
3. Keeley EC, Boura JA, Grines CL. Primary angioplasty versus intravenous thrombolytic therapy for acute myocardial infarction: a quantitative review of 23 randomised trials. Lancet 2003; 361:13–20.
4. Collaborative metaanalysis of randomised trials of antiplatelet therapy for prevention of death, myocardial infarction, and stroke in high risk patients. Antithrombotic Trialists' Collaboration. BMJ 2002; 324:71–86.
5. Antman EM, Anbe DT, Armstrong PW, et al. ACC/AHA guidelines for the management of patients with ST-elevation myocardial infarction; A report of the American College of Cardiology/American Heart Association Task Force on Practice Guidelines (Committee to Revise the 1999 Guidelines for the Management of patients with acute myocardial infarction). J Am Coll Cardiol 2004; 44:E1–E211.
6. Patrono C, Bachmann F, Baigent C, et al. Expert consensus document on the use of antiplatelet agents. The task force on the use of antiplatelet agents in patients with atherosclerotic cardiovascular disease of the European society of cardiology. Eur Heart J 2004; 25:166–181.

7. Montalescot G, Andersen HR, Antoniucci D, et al. Recommendations on percutaneous coronary intervention for the reperfusion of acute ST elevation myocardial infarction. Heart 2004; 90:e37.
8. Silber S, Albertsson P, Aviles FF, et al. Guidelines for percutaneous coronary interventions. The Task Force for Percutaneous Coronary Interventions of the European Society of Cardiology. Eur Heart J 2005; 26:804–847.
9. Popma JJ, Berger P, Ohman EM, et al. Antithrombotic therapy during percutaneous coronary intervention: the Seventh ACCP Conference on Antithrombotic and Thrombolytic Therapy. Chest 2004; 126:576S–599S.
10. Menon V, Harrington RA, Hochman JS, et al. Thrombolysis and adjunctive therapy in acute myocardial infarction: the Seventh ACCP Conference on Antithrombotic and Thrombolytic Therapy. Chest 2004; 126:549S–575S.
11. Schomig A, Neumann FJ, Kastrati A, et al. A randomized comparison of antiplatelet and anticoagulant therapy after the placement of coronary-artery stents. N Engl J Med 1996; 334:1084–1089.
12. Hass WK, Easton JD, Adams HPJr., et al. A randomized trial comparing ticlopidine hydrochloride with aspirin for the prevention of stroke in high-risk patients. Ticlopidine Aspirin Stroke Study Group. N Engl J Med 1989; 321:501–507.
13. Montalescot G, Sideris G, Meuleman C, et al. A randomized comparison of high clopidogrel loading-doses in patients with non-ST-elevation acute coronary syndromes: The ALBION (Assessment of the Best Loading Dose of Clopidgrel to Blunt Platelet Activation, Inflammatin, and Ongoing Necrosis) trial. J Am Coll Cardiol 2006; 48:93–98.
14. Kandzari DE, Berger PB, Kastrati A, et al. Influence of treatment duration with a 600-mg dose of clopidogrel before percutaneous coronary revascularization. J Am Coll Cardiol 2004; 44:2133–2136.
15. Kastrati A, von Beckerath N, Joost A, et al. Loading with 600 mg clopidogrel in patients with coronary artery disease with and without chronic clopidogrel therapy. Circulation 2004; 110:1916–1919.
16. Bhatt DL, Bertrand ME, Berger PB, et al. Meta-analysis of randomized and registry comparisons of ticlopidine with clopidogrel after stenting. J Am Coll Cardiol 2002; 39:9–14.
17. Bertrand ME, Rupprecht HJ, Urban P, et al. Double-blind study of the safety of clopidogrel with and without a loading dose in combination with aspirin compared with ticlopidine in combination with aspirin after coronary stenting: the clopidogrel aspirin stent international cooperative study (CLASSICS). Circulation 2000; 102:624–629.
18. Steinhubl SR, Berger PB, Mann JT3rd, , et al. Early and sustained dual oral antiplatelet therapy following percutaneous coronary intervention: a randomized controlled trial. JAMA 2002; 288:2411–2420.
19. Mehta SR, Yusuf S, Peters RJ, et al. Effects of pretreatment with clopidogrel and aspirin followed by long-term therapy in patients undergoing percutaneous coronary intervention: the PCI-CURE study. Lancet 2001; 358:527–533.
20. Karvouni E, Katritsis DG, Ioannidis JP. Intravenous glycoprotein IIb/IIIa receptor antagonists reduce mortality after percutaneous coronary interventions. J Am Coll Cardiol 2003; 41:26–32.
21. Heeschen C, Hamm CW. Difficulties with oral platelet glycoprotein IIb/IIIa receptor antagonists. Lancet 2000; 355:330–331.
22. The SYMPHONY Investigators, . Comparison of sibrafiban with aspirin for prevention of cardiovascular events after acute coronary syndromes: a randomised trial. Lancet 2000; 355:337–345.
23. De Luca G, Suryapranata H, Zijlstra F, et al. Symptom-onset-to-balloon time and mortality in patients with acute myocardial infarction treated by primary angioplasty. J Am Coll Cardiol 2003; 42:991–997.
24. Antoniucci D, Valenti R, Migliorini A, et al. Relation of time to treatment and mortality in patients with acute myocardial infarction undergoing primary coronary angioplasty. Am J Cardiol 2002; 89:1248–1252.
25. Cannon CP, Gibson CM, Lambrew CT, et al. Relationship of symptom-onset-to-balloon time and door-to-balloon time with mortality in patients undergoing angioplasty for acute myocardial infarction. JAMA 2000; 283:2941–2947.

26. Van de Werf F, Ardissino D, Betriu A, et al. Management of acute myocardial infarction in patients presenting with ST-segment elevation. The Task Force on the Management of Acute Myocardial Infarction of the European Society of Cardiology. Eur Heart J 2003; 24:28–66.
27. Boersma E, Harrington RA, Moliterno DJ, et al. Platelet glycoprotein IIb/IIIa inhibitors in acute coronary syndromes: a meta-analysis of all major randomised clinical trials. Lancet 2002; 359:189–198.
28. Montalescot G, Barragan P, Wittenberg O, et al. Platelet glycoprotein IIb/IIIa inhibition with coronary stenting for acute myocardial infarction. N Engl J Med 2001; 344:1895–1903.
29. Neumann FJ, Blasini R, Schmitt C, et al. Effect of glycoprotein IIb/IIIa receptor blockade on recovery of coronary flow and left ventricular function after the placement of coronary-artery stents in acute myocardial infarction. Circulation 1998; 98:2695–2701.
30. Tcheng JE, Kandzari DE, Grines CL, et al. Benefits and risks of abciximab use in primary angioplasty for acute myocardial infarction: the Controlled Abciximab and Device Investigation to Lower Late Angioplasty Complications (CADILLAC) trial. Circulation 2003; 108:1316–1323.
31. Brener SJ, Barr LA, Burchenal JE, et al. Randomized, placebo-controlled trial of platelet glycoprotein IIb/IIIa blockade with primary angioplasty for acute myocardial infarction. ReoPro and Primary PTCA Organization and Randomized Trial (RAPPORT) Investigators. Circulation 1998; 98:734–741.
32. Stone GW, Grines CL, Cox DA, et al. Comparison of angioplasty with stenting, with or without abciximab, in acute myocardial infarction. N Engl J Med 2002; 346:957–966.
33. Antoniucci D, Rodriguez A, Hempel A, et al. A randomized trial comparing primary infarct artery stenting with or without abciximab in acute myocardial infarction. J Am Coll Cardiol 2003; 42:1879–1885.
34. De Luca G, Suryapranata H, Stone G, et al. Abciximab as adjunctive therapy to reperfusion in acute ST-segment elevation myocardial infarction: a meta-analysis of randomized trials. JAMA 2005; 293:1759–1765.
35. Kaul U, Gupta RK, Haridas KK, et al. Platelet glycoprotein IIb/IIIa inhibition using eptifibatide with primary coronary stenting for acute myocardial infarction: a 30-day follow-up study. Catheter Cardiovasc Interv 2002; 57:497–503.
36. Steen H, Lehrke S, Wiegand UK, et al. Very early cardiac magnetic resonance imaging for quantification of myocardial tissue perfusion in patients receiving tirofiban before percutaneous coronary intervention for ST-elevation myocardial infarction. Am Heart J 2005; 149:564.e1–e7.
37. Danzi GB, Sesana M, Capuano C, et al. Comparison in patients having primary coronary angioplasty of abciximab versus tirofiban on recovery of left ventricular function. Am J Cardiol 2004; 94:35–39.
38. Gersh BJ, Anderson JL. Thrombolysis and myocardial salvage. Results of clinical trials and the animal paradigm—paradoxic or predictable? Circulation 1993; 88:296–306.
39. Reimer KA, Jennings RB. The "wavefront phenomenon" of myocardial ischemic cell death. II. Transmural progression of necrosis within the framework of ischemic bed size (myocardium at risk) and collateral flow. Lab Invest 1979; 40:633–644.
40. Berger PB, Ellis SG, Holmes DR Jr., et al. Relationship between delay in performing direct coronary angioplasty and early clinical outcome in patients with acute myocardial infarction: results from the Global Use of Strategies to Open Occluded Arteries in Acute Coronary Syndromes (GUSTO-IIb) trial. Circulation 1999; 100:14–20.
41. Brodie BR, Stone GW, Morice MC, et al. Importance of time to reperfusion on outcomes with primary coronary angioplasty for acute myocardial infarction (results from the Stent Primary Angioplasty in Myocardial Infarction Trial). Am J Cardiol 2001; 88:1085–1090.
42. Stone GW, Cox D, Garcia E, et al. Normal flow (TIMI-3) before mechanical reperfusion therapy is an independent determinant of survival in acute myocardial infarction: analysis from the primary angioplasty in myocardial infarction trials. Circulation 2001; 104:636–641.

43. Bax M, de Winter RJ, Schotborgh CE, et al. Short- and long-term recovery of left ventricular function predicted at the time of primary percutaneous coronary intervention in anterior myocardial infarction. J Am Coll Cardiol 2004; 43:534–541.
44. Beygui F, Le Feuvre C, Helft G, et al. Myocardial viability, coronary flow reserve, and in-hospital predictors of late recovery of contractility following successful primary stenting for acute myocardial infarction. Heart 2003; 89:179–183.
45. Cutlip DE, Ricciardi MJ, Ling FS, et al. Effect of tirofiban before primary angioplasty on initial coronary flow and early ST-segment resolution in patients with acute myocardial infarction. Am J Cardiol 2003; 92:977–980.
46. Mesquita Gabriel H, Oliveira J, Canas da Silva P, et al. Early administration of abciximab bolus in the emergency room improves microperfusion after primary percutaneous coronary intervention, as assessed by TIMI frame count: results of the ERAMI trial. Eur Heart J 2003; 24(abstr suppl):543.
47. Zorman S, Zorman D, Noc M. Effects of abciximab pretreatment in patients with acute myocardial infarction undergoing primary angioplasty. Am J Cardiol 2002; 90:533–536.
48. Zeymer U, Zahn R, Schiele R, et al. Early eptifibatide improves TIMI 3 patency before primary percutaneous coronary intervention for acute ST elevation myocardial infarction: results of the randomized integrilin in acute myocardial infarction (INTAMI) pilot trial. Eur Heart J 2005; 26:1971–1977.
49. van't Hof AW, Ernst N, de Boer MJ, et al. Facilitation of primary coronary angioplasty by early start of a glycoprotein 2b/3a inhibitor: results of the ongoing tirofiban in myocardial infarction evaluation (On-TIME) trial. Eur Heart J 2004; 25:837–846.
50. Arntz HR, Schroder JF, Pels K, et al. Prehospital versus periprocedural administration of abciximab in STEMI: early and late results from the randomised REOMOBILE-study. Eur Heart J 2003; 24(abstr suppl):268.
51. Lee DP, Herity NA, Hiatt BL, et al. Adjunctive platelet glycoprotein IIb/IIIa receptor inhibition with tirofiban before primary angioplasty improves angiographic outcomes: results of the TIrofiban Given in the Emergency Room before Primary Angioplasty (TIGER-PA) pilot trial. Circulation 2003; 107:1497–1501.
52. Gyongyosi M, Domanovits H, Benzer W, et al. Use of abciximab prior to primary angioplasty in STEMI results in early recanalization of the infarct-related artery and improved myocardial tissue reperfusion - results of the Austrian multi-centre randomized ReoPro-BRIDGING Study. Eur Heart J 2004; 25:2125–2133.
53. Montalescot G, Borentain M, Payot L, et al. Early vs late administration of glycoprotein IIb/IIIa inhibitors in primary percutaneous coronary intervention of acute ST-segment elevation myocardial infarction: a meta-analysis. JAMA 2004; 292:362–366.
54. Keeley EC, Boura JA, Grines CL. Comparison of primary and facilitated percutaneous coronary interventions for ST-elevation myocardial infarction: quantitative review of randomised trials. Lancet 2006; 367:579–588.
55. Brown DL, Fann CS, Chang CJ. Meta-analysis of effectiveness and safety of abciximab versus eptifibatide or tirofiban in percutaneous coronary intervention. Am J Cardiol 2001; 87:537–541.
56. Topol EJ, Moliterno DJ, Herrmann HC, et al. Comparison of two platelet glycoprotein IIb/IIIa inhibitors, tirofiban and abciximab, for the prevention of ischemic events with percutaneous coronary revascularization. N Engl J Med 2001; 344:1888–1894.
57. Godicke J, Flather M, Noc M, et al. Early versus periprocedural administration of abciximab for primary angioplasty: a pooled analysis of 6 studies. Am Heart J 2005; 150:1015.e11–e17.
58. Kastrati A, Mehilli J, Schlotterbeck K, et al. Early administration of reteplase plus abciximab vs abciximab alone in patients with acute myocardial infarction referred for percutaneous coronary intervention: a randomized controlled trial. JAMA 2004; 291:947–954.
59. Facilitated percutaneous coronary intervention for acute ST-segment elevation myocardial infarction: results from the prematurely terminated ADdressing the Value of facilitated ANgioplasty after Combination therapy or Eptifibatide monotherapy in acute Myocardial Infarction (ADVANCE MI) trial. Am Heart J 2005; 150:116–122.

60. Bonnefoy E, Lapostolle F, Leizorovicz A, et al. Primary angioplasty versus prehospital fibrinolysis in acute myocardial infarction: a randomised study. Lancet 2002; 360:825–829.
61. Steg PG, Bonnefoy E, Chabaud S, et al. Impact of time to treatment on mortality after prehospital fibrinolysis or primary angioplasty: data from the CAPTIM randomized clinical trial. Circulation 2003; 108:2851–2856.
62. Svensson L, Aasa M, Dellborg M, et al. Comparison of very early treatment with either fibrinolysis or percutaneous coronary intervention facilitated with abciximab with respect to ST recovery and infarct-related artery epicardial flow in patients with acute ST-segment elevation myocardial infarction: the Swedish Early Decision (SWEDES) reperfusion trial. Am Heart J 2006; 151:798 e1–e7.
63. Chen ZM, Jiang LX, Chen YP, et al. Addition of clopidogrel to aspirin in 45,852 patients with acute myocardial infarction: randomised placebo-controlled trial. Lancet 2005; 366:1607–1621.
64. Sabatine MS, Cannon CP, Gibson CM, et al. Addition of clopidogrel to aspirin and fibrinolytic therapy for myocardial infarction with ST-segment elevation. N Engl J Med 2005; 352:1179–1189.
65. Sabatine MS, Cannon CP, Gibson CM, et al. Effect of clopidogrel pretreatment before percutaneous coronary intervention in patients with ST-elevation myocardial infarction treated with fibrinolytics: the PCI-CLARITY study. JAMA 2005; 294:1224–1232.
66. Collet JP, Montalescot G, Lesty C, et al. Disaggregation of in vitro preformed platelet-rich clots by abciximab increases fibrin exposure and promotes fibrinolysis. Arterioscler Thromb Vasc Biol 2001; 21:142–148.
67. Collet JP, Montalescot G, Lesty C, et al. Effects of Abciximab on the architecture of platelet-rich clots in patients with acute myocardial infarction undergoing primary coronary intervention. Circulation 2001; 103:2328–2331.
68. Collet JP, Montalescot G, Lesty C, et al. A structural and dynamic investigation of the facilitating effect of glycoprotein IIb/IIIa inhibitors in dissolving platelet-rich clots. Circ Res 2002; 90:428–434.
69. Antman EM, Gibson CM, de Lemos JA, et al. Combination reperfusion therapy with abciximab and reduced dose reteplase: results from TIMI 14. The Thrombolysis in Myocardial Infarction (TIMI) 14 Investigators. Eur Heart J 2000; 21:1944–1953.
70. Brener SJ, Zeymer U, Adgey AA, et al. Eptifibatide and low-dose tissue plasminogen activator in acute myocardial infarction: the integrilin and low-dose thrombolysis in acute myocardial infarction (INTRO AMI) trial. J Am Coll Cardiol 2002; 39:377–386.
71. Topol EJ. Reperfusion therapy for acute myocardial infarction with fibrinolytic therapy or combination reduced fibrinolytic therapy and platelet glycoprotein IIb/IIIa inhibition: the GUSTO V randomised trial. Lancet 2001; 357:1905–1914.
72. Lincoff AM, Califf RM, Van de Werf F, et al. Mortality at 1 year with combination platelet glycoprotein IIb/IIIa inhibition and reduced-dose fibrinolytic therapy vs conventional fibrinolytic therapy for acute myocardial infarction: GUSTO V randomized trial. JAMA 2002; 288:2130–2135.
73. Efficacy and safety of tenecteplase in combination with enoxaparin, abciximab, or unfractionated heparin: the ASSENT-3 randomised trial in acute myocardial infarction. Lancet 2001; 358:605–613.
74. Antman EM, Louwerenburg HW, Baars HF, et al. Enoxaparin as adjunctive antithrombin therapy for ST-elevation myocardial infarction: results of the ENTIRE-Thrombolysis in Myocardial Infarction (TIMI) 23 Trial. Circulation 2002; 105:1642–1649.
75. Ellis SG, Armstrong P, Betriu A, et al. Facilitated percutaneous coronary intervention versus primary percutaneous coronary intervention: design and rationale of the Facilitated Intervention with Enhanced Reperfusion Speed to Stop Events (FINESSE) trial. Am Heart J 2004; 147:E16.
76. Neumann FJ, Kastrati A, Schmitt C, et al. Effect of glycoprotein IIb/IIIa receptor blockade with abciximab on clinical and angiographic restenosis rate after the placement of coronary stents following acute myocardial infarction. J Am Coll Cardiol 2000; 35:915–921.
77. Petronio AS, Musumeci G, Limbruno U, et al. Abciximab improves 6-month clinical outcome after rescue coronary angioplasty. Am Heart J 2002; 143:334–341.

78. Petronio AS, Rovai D, Musumeci G, et al. Effects of abciximab on microvascular integrity and left ventricular functional recovery in patients with acute infarction treated by primary coronary angioplasty. Eur Heart J 2003; 24:67–76.
79. Herrmann HC, Moliterno DJ, Ohman EM, et al. Facilitation of early percutaneous coronary intervention after reteplase with or without abciximab in acute myocardial infarction: results from the SPEED (GUSTO-4 Pilot) Trial. J Am Coll Cardiol 2000; 36:1489–1496.
80. Roe MT, Green CL, Giugliano RP, et al. Improved speed and stability of ST-segment recovery with reduced-dose tenecteplase and eptifibatide compared with full-dose tenecteplase for acute ST-segment elevation myocardial infarction. J Am Coll Cardiol 2004; 43:549–556.
81. Ohman EM, Kleiman NS, Gacioch G, et al. Combined accelerated tissue-plasminogen activator and platelet glycoprotein IIb/IIIa integrin receptor blockade with Integrilin in acute myocardial infarction. Results of a randomized, placebo-controlled, dose-ranging trial. IMPACT-AMI Investigators. Circulation 1997; 95:846–854.
82. Ohman EM, Van de Werf F, Antman EM, et al. Tenecteplase and tirofiban in ST-segment elevation acute myocardial infarction: results of a randomized trial. Am Heart J 2005; 150:79–88.

Anticoagulant Agents

E. Marc Jolicoeur and Christopher B. Granger
*Duke Clinical Research Institute and Duke University Medical Center,
Durham, North Carolina, U.S.A.*

INTRODUCTION

Anticoagulant agents are used as adjuncts to reperfusion therapy to enhance the rates of infarct artery patency and to prevent reocclusion. The link between better and persistent epicardial flow, smaller infarct size, improved ventricular function, and prolonged survival has stimulated a series of trials intended to improve antithrombotic therapy for acute myocardial infarction (MI) (Fig. 1) (1). This chapter reviews the efficacy of anticoagulant agents in the settings of fibrinolytic therapy and primary percutaneous coronary intervention (PCI).

Limitations of fibrinolytic therapy include incomplete reperfusion and coronary reocclusion. While the clinical evidence that anticoagulants improve reperfusion rates is lacking (2–8), anticoagulants prevent reocclusion and reinfarction in the early days following fibrinolytic therapy, events that are associated with higher mortality. In a pooled analysis of the Thrombolysis and Angioplasty in Myocardial Infarction (TAMI) trials, Ohman et al. reported that coronary reocclusion early after successful fibrinolysis was associated with a striking increase in in-hospital mortality (4.5% in patients with a patent artery vs. 11% in patients with reocclusion, $p = 0.01$), and predicted worse left ventricular (LV) function among survivors (9). With the available antithrombotic regimens today, post-fibrinolytic reinfarction rates have dropped below 6% (10–13). Not only is the choice of anticoagulant important, but also the duration of anticoagulant administration (13–18) and the rates of early coronary angiography are important (19,20).

Avoidance of Bleeding

In recent trials, 30-day mortality for ST-elevation myocardial infarction (STEMI) has been as low as 4%, even in populations selected for high-risk features (21). Safety, and bleeding in particular, has become an important feature that may distinguish antithrombotic regimens. The choice of agent, dose, and combination that results in the best balance of antithrombotic efficacy and bleeding risk is an important goal (22,23).

Non-cerebral bleeding among patients with acute coronary syndromes (ACS) has long been considered a "nuisance" occurrence that is reversible and treatable by transfusion and anticoagulant discontinuation. However, we now know that bleeding is strongly related to adverse outcomes, including death, stroke, and MI (24). In STEMI populations, major bleeding occurs in about 5% of patients and is associated with a three-fold increase in the risk of death (from 7.0% to 22.8%, $p < 0.001$) (25). A growing body of evidence suggests that blood transfusion itself may have adverse effects in patients with ischemic heart disease (26,27). Thus, as an increasing number of antithrombotic drugs have become available and used in management of STEMI, estimation of bleeding risk and careful use of potent

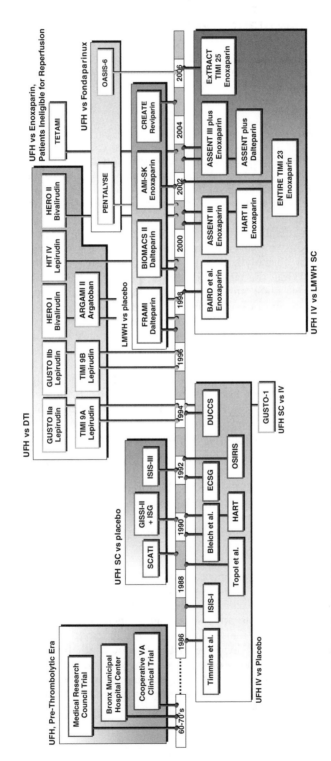

FIGURE 1 Landmark trials of adjunctive anticoagulation therapy with fibrinolysis.

TABLE 1 The Clinical Predictors of Bleeding in Patients with ST-Elevation Myocardial Infarction

Variable	Adjusted OR	95% CI	p value
Age (per 10-yr increase)	1.25	1.14–1.38	<0.0001
Female sex	1.71	1.35–2.17	<0.0001
History of bleeding	2.37	1.18–4.77	0.015
Killip class IV	1.73	1.05–2.86	0.03
Diuretics	1.45	1.12–1.87	0.005
LMWH only[a]	0.60	0.42–0.85	0.004
Thrombolytics only	1.45	1.07–1.97	0.017
GP IIb/IIIa blockers only	1.95	1.40–2.70	<0.0001
Thrombolytics and GP IIb/IIIa blockers	2.09	1.35–3.23	0.0009
IV inotropic agents	1.85	1.38–2.49	<0.0001
Other vasodilators	1.50	1.04–2.15	0.030
Right-heart catheterization	2.79	2.01–3.89	<0.0001
Percutaneous coronary intervention	1.63	1.24–2.15	0.0005

[a]Referent groups: male gender; UFH for LMWH only, both LMWH and UFH; neither thrombolytics nor GP IIb/IIIa blockers for fibrinolytic only, GP IIb/IIIa blockers only, and both thrombolytics and GP IIb/IIIa blockers; no for other variables. Hosmer-Lemeshow goodness-or-fit test p value = 0.99; C-statistic = 0.74.
Abbreviations: Gp, glycoprotein; LMWH, low molecular weight heparin; UFH, unfractionated heparin.
Source: From Ref. 25.

combinations of antithrombotics in high-risk populations is important. The clinical predictors of major bleeding in the STEMI population are summarized in Table 1.

UNFRACTIONATED HEPARIN

Unfractionated heparin (UFH) has been known to exert an anticoagulant effect for nearly 100 years (28). The first clinical trial testing the efficacy of UFH in MI was reported in 1949 (29), but the rationale for anticoagulation with reperfusion therapy was not studied until the early 1980s, when angiographic studies demonstrated that the infarct artery was nearly always occluded by thrombus in the early hours of STEMI (30).

Mechanism of Action

UFH is a heterogeneous mixture of glycosaminoglycans with various molecular size and anticoagulant activity (31). Functionally, heparins can be described as saccharide chains of heterogeneous lengths. UFH acts simultaneously at different levels of the anticoagulation cascade, but its main anticoagulation effect results from the indirect inhibition of factor Xa and thrombin (Fig. 2A). UFH binds and changes the conformation of antithrombin (AT) III (Fig. 2B). As a result, AT III can bind and inhibit coagulant factors Xa and thrombin. UFH has adequate saccharide chain length to simultaneously bind AT III and thrombin (32), as well as Xa. By inhibiting these factors, UFH impedes thrombin from catalyzing the conversion of fibrinogen to fibrin (33). Additionally, UFH prevents the thrombin-related activation of platelets and coagulation factors V and VIII (34).

As for PCI, the superiority of UFH over fondaparinux to prevent catheter-related thrombosis (14,35) has recently highlighted the contact system, a series of coagulation factors (factors XIIa, prekallikrein, high molecular weight kininogen, and C-inhibitor) that exert protective antithrombotic effects on the local vasculature (36). The contact system is activated by negatively charged synthetic material (such as guide wires) and helps prevent the development of thrombi on the surface of artificial materials. UFH has a minimal effect on factor XIIa and other constituents of the contact system (37). This absence of action on the contact system may explain the superiority of UFH in the setting of PCI (38).

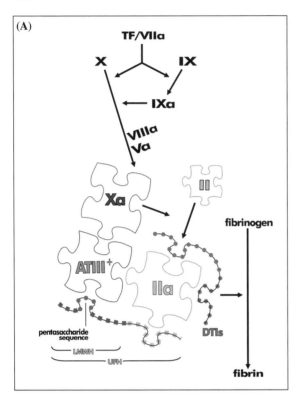

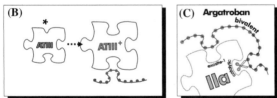

FIGURE 2 The coagulation cascade and the anticoagulant agents. (**A**) UHF, LMWHs, and penta-saccharide agents (fondaparinux) exert their antithrombotic effect indirectly by binding the inhibitory factor ATIII. ATIII neutralizes factor Xa that can no longer catalyze the conversion of factor II to thrombin. Only UFH has sufficient saccharide chain length to bridge ATIII and thrombin. This resulting inhibitory complex blocks the catalytic activity of thrombin, which catalyzes the conversion of fibrinogen to fibrin. DTIs exert their anticoagulant effect by binding the thrombin catabolic site responsible for facilitating the conversion of fibrinogen to fibrin. (**B**) The pentasaccharide sequence (*in pink*) shared by UFH, LMWHs, and pentasaccharide agents is the key sequence that selectively binds to ATIII to change its confor-mation. This conformational change inhibits the binding of ATIII to factor Xa. (**C**) Unlike univalent agents, bivalent DTIs (lepirudin, bivalirudin) simultaneously bind thrombin's exosite-1 and catalytic site. In contrast to lepirudin, bivalirudin transiently inhibits thrombin; after binding to thrombin, the active moiety of bivalirudin is rapidly cleaved by the catalytic site. *Abbreviations*: ATIII, antithrombin III; UFH, unfractionated heparin; DTI, direct thrombin inhibitor; LMWH, low molecular weight heparin.

Adjunctive UFH with Fibrinolytic Agents

Well before the use of fibrinolytic therapy, three large randomized trials assessed the role of UFH in MI (39–41). These trials tested whether UFH could prevent the progression of coronary thrombosis, limit myocardial infarct size, and thus improve survival. Although the mortality rates were numerically lower in each of these trials, only the Bronx Municipal Hospital Center trial showed a statistically significant benefit (40). These trials also showed reduced rates of in-hospital stroke and pulmonary embolism, a finding that remains relevant today (42). A contemporary review of these trials suggests that a significant proportion of the enrolled patients were probably not anticoagulated adequately, which suggests that the therapeutic benefit of UFH could have been underestimated (43).

Subcutaneous Heparin

A series of large trials established the efficacy fibrinolytic therapy (44–48) and beta-blockade (49) in the treatment of MI. The landmark International Study of Infarct Survival (ISIS)-2 trial showed a reduction in mortality with aspirin and streptokinase (SK), with additive effects (45). While UFH has been widely used with fibrinolytic agents, the role of adjunctive UFH in improving outcome has been controversial (50–52). Trials have tested different UFH strategies: immediate versus delayed after fibrinolysis, subcutaneous (SC) versus intravenous (IV) administration, low versus high doses, and use with SK versus fibrin-specific fibrinolytic agents.

Before the publication of the Gruppo Italiano per lo Studio della Sopravvivenze nell'Infarcto Miocardico (GISSI-II) and ISIS-3 trials, SC UFH was considered preferable to IV UFH because it did not require monitoring and was unlikely to lead to excessive anticoagulation (53). The moderate activated partial thromboplastin time (aPTT) prolongation obtained with SC UFH (35–50 seconds) was considered a safe target, especially in the early hours post-SK (54). However, in GISSI-II, a dose of UFH 12,500 IU SC twice daily and started several hours after SK or tissue-type plasminogen activator (t-PA), did not favorably affect the combined outcome of death and severe LV dysfunction, despite enrolling 12,490 patients (55). The International Study Group trial confirmed the finding of GISSI-II and even demonstrated a small, albeit significant, excess in major bleeding with SC UFH (1.0% vs. 0.5%, risk ratio (RR) = 1.79, 95% confidence interval (CI), 1.31–2.45) (56).

Using a design similar to GISSI-II, the ISIS-III trial compared UFH 12,500 IU SC twice daily with placebo in 41,299 patients randomized to SK, t-PA, or anisoylated plasminogen–SK activator complex (APSAC). Unlike GISSI-II however, UFH was started early (4 hours after randomization) and continued for seven days. In spite of this, no beneficial effect on reinfarction (3.2% vs. 3.5%, $p = 0.09$) or death (10.3% vs. 10.6%, $p = $ NS) was observed at 35 days with the anticoagulant (57). SC UFH was associated with excess transfusion rates when compared with placebo (1.0% vs. 0.8%, $p < 0.01$). Pooled analysis of the GISSI-II and ISIS-III trial suggested a transient and modest mortality benefit of SC UFH during the active treatment period (6.8% vs. 7.3%. $p < 0.01$). At 35 days, the mortality benefit was no longer significant (57).

UFH through the SC route is limited by variable bioavailability and a dose-dependent absorption. At a dose of 5000 IU SC, less than a quarter of the drug is absorbed (58,59). The delayed SC administration of UFH up to 12 hours after fibrinolysis may have limited this approach, and more intensive, early IV UFH adjunctive regimens were tested.

Intravenous Heparin

Thrombin generation and activity paradoxically increase within the 30 minutes following the administration of fibrinolytic therapy (60–62). Because IV UFH prevents this paradoxic augmentation, it was thought to be a promising treatment to prevent coronary reocclusion after successful fibrinolysis.

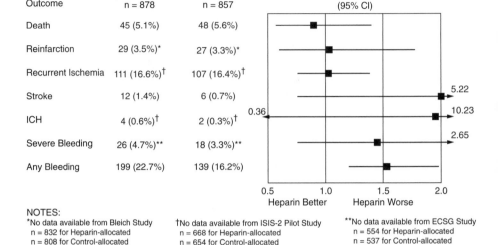

FIGURE 3 Overview of the randomized trials comparing adjunctive intravenous heparin to placebo with fibrinolytic therapy. *Abbreviations*: ECSG, European Cooperation Study Group; ICH, intracranial hemorrhage; ISIS-2, International Study of Infarct Survival; Severe bleeding, bleeding associated with hemodynamic compromise or requiring blood transfusion. *Source*: From Ref. 52.

Despite a strong biologic rationale, there is no compelling evidence of the superiority of IV UFH over placebo at reducing mortality after fibrinolysis. Various estimates suggested that between 20,000 and 50,000 patients would be required in a randomized trial to resolve this issue (51,52). In a systematic overview using the key randomized trials comparing IV UFH with placebo during fibrinolytic therapy, Mahaffey et al. could neither support nor refute the presumed benefit associated with UFH with regard to death, reinfarction, or recurrent ischemia (Fig. 3) (63–67). The in-hospital mortality rates in patients treated with IV UFH were similar to placebo-treated patients (5.1 % vs. 5.6%, odds ratio (OR) = 0.91, 95% CI, 0.59–1.39). In the subgroup of patients treated with t-PA, the same nonsignificant trend was observed (OR = 0.84, 95% CI, 0.43–1.64). Not surprisingly, bleeding was significantly more frequent in patients receiving UFH (OR = 1.55, 95% CI, 1.21–1.98) (52).

The SC and IV UFH regimens were directly compared in the Global Use of Streptokinase and Tissue Plasminogen Activator for Occluded Coronary Artery (GUSTO-1) trial. The trial was designed to test whether early and sustained infarct artery patency was associated with superior survival rates in STEMI. GUSTO-1 compared the efficacy of four fibrinolytic strategies: SK + SC UFH, SK + IV UFH, accelerated t-PA + IV UFH, and SK + t-PA + IV UFH. Per protocol, SC UFH was initiated four hours post-fibrinolysis (12,500 IU twice daily for 7 days) whereas IV UFH was initiated simultaneously with fibrinolytic therapy (bolus: 5000 IU and perfusion: 1000 IU/hr, target aPTT: 60–85 seconds, for 48 hours) (68). The IV route was not superior to the SC route among SK-treated patients; no significant mortality difference was observed at 30 days (7.2% vs. 7.3%, respectively, p = 0.73). Similarly, infarct artery flow at 90 minutes was comparable between the groups

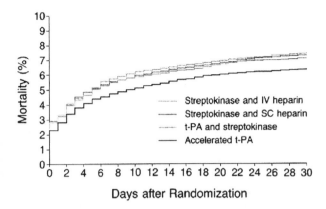

FIGURE 4 Thirty-day mortality with four fibrinolytic strategies. When compared with therapeutic strategies of streptokinase and UFH (either IV or SC), the combination of accelerated t-PA and IV UFH significantly reduced mortality at 30 days (from 7.4% to 6.3%, $p = 0.001$). *Abbreviation*: UFH, unfractionated heparin. *Source*: Adapted from Ref. 68.

[Thrombolysis in Myocardial Infarction (TIMI)-2 and TIMI-3 flows of 54% SC and 60% IV, $p = $ NS] (6). These observations, combined with the GISSI and ISIS trials, challenged the role of either SC or IV UFH in patients treated with SK.

The most important finding of GUSTO-1, however, was the improved survival of patients treated with accelerated t-PA and IV UFH, which also resulted in improved early infarct artery perfusion. The combination significantly reduced mortality at 30 days when compared with SK and SC or IV UFH (10 lives saved per 1000 patients treated; relative risk reduction 14%; 95% CI, 5.9–21.3, $p = 0.001$) (Fig. 4) (6). In terms of safety, an increased number of hemorrhagic strokes was observed in the overall, t-PA-treated patients population (0.72% vs. 0.43%, $p = 0.03$; vs. SK). This increase in hemorrhagic strokes was especially prominent in patients over 75 years of age.

In spite of the benefits seen in GUSTO-1 with combination t-PA and UFH, the contribution of IV UFH was not directly studied. Based on experimental evidence suggesting synergy of action and reduced reocclusion (69,70), adjunctive UFH has been used with fibrin-specific fibrinolytic agents since the first MI trials (71–73), with few exceptions (65,67,74,75). Therefore, it is unknown whether adjunctive IV UFH is superior to SC UFH or even placebo with fibrin-specific fibrinolytic agents. It is also unknown whether the immediate administration of IV UFH is superior to a delayed strategy. The TAMI group studied a modest number of patients treated with t-PA and randomized to either a single high-dose bolus of UFH (10,000 IU) or a placebo. Ninety minutes after fibrinolysis, the rates of infarct artery patency were identical (79%) in the two groups (75). While this trial did not address the need for systemic anticoagulation after fibrinolytic therapy, it at least suggested that UFH did not have a major impact on early reperfusion.

Target aPTT

With fibrin-specific lytic agents, careful dosing to avoid early excessive aPTT prolongation appears to be important to reduce the risk of bleeding, including intracranial hemorrhage. An initial bolus of 60 U/kg (maximum of 4000 U) and an initial infusion of 12 U/kg/hr (maximum of 1000 U/hr) should be used (76). Monitoring strategies using aPTT as early as three hours after treatment initiation has been associated with reduced bleeding complications (77). With SK, if IV UFH is used, the aPTT should not be used within six hours of fibrinolysis to titrate UFH. The systemic fibrinolytic state, with the degradation of fibrinogen, factors V and VIII, and the rise in fibrin degradation products observed after fibrinolysis, all prolong the aPTT (78). Twelve hours post-fibrinolysis, the aPTT should be targeted between 50 to 70 seconds, the interval associated with the lowest 30-day death, stroke, and bleeding rates (53). APTTs above 70 seconds are associated with increased likelihood of adverse clinical outcomes, including death and bleeding. In GUSTO-1, for instance, patients with 12-hour aPTTs above 150 seconds had a 50% increased risk of 30-day mortality compared with patients with aPTTs of 60 seconds. Of interest, aPTTs above 70 seconds are also associated with higher reinfarction rates, a paradox potentially related to the augmented bleeding rate with excessive anticoagulation. In ACS populations, bleeding is an independent predictor of reinfarction that may partly relate to the abrupt discontinuation of anticoagulant and antiplatelet agents (24,26,27,79).

UFH with Primary PCI

UFH has been used since the beginning of PCI to prevent catheter-related thrombosis. UFH remains the favorite anticoagulant when primary PCI is performed (80,81). Except for bivalirudin, no other anticoagulant has been studied for this indication (14,35,82,83). Three methods are commonly used to monitor the activity of UFH: the bleeding time, the aPTT, and the activated clotting time (ACT). In the catheterization laboratory, ACT is preferred because it is more discriminative to the variation of UFH doses, especially when higher levels of anticoagulation are used. The two ACT monitoring devices used are the Hemochron (International Technidyne Corporation, Edison, New Jersey, U.S.) and the HemoTec (Medtronic-HemoTec, Johnston, Rhode Island, U.S.) (84,85). The Hemochron readings consistently exceed the HemoTec ACT, by 100 ± 86 seconds (86).

While randomized data are lacking to guide optimal targets of ACT during PCI (87–91), it is generally agreed that very high levels of periprocedural ACTs (above 400 seconds) are associated with higher hemorrhagic and ischemic event rates (87,92). Dose-adjusted UFH regimens (70–100 IU/kg IV) should be used to avoid excessive anticoagulation (81). When glycoprotein (GP) IIb–IIIa inhibitors are not used, sufficient UFH should be given to reach ACTs ranging from 250 seconds to 300 seconds (with the HemoTec device) or from 300 seconds to 350 seconds (with the Hemochron device). When GP IIb–IIIa inhibitors are used, target ACT above 200 seconds are recommended (80,81).

After successful PCI, UHF can be discontinued, unless an indication for systemic anticoagulation is present, such as anterior MI with aneurysm, LV thrombus, or atrial fibrillation (93–95).

Conclusion

A variety of regimens of adjunctive UFH have been studied, including delayed versus early, SC versus IV, and low dose versus high dose, in association with fibrinolytic therapy and primary PCI. Neither SC nor IV UFH seems to enhance the fibrinolytic efficacy of SK when used with aspirin. Because UFH has been systematically employed with fibrin-specific lytic agents, and their relative benefits may partly relate to UFH use, carefully dosed IV UFH is standard. Together, these trials suggest that rather than accelerating reperfusion, the benefit of UFH anticoagulation is to reduce reinfarction.

LOW MOLECULAR WEIGHT HEPARIN

Low molecular weight heparins (LMWH) are replacing UFH for many clinical indications, except in cardiology. Clinical trials assessing LMWH have been designed to address several of the limitations encountered with the use of UFH. In most of these trials, adjunctive LMWH has been used for a prolonged period (up to 7 days) after fibrinolysis to extend the protection offered by short-term UFH therapy.

Mechanism of Action

LMWHs are a mixture of saccharide chains of varying lengths, many shorter than UFH, that possess the critical pentasaccharide segment responsible for binding to AT III (Fig. 2A). Like UFH, LMWHs mediate their anti-Xa activity via their conformational change of AT III to increase its binding affinity to Xa. In contrast to UFH, LMWHs have a relative lack of additional saccharide residues required to cross-link thrombin and form a ternary heparin/AT/thrombin inhibitory complex (32,96). The relative inability of LMWHs to link thrombin explains their high anti-Xa/anti-IIa ratio. The different LMWH preparations tested in patients with ischemic heart disease vary in terms of anti-Xa/anti-IIa ratio, ionic nature, and release profile of tissue factor pathway inhibitors (97). Depending on the agent used, the maximal values for anti-Xa to anti-IIa activity may vary twofold to threefold (98).

Advantages of LMWH

An impressive list of the pharmacokinetic and pharmacodynamic advantages has been proposed for LMWHs (Table 2). LMWHs have an excellent (>90%) SC bioavailability, a longer half-life, and little nonspecific plasma protein and cellular binding (97). As a result, LMWHs are easy to administer SC, provide a reliable level of anticoagulation, and do not require therapeutic monitoring. LMWHs also present interesting pharmacodynamic properties that, theoretically, result in a superior anticoagulation profile, when compared with UFH (Table 2). LMWHs have a greater capacity for inactivating factor Xa compared with factor IIa (anti-Xa/anti-IIa ratio). Similarly, enoxaparin appears superior to UFH in blunting the von Willebrand factor surge that occurs in the acute phase response of ACS (99,100). These effects on early mediators of the coagulation cascade may explain the better inhibition of platelet function and thrombin generation (99–102). Unlike the high molecular weight fraction of UFH, LMWHs appear less likely to activate platelets (103). LMWHs are less frequently responsible for the anti-platelet factor 4 (anti-PF4) antibody seroconversion associated with heparin-induced thrombocytopenia (HIT) (104).

Due to a lack of clinical experience and uncertain dosing, the use of LMWHs is limited in several situations such as renal insufficiency, obesity, and advanced age. Practice guidelines currently recommend limiting the use of enoxaparin to

TABLE 2 Theoretical Pharmacodynamic Advantages and Limitations of Adjunctive Anticoagulant Agents

Agents	Advantages (references)	Limitations (references)
UFH	1. Partial inhibition of thrombin generation (140,141,190,191) 2. Partial inhibition of thrombin surge induced by thrombolytic agents (78,167) 3. Favorable effect on the coagulation contact system to prevent catheter-related thrombosis (37,36)	1. Binding to platelet and endothelium proteins result in an unpredictable anticoagulant activity. 2. Therapeutic concentration of UFH are associated with platelet activation (103). 3. Interaction with platelet factor 4 (PF4): reduced antithrombotic activity (193). 4. Heparin-induced thrombocytopenia
LMWH	1. Favorable anti-Xa; anti-IIa activity ratio; strong inhibition of thrombin generation (97). 2. Enhanced inhibition of vWF plasmatic surge during acute phase response of ACS (99,101) 3. Less platelet activation than UFH (103,108).	1. Less well proven prevention of thrombin activation induced by fibrinolytic therapy. 2. Heparin-induced thrombocytopenia (less likely than with UFH)
DTI	1. Strong inhibition of thrombin activation, with specific inactivation of fibrin-bound thrombin: accelerated thrombolysis of occlusive platelet-rich thrombosis (190,191) 2. Superior inhibition of vWF plasma surge usually present in the acute phase response of ACS (100)	1. Theoretically less inhibition of thrombin generation (140,141,190,191)
Penta	1. Inhibition of thrombin generation during active coagulation process (152,157); enhanced protection against thrombolytic-induced thrombin generation 2. Resistance to platelet factor 4	1. Less activity against activated thrombin (157) 2. Anti-Xa activity below 5% required before decreasing thrombin synthesis (161) 3. Lack of inhibition of contact (i.e., catheter-induced) thrombosis

Abbreviations: ACS, acute coronary syndrome; DTI, direct thrombin inhibitor; LMWH, low molecular weight heparin; Penta, pentasaccharides; UFH, unfractionated heparin; vWF, von Willebrand factor.

patients with preserved renal function (serum creatinine lower than 2.5 mg/dL in men or 2.0 mg/dL in women) (76,95). The Enoxaparin and Thrombolysis Reperfusion for Acute Myocardial Infarction Treatment (ExTRACT) TIMI-25 trial provides important data to support a lower dose of enoxaparin in patients more than 75 years of age. In elderly patients, enoxaparin was administered without an initial bolus and at 0.75 mg/kg SC every 12 hours, and resulted in a lower incidence of bleeding and intracranial hemorrhage (Table 3).

Adjunctive LMWH with Fibrinolytic Agents
LMWH Vs. Placebo
The failure of SC UFH to improve outcome after SK and aspirin in GISSI-II, ISIS-III, and GUSTO-1 opened the door to dalteparin and enoxaparin for use as adjunctive therapy with fibrinolytic therapy (55,57,68) (Table 4). Most of the early trials assessed the effect of LMWHs in combination with fibrinolytic agents on infarct artery patency, and none provided convincing evidence that the combination could effectively reduce the rates of death and MI (3,17,105).

TABLE 3 Dose-Adjusted Enoxaparin Regimens in the Susceptible Patients

Population	Enoxaparin dose adjustment[a]
Patients < 75 yr	IV Bolus: 30 mg IV[b] SC injection: 1.0 mg/kg q. 12 hr Maximum 100 mg for the first 2 injections
Patients ≥ 75 yr	IV Bolus: None SC injection: 0.75 mg/kg q. 12 hr Maximum 75 mg for the first 2 injections
Creatine clearance < 30 cc/min	IV Bolus: 30 mg IV[b] SC injection: 1 mg/kg q. 24 hr

[a]UFH Bolus: 60 mg/kg (maximum, 4000 U), followed by an infusion of 12 U/kg/hr adjusted to maintain an activated partial-thromboplastin time of 1.5 to 2 times the control value, for 48 hours.
[b] The first dose of enoxaparin was administered between 15 minutes before up to 30 minutes after the initiation of fibrinolytic therapy.
Source: Adapted from Ref. 13.

TABLE 4 Randomized Trials Comparing Adjunctive Low Molecular Weight Heparin to Placebo in Patients Treated with Fibrinolytic Therapy for Acute Myocardial Infarction

Trial (reference)	Lytic	LMWH	1° End point	Safety	Comments
FRAMI n = 776 1997 (105)	SK 1.5 MU	**Dalteparin** 150 IU/kg SC q. 12 hr in-hospital	↓of LV thrombus (14.2% vs. 21.9%, p = 0.03) at 9 days	Major bleeds: 2.9% vs. 0.3% (p = 0.006)	No effect on arterial embolism, reinfarction and death
BIOMACS II, n = 101 1999 (3)	SK 1.5 MU	**Dalteparin** 100 IU/kg SC pre-SK, 120 IU/kg 12 hr post- SK once	Trend toward ↑ 24 hr-TIMI-3 flow in IRA (68% vs. 51%, p = 0.10)	Major bleeds: 3.7% vs. 0% (p = NS)	Pilot/angiographic study. Dalteparin ↓ the ischemic episodes on continuous ECG
AMI-SK n = 496 2002 (17)	SK 1.5 MU	**Enoxaparin** B: 30 mg then 1 mg/kg SC q. 12 hr × 3–8 days	↑day 8-TIMI-3 flow in IRA (70% vs. 58%, p = 0.01)	Major bleeds: 4.8% vs. 2.5% (p = 0.2)	Angiographic study. ↓ death/re-MI/ recurrent ischemia at 30 days (13% vs. 21%, p = 0.03)
CREATE n = 15,570 2005 (193)	Lytics: 73%1° PCI: 6% None: 21%	**Reviparin** Weight adjusted (3,436 IU to 6,871 IU) SC q. 12 hr × 7 days	↓Death/MI/ strokes at day 7 (9.6% vs. 11.0%, p = 0.005). Persistent effect at 30 days	Major bleeds: 0.9% vs. 0.4% (p < 0.001)	Reviparin tested in a resource-poor setting. No other anticoagulant allowed, unless clinically indicated

Abbreviations: B, bolus; ECG, electrocardiogram; IRA, infarct-related artery; LV, left ventricle; MI, myocardial infarction; MU, million unit; NS, nonsignificant; PCI, percutaneous coronary intervention; SC, subcutaneous; SK, streptokinase; TIMI, thrombolysis in myocardial infarction.

Reviparin has a high anti-Xa activity and an anti-Xa/anti-IIa ratio similar to enoxaparin (106). The agent was compared with placebo in the CREATE trial involving 15,570 STEMI patients from India and China (Table 4). A significant proportion of the patients in the trial received no reperfusion therapy (21%). In this context, reviparin significantly reduced the combined end point of death, MI, and stroke at seven days (9.6% vs. 11.0%, hazard ratio (HR) = 0.87, 95% CI. 0.79–0.96, $p = 0.005$), a protective effect that persisted at 30 days. Interestingly, the agent showed a modest, albeit significant, reduction in all-cause mortality.

In an overview including the CREATE trial, a significant reduction of mortality in LMWH-treated patients compared with placebo is observed at 30 days (OR = 0.86, 95% CI, 0.78–0.95), at the price of a small, but significant, excess of major bleeding (1.1% vs. 0.4%, OR = 2.70, 95% CI, 1.83–3.99) (107). This reduction in mortality was driven by the CREATE trial results (51), which may not be directly applicable to western hemisphere health care systems. In summary, it appears that LMWH, and especially enoxaparin and reviparin, can facilitate early coronary reperfusion and reduce the risk of reocclusion, providing that the LMWH is continued for more than 48 hours after fibrinolysis.

LMWH Vs. UFH

In the current era, only two LMWHs have undergone direct comparison with UFH: enoxaparin and dalteparin. Dalteparin was assessed in the Assessment of the Safety and Efficacy of a New Thrombolytic (ASSENT)-Plus trial, which was mainly an angiographic study that compared the effect of dalteparin (4–7 days) and UFH (48 hour) on post-fibrinolysis coronary blood flow (7). In combination with t-PA, dalteparin and UFH resulted in similar rates of predischarge TIMI-3 coronary flow (69.3% vs. 62.5%, OR = 1.11, 95% CI, 0.96–1.28, $p = 0.16$). During the initial seven days of treatment with dalteparin, there were significantly lower rates of reinfarction when compared with UFH. Interestingly, after discontinuation of dalteparin, there was a "rebound" of reinfarction similar to what has been reported with UFH (Fig. 5), so that no discernable benefit in favor of dalteparin was present at 30 days.

Prior to the series of larger trials from the ASSENT and the TIMI groups, two small trials compared the efficacy of enoxaparin and UFH with SK (108) or t-PA (5) (Table 5). The angiographic Heparin and Aspirin Reperfusion Therapy (HART)-II study demonstrated that enoxaparin used in conjunction with t-PA was non-inferior to UFH in achieving infarct artery patency 90 minutes after fibrinolysis. The overall rates of TIMI-2 or 3 flows were 80.1% for enoxaparin and 75.1% for UFH (lower bound of 1-sided 95% CI of difference is −2%, $p < 0.05$) (5). Baird et al. were the first to suggest a clinical benefit of LMWH over UFH when used in combination with fibrinolytic agents. Adjunctive enoxaparin appeared better than UFH at reducing the 90-day combined end point of death, reinfarction, and hospitalization for unstable angina.

ASSENT-III was the first properly sized trial to compare LMWH and UFH with fibrinolytic treatment in STEMI (18). ASSENT-III compared three adjunctive strategies used with tenecteplase (TNK): weight-adjusted UFH for 48 hour, enoxaparin for seven days, or abciximab for 12 hour (with UFH and half-dose TNK). Enoxaparin was better than UFH in reducing the composite primary end point of death, in-hospital reinfarction, and refractory ischemia at 30 days (11.4% vs. 15.4%, $p < 0.001$), by reducing the incidence of ischemic complications. Enoxaparin resulted in a nonsignificant trend for an increase in major bleeding. Interestingly, there was a net beneficial effect, even in the elderly, with a 30 mg IV bolus followed by 1 mg/kg SC every 12 hours.

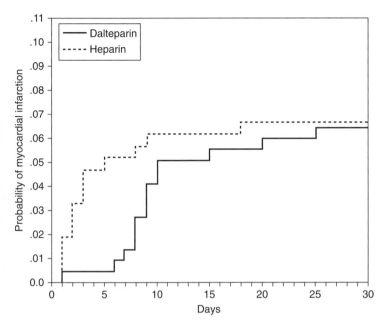

FIGURE 5 Rebound effect with dalteparin? This figure proposes that both UFH and dalteparin may cause a rebound thrombotic activation after their discontinuation. *Abbreviation*: UFH, unfractionated heparin. *Source*: From Ref. 7.

As an extension of ASSENT-III, the ASSENT-III-Plus trial explored the efficacy and safety of TNK in combination with enoxaparin or UFH in a prehospital setting. In ASSENT-III-Plus, more than 50% of the patients enrolled received the fibrinolytic within two hours of symptom onset (109). There was an increase in bleeding, and particularly in ICH (2.20% vs. 0.97%, $p = 0.047$), along with an absence of significant difference in the combined incidence of death, in-hospital reinfarction, and refractory ischemia between enoxaparin and UFH (14.2% vs. 17.4%. $p = 0.08$). Increased bleeding and ICH with enoxaparin was seen in patients more than 75 years of age. This led the authors to recommend that UFH, not enoxaparin, should be used with TNK in the prehospital setting, at least until more data were available. In a pooled analysis of the two trials, the TNK-enoxaparin combination showed a consistent reduction in reinfarction and refractory angina, at a cost of increased bleeding, and with no reduction in mortality (110).

Enoxaparin was further examined by the TIMI group with the Enoxaparin and TNK-tPA with or Without GP IIb/IIIa Inhibitor as Reperfusion Strategy (ENTIRE) and ExTRACT trials. In association with TNK, adjunctive enoxaparin was not superior to UFH in achieving early infarct artery patency (51% vs. 52% at 60 minutes), but effectively protected against recurrent ischemic events.

The excessive bleeding reported with enoxaparin in ASSENT-III called for a safer method of administration. ExTRACT TIMI-25 was a large trial of enoxaparin versus UFH with fibrinolytic therapy, with death and recurrent MI at 30 days as the primary end point. The dose of enoxaparin was modified in the elderly, withholding the bolus and giving 0.75 mg/kg SC every 12 hours for patients more than 75 years old (Table 3) (76,111). The seven-day administration of enoxaparin

TABLE 5 Randomized Trials Comparing Adjunctive Low Molecular Weight Heparin and Unfractionated Heparin in Patients Treated with Fibrinolytic Therapy for Acute Myocardial Infarction

Trial (reference)	Lytic[a]	(Randomized treatment)		LMWH vs. UFH		
		LMWH	UFH	1° End point	Safety	Comments
ASSENT-III $n = 4078$ 2001 (18)	TNK 30–50 mg (weight adjusted)	**Enoxaparin** B: 30 mg then 1 mg/kg SC q. 12 hr × 7 days	B: 60 U/kg I: 12 U/kg/hr × 48 hr (aPTT 50–70 sec)	↓ death/re-MI/ischemia at 30 days: 11.4% vs. 15.4% ($p < 0.001$)	Major bleeds: 3.0% vs. 2.2% ($p =$ NS) ICH: 0.9% vs. 0.9% ($p =$ NS)	Not powered to examine mortality. Anticoagulant given prior to TNK. Benefit appears within 48 hr of enoxaparin
HART-II $n = 400$ 2001 (5)	t-PA ≤ 100 mg	**Enoxaparin** B: 30 mg then 1 mg/kg SC q. 12 hr, unspecified length	B: 4000–5000 IU, I: 15 IU/kg/hr × 3 days (aPTT 2–2.5×)	Non inferior 90-min TIMI-2/3 flow: 80.1% vs. 75.1%	Major bleeds: 3.6% vs. 3.0% ($p =$ NS) ICH: 1.0% vs. 1.0% ($p =$ NS)	Noninferiority angiographic study. Reocclusion rate at follow-up angiogram: enox = 5.9% vs. UFH = 9.8% ($p = 0.26$)
Baird et al. $n = 300$ 2002 (108)	SK 1.5 MU or APSAC 30 IU or t-PA ≤ 100 mg	**Enoxaparin** B: 40 mg then 40 mg SC q. 8 hr × 4 days	B: 5,000 IU, I: 30,000 IU/24 hr × 4 days (aPTT 2–2.5×)	90-day death/re-MI/UA: 36.4% vs. 25.5% ($p = 0.04$)	Major bleeds: 3% vs. 4% ($p =$ NS). No ICH reported	Aspirin (75–300 mg/days) started 4 days after index MI. Patients with anterior MI received UFH for an additional 3 days
ENTIRE/TIMI-23 $n = 242$ 2002 (2)	TNK 0.53 mg/kg	**Enoxaparin** B: 30 mg (optional) then 1 mg/kg SC q. 12 hr, × 8 days	B: 60 U/kg I: 12 U/kg/hr ≥36 hr (aPTT 1.5–2.5×)	60-min TIMI-3 flow[b]: 48% without enox bolus, 51% with enox bolus vs. 52% with UFH	Major bleeds: 2.4% vs. 1.9% ($p =$ NS) ICH: 0.6% vs. 0% ($p =$ NS)	Angiographic study. Factorial design co-assessing half-dose TNK + abciximab. Combined end point mortality/MI at 30 days: enox = 4.4% vs. UFH = 15.9% ($p = 0.005$)

Study	Fibrinolytic	LMWH regimen	UFH regimen	Efficacy	Major bleeds[b]	Comments
ASSENT-Plus n = 439 2003 (7)	t-PA ≤ 100 mg	**Dalteparin** B: 30 anti-Xa IU/kg IV then 120 IU/kg q. 12 hr × 4–7 days	B: 4,000–5,000 IU, I: 800–1,000 IU/hr × 48 hr (aPTT 50–75 sec)	Similar TIMI-3 flow at day 4–7: 69.3% vs. 62.5% (p = 0.16)	Major bleeds[b]: 3.6% vs. 5.2% ICH: 0.5% vs. 1.9%	Trend toward ↓ death/MI favoring dalteparin in the first 7 days (3.6 vs. 8.1%, p = 0.059), but similar at 30 days (9.1% vs. 10.6% p = NS)
ASSENT-III Plus n = 1,639 2003 (109)	Prehospital TNK 30–50 mg (weight adjusted)	**Enoxaparin** B: 30 mg then 1 mg/kg SC q. 12 hr × 7 days	B: 60 U/kg I: 12U/kg/hr × 48 hr (aPTT 50–70 sec)	Nonsignificant ↓ of 30-day death/re-MI/ischemia: 14.2% vs. 17.4% (p = 0.08).	Major bleeds: 4.0% vs. 2.8% (p = 0.18). ICH: 2.2% vs. 1.0% (p = 0.05)	Prehospital extension of ASSENT-III trial. Trend toward ↑ mortality in the enox group, mainly driven by excess ICH, especially in the elderly
ExTRACT/TIMI-25 n = 20,506 2006 (13)	TNK 0.53 mg/kg	**Enoxaparin**[c] B: 30 mg then 1 mg/kg SC q. 12 hr × 7 days	B: 60 U/kg I: 12 U/kg/hr × 48 hr (aPTT 1.5–2.0×)	Significant reduction of death/re-MI: 9.9% vs. 12.0% (p < 0.001)	Major bleeds: 2.1% vs. 1.4% (p < 0.001) ICH: 0.8% vs. 0.7% (p = 0.14)	Double-blind double-dummy trial. Not powered to assess 30-day mortality, which was nonsignificantly affected: 3.7% vs. 3.8% (p = 0.76)

[a]SK given over 60 minutes or accelerated t-PA.
[b]No statistical comparison performed.
[c]Enoxaparin was adjusted for age and renal function (Table 3).

Abbreviations: AAS, aspirin; APSAC, anisoylated plasminogen-streptokinase activator complex (anistreplase); aPTT, activated partial thromboplastin time; B, intravenous bolus; I, intravenous infusion; ICH, intracranial hemorrhage; IV, intravenous; Enox, enoxaparin; LMWH, low molecular weight heparin; Re-MI, reinfarction; rt-PA, recombinant tissue plasminogen activator; SK, streptokinase; TNK, tenecteplase; tPA, tissue-plasminogen activator; UA, unstable angina; UFH, unfractionated heparin.

Death through Day 180

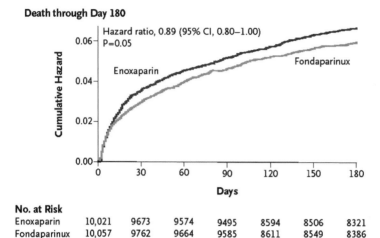

No. at Risk

Enoxaparin	10,021	9673	9574	9495	8594	8506	8321
Fondaparinux	10,057	9762	9664	9585	8611	8549	8386

FIGURE 6   A prolonged administration of enoxaparin is superior to unfractionated heparin at pre-venting death and recurrent myocardial infarction. Enoxaparin for seven days protected significantly better than fondaparinux labels for 48 hours against death and recurrent MI at 30 days (9.9% vs. 12.0%, $p < 0.001$). The mortality was not significantly affected: 3.7% vs. 3.8% ($p = 0.76$) (data not shown). *Abbreviations*: UFH, unfractionated heparin; MI, myocardial infarction. *Source*: From Ref. 13.

compared with standard 48-hour UFH significantly reduced death and reinfarction rates at day 30 (RR = 0.83, 95% CI, 0.77–0.90, $p < 0.001$). However, mortality was not significantly reduced (RR = 0.92, 95% CI, 0.84–1.02) (Fig. 6), and major bleeding was modestly increased (2.1% vs. 1.4%, $p < 0.001$) (13). The problem of higher rates of ICH in the elderly with enoxaparin vs. UFH was not observed with the modified dosing. Interestingly, the absolute benefit tended to be greater in women, possibly because of their higher risk profile at presentation (112,113). In terms of clinical benefit, the number needed to treat with enoxaparin to prevent one death/nonfatal MI was about 50: the number needed to harm with major bleeding was about 150 patients (114). Renal function remained a major predictor of hemorrhagic complications and higher bleeding rates with enoxaparin appeared with creatinine clearance as high as 90 mL/min. At creatinine clearance below 60 mL/min, enoxaparin no longer showed a clinical benefit, partially because of the excessive bleeding in this population (3.5% compared to 1.9% with UFH, $p < 0.01$) (115). Until alternative dosing regimens are proven safe, enoxaparin should be used with caution in patients with low creatinine clearance (2).

In both ExTRACT and ASSENT-III, about half of the benefit of enoxaparin was observed in the first 48 hours (during treatment with both enoxaparin and UFH), and half after UFH was stopped (Fig. 6). These trials confirmed that the prolonged administration of an adjunctive anticoagulant can prevent the recur-rence of ischemic events (13,110). Even with limitations of postrandomization subgroup analysis, it is interesting that enoxaparin appeared better than UFH at preventing death and recurrent MI (14.2% vs. 18.9%, OR = 0.68, $p = 0.002$) in the group of patients undergoing PCI during the active treatment phase, where both enoxaparin and UFH had been administered for similar times (116).

The advantage of enoxaparin as an adjunct to fibrinolytic therapy needs to be interpreted in the context of the growing use of clopidogrel (12,117) and early PCI

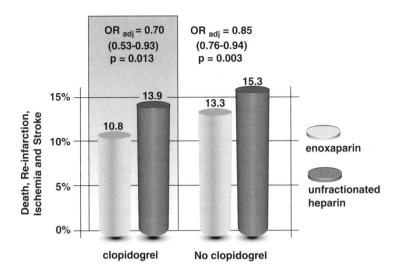

FIGURE 7 After fibrinolysis, clopidogrel and enoxaparin are associated with the best outcomes. Extract TIMI-25 was designed and initiated prior to the release of CLARITY TIMI-28 (12) and the COMMIT trial (117). After stratification by clopidogrel use, the benefit of enoxaparin was still evident in both strata. The best outcomes were observed in patients treated with enoxaparin and clopidogrel. *Abbreviations*: TIMI, Thrombolysis in Myocardial Infarction; CLARITY TIMI, Clopidogrel as Adjunctive Reperfusion Therapy–Thrombolysis in Myocardial Infarction; COMMIT, Clopidogrel and Metoprolol in Myocardial Infarction Trial; OR, odds ratio. *Source*: Adapted from Ref. 121.

(19,20,80,118–120) in this population. In the ExTRACT trial, the therapeutic advantage of enoxaparin over UFH was consistent in the subgroup of patients treated with clopidogrel, where a significant reduction of death, MI, and stroke was observed (10.8% vs. 13.9%, OR = 0.70, $p = 0.013$) (Fig. 7). Interestingly, the combination of the two agents appeared safe, as the increased risk of major bleeding was numerically, but not statistically, higher in clopidogrel-treated patients (2.7% vs. 1.0%) compared with those who were not treated with clopidogrel (2.1% vs. 1.2%, p(interaction) = 0.61) (121). Thus, the combined use of enoxaparin and clopidogrel in patients treated with fibrinolytic therapy appears reasonable.

LMWH with Primary PCI
LMWHs in general, and enoxaparin in particular, have an extensive efficacy and safety record for the treatment of non-STEMI (NSTEMI), including use with an early invasive strategy (122–124). In the GRACE registry, LMWHs were used more frequently and were associated with a reduced risk of death, irrespective of whether patients were treated conservatively or invasively (125). However, the use of LMWH anticoagulation during primary PCI has not been systematically evaluated in randomized controlled trials. As a result, the American and European guidelines do not recommend LMWHs as a primary agent for this indication (80,81).

Pharmacologic studies performed in steady conditions have demonstrated that an appropriate level of anticoagulation (anti-factor Xa > 0.5 IU/mL) can be reached within 60 minutes of a single SC enoxaparin injection (98). However, evidence suggests that this pharmacologic data may not be applicable to STEMI patients treated with primary PCI (126,127). As part of the Which Early ST-Elevation Therapy

(WEST) trial, concerning rates of catheter-related thrombosis were reported among primary PCI patients who received one dose of SC enoxaparin (1 mg/kg) at earliest point of care (on average 70 minutes before the beginning of the primary PCI) (35). Pharmacokinetic data from this trial showed that plasma anti-Xa levels were often below the target range at the time of primary PCI: 85% of patients (28/33) were less than 0.5 U/mL (128). Poor skin perfusion experienced by some patients might alter the absorption rate of enoxaparin (through high sympathetic tone and SC vaso-constriction) and thus result in an insufficient level of anticoagulation at the time of PCI (35). However, supplemental IV enoxaparin (0.3–0.5 mg/kg) at the time of PCI resulted in adequate anti-Xa levels in all patients with few having levels greater than 1.5 IU/mL. It is currently recommended that PCI with enoxaparin should be per-formed only after a steady state of anticoagulation has been reached (129). Using the SC route, this steady state is generally obtained after the second LMWH injection. In the setting of primary PCI, where time is restricted, an IV enoxaparin supplement (0.3–0.5 mg/kg) to the usual SC dose (1 mg/kg) should be used. Although recom-mended by some (130), the monitoring of anti-Xa activity during PCI is not currently available in most centers. The relatively limited experience with LMWH in the catheterization laboratory, and especially for primary PCI, may explain the tendency of the interventional cardiologist to switch to UFH during procedures (129). More data are needed regarding use of enoxaparin during primary PCI.

DIRECT THROMBIN INHIBITORS

Mechanism of Action

During the coagulation process, thrombin cleaves fibrinogen into fibrin which generates a matrix for the thrombus. As the thrombus progresses, thrombin binds to soluble fibrin. This binding maintains thrombin's enzymatic activity by pro-tecting it from the inhibitory action of UFH (131). This "clot-bound" thrombin may be an important target for alternative anticoagulants, including direct thrombin inhibitors (DTIs) that can inhibit clot-bound thrombin (132) (Table 2).

DTIs bind the serine-protease catalytic site of thrombin and prevent the con-version of fibrinogen to fibrin (Fig. 2A). DTIs are classified as either univalent agents, which exclusively bind the catalytic site, or as bivalent agents, which simultaneously bind the catalytic site and the thrombin substrate recognition exosite-1. In ACS, the bivalent agents appear to have stronger evidence for clinical benefit (133).

There are currently three DTIs commercially available (Table 6). Argatroban is a univalent agent approved for the treatment of HIT. Its use is not approved for general STEMI patients (81). Lepirudin (recombinant hirudin) is a potent and selective bivalent agent that forms a 1:1 stoichiometric slowly reversible complex with thrombin as a noncompetitive inhibitor (134). Bivalirudin also forms a 1:1 stoichiometric complex with thrombin. Unlike other DTIs, however, bivalirudin only binds transiently to thrombin; soon after its binding, bivalirudin's amino-terminal active moiety is cleaved apart from the catalytic site of thrombin (135,136) (Fig. 2C). This transient binding, along with its short half-life, may explain the lower risk of bleeding observed in some clinical trials with bivalirudin (131,133,137).

Adjunctive DTIs with Fibrinolytic Agents

Post-fibrinolysis angiographic studies have shown superior coronary patency rates with DTIs when compared with UFH (4,8,138). Despite this, no single large scale

TABLE 6 The Direct Thrombin Inhibitors

	Argatroban	Lepirudin	Bivalirudin
Thrombin inhibition	Transient	Noncompetitive inhibitor (slowly reversible)	Transient
Agent	Univalent	Bivalent	Bivalent
Elimination	Hepatic	Renal	Enzymatic 80% and renal (20%)
Half-life (normal volunteers)	39–51 min	1–3 hr	25 min
Approved for ACS	No	Yes	Yes
Approved for HIT	Yes	Yes	No[a]
Approved for PCI	No	No	Yes
PCI dose	**B**: 350 µg/kg **I**: 25–30 µg/kg/min ACT: 300–450 sec (150)3)	Repeated boluses of 0.4–0.8 mg/kg, no infusion ACT: 300–350 sec (82,194)0)	B: 0.75 mg/kg I: 1.75 mg/kg/hr × 4 hr, then 0.2 mg/kg/hr for 20 hr, ACT: >300 sec (27)

[a]Bivalirudin is not approved for the medical treatment of HIT patients, but is approved for PCI in the setting of a recent HIT.
Abbreviations: ACT, activated clotting time; aPTT, activated partial thromboplastin time; B, bolus; HIT, heparin-induced thrombocytopenia; I, infusion; INR, international normalized ratio; PCI, percutaneous coronary intervention.
Source: Adapted from Ref. 151.

trial has clearly demonstrated the clinical superiority of DTIs over UFH as adjunctive therapy with fibrinolytic agents during STEMI. A meta-analysis showed that compared with UFH, DTIs reduce the risk of death and reinfarction at 30 days (7.4% vs. 8.2%, OR = 0.91, 95% CI, 0.84–0.99). Interestingly, similar rates of major bleeding were observed (2.9% vs. 3.3%, OR = 0.89, 95% CI, 0.71–1.11) (Five trials, n = 9947) (133).

Argatroban
The clinical experience with argatroban in MI is limited to small or incomplete trials. The ARGAMI-II trial was stopped prematurely after 1001 patients were enrolled due to a lack of efficacy of argatroban compared with UFH (139).

Lepirudin
GUSTO-IIa and TIMI-9a were the first major trials to explore the efficacy and the safety of lepirudin in ACS. Both trials employed the same relatively high doses of lepirudin and UFH, and both trials were prematurely stopped after unacceptable rates of major bleeding (up to 13.9%) and ICH were observed (22,23) (Table 7), especially in the lepirudin arms. Indeed, the safety lessons learned from these trials were applied to the GUSTO-IIb and TIMI-9b trials, which were initiated using reduced anticoagulant doses with careful aPTT monitoring.

As an adjunct to fibrinolytic therapy, lepirudin offers a modest reduction of reinfarction at 48 hours compared with UFH (140). In both GUSTO-IIb and TIMI-9b, the 30-day rate of death and MI were similar between lepirudin and UFH (Table 7). Importantly, neither GUSTO IIb nor TIMI-9b demonstrated significantly excessive bleeding. This absence of sustained benefit with lepirudin may relate to a rebound hypercoagulability after its discontinuation (140,141).

TABLE 7 Selected Randomized Trials Comparing Adjunctive Direct Thrombin Inhibitors to Unfractionated Heparin in Patients Treated with Fibrinolytic Therapy for Acute Myocardial Infarction

Trial (reference)	Lytic[a]	DTI	UFH	1° End point	Safety	Comments
TIMI-9a n = 757 1994 (22)	SK 1.5 MU or t-PA ≤ 100 mg	**Lepirudin** B: 0.6 mg/kg I: 0.2 mg/kg/hr × 4 days (aPTT: unadjusted)	B: 5,000 IU I: 1,000–1,300 IU/hr × 4 days (aPTT: 55–85 sec)	Stopped early, not reported	Major bleeds: 13.9% vs. 10.1% (p = NS)ICH: 1.7% vs. 1.9% (p = NS)	Trial suspended prematurely because of excessive hemorrhage rates
GUSTO-IIa n = 2,564 1994 (23)	SK 1.5 MU or t-PA ≤ 100 mg	**Lepirudin** B: 0.6 mg/kg I: 0.2 mg/kg/hr × 3–5 days (aPTT: 60–90 sec)	B: 5,000 IU I: 1,000–1,300 IU/hr × 3–5 days (aPTT: 60–90 sec)	Stopped early, not reported	Major bleeds: not reported ICH: 1.3% vs. 0.7% (p = 0.11)	Trial suspended prematurely because of an overall excess in intracranial hemorrhage
TIMI-9b n = 3,002 1996 (141)	SK 1.5 MU or t-PA ≤ 100 mg	**Lepirudin** B: 0.1 mg/kg I: 0.1 mg/kg/hr × 4 days (aPTT: 55–85 sec)	B: 5,000 IU I: 1,000 IU/hr × 4 days (aPTT: 60–90 sec)	No difference in death/ re-MI/CHF/shock at 30 days: 12.9% vs. 11.9% (p = NS)	Major bleeds: 4.6% vs. 5.3% (p = NS)	Post hoc analyses did not identify a subgroup of patients where adjunctive lepirudin appeared beneficial
GUSTO-IIb n = 4,131[b] 1996 (140)	SK 1.5 MU or t-PA ≤100 mg	**Lepirudin** B: 0.1 mg/kg I: 0.1 mg/kg/hr × 3–5 days (aPTT: 60–80 sec)	B: 5,000 IU I: 1,000 IU/hr × 60 hr (aPTT: 60–80 sec)	In STEMI subpopulation, no significant effect on death/re-MI at 30 days: 9.9% vs. 11.3% (p = 0.13)	Major bleeds: 1.1% vs. 1.5% (p = 0.2) ICH: 0.4% vs. 0.9% (p = NS)	Adjunctive therapy given 35 min after lytics (median)

Trial	Thrombolytic	DTI dosing	Comparator dosing	Efficacy	Bleeding	Comments
HERO-I n = 412 1997 (8)	SK 1.5 MU	**Bivalirudin** High dose: as HERO-II low dose: ½ high dose, × 60 hr (aPTT: <120 sec)	B: 5,000 IU I: 1,000–1,200 IU/hr × 60 hr (aPTT: normogram)	↑ 90-min TIMI-3 flow: 48% for high dose vs. 35% for UFH (p = 0.03).	Major bleeds: 19% high dose, 14% low dose vs. 27% with UFH (p < 0.01) no ICH reported	Angiographic study. No effect of LVEF. Trend toward ↓ reocclusion at 48 hr with bivalirudin (1% vs. 7%, p = NS)
HIT-IV n = 1208 1999 (4)	SK 1.5 MU	**Lepirudin** B: 0.2 mg/kg IV then 0.5 mg/kg q. 12 hr SC × 5–7 days (aPTT: 1.5–2.5×)	B: 0.2 mg/kg IV then 12,500 IU q. 12 hr SC × 5–7 days (aPTT: 1.5–2.5×)	No effect on 90-min TIMI-3 flow: 40.7% vs. 33.5% (p = 0.16)	Major bleeds: 3.3% vs. 3.5% (p = NS) ICH: 0.2% vs. 0.3% (p = NS)	Lepirudin/UFH given pre-SK. No effect on 30-day death/re-MI/stroke despite ↑ early ST-segment resolution with lepirudin (28% vs. 22%, p = 0.05)
HERO-II n = 17,073 2001 (144)	SK 1.5 MU	**Bivalirudin** B: 0.25 mg/kg I: 0.5 mg/kg/hr × 12 hr, 0.25 mg/kg/hr × 36 hr (aPTT: <120 sec)	B: 5,000 IU I: 800–1,000 U/hr × 48 hr. (aPTT: 50–75 sec)	No effect on 30-day mortality: 10.8% vs. 10.9% (p = 0.85)	Major bleeds: 0.7% vs. 0.5% (p = 0.07) ICH: 0.6% vs. 0.4% (p = 0.09)	Bivalirudin/UFH given pre-SK. Bivalirudin ↓ /within 96 hr: 1.6% vs. 2.3% (p = 0.001) but ↑ moderate bleeding (higher aPTTs)

[a]SK given over 60 minutes and accelerated t-PA.
[b]STEMI subgroup only.

Abbreviations: ACS, acute coronary syndrome; Aptt, activated partial thromboplastin time; CHF, congestive heart failure; B, bolus; DTI, direct thrombin inhibitor; I, infusion; IRA, infarct-related artery; LVEF, left ventricular ejection fraction; MU, million unit; SK, streptokinase; STEMI, ST-elevation myocardial infarction; TIMI, thrombolysis in myocardial infarction; UFH, unfractionated heparin.

The body of evidence collected for lepirudin suggests a narrow therapeutic window with the agent. The risk-to-benefit ratio of lepirudin appears to be dose dependent: higher doses are linked to an unacceptable rate of bleeding complication (22,23) and lower doses are associated with less antithrombotic efficacy (140,141). Lepirudin accumulates in patients with renal insufficiency and therefore should be avoided in these patients (127,142). With hope of refining the safety profile of adjunctive lepirudin, SC instead of IV injection was tested in the HIT-4 trial. Using the SC strategy, lepirudin caused similar in-hospital major bleeding when compared with IV UFH (3.3% for lepirudin vs. 3.5% for UFH, p = NS). Death and reinfarction rates were similar at 30 days (4).

Bivalirudin
Bivalirudin without GP IIb/IIIa inhibitors is of similar effectiveness as heparin plus IIb/IIIa inhibitors in the prevention of thrombotic events in non ST-elevation ACS (84,133,137,143), although there is some controversy about how convincing the evidence is for non-inferiority. The principal advantage of bivalirudin lies in its safety profile, as it appears to reduce bleeding. In a meta-analysis of six non STACS trials (n = 5674), bivalirudin was associated with a significant reduction in recurrent MI at 30–50 days (OR = 0.73, 95% CI, 0.55–0.97, p = 0.04), and there was a substantial reduction of major hemorrhage (OR = 0.41, 95% CI, 0.32–0.52, p = 0.04), representing 8 fewer events per 1000 patients treated with bivalirudin (137). The data supporting the use of bivalirudin is less convincing in STEMI, treated with either fibrinolytic therapy or primary PCI.

The HERO-I and HERO-II trials compared bivalirudin with UFH as adjunctive therapies to SK and aspirin in STEMI. While HERO-I established the superiority of bivalirudin to achieve early and complete patency of the infarct artery, HERO-II showed no reduction in 30-day mortality (10.8% vs. 10.9%, p = 0.85) and a tendency for more major bleeding (0.7% vs. 0.5%, p = 0.07) (8144). Similar to lepirudin in GUSTO-IIb, there was significantly less in-hospital reinfarction with bivalirudin (1.6% vs. 2.3%, p = 0.001) (144). During the active anticoagulation period, patients randomized to bivalirudin had significantly higher aPTTs.

Thus, in spite of the theoretic benefits, the use of DTIs with fibrinolytic therapy is restricted to patients with contraindications to UFH, including HIT (81). Because of its wider therapeutic window, bivalirudin (with SK) is favored over lepirudin in this setting (144).

DTIs with Primary PCI
DTIs are effective compared with UFH for NSTEMI patients undergoing PCI (82,133,145–147). However, the use of DTIs during primary PCI has not been studied in clinical outcome trials. Some data nonetheless suggest that they may be beneficial in this context. In a recent meta-analysis from the DTI Trialists' Collaborative Group, ACS patients undergoing unplanned early PCI after fibrinolysis had a 10% lower risk of death or reinfarction at 30 days with DTIs versus UFH (HR = 0.90, 95% CI, 0.84–0.97). The protective effect of DTIs persisted after adjustment of baseline characteristics and propensity to undergo PCI. Interestingly, DTIs were associated with a lower incidence of major bleeding (2.6% vs. 7.5%, p < 0.001) (145).

Bivalirudin appears to be the most promising DTI for primary PCI. In the Acute Catheterization and Urgent Intervention Triage strategY (ACUITY) trial, in which the majority of ACS patients underwent early PCI, bivalirudin as monotherapy compared with UFH plus GP IIb/IIIa inhibitor was associated with a significantly lower rate of bleeding (3.0% vs. 5.7%, $p < 0.0001$) (83). In a recent pooled analysis of PCI trials, the combined incidence of death, MI, revascularization, and major bleeding at 48 hours was significantly reduced in the bivalirudin group compared with UFH (1.1% vs. 7.8%, $p < 0.01$). The reduction in major bleeding events was the main driver of this combined effect (2.7% vs. 5.8%, $p < 0.01$) (146). It also appears that patients can be switched from UFH or enoxaparin to bivalirudin prior to PCI without increasing the bleeding risk (148,149). However encouraging these data may be, direct evidence in a prospective trial dedicated to primary PCI is still required before any recommendation on bivalirudin use can be formulated. To date, the role of DTIs in MI is limited to HIT (80,81,150,151).

PENTASACHARIDES

Mechanism of Action
Although several molecules of the pentasaccharide family are currently undergoing clinical testing, fondaparinux is the only agent that has been studied in clinical outcome trials in ischemic heart disease. Fondaparinux is a synthetic analogue of the pentasaccharide sequence of UFH. Pentasaccharides are indirect inhibitors of factor Xa through AT III. Like UFH and LMWHs, pentasaccharide agents induce a conformational change of AT III, which enhances its affinity for factor Xa (Fig. 2) (152,153). Unlike heparins, however, fondaparinux is too short to bridge AT to thrombin and thus has no AT activity. Ultimately, fondaparinux inhibits the generation of new thrombin, but does not affect thrombin once activated (152). This absence of thrombin inhibition may explain, at least in part, the safer profile of fondaparinux in comparison with UFH or LMWH in the treatment of ACS (14,154).

Fondaparinux does not interact with plasma proteins and thus has a predictable dose-response effect. The anticoagulant has an excellent SC bioavailability and because of its rather long half-life (15–20 hours), it can be administered once daily (155). Fondaparinux neither affects the prothrombin time (PT), nor the aPTT, or the bleeding time. Although fondaparinux activity can be assessed using a factor Xa activity assay, laboratory monitoring has not been used in its clinical development. Fondaparinux is renally excreted and the single fixed dose of 2.5 mg SC once daily has been used safely across a broad range of creatinine levels (14,154). However, it should be avoided with creatinine clearance less than 30 cc/min. Fondaparinux has been promising in the treatment of deep vein thrombosis and pulmonary embolism (156). Fondaparinux has now been studied in more than 35,000 ACS patients and has been safe, effective, and easy to use, although it has limitations for use during PCI.

Adjunctive Pentasaccharides with Fibrinolytic Agents
The synthetic PENTasaccharide as an Adjunct to fibrinoLYsis in ST-Elevation acute myocardial infarction (PENTALYSE) angiographic study assessed the efficacy of escalating fondaparinux doses (4 mg, 8 mg, and 12 mg IV) compared with IV UFH given before t-PA in STEMI patients. While the coadministration of adjunctive fondaparinux resulted in similar rates of coronary patency at 90 minutes when compared with UFH (TIMI-3 flow: 64% vs. 68%, $p = 0.6$), its prolonged SC

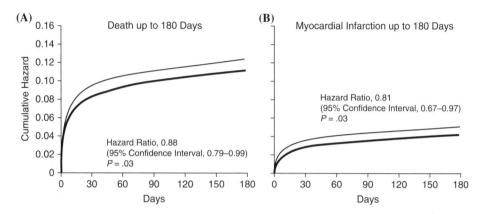

FIGURE 8 Long-term efficacy of adjunctive fondaparinux versus standard medical therapy with fibrinolysis in acute myocardial infarction. Fondaparinux was associated with a reduction of death (10.5% vs. 11.6%, $p = 0.03$) and myocardial infarction (3.8% vs. 4.6%, $p = 0.03$) at 180 days when compared with standard medical therapy. The bold line illustrates fondaparinux. *Source*: From Ref. 14.

administration (5–7 days) was associated with a trend of less infarct artery reocclusion (0.9% vs. 7.0%, $p = 0.065$) (157).

The efficacy of fondaparinux on clinical outcomes was assessed by the Organization to Assess Strategies for Ischemic Syndromes (OASIS)-6 trial study that compared eight days of fondaparinux (2.5 mg SC daily) with either UFH or no anticoagulation in 12,092 STEMI patients. Of note, among the patients treated with UFH, 75% received the anticoagulant for less than 48 hours, according to standard practice. Nearly 50% of the patients in the control group, mostly patients treated with SK, did not receive any adjunctive anticoagulation. In this context, fondaparinux showed a reduction in death and reinfarction at 30-day (9.7% vs. 11.2%, HR $= 0.86$, 95% CI, 0.77–0.96, $p = 0.008$) without increasing the incidence of hemorrhagic stroke or major bleeding (1.0% vs. 1.3%, HR $= 0.77$, 95% CI, 0.55–1.08, $p = 0.13$) (14). These benefits persisted at 180 days (Fig. 8).

The prolonged fondaparinux administration employed during OASIS-6 (8-day course) compared with standard use of UFH (48 hours) or even placebo emphasizes the importance of the strategy employed. Together with enoxaparin in the ExTRACT TIMI-25 trial, the positive finding of OASIS-6 raises the question as to whether UFH for 48 hours after fibrinolysis is an adequate anticoagulant duration (158,159). Arguably, much of the benefit of fondaparinux may be due to its prolonged administration after fibrinolysis rather than its superiority as an anticoagulant. This is supported by a post hoc analysis of OASIS-6 showing that most of the benefit of fondaparinux occurred after the active treatment period of UFH (158).

Pentasaccharides with Primary PCI
The pilot Arixtra Study in Percutaneous Coronary Intervention: A Randomized Evaluation (ASPIRE) assessed the feasibility of using fondaparinux during PCI and compared IV fondaparinux 2.5 mg and 5.0 mg with UFH (160). Although the study was open to STEMI patients, fewer than 5% of the 350 patients were enrolled for

primary PCI. In this context, fondaparinux was associated with a nonsignificant reduction in total bleeding risk (6.4% vs. 7.7%, HR = 0.81, 95% CI, 0.35–1.84, $p = 0.61$), again with a nonsignificant trend toward lower bleeding risk with fondaparinux 2.5 mg compared with fondaparinux 5 mg (3.4% vs. 9.6%, $p = 0.06$). The composite efficacy outcome of death, MI, urgent revascularization, and the need for bail out GP IIb/IIIa inhibitors was similar between UFH and fondaparinux (6.0% vs. 6.0%, HR = 1.02, 95% CI, 0.41–2.52), with no obvious dose response between the two fondaparinux groups. Interestingly, a signal for increased rates of catheter-related thrombosis was reported in this study, especially with fondaparinux 2.5 mg (7.6% vs. 1.8%, compared to UFH). A similar catheter-related thrombosis problem was reported in the OASIS-5 trial where fondaparinux was compared with enoxaparin in ACS (154).

The favorable findings of fondaparinux in OASIS-6 did not extend to patients treated with primary PCI. While significant benefits with fondaparinux were observed at 30 days among nonreperfused patients (12.2% vs. 15.1%, HR = 0.80, 95% CI, 0.65–0.98, $p = 0.003$) and among patients treated with fibrinolytic therapy (10.9% vs. 13.6%, HR = 0.79, 95% CI, 0.68–0.92, $p = 0.003$), no benefit was observed in primary PCI patients (6.0% vs. 4.9%, HR = 1.24, 95% CI, 0.95–1.63, $p = 0.12$). As noted in ASPIRE, coronary complications such as abrupt coronary artery closure and the no-reflow phenomenon were more frequent among patients treated with fondaparinux. Interestingly, these coronary complications were no longer noted in fondaparinux patients who received UFH prior to randomization. In vitro cell-based models of coagulation suggests that factor X levels as low as 1% to 5% are required before thrombin generation is significantly affected (161). Given the absence of monitoring of factor Xa activity in ASPIRE and OASIS-6, the possibility of an insufficient level of anticoagulation with IV doses up to 5 mg cannot be excluded, and contact activation of the coagulation system may not be effectively prevented with anti-Xa inhibition alone.

SPECIAL POPULATIONS AND CIRCUMSTANCES

The Rebound/Reactivation Phenomenon

A rebound in clinical thrombosis upon discontinuation of UFH in ACS patients was originally described by Theroux et al. (162). In GUSTO-1, where aspirin was systematically used, the likelihood of reinfarction after IV UFH discontinuation was highest two to four hours after discontinuation, with a third of 30-day reinfarctions occurring within 10 hours (78). Similar clusters of thrombotic events upon UFH discontinuation have been described with dalteparin in the Fragmin during Instability in Coronary Artery Disease (FRISC) and the ASSENT-Plus studies (7,163), with enoxaparin in Efficacy and Safety of Subcutaneous Enoxaparin in Non-Q-Wave Coronary Events (ESSENCE) and TIMI-11B studies (159,164,165), and with the univalent DTI inogatran in the Thrombin inhibition in Myocardial Ischemia (TRIM) study (166).

A worrisome aspect of the rebound phenomenon is that it may occur in patients considered stable and potentially eligible for hospital discharge. Consequently, certain high-risk patients should be carefully monitored in the early hours after the discontinuation of anticoagulant agents. The progressive weaning of the dose of anticoagulants has been proposed as an alternative solution, but the strategy is unproven (168).

Postinfarction Mural Thrombus and Stroke

Another target for anticoagulant therapy is to prevent LV thrombus formation, a complication frequently encountered in anterior MI and associated with an increased risk of systemic emboli (169). In the original autopsy series, the prevalence of LV mural thrombus after MI was 40% to 50% (170). UFH trials prior to the use of fibrinolytics showed that systemic anticoagulation could significantly reduce stroke rates (39–41). In patients with anterior MI treated with fibrinolysis, LV thrombus has been identified by echocardiography in up to 30% of patients (105,171,172). In the fibrinolytic era, the use of systemic anticoagulation has also been associated with a significant reduction in arterial embolization (OR = 0.14, 95% CI, 0.04–0.52) (169). In spite of this, longer-term anticoagulation is uncommonly used.

Prior to the publication of GISSI-II, two trials demonstrated a 21% absolute risk reduction of mural thrombus development using a fixed dose of SC UFH (12,500 IU every 12 hr) after MI (54,173). Using the exact same UFH regimen, GISSI-II could not replicate this finding (27% vs. 30% in the placebo-treated patients, p = NS) (55). The concomitant use of aspirin and fibrinolytic therapy in GISSI-II may explain the differences observed between the trials. In the Fragmin in Acute Myocardial Infarction (FRAMI) trial, despite the efficacy of dalteparin at reducing the incidence of LV thrombus when compared with placebo (OR = 0.63, 95% CI, 0.43–0.92, p = 0.02), no reduction in arterial embolism was observed at nine days, with stroke rates of 1.5% vs. 1.3%, p = NS (105). In the current era of aggressive reperfusion therapy (174) and imaging tools (175), the prevalence of LV thrombus and the value of its prevention need to be reassessed.

Patients Not Eligible for Reperfusion

A significant proportion of STEMI patients will not receive reperfusion therapy, often because of delayed presentation, advanced age, or major contraindication (176,177). In this context, anticoagulants are frequently used, assuming that the evidence of benefit in non-ST-segment elevation ACS is relevant to this population. However, relatively few contemporary studies have investigated the efficacy of anticoagulants in this population and as a result, there is no clear consensus on their use (76,80).

In the Studio sulla Calciparina nell'Angina e nella Thombosi Ventricolare nell'Infarto (SCATI) trial, the subgroup of patients with delayed hospital presentation (more than 6 hours after the initiation of the symptoms) who were not treated with a fibrinolytic agent did not appear to benefit from UFH (given as an 2000 IU IV bolus, followed by 12,500 IU SC twice daily), either in terms of mortality or reinfarction. If anything, anticoagulation reduced the rate of LV thrombus formation, but without significantly affecting the rate of arterial embolic episodes (173). To some extent, the SCATI trial is similar to the clinical trials performed in the 1970s when aspirin and fibrinolytic therapy were not systematically employed (39–41). In a post hoc analysis of the TIMI-11B and ESSENCE trials, the patients initially identified as NSTEMI who were subsequently found to have Q-wave MI had a more favorable outcome when treated with enoxaparin compared with UFH. A 28% reduction of the composite outcome of death/MI/recurrent angina at 30 days was found between the two groups (178). In the OASIS-6 trial, 23.4% of patients with STEMI had no reperfusion therapy within the first 24 hours of presentation. The benefit of fondaparinux among patients not receiving reperfusion therapy was consistent with the overall trial and with the fibrinolytic-treated population (death and reinfarction, 15.1% in control vs. 12.2% with fondaparinux, HR = 0.80, 95% CI, 0.65–0.98, p = 0.003) (179).

Treatment of Acute ST-segment Elevation Myocardial Infarction Patients Ineligible for Reperfusion (TETAMI) is the only trial designed to prospectively and exclusively assess various anticoagulation strategies in STEMI patients not eligible for early reperfusion therapy. The primary aim of TETAMI study was to investigate the efficacy and safety of treatment with enoxaparin or tirofiban, alone or in combination. Using a factorial design, enoxaparin and tirofiban were compared with UFH and placebo, respectively (180). The anticoagulant agents were administered for a mean duration of 2.5 days. Enoxaparin and UFH were similar in terms of death, reinfarction, or recurrent angina at 30 days (15.7% vs. 17.3%, respectively, OR = 0.89, 95% CI, 0.66–1.21, p = NS) (176). The addition of tirofiban to either UFH or enoxaparin did not influence the outcome. As highlighted by the authors, future trials with more statistical power are required to detect treatment benefit in this important population.

HIT

HIT is a syndrome involving antibodies directed against the PF4 heparin complex. The resultant antibody complexes bind to and activate platelets, which in return secrete more PF4 and procoagulants and amplify the coagulation process (181).

Immunologically mediated HIT (182) is characterized by the presence of unexplained thrombocytopenia, with an absolute platelet count drop below 150 × 10^9/L (or a relative platelet count drop greater than 50% from baseline) and serologic evidence of anti-PF4 antibody, all in the context of recent UFH exposure (104). In the cardiology population, the differential diagnosis should include drug-related (GP IIb/IIIa inhibitors and thienopyridines) and mechanically induced (intra-aortic balloon pump) thrombocytopenia. Bovine UFH is more likely to cause HIT than UFH derived from porcine intestinal mucosa (183). Similarly, UFH is more likely to cause HIT than LMWHs, essentially because of the greater immunogenicity of the long polysaccharide chain of UFH (184). HIT uncommonly manifests itself by coronary thrombosis. In large clinical series, MI usually represents less that 5% of all HIT-related thrombotic complications (185).

Whenever HIT is suspected, UFH should immediately be stopped and alternative anticoagulation should be initiated and continued until the confirmatory antibody assays are available. DTIs appear as the logical choice of alternative anticoagulation, at least in the cardiac population (186). Fondaparinux theoretically may be a reasonable choice, although it has not been well studied. Because of the thrombocytopenia associated with acute HIT, primary PCI may be the best reperfusion option. In this context, bivalirudin may be the best choice during and after the procedure (83,150,151,187).

Elderly Patients

Adjunctive anticoagulation must be carefully administered to elderly patients because of their increased risk for bleeding, and particularly hemorrhagic stroke. Patients older than 75 years of age have sometimes been excluded from clinical trials, either explicitly on the basis of age or indirectly because of other comorbid factors (188). As a consequence, reperfusion strategies employing adjunctive anticoagulants have been less well studied in this population. Enoxaparin has been shown to increase intracranial hemorrhage compared with UFH (6.7% vs. 1.2%, $p = 0.01$) (Table 5) (109). Pharmacodynamic studies performed in acute MI patients suggest that elderly patients have an anti-Xa activity clearance at least 20% less than younger patients (189). On the basis of this concept, the ExTRACT TIMI-25 trial has tested a novel modified regimen of enoxaparin in patients older than 75 years (Table 3) (13). By simply avoiding the initial enoxaparin bolus and by reducing the maintenance dose by 25%, the new regimen appeared to prevent the excessive enoxaparin-related bleeding previously observed. Death and recurrent MI were decreased in the population, consistent with the overall ExTRACT TIMI-25 results (24.8% vs. 26.3%, RR = 0.94, 95% CI, 0.82–1.08, p(interaction) = 0.10) (189).

Fondaparinux was recently demonstrated superior to standard medical therapy in STEMI patients (14). In a prespecified post hoc analysis of OASIS-6, fondaparinux remained significantly more effective among patients older than 62 years of age (primary end point 14.1% vs. 16.8, $p < 0.05$), with less major bleeding. Despite the interesting profile presented by bivalirudin, no data specifically addressing the safety issues are available for elderly patients (83,144).

CONCLUSION

The use of adjunctive anticoagulant therapy with fibrinolytic therapy does not translate into superior early infarct artery patency, but protects against the paradoxical activation of the coagulation system. The continued administration of an anticoagulant for longer than 48 to 72 hours appears to protect against recurrent ischemic events. When compared with standard medical therapy, the prolonged administration of enoxaparin or fondaparinux after fibrinolysis for STEMI is associated with a reduction in death and recurrent MI. During primary PCI, UFH still remains the preferred agent, as the use of LMWHs and DTIs has not been adequately studied in this setting. Fondaparinux should be avoided as monotherapy when a PCI is performed.

Many questions remain with adjunctive anticoagulation, particularly regarding the optimal combination and timing of antiplatelet and anticoagulant therapies according to various reperfusion and revascularization strategies. While early and routine use of angiography is increasing, it remains to be proven that this approach is superior to the more conservative approach of prolonged anticoagulation combined with an ischemia-driven revascularization strategy.

With the use evidence-based treatment, including fibrin-specific fibrinolytic agents, primary PCI, and thienopyridines, the prognosis of MI has significantly improved. Because of this remarkable progress, safety in general and bleeding in particular are becoming key factors guiding the choice of the best anticoagulant regimen. Age-adjusted enoxaparin dosing, fondaparinux, and bivalirudin hold promise in achieving this goal. More than ever, strategies directed at balancing effective anticoagulation with low bleeding rates are required.

REFERENCES

1. Ross AM, Coyne KS, Moreyra E, et al. Extended mortality benefit of early postinfarction reperfusion. Circulation 1998; 97:1549–1556.
2. Antman EM, Louwerenburg HW, Baars HF, et al. Enoxaparin as adjunctive antithrombin therapy for ST-elevation myocardial infarction: results of the ENTIRE-Thrombolysis in Myocardial Infarction (TIMI) 23 trial. Circulation 2002; 105:1642–1649.

3. Frostfeldt G, Ahlberg G, Gustafsson G, et al. Low molecular weight heparin (dalteparin) as adjuvant treatment to thrombolysis in acute myocardial infarction—a pilot study: Biochemical Markers in Acute Coronary Syndromes (BIOMACS II). J Am Coll Cardiol 1999; 33:627–633.
4. Neuhaus KL, Molhoek GP, Zeymer U, et al. Recombinant hirudin (lepirudin) for the improvement of thrombolysis with streptokinase in patients with acute myocardial infarction: results of the HIT-4 trial. J Am Coll Cardiol 1999; 34:966–973.
5. Ross AM, Molhoek P, Lundergan C, et al. Randomized comparison of enoxaparin, a low-molecular-weight heparin, with unfractionated heparin adjunctive to recombinant tissue plasminogen activator thrombolysis and aspirin: second trial of Heparin and Aspirin Reperfusion Therapy (HART II). Circulation 2001; 104:648–652.
6. The GUSTO Angiographic Investigators. The effects of tissue plasminogen activator, streptokinase, or both on coronary artery patency, ventricular function, and survival after acute myocardial infarction. N Engl J Med 1993; 329:1615–1622.
7. Wallentin L, Bergstrand L, Dellborg M, et al. Low molecular weight heparin (dalteparin) compared to unfractionated heparin as an adjunct to rt-PA (alteplase) for improvement of coronary artery patency in acute myocardial infarction—the ASSENT Plus study. Eur Heart J 2003; 24:897–908.
8. White HD, Aylward PE, Frey MJ, et al. Randomized, double-blind comparison of hirulog versus heparin in patients receiving streptokinase and aspirin for acute myocardial infarction (HERO). Circulation 1997; 96:2155–2161.
9. Ohman EM, Califf RM, Topol EJ, et al. Consequences of reocclusion after successful reperfusion therapy in acute myocardial infarction. Circulation 1990; 82:781–791.
10. Gibson CM, Karha J, Murphy SA, et al. Early and long-term clinical outcomes associated with reinfarction following fibrinolytic administration in the thrombolysis in myocardial infarction trials. J Am Coll Cardiol 2003; 42:7–16.
11. Hudson MP, Granger CB, Topol EJ, et al. Early reinfarction after fibrinolysis: experience from the global utilization of streptokinase and tissue plasminogen activator (alteplase) for occluded coronary arteries (GUSTO I) and global use of strategies to open occluded coronary arteries (GUSTO III) trials. Circulation 2001; 104:1229–1235.
12. Sabatine MS, Cannon CP, Gibson CM, et al. Addition of clopidogrel to aspirin and fibrinolytic therapy for myocardial infarction with ST-segment elevation. N Engl J Med 2005; 352:1179–1189.
13. Antman EM, Morrow DA, McCabe CH, et al. Enoxaparin versus unfractionated heparin with fibrinolysis for ST-elevation myocardial infarction. N Engl J Med 2006; 354: 1477–1488.
14. Yusuf S, Mehta SR, Chrolavicius S, et al. Effects of fondaparinux on mortality and reinfarction in patients with acute ST-segment elevation myocardial infarction: the OASIS-6 randomized trial. JAMA 2006; 295:1519–1530.
15. Wallentin L, Goldstein P, Armstrong PW, et al. Efficacy and safety of tenecteplase in combination with the low-molecular-weight heparin enoxaparin or unfractionated heparin in the prehospital setting: The Assessment of the Safety and Efficacy of a New Thrombolytic Regimen (ASSENT)-3 PLUS randomized trial in acute myocardial infarction. Circulation 2003; 108:135–142.
16. The CREATE Trial Group, . Effects of reviparin, a low-molecular-weight heparin, on mortality, reinfarction, and strokes in patients with acute myocardial infarction presenting with ST-segment elevation. JAMA 2005; 293:427–435.
17. Simoons ML, Krzeminska-Pakula M, Alonso A, et al. Improved reperfusion and clinical outcome with enoxaparin as an adjunct to streptokinase thrombolysis in acute myocardial infarction. The AMI-SK study. Eur Heart J 2002; 23:1282–1290.
18. Efficacy and safety of tenecteplase in combination with enoxaparin, abciximab, or unfractionated heparin: the ASSENT-3 randomised trial in acute myocardial infarction. Lancet 2001; 358:605–613.
19. Armstrong PW. A comparison of pharmacologic therapy with/without timely coronary intervention vs. primary percutaneous intervention early after ST-elevation myocardial infarction: the WEST (Which Early ST-elevation myocardial infarction Therapy) study. Eur Heart J 2006; 27:1530–1538.

20. Le May MR, Wells GA, Labinaz M, et al. Combined angioplasty and pharmacological intervention versus thrombolysis alone in acute myocardial infarction (CAPITAL AMI study). J Am Coll Cardiol 2005; 46:417–424.
21. The Apex AMI Investigators, . Pexelizumab for acute ST-elevation myocardial infarction in patients undergoing primary percutaneous coronary intervention: a randomized controlled trial. JAMA 2007; 297:43–51.
22. Antman EM. Hirudin in acute myocardial infarction. Safety report from the Thrombolysis and Thrombin Inhibition in Myocardial Infarction (TIMI) 9A Trial. Circulation 1994; 90: 1624–1630.
23. Randomized trial of intravenous heparin versus recombinant hirudin for acute coronary syndromes. The Global Use of Strategies to Open Occluded Coronary Arteries (GUSTO) IIa Investigators. Circulation 1994; 90:1631–1637.
24. Eikelboom JW, Hirsh J. Bleeding and management of bleeding. Eur Heart J Suppl 2006; 8:G38–G45.
25. Moscucci M, Fox KA, Cannon CP, et al. Predictors of major bleeding in acute coronary syndromes: the Global Registry of Acute Coronary Events (GRACE). Eur Heart J 2003; 24:1815–1823.
26. Rao SV, Jollis JG, Harrington RA, et al. Relationship of blood transfusion and clinical outcomes in patients with acute coronary syndromes. JAMA 2004; 292:1555–1562.
27. Rao SV, Eikelboom JA, Granger CB, et al. Bleeding and blood transfusion issues in patients with non-ST-segment elevation acute coronary syndromes. Eur Heart J 2007; 28:1193–1204.
28. Barratt JO. The action of anticoagulants. J Physiol 1937; 90:377–384.
29. Wright IS, Marple CD. The use of anticoagulants in the treatment of myocardial infarction. Mod Concepts Cardiovasc Dis 1949; 18:55.
30. DeWood MA, Spores J, Notske R, et al. Prevalence of total coronary occlusion during the early hours of transmural myocardial infarction. N Engl J Med 1980; 303:897–902.
31. Hirsh J, Raschke R. Heparin and low-molecular-weight heparin: the Seventh ACCP Conference on Antithrombotic and Thrombolytic Therapy. Chest 2004; 126:188S–203S.
32. Danielsson A, Raub E, Lindahl U, Bjork I. Role of ternary complexes, in which heparin binds both antithrombin and proteinase, in the acceleration of the reactions between antithrombin and thrombin or factor Xa. J Biol Chem 1986; 261:15467–15473.
33. Rosenberg RD, Lam L. Correlation between structure and function of heparin. Proc Natl Acad Sci U S A 1979; 76:1218–1222.
34. Beguin S, Lindhout T, Hemker HC. The mode of action of heparin in plasma. Thromb Haemost 1988; 60:457–462.
35. Buller CE, Pate GE, Armstrong PW, et al. Catheter thrombosis during primary percutaneous coronary intervention for acute ST elevation myocardial infarction despite subcutaneous low-molecular-weight heparin, acetylsalicylic acid, clopidogrel and abciximab pretreatment. Can J Cardiol 2006; 22:511–515.
36. Colman RW, Schmaier AH. Contact system: a vascular biology modulator with anticoagulant, profibrinolytic, antiadhesive, and proinflammatory attributes. Blood 1997; 90:3819–3843.
37. Pixley RA, Schapira M, Colman RW. Effect of heparin on the inactivation rate of human activated factor XII by antithrombin III. Blood 1985; 66:198–203.
38. Mahaffey KW, Becker RC. The scientific community's quest to identify optimal targets for anticoagulant pharmacotherapy. Circulation 2006; 114:2313–2316.
39. Assessment of short-anticoagulant administration after cardiac infarction. Report of the Working Party on Anticoagulant Therapy in Coronary Thrombosis to the Medical Research Council. BMJ 1969; 1:335–342.
40. Drapkin A, Merskey C. Anticoagulant therapy after acute myocardial infarction. Relation of therapeutic benefit to patient's age, sex, and severity of infarction. JAMA 1972; 222:541–548.
41. Anticoagulants in acute myocardial infarction. Results of a cooperative clinical trial. JAMA 1973; 225:724–729.
42. Menon V, Harrington RA, Hochman JS, et al. Thrombolysis and adjunctive therapy in acute myocardial infarction: The Seventh ACCP Conference on Antithrombotic and Thrombolytic Therapy. Chest 2004; 126:549S–557S.

43. Goldberg RJ, Gore JM, Dalen JE. The role of anticoagulant therapy in acute myocardial infarction. Am Heart J 1984; 108:1387–1393.
44. Effectiveness of intravenous thrombolytic treatment in acute myocardial infarction. Gruppo Italiano per lo Studio della Streptochinasi nell'Infarto Miocardico (GISSI). Lancet 1986; 1:397–402.
45. Randomised trial of intravenous streptokinase, oral aspirin, both, or neither among 17,187 cases of suspected acute myocardial infarction: ISIS-2. ISIS-2 (Second International Study of Infarct Survival) Collaborative Group. Lancet 1988; 2:349–360.
46. Effect of intravenous APSAC on mortality after acute myocardial infarction: preliminary report of a placebo-controlled clinical trial. AIMS Trial Study Group. Lancet 1988; 1:545–549.
47. Sheehan FH, Braunwald E, Canner P, et al. The effect of intravenous thrombolytic therapy on left ventricular function: a report on tissue-type plasminogen activator and streptokinase from the Thrombolysis in Myocardial Infarction (TIMI Phase I) trial. Circulation 1987; 75:817–829.
48. Wilcox RG, von der LG, Olsson CG, et al. Trial of tissue plasminogen activator for mortality reduction in acute myocardial infarction. Anglo-Scandinavian Study of Early Thrombolysis (ASSET). Lancet 1988; 2:525–530.
49. Randomised trial of intravenous atenolol among 16,027 cases of suspected acute myocardial infarction: ISIS-1. First International Study of Infarct Survival Collaborative Group. Lancet 1986; 2:57–66.
50. Collins R, MacMahon S, Flather M, et al. Clinical effects of anticoagulant therapy in suspected acute myocardial infarction: systematic overview of randomised trials. BMJ 1996; 313:652–659.
51. Eikelboom JW, Quinlan DJ, Mehta SR, et al. Unfractionated and low-molecular-weight heparin as adjuncts to thrombolysis in aspirin-treated patients with ST-elevation acute myocardial infarction: a meta-analysis of the randomized trials. Circulation 2005; 112:3855–3867.
52. Mahaffey KW, Granger CB, Collins R, et al. Overview of randomized trials of intravenous heparin in patients with acute myocardial infarction treated with thrombolytic therapy. Am J Cardiol 1996; 77:551–556.
53. Granger CB, Hirsch J, Califf RM, et al. Activated partial thromboplastin time and outcome after thrombolytic therapy for acute myocardial infarction: results from the GUSTO-I trial. Circulation 1996; 93:870–878.
54. Turpie AG, Robinson JG, Doyle DJ, et al. Comparison of high-dose with low-dose subcutaneous heparin to prevent left ventricular mural thrombosis in patients with acute transmural anterior myocardial infarction. N Engl J Med 1989; 320:352–357.
55. GISSI-2: a factorial randomised trial of alteplase versus streptokinase and heparin versus no heparin among 12,490 patients with acute myocardial infarction. Gruppo Italiano per lo Studio della Sopravvivenza nell'Infarto Miocardico. Lancet 1990; 336:65–71.
56. In-hospital mortality and clinical course of 20,891 patients with suspected acute myocardial infarction randomised between alteplase and streptokinase with or without heparin. The International Study Group. Lancet 1990; 336:71–75.
57. ISIS-3: a randomised comparison of streptokinase vs tissue plasminogen activator vs anistreplase and of aspirin plus heparin vs aspirin alone among 41,299 cases of suspected acute myocardial infarction. ISIS-3 (Third International Study of Infarct Survival) Collaborative Group. Lancet 1992; 339:753–770.
58. Dawes J, Prowse CV, Pepper DS. Absorption of heparin, LMW heparin and SP54 after subcutaneous injection, assessed by competitive binding assay. Thromb Res 1986; 44:683–693.
59. Kroon C, ten Hove WR, de Boer A, et al. Highly variable anticoagulant response after subcutaneous administration of high-dose (12,500 IU) heparin in patients with myocardial infarction and healthy volunteers. Circulation 1992; 86:1370–1375.
60. Nilsen DW, Goransson L, Larsen AI, et al. Systemic thrombin generation and activity resistant to low molecular weight heparin administered prior to streptokinase in patients with acute myocardial infarction. Thromb Haemost 1997; 77:57–61.
61. Galvani M, Abendschein DR, Ferrini D, et al. Failure of fixed dose intravenous heparin to suppress increases in thrombin activity after coronary thrombolysis with streptokinase. J Am Coll Cardiol 1994; 24:1445–1452.

62. Leopold JA, Loscalzo J. Platelet activation by fibrinolytic agents: a potential mechanism for resistance to thrombolysis and reocclusion after successful thrombolysis. Coron Artery Dis 1995; 6:923–929.
63. Hsia J, Hamilton WP, Kleiman N, et al. A comparison between heparin and low-dose aspirin as adjunctive therapy with tissue plasminogen activator for acute myocardial infarction. Heparin-Aspirin Reperfusion Trial (HART) Investigators. N Engl J Med 1990; 323:1433–1437.
64. O'Connor CM, Meese R, Carney R, et al. A randomized trial of intravenous heparin in conjunction with anistreplase (anisoylated plasminogen streptokinase activator complex) in acute myocardial infarction: the Duke University Clinical Cardiology Study (DUCCS) 1. J Am Coll Cardiol 1994; 23:11–18.
65. de Bono DP, Simoons ML, Tijssen J, et al. Effect of early intravenous heparin on coronary patency, infarct size, and bleeding complications after alteplase thrombolysis: results of a randomised double blind European Cooperative Study Group trial. Br Heart J 1992; 67:122–128.
66. ISIS (International Studies of Infarct Survival) Pilot Study Investigation. Randomized factorial trial of high-dose intravenous streptokinase, of oral aspirin and of intravenous heparin in acute myocardial infarction. Eur Heart J 1987; 8:634–642.
67. Bleich SD, Nichols TC, Schumacher RR, et al. Effect of heparin on coronary arterial patency after thrombolysis with tissue plasminogen activator in acute myocardial infarction. Am J Cardiol 1990; 66:1412–1417.
68. The GUSTO Investigators. An international randomized trial comparing four thrombolytic strategies for acute myocardial infarction. N Engl J Med 1993; 329:673–682.
69. Cercek B, Lew AS, Hod H, et al. Enhancement of thrombolysis with tissue-type plasminogen activator by pretreatment with heparin. Circulation 1986; 74:583–587.
70. Andrade-Gordon P, Strickland S. Interaction of heparin with plasminogen activators and plasminogen: effects on the activation of plasminogen. Biochemistry 1986; 25:4033–4040.
71. Williams DO, Borer J, Braunwald E, et al. Intravenous recombinant tissue-type plasminogen activator in patients with acute myocardial infarction: a report from the NHLBI thrombolysis in myocardial infarction trial. Circulation 1986; 73:338–346.
72. The Thrombolysis in Myocardial Infarction (TIMI) Trial. Phase I findings. TIMI Study Group. N Engl J Med 1985; 312:932–936.
73. Topol EJ, Califf RM, George BS, et al. A randomized trial of immediate versus delayed elective angioplasty after intravenous tissue plasminogen activator in acute myocardial infarction. N Engl J Med 1987; 317:581–588.
74. Guerci AD, Gerstenblith G, Brinker JA, et al. A randomized trial of intravenous tissue plasminogen activator for acute myocardial infarction with subsequent randomization to elective coronary angioplasty. N Engl J Med 1987; 317:1613–1618.
75. Topol EJ, George BS, Kereiakes DJ, et al. A randomized controlled trial of intravenous tissue plasminogen activator and early intravenous heparin in acute myocardial infarction. Circulation 1989; 79:281–286.
76. Antman EM, Anbe DT, Armstrong PW, et al. ACC/AHA guidelines for the management of patients with ST-elevation myocardial infarction: a report of the American College of Cardiology/American Heart Association Task Force on Practice Guidelines (Committee to Revise the 1999 Guidelines for the Management of Patients with Acute Myocardial Infarction). Circulation 2004; 110:e82–e292.
77. Curtis JP, Alexander JH, Huang Y, et al. Efficacy and safety of two unfractionated heparin dosing strategies with tenecteplase in acute myocardial infarction (results from Assessment of the Safety and Efficacy of a New Thrombolytic Regimens 2 and 3). Am J Cardiol 2004; 94:279–283.
78. Granger CB, Becker R, Tracy RP, et al. Thrombin generation, inhibition and clinical outcomes in patients with acute myocardial infarction treated with thrombolytic therapy and heparin: results from the GUSTO-I trial. J Am Coll Cardiol 1998; 31:497–505.
79. Eikelboom JW, Mehta SR, Anand SS, et al. Adverse impact of bleeding on prognosis in patients with acute coronary syndromes. Circulation 2006; 114:774–782.
80. Silber S, Albertsson P, Aviles FF, et al. Guidelines for percutaneous coronary interventions. The Task Force for Percutaneous Coronary Interventions of the European Society of Cardiology. Eur Heart J 2005; 26:804–847.

81. Smith SC Jr., Feldman TE, Hirshfeld JW Jr., et al. ACC/AHA/SCAI 2005 guideline update for percutaneous coronary intervention: a report of the American College of Cardiology/American Heart Association Task Force on Practice Guidelines (ACC/AHA/SCAI Writing Committee to Update 2001 Guidelines for Percutaneous Coronary Intervention). Circulation 2006; 113:e166–e286.

82. Roe MT, Granger CB, Puma JA, et al. Comparison of benefits and complications of hirudin versus heparin for patients with acute coronary syndromes undergoing early percutaneous coronary intervention. Am J Cardiol 2001; 88:1403–1406.

83. Stone GW, McLaurin BT, Cox DA, et al. Bivalirudin for patients with acute coronary syndromes. N Engl J Med 2006; 355:2203–2216.

84. Dougherty KG, Gaos CM, Bush HS, et al. Activated clotting times and activated partial thromboplastin times in patients undergoing coronary angioplasty who receive bolus doses of heparin. Cathet Cardiovasc Diagn 1992; 26:260–263.

85. Bowers J, Ferguson JJ III. The use of activated clotting times to monitor heparin therapy during and after interventional procedures. Clin Cardiol 1994; 17:357–361.

86. Avendano A, Ferguson JJ. Comparison of Hemochron and HemoTec activated coagulation time target values during percutaneous transluminal coronary angioplasty. J Am Coll Cardiol 1994; 23:907–910.

87. Popma JJ, Satler LF, Pichard AD, et al. Vascular complications after balloon and new device angioplasty. Circulation 1993; 88:1569–1578.

88. Narins CR, Hillegass WB Jr., Nelson CL, et al. Relation between activated clotting time during angioplasty and abrupt closure. Circulation 1996; 93:667–671.

89. Frierson JH, Dimas AP, Simpfendorfer CC, et al. Is aggressive heparinization necessary for elective PTCA? Cathet Cardiovasc Diagn 1993; 28:279–282.

90. Tolleson TR, O'Shea JC, Bittl JA, et al. Relationship between heparin anticoagulation and clinical outcomes in coronary stent intervention: observations from the ESPRIT trial. J Am Coll Cardiol 2003; 41:386–393.

91. Brener SJ, Moliterno DJ, Lincoff AM, et al. Relationship between activated clotting time and ischemic or hemorrhagic complications: analysis of 4 recent randomized clinical trials of percutaneous coronary intervention. Circulation 2004; 110:994–998.

92. Chew DP, Bhatt DL, Lincoff AM, et al. Defining the optimal activated clotting time during percutaneous coronary intervention: aggregate results from 6 randomized, controlled trials. Circulation 2001; 103:961–966.

93. Friedman HZ, Cragg DR, Glazier SM, et al. Randomized prospective evaluation of prolonged versus abbreviated intravenous heparin therapy after coronary angioplasty. J Am Coll Cardiol 1994; 24:1214–1219.

94. Rabah M, Mason D, Muller DW, et al. Heparin after percutaneous intervention (HAPI): a prospective multicenter randomized trial of three heparin regimens after successful coronary intervention. J Am Coll Cardiol 1999; 34:461–467.

95. Menon V, Harrington RA, Hochman JS, et al. Thrombolysis and adjunctive therapy in acute myocardial infarction: the Seventh ACCP Conference on Antithrombotic and Thrombolytic Therapy. Chest 2004; 126:549S–575S.

96. Jordan RE, Oosta GM, Gardner WT, et al. The kinetics of hemostatic enzyme-antithrombin interactions in the presence of low molecular weight heparin. J Biol Chem 1980; 255: 10081–10090.

97. Antman EM. The search for replacements for unfractionated heparin. Circulation 2001; 103:2310–2314.

98. Samama MM, Gerotziafas GT. Comparative pharmacokinetics of LMWHs. Semin Thromb Hemost 2000; 26(suppl 1):31–38.

99. Montalescot G, Philippe F, Ankri A, et al. Early increase of von Willebrand Factor predicts adverse outcome in unstable coronary artery disease: beneficial effects of enoxaparin. Circulation 1998; 98:294–299.

100. Montalescot G, Collet JP, Lison L, et al. Effects of various anticoagulant treatments on von Willebrand factor release in unstable angina. J Am Coll Cardiol 2000; 36:110–114.

101. Beguin S, Mardiguian J, Lindhout T, et al. The mode of action of low molecular weight heparin preparation (PK10169) and two of its major components on thrombin generation in plasma. Thromb Haemos 1989; 61:30–34.

102. Antman EM, Cohen M, Radley D, et al. Assessment of the treatment effect of enoxaparin for unstable angina/non-Q-wave myocardial infarction: TIMI 11B-ESSENCE meta-analysis. Circulation 1999; 100:1602–1608.
103. Xiao Z, Theroux P. Platelet activation with unfractionated heparin at therapeutic concentrations and comparisons With a low-molecular-weight heparin and with a direct thrombin inhibitor. Circulation 1998; 97:251–256.
104. Warkentin TE. Heparin-induced thrombocytopenia: pathogenesis and management. Br J Haematol 2003; 121:535–555.
105. Kontny F, Dale J, Abildgaard U, et al. Randomized trial of low molecular weight heparin (dalteparin) in prevention of left ventricular thrombus formation and arterial embolism after acute anterior myocardial infarction: the Fragmin in Acute Myocardial Infarction (FRAMI) study. J Am Coll Cardiol 1997; 30:962–969.
106. Fareed J, Jeske W, Hoppensteadt D, et al. Low-molecular-weight heparins: pharmacologic profile and product differentiation. Am J Cardiol 1998; 82:3L–10L.
107. Yusuf S, Mehta SR, Diaz R, et al. Challenges in the conduct of large simple trials of important generic questions in resource-poor settings: the CREATE and ECLA trial program evaluating GIK (glucose, insulin and potassium) and low-molecular-weight heparin in acute myocardial infarction. Am Heart J 2004; 148:1068–1078.
108. Baird SH, Menown IBA, Mcbride SJ, et al. Randomized comparison of enoxaparin with unfractionated heparin following fibrinolytic therapy for acute myocardial infarction. Eur Heart J 2002; 23:627–632.
109. Wallentin L, Goldstein P, Armstrong PW, et al. Efficacy and safety of tenecteplase in combination with the low-molecular-weight heparin enoxaparin or unfractionated heparin in the prehospital setting: the Assessment of the Safety and Efficacy of a New Thrombolytic Regimen (ASSENT)-3 PLUS randomized trial in acute myocardial infarction. Circulation 2003; 108:135–142.
110. Armstrong PW, Chang WC, Wallentin L, et al. Efficacy and safety of unfractionated heparin versus enoxaparin: a pooled analysis of ASSENT-3 and -3 PLUS data. CMAJ 2006; 174:1421–1426.
111. Van de WF, Ardissino D, Betriu A, et al. Management of acute myocardial infarction in patients presenting with ST-segment elevation. The Task Force on the Management of Acute Myocardial Infarction of the European Society of Cardiology. Eur Heart J 2003; 24:28–66.
112. Mega JL, Morrow DA, Ostor E, et al. Outcomes and optimal antithrombotic therapy in women undergoing fibrinolysis for ST-elevation myocardial infarction. Circulation 2007; 115:2822–2828.
113. Harrington RA. Women, acute ischemic heart disease, and antithrombotic therapy: challenges and opportunities. Circulation 2007; 115:2796–2798.
114. Gibbons RJ, Fuster V. Therapy for patients with acute coronary syndromes—new opportunities. N Engl J Med 2006; 354:1524–1527.
115. Fox KAA, Antman EM, Montalescot G, et al. The impact of renal dysfunction on outcomes in the ExTRACT-TIMI 25 trial. J Am Coll Cardiol 2007; 49:2249–2255.
116. Gibson CM, Murphy SA, Montalescot G, et al. Percutaneous coronary intervention in patients receiving enoxaparin or unfractionated heparin after fibrinolytic therapy for ST-segment elevation myocardial infarction in the ExTRACT-TIMI 25 trial. J Am Coll Cardiol 2007; 49:2238–2246.
117. Chen ZM, Jiang LX, Chen YP, et al. Addition of clopidogrel to aspirin in 45,852 patients with acute myocardial infarction: randomised placebo-controlled trial. Lancet 2005; 366:1607–1621.
118. Fernandez-Aviles F, Alonso JJ, Castro-Beiras A, et al. Routine invasive strategy within 24 hours of thrombolysis versus ischaemia-guided conservative approach for acute myocardial infarction with ST-segment elevation (GRACIA-1): a randomised controlled trial. Lancet 2004; 364:1045–1053.
119. Scheller B, Hennen B, Hammer B, et al. Beneficial effects of immediate stenting after thrombolysis in acute myocardial infarction. J Am Coll Cardiol 2003; 42:634–641.
120. Thiele H, Engelmann L, Elsner K, et al. Comparison of pre-hospital combination-fibrinolysis plus conventional care with pre-hospital combination-fibrinolysis plus

facilitated percutaneous coronary intervention in acute myocardial infarction. Eur Heart J 2005; 26:1956–1963.

121. Sabatine MS, Morrow DA, Dalby A, et al. Efficacy and safety of enoxaparin versus unfractionated heparin in patients with ST-segment elevation myocardial infarction also treated with clopidogrel. J Am Coll Cardiol 2007; 49:2256–2263.

122. Fox KAA, Poole-Wilson PA, Henderson RA, et al. Interventional versus conservative treatment for patients with unstable angina or non-ST-elevation myocardial infarction: the British Heart Foundation RITA 3 randomised trial. Lancet 2002; 360:743–751.

123. Invasive compared with non-invasive treatment in unstable coronary-artery disease: FRISC II prospective randomised multicentre study. Lancet 1999; 354:708–715.

124. Ferguson JJ, Califf RM, Antman EM, et al. Enoxaparin vs unfractionated heparin in high-risk patients with non-ST-segment elevation acute coronary syndromes managed with an intended early invasive strategy: primary results of the SYNERGY randomized trial. JAMA 2004; 292:45–54.

125. Brieger D, Van de WF, Avezum A, et al. Interactions between heparins, glycoprotein IIb/IIIa antagonists, and coronary intervention. The Global Registry of Acute Coronary Events (GRACE). Am Heart J 2007; 153:960–969.

126. Argenti D, Hoppensteadt D, Heald D, et al. Pharmacokinetics of enoxaparin in patients undergoing percutaneous coronary intervention with and without glycoprotein IIb/IIIa therapy. Am J Ther 2003; 10:241–246.

127. Gerotziafas GT, Zafiropoulos A, Van DP, et al. Inhibition of factor VIIa generation and prothrombin activation by treatment with enoxaparin in patients with unstable angina. Br J Haematol 2003; 120:611–617.

128. Welsh RC, Gordon P, Westerhout CM, et al. A novel enoxaparin regime for ST elevation myocardial infarction patients undergoing primary percutaneous coronary intervention: A WEST sub-study. Catheter Cardiovasc Interv 2007; 70:341–348.

129. Kereiakes DJ, Montalescot G, Antman EM, et al. Low-molecular-weight heparin therapy for non-ST-elevation acute coronary syndromes and during percutaneous coronary intervention: An expert consensus. Am Heart J 2002; 144:615–624.

130. Moliterno DJ, Hermiller JB, Kereiakes DJ, et al. A novel point-of-care enoxaparin monitor for use during percutaneous coronary intervention. Results of the Evaluating Enoxaparin Clotting Times (ELECT) Study. J Am Coll Cardiol 2003; 42:1132–1139.

131. Bates SM, Weitz JI. Direct thrombin inhibitors for treatment of arterial thrombosis: potential differences between bivalirudin and hirudin. Am J Cardiol 1998; 82: 12P–18P.

132. Weitz JI, Hudoba M, Massel D, et al. Clot-bound thrombin is protected from inhibition by heparin-antithrombin III but is susceptible to inactivation by antithrombin III-independent inhibitors. J Clin Invest 1990; 86:385–391.

133. Direct thrombin inhibitors in acute coronary syndromes: principal results of a meta-analysis based on individual patients' data. Lancet 2002; 359:294–302.

134. Rydel TJ, Ravichandran KG, Tulinsky A, et al. The structure of a complex of recombinant hirudin and human alpha-thrombin. Science 1990; 249:277–280.

135. Parry MA, Maraganore JM, Stone SR. Kinetic mechanism for the interaction of Hirulog with thrombin. Biochemistry 1994; 33:14807–14814.

136. Witting JI, Bourdon P, Brezniak DV, et al. Thrombin-specific inhibition by and slow cleavage of hirulog-1. Biochem J 1992; 283(pt 3):737–743.

137. Kong DF, Topol EJ, Bittl JA, et al. Clinical outcomes of bivalirudin for ischemic heart disease. Circulation 1999; 100:2049–2053.

138. Jang IK, Brown DF, Giugliano RP, et al. A multicenter, randomized study of argatroban versus heparin as adjunct to tissue plasminogen activator (TPA) in acute myocardial infarction: myocardial infarction with novastan and TPA (MINT) study. J Am Coll Cardiol 1999; 33:1879–1885.

139. Alderman EL. Results from late-breaking clinical trials sessions at ACC '98. American College of Cardiology. J Am Coll Cardiol 1998; 32:1–7.

140. A comparison of recombinant hirudin with heparin for the treatment of acute coronary syndromes. The Global Use of Strategies to Open Occluded Coronary Arteries (GUSTO) IIb Investigators. N Engl J Med 1996; 335:775–782.

141. Antman EM. Hirudin in acute myocardial infarction: Thrombolysis and Thrombin Inhibition in Myocardial Infarction (TIMI) 9B trial. Circulation 1996; 94:911–921.
142. Tardy B, Lecompte T, Boelhen F, et al. Predictive factors for thrombosis and major bleeding in an observational study in 181 patients with heparin-induced thrombocytopenia treated with lepirudin. Blood 2006; 108:1492–1496.
143. Stone GW, Bertrand ME, Moses JW, et al. Routine upstream initiation vs deferred selective use of glycoprotein IIb/IIIa inhibitors in acute coronary syndromes: the ACUITY timing trial. JAMA 2007; 297:591–602.
144. White H. Thrombin-specific anticoagulation with bivalirudin versus heparin in patients receiving fibrinolytic therapy for acute myocardial infarction: the HERO-2 randomised trial. Lancet 2001; 358:1855–1863.
145. Sinnaeve PR, Simes J, Yusuf S, et al. Direct thrombin inhibitors in acute coronary syndromes: effect in patients undergoing early percutaneous coronary intervention. Eur Heart J 2005; 26:2396–2403.
146. Ebrahimi R, Lincoff AM, Bittl JA, et al. Bivalirudin vs heparin in percutaneous coronary intervention: a pooled analysis. J Cardiovasc Pharmacol Ther 2005; 10:209–216.
147. Mehta SR, Eikelboom JW, Rupprecht HJ, et al. Efficacy of hirudin in reducing cardiovascular events in patients with acute coronary syndrome undergoing early percutaneous coronary intervention. Eur Heart J 2002; 23:117–123.
148. Waksman R, Wolfram RM, Torguson RL, et al. Switching from enoxaparin to bivalirudin in patients with acute coronary syndromes without ST-segment elevation who undergo percutaneous coronary intervention. Results from SWITCH–a multicenter clinical trial. J Invasive Cardiol 2006; 18:370–375.
149. Gibson CM, Ten Y, Murphy SA, et al. Association of prerandomization anticoagulant switching with bleeding in the setting of percutaneous coronary intervention (A REPLACE-2 Analysis). Am J Cardiol 2007; 99:1687–1690.
150. Lewis BE, Matthai WH Jr., Cohen M, et al. Argatroban anticoagulation during percutaneous coronary intervention in patients with heparin-induced thrombocytopenia. Catheter Cardiovasc Interv 2002; 57:177–184.
151. Jolicoeur EM, Wang T, Lopes RD, et al. Percutaneous coronary interventions in patients with heparin-induced thrombocytopenia. Curr Cardiol Rep 2007; 9:396–405.
152. Walenga JM, Jeske WP, Bara LS, et al. Biochemical and pharmacologic rationale for the development of a synthetic heparin pentasaccharide. Thromb Res 1997; 86:1–36.
153. Bauer KA, Hawkins DW, Peters PC, et al. Fondaparinux, a synthetic pentasaccharide: the first in a new class of antithrombotic agents—the selective factor Xa inhibitors. Cardiovasc Drug Rev 2002; 20:37–52.
154. Yusuf S, Mehta SR, Chrolavicius S, et al. Comparison of fondaparinux and enoxaparin in acute coronary syndromes. N Engl J Med 2006; 354:1464–1476.
155. Boneu B, Necciari J, Cariou R, et al. Pharmacokinetics and tolerance of the natural pentasaccharide (SR90107/Org31540) with high affinity to antithrombin III in man. Thromb Haemost 1995; 74:1468–1473.
156. Bates SM, Weitz JI. The status of new anticoagulants. Br J Haematol 2006; 134:3–19.
157. Coussement PK, Bassand JP, Convens C, et al. A synthetic factor-Xa inhibitor (ORG31540/SR9017A) as an adjunct to fibrinolysis in acute myocardial infarction. The PENTALYSE study. Eur Heart J 2001; 22:1716–1724.
158. Califf RM. Fondaparinux in ST-segment elevation myocardial infarction: the drug, the strategy, the environment, or all of the above? JAMA 2006; 295:1579–1580.
159. Bijsterveld NR, Peters RJG, Murphy SA, et al. Recurrent cardiac ischemic events early after discontinuation of short-term heparin treatment in acute coronary syndromes: results from the thrombolysis in myocardial infarction (TIMI) 11B and efficacy and safety of subcutaneous enoxaparin in Non-Q-Wave coronary events (ESSENCE) studies. J Am Coll Cardiol 2003; 42:2083–2089.
160. Mehta SR, Steg PG, Granger CB, et al. Randomized, blinded trial comparing fondaparinux with unfractionated heparin in patients undergoing contemporary percutaneous coronary intervention: Arixtra Study in Percutaneous Coronary Intervention: a randomized evaluation (ASPIRE) pilot trial. Circulation 2005; 111:1390–1397.

161. Monroe DM, Hoffman M. What does it take to make the perfect clot? Arterioscler Thromb Vasc Biol 2006; 26:41–48.
162. Theroux P, Waters D, Lam J, et al. Reactivation of unstable angina after the discontinuation of heparin. N Engl J Med 1992; 327:141–145.
163. Low-molecular-weight heparin during instability in coronary artery disease, Fragmin during Instability in Coronary Artery Disease (FRISC) study group. Lancet 1996; 347:561–568.
164. Cohen M, Demers C, Gurfinkel EP, et al. A comparison of low-molecular-weight heparin with unfractionated heparin for unstable coronary artery disease. Efficacy and Safety of Subcutaneous Enoxaparin in Non-Q-Wave Coronary Events Study Group. N Engl J Med 1997; 337:447–452.
165. Antman EM, McCabe CH, Gurfinkel EP, et al. Enoxaparin prevents death and cardiac ischemic events in unstable angina/non-Q-wave myocardial infarction. Results of the thrombolysis in myocardial infarction (TIMI) 11B trial. Circulation 1999; 100:1593–1601.
166. A low molecular weight, selective thrombin inhibitor, inogatran, vs heparin, in unstable coronary artery disease in 1209 patients. A double-blind, randomized, dose-finding study. Thrombin inhibition in Myocardial Ischaemia (TRIM) study group. Eur Heart J 1997; 18:1416–1425.
167. Granger CB, Miller JM, Bovill EG, et al. Rebound increase in thrombin generation and activity after cessation of intravenous heparin in patients with acute coronary syndromes. Circulation 1995; 91:1929–1935.
168. Becker RC, Spencer FA, Li Y, et al. Thrombin generation after the abrupt cessation of intravenous unfractionated heparin among patients with acute coronary syndromes: potential mechanisms for heightened prothrombotic potential. J Am Coll Cardiol 1999; 34:1020–1027.
169. Vaitkus PT, Barnathan ES. Embolic potential, prevention and management of mural thrombus complicating anterior myocardial infarction: a meta-analysis. J Am Coll Cardiol 1993; 22:1004–1009.
170. Chesebro JH, Fuster V. Antithrombotic therapy for acute myocardial infarction: mechanisms and prevention of deep venous, left ventricular, and coronary artery thromboembolism. Circulation 1986; 74:III1–III10.
171. Yilmaz R, Celik S, Baykan M, et al. Pulsed wave tissue Doppler-derived myocardial performance index for the assessment of left ventricular thrombus formation risk after acute myocardial infarction. Am Heart J 2004; 148:1102–1108.
172. Vecchio C, Chiarella F, Lupi G, et al. Left ventricular thrombus in anterior acute myocardial infarction after thrombolysis. A GISSI-2 connected study. Circulation 1991; 84:512–519.
173. Randomised controlled trial of subcutaneous calcium-heparin in acute myocardial infarction, . The SCATI (Studio sulla Calciparina nell'Angina e nella Trombosi Ventricolare nell'Infarto) Group. Lancet 1989; 2:182–186.
174. Porter A, Kandalker H, Iakobishvili Z, et al. Left ventricular mural thrombus after anterior ST-segment-elevation acute myocardial infarction in the era of aggressive reperfusion therapy–still a frequent complication. Coron Artery Dis 2005; 16:275–279.
175. Srichai MB, Junor C, Rodriguez LL, et al. Clinical, imaging, and pathological characteristics of left ventricular thrombus: a comparison of contrast-enhanced magnetic resonance imaging, transthoracic echocardiography, and transesophageal echocardiography with surgical or pathological validation. Am Heart J 2006; 152:75–84.
176. Cohen M, Gensini GF, Maritz F, et al. The safety and efficacy of subcutaneous enoxaparin versus intravenous unfractionated heparin and tirofiban versus placebo in the treatment of acute ST-segment elevation myocardial infarction patients ineligible for reperfusion (TETAMI): a randomized trial. J Am Coll Cardiol 2003; 42:1348–1356.
177. Eagle KA, Goodman SG, Avezum A, et al. Practice variation and missed opportunities for reperfusion in ST-segment-elevation myocardial infarction: findings from the Global Registry of Acute Coronary Events (GRACE). Lancet 2002; 359:373–377.
178. Cohen M, Antman EM, Gurfinkel E, et al. Impact of enoxaparin low molecular weight heparin in patients with Q-wave myocardial infarction. Am J Cardiol 2000; 86:553–556, A9.

179. The OASI. Effects of fondaparinux on mortality and reinfarction in patients with acute ST-segment elevation myocardial infarction: the OASIS-6 randomized trial. JAMA 2006; 295:1519–1530.
180. Cohen M, Maritz F, Gensini GF, et al. The TETAMI trial: the safety and efficacy of subcutaneous enoxaparin versus intravenous unfractionated heparin and of tirofiban versus placebo in the treatment of acute myocardial infarction for patients not thrombolyzed: methods and design. J Thromb Thrombolysis 2000; 10:241–246.
181. Warkentin TE. Heparin-induced thrombocytopenia: IgG-mediated platelet activation, platelet microparticle generation, and altered procoagulant/anticoagulant balance in the pathogenesis of thrombosis and venous limb gangrene complicating heparin-induced thrombocytopenia. Transfus Med Rev 1996; 10:249–258.
182. Warkentin TE, Kelton JG. Temporal aspects of heparin-induced thrombocytopenia. N Engl J Med 2001; 344:1286–1292.
183. Warkentin TE. Pork or beef? Ann Thorac Surg 2003; 75:15–16.
184. Warkentin TE, Levine MN, Hirsh J, et al. Heparin-induced thrombocytopenia in patients treated with low-molecular-weight heparin or unfractionated heparin. N Engl J Med 1995; 332:1330–1335.
185. Warkentin TE, Kelton JG. A 14-year study of heparin-induced thrombocytopenia. Am J Med 1996; 101:502–507.
186. Warkentin TE, Greinacher A. Heparin-induced thrombocytopenia: recognition, treatment, and prevention: the Seventh ACCP Conference on Antithrombotic and Thrombolytic Therapy. Chest 2004; 126:311S–337S.
187. Mahaffey KW, Lewis BE, Wildermann NM, et al. The anticoagulant therapy with bivalirudin to assist in the performance of percutaneous coronary intervention in patients with heparin-induced thrombocytopenia (ATBAT) study: main results. J Invasive Cardiol 2003; 15:611–616.
188. Alexander KP, Newby LK, Armstrong PW, et al. Acute coronary care in the elderly, part II: ST-segment-elevation myocardial infarction: a scientific statement for healthcare professionals from the American Heart Association Council on Clinical Cardiology: in collaboration with the Society of Geriatric Cardiology. Circulation 2007; 115:2570–2589.
189. White HD, Braunwald E, Murphy SA, et al. Enoxaparin vs. unfractionated heparin with fibrinolysis for ST-elevation myocardial infarction in elderly and younger patients: results from ExTRACT-TIMI 25. Eur Heart J 2007; 28:1066–1071.
190. Mruk JS, Zoldhelyi P, Webster MW, et al. Does antithrombotic therapy influence residual thrombus after thrombolysis of platelet-rich thrombus? Effects of recombinant hirudin, heparin, or aspirin. Circulation 1996; 93:792–799.
191. Rao AK, Sun L, Chesebro JH, et al. Distinct effects of recombinant desulfatohirudin (Revasc) and heparin on plasma levels of fibrinopeptide A and prothrombin fragment F1.2 in unstable angina: a multicenter trial. Circulation 1996; 94:2389–2395.
192. Hirsh J. Heparin. N Engl J Med 1991; 324:1565–1574.
193. Yusuf S, Mehta SR, Xie C, et al. Effects of reviparin, a low-molecular-weight heparin, on mortality, reinfarction, and strokes in patients with acute myocardial infarction presenting with ST-segment elevation. JAMA 2005; 293:427–435.
194. Cochran K, DeMartini TJ, Lewis BE, et al. Use of lepirudin during percutaneous vascular interventions in patients with heparin-induced thrombocytopenia. J Invasive Cardiol 2003; 15:617–621.

14 Myocyte Protection by Pharmacological Therapy

David Faxon
*Department of Medicine, Brigham and Women's Hospital, Harvard Medical School,
Boston, Massachusetts, U.S.A.*

INTRODUCTION

Acute myocardial infarction (AMI) occurs in an estimated 500,000 Americans each year (1). Early reperfusion with fibrinolytic therapy or percutaneous coronary intervention (PCI) has been shown to significantly reduce mortality by salvaging ischemic myocardium and reducing infarct size (2). Reperfusion remains the most powerful method to reduce infarct size and the earlier that reperfusion occurs after coronary occlusion, the smaller the infarct size, the better the left ventricular function, and the lower the long-term mortality. Numerous clinical trials have also demonstrated that the degree of restoration of blood flow and myocardial perfusion is important (3). When complete and normal blood flow to the microcirculation is obtained, outcome is further improved. To date, PCI with adjunctive pharmacological therapy is most effective in restoring rapid and complete blood flow in the infarct artery (4). However, despite successful reperfusion, a significant number of patients fail to demonstrate benefit. Animal studies have demonstrated that reperfusion itself can result in adverse consequences that can lead to further myocyte death that might be avoided with adjunctive therapy (5,6). This chapter will discuss the proposed mechanisms for ischemia/reperfusion injury and the results of the clinical trials of various pharmacological agents that have been conducted to enhance myocyte salvage.

MECHANISMS OF REPERFUSION INJURY

Animal studies have shown that following prolonged ischemia, reperfusion itself is associated with further myocyte death (6). Clinical evidence for reperfusion injury includes myocardial stunning, microvascular dysfunction and no-reflow, and arrhythmias (Fig. 1). Following reperfusion, myocardial function can recover rapidly if the duration of ischemia is brief. However, in the majority of patients, it remains depressed despite restoration of normal blood flow to viable myocardium. Prolonged postischemic dysfunction of viable myocardium in the presence of normal blood flow is referred to as myocardial stunning (7). While reperfusion is the most powerful means to restore myocardial function and salvage ischemic myocardium, reperfusion injury can lead to further cell death. Experimentally, techniques that reduce reperfusion injury lead to greater degrees of myocardial salvage, improved microvascular flow, and reduction in reperfusion arrhythmias (8).

The mechanisms of reperfusion injury are complex and multifactorial (Fig. 2) (5,8). Ischemia results in loss of mitochondrial oxidative phosphorylation, depletion of high-energy phosphates (ATP), a compensatory shift to anaerobic glycolysis, and accumulation of hydrogen ions and lactate. The result is a decrease in cytosolic pH (5). Acidosis inhibits glycolysis, impairs contraction, and alters ion transport through accumulation of oxygen-free radicals (9,10). The myocytes have a

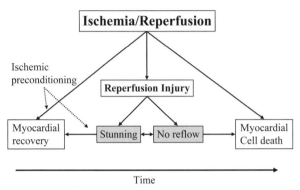

FIGURE 1 The principal clinical manifestations of reperfusion injury. Myocardial stunning and the no-reflow phenomenon are manifestations of reperfusion injury that can result in recovery or further myocardial cell death. Ischemic preconditioning reduces the likelihood of cell death and promotes myocardial recovery.

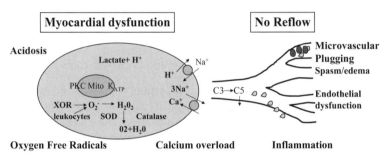

FIGURE 2 The principal mechanisms of reperfusion injury. These include myocardial dysfunction due to acidosis, generation of oxygen-free radicals, and calcium overload, as well as no-reflow due to endothelial dysfunction, microvascular plugging, and inflammation. (See text for detail.)

number of mechanisms to deal with this cellular insult. Oxygen-free radical scavengers, such as superoxide dismutase, reduce free radical stress. Heat shock protein is released, which facilitates the removal and degradation of damaged proteins. Initially, there is an efflux of potassium ions and an influx of sodium ions due to interruption of the sodium/potassium ATPase pump. The resulting influx of sodium results in cell swelling. Acidosis with accumulation of hydrogen is exchanged for sodium through the sodium/hydrogen exchanger (NHE) and the sodium in turn is exchanged for calcium (11). As a consequence of ion channel dysfunction, there is accumulation of intracellular calcium, further reducing contraction and contributing to ultimate cell death. Accumulation of free fatty acids (FFA) and phospholipid depletion further impair membrane integrity. Cell death is a result of both oncosis and apoptosis (12). In addition to direct myocyte damage and cell death, prolonged ischemia causes vascular endothelial damage leading to microvascular dysfunction.

Reperfusion can salvage myocytes that have not been irreversibly injured, but fails to salvage those that have died or are destined to die. A group of cells largely on the border zones of the infarct are salvageable, but vulnerable to reperfusion injury. During reperfusion, reactive oxygen species are generated from the increase in acidosis and inflammation (13). Contributing to reperfusion injury is the no-reflow phenomenon that is felt to be due to a reduction in microvascular flow (14).

Microvascular dysfunction is another manifestation of reperfusion injury. Endothelial damage combined with myocyte death causes a release of inflammatory cells (15). The infiltration of inflammatory cells results in microvascular plugging, thrombosis, and microvascular vasospasm. One protective mechanism is the generation of nitric oxide (NO) through activation of hypoxia-inducible factor-1 activation (16). NO release results in vasodilatation and stabilization of the mitochondria.

One of the most powerful factors known to reduce reperfusion injury is ischemic preconditioning (17,18). In experimental animals, repeated brief ischemic periods prior to prolonged ischemia can reduce infarct size by 25%. The beneficial effect of ischemic preconditioning disappears if the interval between the periods of brief ischemia and the prolonged ischemia is longer than three to four hours. However, a second window of protection can be realized after 24 hours. The mechanisms responsible for preconditioning are not completely understood. Experimental studies suggest that it is due, in part, to the release of adenosine and bradykinin that activate cardiac myocyte signal transduction pathways including p13k-AKT, ERK-1, and ERK-2. These kinases restore ATP-dependent mitochondrial potassium channels and activate protein kinase C that in turn protects mitochondrial function and intracellular potassium levels and delays cell death. If ischemia is brief, then recovery is possible, but with prolonged ischemia, cell death occurs despite preconditioning. Ischemic preconditioning can result in smaller infarct size, reduced incidence of no-reflow, and fewer arrhythmias. Clinically, preinfarction angina is also associated with reduction in ventricular dysfunction, no-reflow, and arrhythmias (19,20). Ischemic postconditioning is the application of alternating episodes of myocardial ischemia and reperfusion at the end of the infarct period. Experimental studies have shown that even three 30-second episodes of alternating reocclusion and reperfusion can substantially reduce infarct size (17). This is consistent with older studies showing that low flow or gradual reperfusion reduces infarct size.

PHARMACOLOGICAL APPROACHES

The goal of adjunctive pharmacological therapy in AMI is to reduce morbidity and mortality by increasing and maintaining infarct artery patency, reducing ventricular enlargement and infarct expansion, and reducing reperfusion injury. Antiplatelet and anticoagulant agents have been shown to be effective in improving patency and reducing mortality and are discussed in chapters 12 and 13. Agents directed at improving remodeling and ventricular function include β-blockers and angiotensin converting enzyme inhibitors. These agents have been extensively reviewed previously and will not be covered here (2). The focus of this chapter will be on agents that are directed toward reducing reperfusion injury. These drugs can be grouped into agents directed at the myocyte (oxygen-free radical scavengers, calcium channel blockers, K_{ATP} channel openers, sodium/potassium exchange inhibitors, and metabolic modulating agents) and agents directed toward improving microvascular flow and reducing inflammation (vasodilators, leukocyte integrin blockers, and complement inhibitors).

Oxygen-Free Radical Scavengers

One of the key mechanisms for reducing the adverse effects of acidosis due to increasing oxygen-free radicals is the production of oxygen-free radical scavengers such as glutathione peroxidase. While antioxidants such as superoxide dismutase, glutathione, bucillamine, and N-acetylcysteine reduce reperfusion injury in animal models, clinical evidence of benefit is lacking (21,22). The Infarct Size Limitation: Acute N-acetylcysteine Defense trial (ISLAND) was a small pilot study of N-acetylcysteine in acute anterior MI. The study randomized 20 patients receiving successful streptokinase therapy to N-acetylcysteine or placebo and compared them to 10 unsuccessfully treated patients (23,24). Those treated with the anti-oxidant showed a smaller infarct size and better left ventricular function. The study was very small and needs to be validated in a larger study. A study using recombinant superoxide following primary PCI was negative (25). Two trials of another antioxidant, trimetazidine, were likewise negative (26,27).

Calcium Channel Blockers

Calcium levels increase in the ischemic myocyte due to a reduction in the sodium/hydrogen pump that increases intracellular sodium, and in turn is exchanged for calcium. Increased intracellular calcium inhibits contraction and leads to mito-chondrial dysfunction (28). The calcium channel antagonist diltiazem, adminis-tered prior to reperfusion, reduced infarct size in animal models (28). However, clinical trials of calcium channel antagonists have been disappointing. Goldbourt et al. randomized 1006 patients with AMI to nifedipine 60 mg or placebo and found an increased mortality in the nifedipine group (29). Theroux demonstrated a reduction in infarct size with intravenous diltiazem in 59 patients receiving tissue-type plasminogen activator (t-PA) (30), a finding confirmed by Pizzetti et al. (31). In the randomized Verapamil Acute Myocardial Infarction trial, a trend toward smaller left ventricular size and a small, but significant, reduction in heart failure at three months were reported (32). In all of these studies, administration of the calcium channel antagonist occurred prior to administration of the fibrinolytic agent. At present, as per the American College of Cardiology/American Heart Association (ACC/AHA) ST-elevation myocardial infarction (STEMI) guidelines, calcium channel antagonists are not indicated in STEMI in the absence of other complications or indications (2). If they are used for control of arrhythmia or for postinfarction angina, amlodipine is the preferred agent since hypotension and depression of left ventricular function is less significant.

K_{ATP} Channel Openers

One of the mechanisms responsible for the benefit of ischemic preconditioning is the opening of the K_{ATP} channels. It is hypothesized that the influx of potassium stabilizes mitochondrial function (33). In experimental studies, K_{ATP} channel openers have been shown to have effects similar to ischemic preconditioning (34,35). One of these agents, nicorandil, has undergone experimental and clinical investigation (36). Nicorandil is a complex drug that is a K_{ATP} channel opener and has a nitrate effect. The largest clinical trial to date has been the Impact Of Nicorandil in Angina (IONA) trial conducted in 5126 patients with stable angina (37). The study showed a significant reduction in the composite end point of car-diovascular death, MI, or rehospitalization for chest pain (13.1% vs. 15.5%; $p = 0.014$) at 1.6 months. However, individual end points were not different. A limited number of trials have been reported in AMI. Sakata et al. demonstrated an improvement in perfusion and myocardial function by echo after nicorandil administration in 10 patients receiving primary PCI (38). Sugimoto showed a reduced cardiovascular event rate in 272 patients in a retrospective analysis (39).

Ikeda also showed earlier resolution of ST-segment elevation in 60 patients with STEMI randomized to nicorandil or placebo (40). In a larger randomized trial of 368 patients undergoing primary PCI, Ishii et al. demonstrated a significant reduction in cardiovascular death and rehospitalization for congestive heart failure at an average follow-up of 2.5 years (6.5% vs. 16.4%; HR $= 0.39$; $p = 0.0058$) (41). A large multicenter trial is currently ongoing.

Sodium/Hydrogen Exchange Inhibitors

Intracellular acidosis is an early consequence of myocardial cell ischemia. As acidosis increases, the NHE exchanges hydrogen ions for sodium, which in turn is exchanged for calcium resulting in an increase in intracellular calcium. Inhibition of this system has been shown to be cardioprotective in animal models of ischemia and reperfusion (42). In a small study by Rupprecht in 100 patients with acute anterior MI, cariporide, a potent and specific inhibitor of NHE, improved left ventricular ejection fraction and reduced enzymatic infarct size at 21 days (43). The Guard During Ischemia Against Necrosis (GUARDIAN) Trial was the first large-scale trial to evaluate cariporide in myocardial ischemia (Fig. 3) (44). A total of 11,590 patients with unstable angina or non-ST-elevation MI or undergoing high-risk revascularization were studied. The primary end point was all-cause mortality or MI at 36 days. No difference in mortality was seen, but at the highest dose, patients undergoing coronary artery bypass graft surgery (CABG) had a 25% risk reduction of the primary end point. In addition, there was reduction in the rate of Q-wave MI, but not non-Q-wave MI. As a result, a separate trial was undertaken in patients undergoing CABG. The Na+/H+ Exchange Inhibition to Prevent Coronary Events in Acute Cardiac Conditions (EXPEDITION) trial enrolled over 7000 patients (54). The study did show a significant reduction in the primary end point of all-cause mortality and non-fatal MI at day 5 and at 6 months (23.9% vs. 20.2%; $p = 0.0005$). However, there was an unexpected and significant increase in cerebrovascular events at day 5 and at 6 months in the cariporide group (4.8% vs. 2.7%),

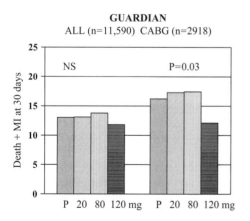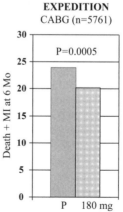

FIGURE 3 The results of the GUARDIAN (44) and EXPEDITION (45) trials of the sodium/hydrogen exchange inhibitor, cariporide. The GUARDIAN trial demonstrated no reduction in death or MI while the EXPEDITION trial in patients undergoing CABG showed a reduction in death and MI at six months, but had an unexpectedly high stroke rate (not shown).

limiting its clinical usefulness. Using another NHE inhibitor, the Evaluation of the Safety and Cardioprotective Effects of Eniporide in Acute Myocardial Infarction (ESCAMI) trial failed to demonstrate a reduction in enzymatic infarct size or clinical outcomes in 1389 patients with AMI largely treated with fibrinolysis (46). Thus, despite convincing experimental data, inhibitors of NHE are yet to be shown to be of clinical benefit in AMI. However, the possible benefit in patients undergoing CABG support further study in this area.

Metabolic Modulation with Glucose-Insulin-Potassium

More than 40 years ago, Sodi-Pollares reported that the intravenous administration of the "polarizing solution" of glucose-insulin-potassium (GIK) improved the electrocardiographic signs of AMI (47). The basis for the benefit of GIK in acute ischemia has been extensively studied (48). During AMI, plasma FFA levels increase rapidly and these levels are toxic to the ischemic myocardium. GIK decreases FFA toxicity and shifts oxidative metabolism away from FFA to glucose, thus replenishing ATP. Experimental studies have shown that even with total coronary occlusion, the ischemic myocardium can metabolize glucose. GIK can also improve the function of the acutely loaded, but not infarcted, region as well. A large number of randomized clinical trials have been published comparing GIK and control (49–51). A meta-analysis of 16 of the trials indicated an 18% reduction in mortality with GIK, but due to the wide confidence limits, the reduction was only marginally positive despite having over 5000 patients (52). High-dose GIK trials, however, showed a greater benefit than low-dose trials. The largest clinical trial to study GIK was the CREATE-ECLA trial that randomized 20,201 patients with AMI from 470 centers worldwide (Fig. 4) (53). The study was the combination of an international study [Clinical Trial of Reviparin and Metabolic Modulation in Acute Myocardial Infarction Treatment Evaluation (CREATE)] and a South American study [Estudios Cardiologicas Latin America Study Group (ECLA) 2 GIK Full Scale Trial]. The primary end point was all-cause mortality at 30 days. Seven hundred and forty five of the patients were treated with fibrinolytic therapy and 9% with primary PCI. The average time from symptom onset to randomization was 3.85 hours. The study showed no significant difference in mortality at 30 days between treatments (10.0% for GIK and 9.7% for control; HR 1.03; $p = 0.45$). Likewise, cardiogenic shock, reinfarction, and heart failure rates were not different. The study has been criticized by some because the GIK was given almost one hour later, often after reperfusion had occurred (54). Experimental studies have shown

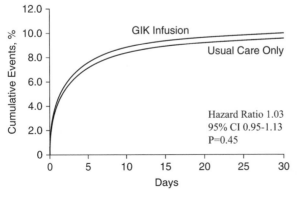

FIGURE 4 The primary end point of the CREATE-ELCA (53) trial. This study of patients with ST segment elevation MI failed to demonstrate a difference in the primary end point of death, cardiac arrest, cardiogenic shock, and reinfarction at 30 days between GIK and placebo.

benefit that only occurs when GIK is given at or before reperfusion. The overall mortality was also high and most of the patients were enrolled in countries where delivery of care might be suboptimal. Despite these concerns, it is unlikely that any further studies will be performed with GIK in AMI.

White Blood Cell Inhibitors

White blood cell counts increase during AMI and have been shown to parallel the size of the infarct as well as predict short- and long-term mortality (55). During reperfusion, white blood cells, particularly neutrophils, attach to damaged endothelium and migrate into the infarct zone (13). The neutrophil releases proteinases, chemokines, leukotrienes, and oxygen-free radicals that contribute to reperfusion injury (56). In addition, in combination with platelets and thrombus, white blood cells contribute to microvascular plugging and the no-reflow phenomenon (57). Experimental studies have shown that inhibition of the CD11 or CD11/CD18 integrin receptor on the white blood cell prevents attachment and migration into the infarct zone, and reduces infarct size when given at the time of reperfusion (58). Two studies have examined these agents (Fig. 5). The Hu23F2G Anti-Adhesion to Limit Cytotoxic Injury Following Acute MI (HALT-MI) trial was a study of a humanized monoclonal antibody against the CD11/CD18 integrin receptor (59). The primary end point was infarct size determined by Single Photon Emission Computed Tomography (SPECT) nuclear imaging at five to seven days after randomization. Four hundred and twenty patients with STEMI, within six hours of symptom onset undergoing primary PCI, were enrolled. Two doses of the antibody were studied. The study showed no differences in SPECT, enzymatic infarct size, or other clinical outcomes. The Limitation of Myocardial Infarction following Thrombolysis in Acute Myocardial Infarction (LIMIT-MI) study evaluated another specific antibody to the CD18 integrin receptor, rhuMAB CD 18 (60). In this study, 413 patients were enrolled within 12 hours of symptom onset and all received t-PA. The primary end point was Thrombolysis in Myocardial Infarction (TIMI) frame

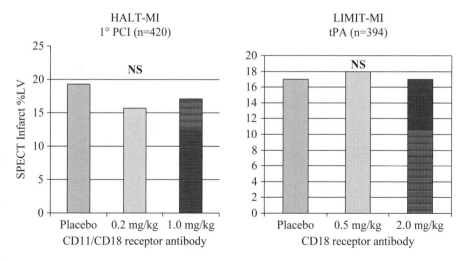

FIGURE 5 Trials of inhibitors of the leukocyte CD11/18 and CD18 integrin receptor. The HALT-MI (59) and LIMIT-MI (60) trials failed to demonstrate a reduction in myocardial infarct size as measured by SPECT imaging. The primary end point of the LIMIT-MI trial was corrected TIMI frame count that was also not significantly different.

count at 90 minutes following fibrinolysis. The study failed to show any differences between control and two doses of the antibody. As in the previous study, other end points were not significantly different. These two studies do not support the benefit of inhibition of white blood cells during reperfusion.

Complement Inhibitors

Complement inhibitor is an important contributor to the inflammatory damage that occurs in AMI (61). Complement activates leukocytes and endothelial cells, directly damages myocardial cells, upregulates cytokine expression, and increases apoptosis. In animals, inhibition of the complement component C5 leads to reduced infarct size (62). Five clinical studies have been conducted with pexelizumab, an anti-C5 complement antibody: the Complement and Reduction of Infarct size after Angioplasty or Lytics (CARDINAL) trials [which included the parallel trials COMPlement inhibition in myocardial infarction trated with thrombyLYtics (COMPLY) (63) and COMplement inhibition in Myocardial infarction treated with Angioplasty (COMMA) (64)], the APEX-MI study (65), and the Pexelizumab for Reduction in Infarction and Mortality in Coronary Artery Bypass Graft surgery (PRIMO-CABG) 1 (66) and PRIMO-CABG 2 trials (Fig. 6). The COMPLY trial evaluated complement inhibition in patients treated with fibrinolysis and the COMMA trial evaluated patients treated with primary PCI. In the COMPLY study, 943 patients with STEMI were randomized to pexelizumab in two doses versus placebo. The primary end point of enzymatic infarct size at 72 hours did not differ between the groups, nor did 90-day clinical events. The COMMA study randomized 960 patients with STEMI and likewise showed no difference in enzymatic infarct size (64). Interestingly, the 90-day mortality was significantly lower in the treatment groups (1.8% vs. 5.9%; $p = 0.014$) (Fig. 7). On the basis of this finding, the APEX-MI trial (65) was designed to randomize 8500 patients undergoing primary PCI with a primary end point of 30-day mortality. Because of the negative result of the PRIMO-CABG trials, this trial was stopped after enrolling 5745 patients. There was no difference in 30-day mortality rates. The composite end points of death, shock, and congestive heart failure

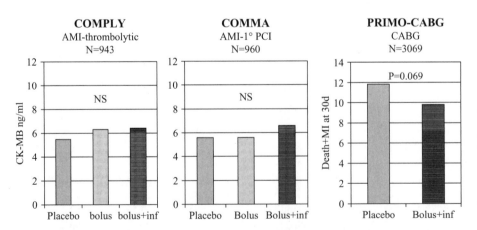

FIGURE 6 The clinical trials of C5 complement inhibitor. Pexelizumab failed to show a significant benefit in the primary end point of infarct size measured by CK-MB curves in the COMPLY (63) and COMMA (64) trials. The PRIMO-CABG (65) trial also failed to show a difference in the primary end point of death or MI at 30 days after CABG.

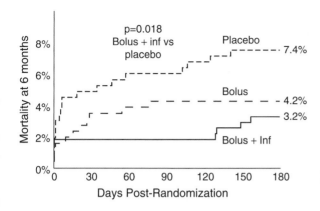

FIGURE 7 The impact of pexelizumab on mortality. The COMMA trial (64) did show a mortality benefit in patients undergoing primary PCI.

were also similar. The PRIMO-CABG 1 trial (66) randomized 3099 patients undergoing CABG. Patients received either placebo or two doses of pexelizumab. The primary end point was death or MI at 30 days. The study failed to demonstrate a significant difference (11.8% for placebo and 9.8% for pexelizumab; RR 18%; $p = 0.07$), but in the overall intention to treat populations (CABG patients with and without concomitant valve surgery), pexelizumab was beneficial ($p = 0.03$). A second trial, the PRIMO-CABG 2 trial with 4250 patients, also failed to demonstrate a benefit in the combined end point of death or MI at 30 days, although there was trend toward benefit. It seems unlikely that this particular complement inhibitor will be marketed in the United States.

Adenosine

Adenosine and adenosine receptor agonists have been shown to induce coronary artery vasodilatation, reverse coronary spasm, replenish high-energy phosphates, and improve cardiac hemodynamics (67,68). Adenosine receptor stimulation is felt to be a key process in ischemic preconditioning. In addition, it inhibits platelet and neutrophil activation. Thus, adenosine should be an ideal agent to reduce reperfusion injury. Numerous experimental studies have confirmed its benefit and seven clinical trials have been conducted (69–71). Garratt et al. studied 45 patients undergoing primary PCI and showed an improvement in myocardial perfusion with adenosine administration (72). The first large trial was the Acute Myocardial Infarction STudy of ADenosine (AMISTAD) trial (Fig. 8) (73). Two hundred and thirty six patients within six hours of AMI were randomized to adenosine or placebo prior to receiving fibrinolysis. The primary end point was myocardial salvage determined by serial SPECT imaging. The study showed a 33% relative reduction in infarct size (13% vs. 19.5%) that occurred primarily in those with anterior MI. There was also a trend toward improved clinical benefit. However, the study has been criticized for the large infarct size seen in the anterior MI group receiving placebo (45.5%), something not seen currently with primary PCI. The ATTenuation by Adenosine of Cardiac Complications (ATTACC) study randomized 608 patients within 12 hours of symptom onset (74). The primary end point of left ventricular function determined by two-dimensional echo was not different between adenosine and placebo. There was a trend toward an improved cardiovascular mortality, however [8.9% vs. 12.1%; OR 0.71 (0.4–1.2); $p = 0.2$]. The AmP574 Delivery for Myocardial Infarction Reduction (ADMIRE) study differed from the prior studies in several ways (75). It used an adenosine A2 receptor agonist and studied its effect in 311 patients undergoing primary PCI. Only balloon

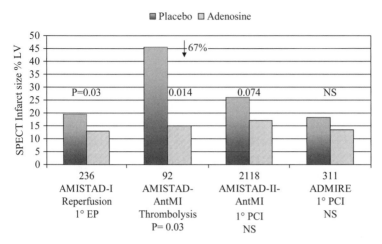

□ Placebo   □ Adenosine

FIGURE 8   The effect of adenosine in STEMI. Adenosine showed a reduction in infarct size in the AMISTAD I trial (73) in patients receiving fibrinolysis which was confined to the group with anterior MI. In the AMISTAD II trial (76) of patients receiving fibrinolysis or primary PCI and in the ADMIRE trials (75) of patients receiving primary PCI, no reduction in infarct size was seen.

angioplasty was used in this study, however. The primary end point of infarct size determined by technetium Tc-99 sestamibi scanning was not different, nor were left ventricular ejection fraction or clinical events. The AMISTAD-II trial was undertaken to test the benefit of adenosine in a larger group of patients undergoing either fibrinolysis or primary PCI and to test two doses of adenosine. Two thousand one hundred and eighteen patients were enrolled and 58% received a lytic agent, while the remainder underwent PCI (76). There was no difference in the primary end point of new or worsening congestive heart failure or death at six months. The pooled adenosine group, however, had a trend toward smaller infarct size as measured by SPECT imaging (17% vs. 27%; $p = 0.07$). In summary, adenosine despite considerable theoretical and experimental data to support its benefit, also has failed to show clinical benefit in multiple clinical trials.

Other Agents

A number of other agents have been studied experimentally and in limited clinical studies with some promise. One of the promising approaches is to increase NO production through administration of nitropruside, nitrites, or L-arginine (77,78). Improvement in oxygen delivery through aqueous oxygen has shown preliminary promise (79,80). Erythropoietin is also cardioprotective, and in an experimental study, it demonstrated a reduction in infarct size (81). A number of new pathways that may contribute to ischemia/reperfusion injury are also being investigated that may lead to new therapeutic approaches (82).

SUMMARY AND FUTURE DIRECTIONS

The efforts to find an effective pharmacological agent to reduce infarct size have spanned more than 40 years and have yet to be realized. The numerous agents discussed above have good rationale and significant experimental data to support a clinical benefit, yet to date, no therapy had consistently shown a reduction in infarct size or improvement in clinical outcome. In part, this may be due to the small size of most studies and the use of surrogate end points, such as infarct size measure by various imaging techniques (83). Most of the current agents that have shown benefit in the clinical arena have been studied in very large trials of 10,000 to 20,000 patients. This may be necessary since the benefit of early reperfusion therapy has now decreased the in-hospital mortality rate of STEMI to less than 5%, and in many studies it is now 1% to 2%. In addition, reperfusion injury is difficult to measure and is likely to be only improved if the agent is administered prior to reperfusion, something that is difficult to do clinically. Also, the process of ischemia-reperfusion injury is multifactorial and it may be necessary to use multiple agents to obtain benefit. This approach has recently been undertaken in cardiac surgery where evaluating pharmacological interventions may be superior, given the controlled circumstances of ischemia and reperfusion. A number of new agents are on the horizon and are likely to be studied in the future. Any means to improve myocardial function and reduce the mortality of AMI will be embraced by the medical community.

REFERENCES

1. Thom T, Haase N, Rosamond W, et al. Heart disease and stroke statistics—2006 update: a report from the American Heart Association Statistics Committee and Stroke Statistics Subcommittee. Circulation 2006; 113:e85–e151.
2. Antman EM, Anbe DT, Armstrong PW, et al. ACC/AHA guidelines for the management of patients with ST-elevation myocardial infarction: a report of the American College of Cardiology/American Heart Association Task Force on Practice Guidelines (committee to revise the 1999 guidelines for the management of patients with acute myocardial infarction). Circulation 2004; 110:e82–e292.
3. Gibson CM, Murphy SA, Morrow DA, et al. Angiographic perfusion score: an angiographic variable that integrates both epicardial and tissue level perfusion before and after facilitated percutaneous coronary intervention in acute myocardial infarction. Am Heart J 2004; 148:336–340.
4. Keeley EC, Boura JA, Grines CL. Primary angioplasty versus intravenous thrombolytic therapy for acute myocardial infarction: a quantitative review of 23 randomised trials. Lancet 2003; 361:13–20.
5. Buja LM. Myocardial ischemia and reperfusion injury. Cardiovasc Pathol 2005; 14:170–175.
6. Ambrosio G, Tritto I. Reperfusion injury: experimental evidence and clinical implications. Am Heart J 1999; 138(2 pt 2):S69–S75.
7. Verma S, Fedak PW, Weisel RD, et al. Fundamentals of reperfusion injury for the clinical cardiologist. Circulation 2002; 105:2332–2336.
8. Cannon RO III. Mechanisms, management and future directions for reperfusion injury after acute myocardial infarction. Nat Clin Pract Cardiovasc Med 2005; 2:88–94.
9. Bolli R, Jeroudi MO, Patel BS, et al. Direct evidence that oxygen-derived free radicals contribute to postischemic myocardial dysfunction in the intact dog. Proc Natl Acad Sci U S A 1989; 86:4695–4699.
10. Jeroudi MO, Hartley CJ, Bolli R. Myocardial reperfusion injury: role of oxygen radicals and potential therapy with antioxidants. Am J Cardiol 1994; 73:2B–7B.
11. Cingolani HE, Ennis IL, Mosca SM. NHE-1 and NHE-6 Activities: ischemic and reperfusion injury. Circ Res 2003; 93:694–696.
12. Eefting F, Rensing B, Wigman J, et al. Role of apoptosis in reperfusion injury. Cardiovasc Res 2004; 61:414–426.
13. Kaminski KA, Bonda TA, Korecki J, et al. Oxidative stress and neutrophil activation—the two keystones of ischemia/reperfusion injury. Int J Cardiol 2002; 86:41–59.
14. Reffelmann T, Kloner RA. The "no-reflow" phenomenon: basic science and clinical correlates. Heart 2002; 87:162–168.

15. Yasuda M, Takeuchi K, Hiruma M, et al. The complement system in ischemic heart disease. Circulation 1990; 81:156–163.
16. Jung F, Palmer LA, Zhou N, et al. Hypoxic regulation of inducible nitric oxide synthase via hypoxia inducible factor-1 in cardiac myocytes. Circ Res 2000; 86:319–325.
17. Yellon DM, Hausenloy DJ. Realizing the clinical potential of ischemic preconditioning and postconditioning. Nat Clin Pract Cardiovasc Med 2005; 2:568–575.
18. Rezkalla SH, Kloner RA. Ischemic preconditioning and preinfarction angina in the clinical arena. Nat Clin Pract Cardiovasc Med 2004; 1:96–102.
19. Kloner RA, Jennings RB. Consequences of brief ischemia: stunning, preconditioning, and their clinical implications: part 2. Circulation 2001; 104:3158–3167.
20. Kloner RA, Jennings RB. Consequences of brief ischemia: stunning, preconditioning, and their clinical implications: part 1. Circulation 2001; 104:2981–2999.
21. Przyklenk K. Oxygen-derived free radicals and "stunned myocardium." Free Radic Biol Med 1988; 4:39–44.
22. Przyklenk K. Pharmacologic treatment of the stunned myocardium: the concepts and the challenges. Coron Artery Dis 2001; 12:363–369.
23. Sochman J. N-acetylcysteine in acute cardiology: 10 years later: what do we know and what would we like to know?! J Am Coll Cardiol 2002; 39:1422–1428.
24. Sochman J, Vrbska J, Musilova B, et al. Infarct size limitation: Acute N-acetylcysteine Defense (ISLAND trial): preliminary analysis and report after the first 30 patients. Clin Cardiol 1996; 19:94–100.
25. Flaherty JT, Pitt B, Gruber JW, et al. Recombinant human superoxide dismutase (h-SOD) fails to improve recovery of ventricular function in patients undergoing coronary angioplasty for acute myocardial infarction. Circulation 1994; 89:1982–1991.
26. Effect of 48-h intravenous trimetazidine on short- and long-term outcomes of patients with acute myocardial infarction, with and without thrombolytic therapy; A double-blind, placebo-controlled, randomized trial. The EMIP-FR Group. European Myocardial Infarction Project—Free Radicals. Eur Heart J 2000; 21:1537–1546.
27. Steg PG, Grollier G, Gallay P, et al. A randomized double-blind trial of intravenous trimetazidine as adjunctive therapy to primary angioplasty for acute myocardial infarction. Int J Cardiol 2001; 77:263–273.
28. Kloner RA, Przyklenk K. Progress in cardioprotection: the role of calcium antagonists. Am J Cardiol 1990; 66:2H–9H.
29. Goldbourt U, Behar S, Reicher-Reiss H, et al. Early administration of nifedipine in suspected acute myocardial infarction. The Secondary Prevention Reinfarction Israel Nifedipine Trial 2 Study. Arch Intern Med 1993; 153:345–353.
30. Theroux P, Gregoire J, Chin C, et al. Intravenous diltiazem in acute myocardial infarction. Diltiazem as adjunctive therapy to activase (DATA) trial. J Am Coll Cardiol 1998; 32:620–628.
31. Pizzetti G, Mailhac A, Li Volsi L, et al. Beneficial effects of diltiazem during myocardial reperfusion: a randomized trial in acute myocardial infarction. Ital Heart J 2001; 2:757–765.
32. Marangelli V, Memmola C, Brigiani MS, et al. Early administration of verapamil after thrombolysis in acute anterior myocardial infarction. Effect on left ventricular remodeling and clinical outcome. VAMI Study Group. Verapamil Acute Myocardial Infarction. Ital Heart J 2000; 1:336–343.
33. Sato T, Marban E. The role of mitochondrial K(ATP) channels in cardioprotection. Basic Res Cardiol 2000; 95:285–289.
34. Schalla S, Higgins CB, Chujo M, et al. Effect of potassium-channel opener therapy on reperfused infarction in hypertrophied hearts: demonstration of preconditioning by using functional and contrast-enhanced magnetic resonance imaging. J Cardiovasc Pharmacol Ther 2004; 9:193–202.
35. Ishida H, Higashijima N, Hirota Y, et al. Nicorandil attenuates the mitochondrial Ca 2+ overload with accompanying depolarization of the mitochondrial membrane in the heart. Naunyn Schmiedebergs Arch Pharmacol 2004; 369:192–197.
36. Tsuchida A, Miura T, Tanno M, et al. Infarct size limitation by nicorandil: roles of mitochondrial K(ATP) channels, sarcolemmal K(ATP) channels, and protein kinase C. J Am Coll Cardiol 16 2002; 40:1523–1530.

37. Effect of nicorandil on coronary events in patients with stable angina: the Impact Of Nicorandil in Angina (IONA) randomised trial. Lancet 2002; 359:1269–1275.
38. Sakata Y, Kodama K, Komamura K, et al. Salutary effect of adjunctive intracoronary nicorandil administration on restoration of myocardial blood flow and functional improvement in patients with acute myocardial infarction. Am Heart J 1997; 133:616–621.
39. Sugimoto K, Ito H, Iwakura K, et al. Intravenous nicorandil in conjunction with coronary reperfusion therapy is associated with better clinical and functional outcomes in patients with acute myocardial infarction. Circ J 2003; 67:295–300.
40. Ikeda N, Yasu T, Kubo N, et al. Nicorandil versus isosorbide dinitrate as adjunctive treatment to direct balloon angioplasty in acute myocardial infarction. Heart 2004; 90:181–185.
41. Ishii H, Ichimiya S, Kanashiro M, et al. Impact of a single intravenous administration of nicorandil before reperfusion in patients with ST-segment-elevation myocardial infarction. Circulation 2005; 112:1284–1288.
42. Allen DG, Xiao XH. Role of the cardiac Na+/H+ exchanger during ischemia and reperfusion. Cardiovasc Res 2003; 57:934–941.
43. Rupprecht H-J, Dahl Jv, Terres W, et al. Cardioprotective effects of the Na+/H+ exchange inhibitor cariporide in patients with acute anterior myocardial infarction undergoing direct PTCA. Circulation 2000; 101:2902–2908.
44. Theroux P, Chaitman BR, Danchin N, et al. Inhibition of the sodium-hydrogen exchanger with cariporide to prevent myocardial infarction in high-risk ischemic situations: main results of the GUARDIAN trial. Circulation 2000; 102:3032–3038.
45. Mentzer RM. EXPEDITION: Sodium-proton exchange inhibition to prevent coronary events in acute cardiac conditions trial. Paper presented at American Heart Association Scientific Sessions 2003; 11/12/2003, 2003; Orlando, Florida.
46. Zeymer U, Suryapranata H, Monassier JP, et al. The Na+/H+ exchange inhibitor eniporide as an adjunct to early reperfusion therapy for acute myocardial infarction: results of the evaluation of the safety and cardioprotective effects of eniporide in acute myocardial infarction (ESCAMI) trial. J Am Coll Cardiol 2001; 38:E1644–E1650.
47. Sodi-Pollaries D, Testelli RM, Fishleder BL. Effects of an intravenous infusion of potassium-glucose-insulin solution on the electrocardiographic signs of myocardial infarction: preliminary clinical report. Am J Cardiol 1962; 9:166–181.
48. Apstein CS. The benefits of glucose-insulin-potassium for acute myocardial infarction (and some concerns). J Am Coll Cardiol 2003; 42:792–795.
49. Diaz R, Paolasso EA, Piegas LS, et al. Metabolic modulation of acute myocardial infarction: the ECLA glucose-insulin-potassium pilot trial. Circulation 1998; 98:2227–2234.
50. van der Horst IC, Timmer JR, Ottervanger JP, et al. Glucose-insulin-potassium and reperfusion in acute myocardial infarction: rationale and design of the Glucose-Insulin-Potassium Study-2 (GIPS-2). Am Heart J 2005; 149:585–591.
51. van der Horst ICC, Zijlstra F, van't Hof AWJ, et al. Glucose-insulin-potassium infusion inpatients treated with primary angioplasty for acute myocardial infarction: the glucose-insulin-potassium study: a randomized trial. J Am Coll Cardiol 2003; 42:784–791.
52. Yusuf S, Mehta SR, Diaz R, et al. Challenges in the conduct of large simple trials of important generic questions in resource-poor settings: the CREATE and ECLA trial program evaluating GIK (glucose, insulin and potassium) and low-molecular-weight heparin in acute myocardial infarction. Am Heart J 2004; 148:1068–1078.
53. Mehta SR, Yusuf S, Diaz R, et al. Effect of glucose-insulin-potassium infusion on mortality in patients with acute ST-segment elevation myocardial infarction: the CREATE-ECLA randomized controlled trial. JAMA 2005; 293:437–446.
54. Apstein CS. Glucose-insulin-potassium infusion and mortality in the CREATE-ECLA trial. JAMA 2005; 293:2596–2597.
55. Patel MR, Mahaffey KW, Armstrong PW, et al. Prognostic usefulness of white blood cell count and temperature in acute myocardial infarction (from the CARDINAL Trial). Am J Cardiol 2005; 95:614–618.
56. Frangogiannis NG. The role of the chemokines in myocardial ischemia and reperfusion. Curr Vasc Pharmacol 2004; 2:163–174.

57. Hansen PR. Role of neutrophils in myocardial ischemia and reperfusion. Circulation 1995; 91:1872–1885.
58. Thiagarajan RR, Winn RK, Harlan JM. The role of leukocyte and endothelial adhesion molecules in ischemia-reperfusion injury. Thromb Haemost 1997; 78:310–314.
59. Faxon DP, Gibbons RJ, Chronos NA, et al. The effect of blockade of the CD11/CD18 integrin receptor on infarct size in patients with acute myocardial infarction treated with direct angioplasty: the results of the HALT-MI study. J Am Coll Cardiol 2002; 40:1199–1204.
60. Baran KW, Nguyen M, McKendall GR, et al. Double-blind, randomized trial of an anti-CD18 antibody in conjunction with recombinant tissue plasminogen activator for acute myocardial infarction: limitation of myocardial infarction following thrombolysis in acute myocardial infarction (LIMIT AMI) study. Circulation 2001; 104:2778–2783.
61. Frangogiannis NG, Smith CW, Entman ML. The inflammatory response in myocardial infarction. Cardiovasc Res 2002; 53:31–47.
62. de Zwaan C, van Dieijen-Visser MP, Hermens WT. Prevention of cardiac cell injury during acute myocardial infarction: possible role for complement inhibition. Am J Cardiovasc Drugs 2003; 3:245–251.
63. Mahaffey KW, Granger CB, Nicolau JC, et al. Effect of pexelizumab, an anti-C5 complement antibody, as adjunctive therapy to fibrinolysis in acute myocardial infarction: the COMPlement inhibition in myocardial infarction treated with thromboLYtics (COMPLY) trial. Circulation 2003; 108:1176–1183.
64. Granger CB, Mahaffey KW, Weaver WD, et al. Pexelizumab, an anti-C5 complement antibody, as adjunctive therapy to primary percutaneous coronary intervention in acute myocardial infarction: the COMplement inhibition in Myocardial infarction treated with Angioplasty (COMMA) trial. Circulation 2003; 108:1184–1190.
65. APEX AMI Investigators, Armstrong PW, Granger CB, et al. Pexelizumab for acute ST-elevation myocaridal infarction in patients undergoing primary percutaneous coronary intervention: a randomized controlled trial. JAMA 2007; 297:43–51.
66. Verrier ED, Shernan SK, Taylor KM, et al. Terminal complement blockade with pexelizumab during coronary artery bypass graft surgery requiring cardiopulmonary bypass: a randomized trial. JAMA 2004; 291:2319–2327.
67. Donato M, Gelpi RJ. Adenosine and cardioprotection during reperfusion: an overview. Mol Cell Biochem 2003; 251:153–159.
68. Glover DK, Riou LM, Ruiz M, et al. Reduction of infarct size and postischemic inflammation from ATL-146e, a highly selective adenosine A2A receptor agonist, in reperfused canine myocardium. Am J Physiol Heart Circ Physiol 2005; 288:H1851–H1858.
69. Przyklenk K, Whittaker P. Cardioprotection with adenosine: "a riddle wrapped in a mystery". Br J Pharmacol 2005; 145:699–700.
70. Quintana M, Kahan T, Hjemdahl P. Pharmacological prevention of reperfusion injury in acute myocardial infarction. A potential role for adenosine as a therapeutic agent. Am J Cardiovasc Drugs 2004; 4:159–167.
71. Xu Z, Mueller RA, Park SS, et al. Cardioprotection with adenosine A2 receptor activation at reperfusion. J Cardiovasc Pharmacol 2005; 46:794–802.
72. Garratt KN, Holmes DR Jr., Molina-Viamonte V, et al. Intravenous adenosine and lidocaine in patients with acute mycocardial infarction. Am Heart J 1998; 136:196–204.
73. Mahaffey KW, Puma JA, Barbagelata NA, et al. Adenosine as an adjunct to thrombolytic therapy for acute myocardial infarction : Results of a multicenter, randomized, placebo-controlled trial: the Acute Myocardial Infarction STudy of ADenosine (AMISTAD) trial. J Am Coll Cardiol 1999; 34:1711–1720.
74. Quintana M, Hjemdahl P, Sollevi A, et al. Left ventricular function and cardiovascular events following adjuvant therapy with adenosine in acute myocardial infarction treated with thrombolysis, results of the ATTenuation by Adenosine of Cardiac Complications (ATTACC) study. Eur J Clin Pharmacol 2003; 59:1–9.
75. Kopecky SL, Aviles RJ, Bell MR, et al. A randomized, double-blinded, placebo-controlled, dose-ranging study measuring the effect of an adenosine agonist on infarct size reduction in patients undergoing primary percutaneous transluminal coronary angioplasty: the ADMIRE (AmP579 Delivery for Myocardial Infarction REduction) study. Am Heart J 2003; 146:146–152.

76. Ross AM, Gibbons RJ, Stone GW, et al. A Randomized, Double-Blinded, Placebo-Controlled Multicenter Trial of Adenosine as an Adjunct to Reperfusion in the Treatment of Acute Myocardial Infarction (AMISTAD-II). J Am Coll Cardiol 2005; 45:1775–1780.
77. Colagrande L, Formica F, Porta F, et al. L-Arginine effects on myocardial stress in cardiac surgery: preliminary results. Ital Heart J 2005; 6:904–910.
78. Duranski MR, Greer JJ, Dejam A, et al. Cytoprotective effects of nitrite during in vivo ischemia-reperfusion of the heart and liver. J Clin Invest 2005; 115:1232–1240.
79. Glazier JJ. Attenuation of reperfusion microvascular ischemia by aqueous oxygen: experimental and clinical observations. Am Heart J 2005; 149:580–584.
80. Burkhoff D, Lefer DJ. Cardioprotection before revascularization in ischemic myocardial injury and the potential role of hemoglobin-based oxygen carriers. Am Heart J 2005; 149:573–579.
81. Bullard AJ, Govewalla P, Yellon DM. Erythropoietin protects the myocardium against reperfusion injury in vitro and in vivo. Basic Res Cardiol 2005; 100:397–403.
82. Hausenloy DJ, Yellon DM. New directions for protecting the heart against ischaemia-reperfusion injury: targeting the reperfusion injury salvage kinase (RISK)-pathway. Cardiovasc Res 2004; 61:448–460.
83. Bolli R, Becker L, Gross G, et al. Myocardial protection at a crossroads: the need for translation into clinical therapy. Circ Res 2004; 95:125–134.

15

Myocyte Protection by Device Therapy

Sanjeevan Pasupati and John G. Webb
Division of Cardiology, St. Paul's Hospital, University of British Columbia, Vancouver, Canada

INTRODUCTION

The importance of early reperfusion in the management of acute ST elevation myocardial infarction (STEMI) is well established. Randomized trials favor primary percutaneous coronary intervention (PCI), when delivered in a timely manner, as the preferred method of reperfusion (1,2). However, despite successful reperfusion with primary PCI, some patients are left with abnormal epicardial coronary flow. Even when normal coronary flow is achieved, normal myocardial perfusion is not guaranteed (3).

Reduced myocardial perfusion is associated with adverse left ventricular remodeling, heart failure, and mortality (4–6). Impaired microvascular perfusion causing myocyte injury is due to microvascular obstruction from distal embolization of atherosclerotic and thrombotic debris from the lesion site, reperfusion injury, and ischemia-induced microvascular damage from endothelial cell edema, leukocyte plugging of postcapillary venules, free oxygen radical generation, and microvascular spasm (7–12). These effects are not transient and may self-propagate over a period of time causing microcirculatory damage and myocyte necrosis (13,14).

Multiple pharmacological and device therapies have been trialed to protect the myocyte from microvascular injury. The pharmacological therapies have been discussed in the previous chapter. Device therapies of current interest in the setting of primary PCI can be listed under four categories: (1) thrombectomy, (2) embolic protection, (3) cooling, and (4) supersaturated oxygen delivery. Thrombectomy and embolic protection devices focus on the prevention of distal embolization, while cooling and supersaturated oxygen reduce the impact of reperfusion injury and ischemia-induced microvascular damage.

Electrocardiography, echocardiography, nuclear SPECT imaging, magnetic resonance imaging (MRI), and coronary angiography have all been used as clinical tools to assess the treatment benefits of the above interventions. When using an echocardiogram, wall motion score index (WMSI) is a more accurate method to look at the recovery of the left ventricular function in the infarct zone than the left ventricular ejection fraction because it is not influenced by the effects of hyperkinesis of the contralateral wall. Infarct size is currently best measured using SPECT or contrast-enhanced MRI. Markers of impaired microvascular perfusion and the investigational tools used to detect them are detailed in Table 1.

THROMBECTOMY DEVICES

Rationale
Thromboembolism with macrovascular and microvascular obstruction may play a significant role in reducing myocardial perfusion (5,15,16). By implication, removal of coronary thrombus at the time of primary PCI has the potential to improve myocardial reperfusion and clinical outcome. Approaches to the management of

TABLE 1 Markers of Impaired Microvascular Perfusion

Test (Ref.)	Marker
1 ECG (96)	ST resolution
2 MCE (94,97,98)	WMSI
	Left ventricular ejection fraction
3 SPECT scan (99,100)	Tracer activity
4 Contrast enhanced MRI (101)	Hypo enhanced area
5 Coronary angiogram (102)	TIMI myocardial perfusionTMP
	TIMI flow rate

Abbreviations: MCE, myocardial contrast echo; WMSI, wall motion score index; TIMI, thrombolysis in myocardial infarction; TMP, TIMI myocardial perfusion.

intracoronary thrombus include anticoagulation or fibrinolysis, proximal or distal embolic protection, and mechanical thrombus removal or thrombectomy. Thrombectomy can by achieved by means of aspiration or mechanical disruption and aspiration.

Device Therapies
Perhaps the simplest approach to thrombectomy is catheter aspiration. The Export™ (Medtronic Inc., Minneapolis, Minnesota, U.S.) and Pronto™ (Vascular Solutions Inc., Minneapolis, Minnesota, U.S.) catheters have been used for this purpose (Fig. 1). Both incorporate a lumen for passage over a standard angioplasty wire and a lumen to allow thrombus aspiration and removal.

The AngioJet™ rheolytic catheter (Possis Medical Inc., Minneapolis, Minnesota, U.S.) (17) incorporates high pressure saline jets and matched aspiration to create a vacuum effect disrupting and evacuating thrombus (Fig. 2). The X-Sizer™ mechanical extraction system (ev3, Plymouth, Minnesota, U.S.) (18) combines a powerful vacuum and a helical cutter at the tip of the catheter that draws in and disrupts thrombus. The Rinspiration™ thrombectomy system (Kerberos Proximal Solutions Inc., MountainView, California, U.S.) allows for simultaneous irrigation and aspiration (19) (Fig. 3). The TriActiv FX™ (Kensey-Nash Inc., Exton, PA) is somewhat similar but also includes a distal occlusion balloon.

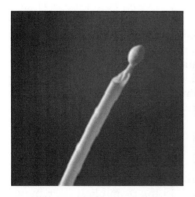 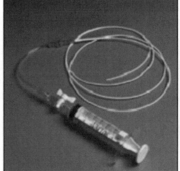

FIGURE 1 Pronto extraction catheter.

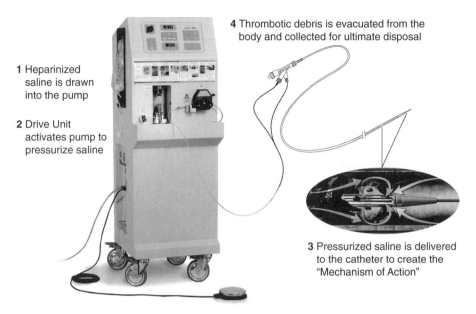

1 Heparinized saline is drawn into the pump

2 Drive Unit activates pump to pressurize saline

4 Thrombotic debris is evacuated from the body and collected for ultimate disposal

3 Pressurized saline is delivered to the catheter to create the "Mechanism of Action"

FIGURE 2 AngioJet™ rheolytic (Possis Medical Inc., Minneapolis, Minnesota, U.S.) device. *Source*: Courtesy of Possis Medical Inc.

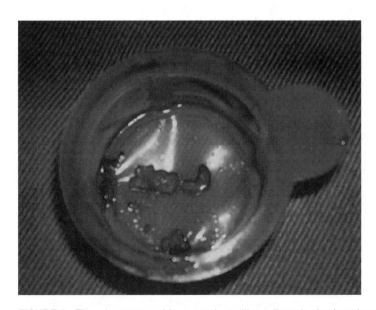

FIGURE 3 Thrombus removed from a patient with cardiogenic shock and an occluded saphenous vein bypass graft using the Kerberos Rinspiration system.

Trials of Thrombectomy

While thrombus removal can be demonstrated with simple aspiration devices such as the Export and Pronto catheters, improved outcome remains to be proven. In the 60-patient DEAR-MI study, the Pronto extraction catheter was associated with a significant improvement in myocardial perfusion (blush score and ST-segment resolution) with primary PCI, but there was no apparent benefit in major adverse cardiac event rates (20).

The thrombectomy devices with the most clinical data are the AngioJet and X-Sizer systems (18). Both have been shown to reduce thrombus burden. However, clinical benefit has not been demonstrated (21–26). The AIMI study showed a paradoxical increase in the infarct size when AngioJet was used with primary PCI (27). Prospective randomized studies that have looked at thrombectomy using the X-Sizer system with primary PCI have similarly failed to show a difference in thrombolysis in myocardial infarction (TIMI) flow or an improvement in major adverse cardiac events (21,23).

EMBOLIC PROTECTION DEVICES

Rationale

Primary PCI is extremely effective at restoring epicardial coronary flow. However, despite restoration of normal TIMI grade 3 flow, myocardial perfusion frequently remains impaired (28–33). Indicators of myocardial perfusion, such as angiographic blush and ST-segment analysis, suggest that normal tissue perfusion is achieved only in the minority of patients after primary PCI. Myocardial perfusion, more so than epicardial flow, is the more important predictor of infarct size, left ventricular function, and clinical outcome (30,34,35).

Diminished myocardial perfusion following PCI is likely multifactorial. Considerable evidence suggests that thromboembolism, atheroembolism, and the corresponding microvascular response are major contributors.

Thromboemboli with capillary block may well be the major contributor to the slow flow and no-reflow phenomenon (impeded blood flow despite a patent artery). Capillary plugging with microemboli composed of platelets, red blood cells, lipoid material, and atheroma (including components of the necrotic core of ruptured atherosclerotic plaque) has been demonstrated after the restoration of normal coronary flow following primary PCI.

Ruptured atheromatous plaque and thrombus play a central role in the pathogenesis of epicardial coronary occlusion in acute STEMI. It is perhaps not surprising that PCI may dislodge atheromatous and thrombotic material from the arterial wall resulting in embolism and microvascular obstruction. The use of embolic protection devices would seem an attractive strategy in this setting.

Device Therapies

Three general types of embolic protection devices have been utilized in the setting of acute MI: (1) a distally placed occlusive balloon in conjunction with an aspiration catheter, (2) a proximally placed occlusive balloon also in conjunction with aspiration, and (3) a distally placed filter.

The initial and greatest experience has been with distal protection using the PercuSurge™ temporary occlusion-aspiration system (Medtronic Inc., Santa Rosa, California, U.S.) (Fig. 4). This consists of an angioplasty guidewire (GuardWire™, Boston Scientific Inc., Natick, Massachusetts, U.S.) incorporating a soft balloon. The

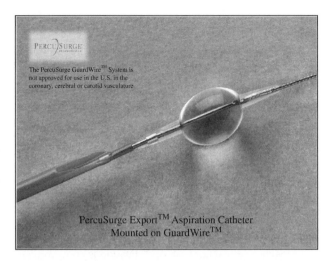

FIGURE 4 PercuSurge GuardWire and Export catheter.

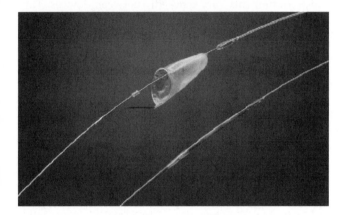

FIGURE 5 FilterWire.

wire is passed through and beyond the culprit lesion where the occlusive balloon is inflated downstream producing a stagnant column of blood. Routine PCI is performed following which a catheter (Export) is advanced down the artery and used to aspirate and remove the column of blood with any blood-borne debris (36–38).

Proximal occlusion devices represent a more recent development (38). The Proxis™ device (Velocimed Inc., Maple Grove, Minnesota, U.S.) consists of an occlusive balloon catheter placed upstream from the culprit lesion to obstruct flow. This catheter allows routine PCI to be accomplished through a central lumen following which embolic debris are aspirated. The major potential advantage unique to this approach is the ability to provide embolic protection during wire and device passage across the culprit lesion.

Distally placed intravascular filters represent the third alternative. The Filter-Wire™ (Boston Scientific Inc., Natick, Massachusetts, U.S.) is typical of these devices (Fig. 5). An angioplasty guidewire incorporates a collapsible filter basket, which is deployed distal to the culprit lesion. Following routine PCI, the filter is removed with its captured embolic debris. The major potential advantage of filters is the ability to maintain continuous perfusion.

Each of these different approaches to prevention of embolism has potential advantages and disadvantages. By way of example, embolism may occur during wiring or downstream placement of a distal protection balloon or filter (36,38). In contrast, proximal occlusion systems can provide protection prior to manipulation of the culprit lesion, a potential advantage in the setting of acute STEMI with bulky thrombus. Occlusive balloons, whether placed proximally or distally, are limited by cessation of normal flow and resultant ischemia. Intermittent reperfusion may be necessary with the attendant temporary loss of embolic protection and the need for redeployment. Filters allow continuous perfusion but may be compromised by large amounts of debris or thrombus or passage of particles smaller than the size of their pores. Distal occlusion balloons may redirect flow and emboli into more proximal side branches. Distal protection with either a balloon or filter presupposes a clear distal landing zone, while proximal protection presupposes a clear proximal landing zone, presenting anatomic constraints on device selection. Positioning of a distal device may be difficult in the setting of STEMI where distal contrast opacification is compromised by coronary occlusion.

Technical and anatomic requirements vary markedly between devices. Time spent deploying an embolic protection device increases time to reperfusion. All devices suffer from an increase in procedural complexity, duration, complications, and cost.

Trials of Embolic Protection

Initial reports of embolic protection in STEMI were encouraging. Early nonrandomized studies with the PercuSurge GuardWire distal occlusion/aspiration system suggested significant clinical benefit (39–44). The interim analysis of the first 188 patients in the RUBY registry suggested that the PercuSurge device was delivered successfully in 87% of the cases during primary PCI (45). Subsequently, the randomized EMERALD trial found that although distal occlusion reduced the incidence of angiographic slow flow and no reflow, there was no benefit in terms of ST-segment resolution, infarct size, or clinical outcome (46) (Fig. 6). Similarly, the Japanese ASPARAGUS study failed to show benefit (47,48). Distal filter protection during primary PCI has also been investigated (49,50). The PROMISE study failed to show improved perfusion or reduced infarct size (51).

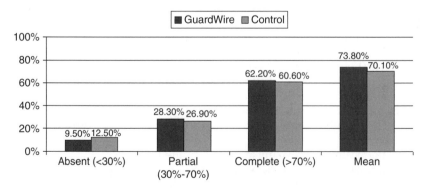

FIGURE 6   EMERALD primary end point of ST segment resolution at 30 minutes.

The proximal balloon occlusion device (Proxis device) has shown similar MACE rates to the GuardWire and FilterWire in saphenous vein graft interventions (52). There are pilot studies and registry data to show this device is safe with excellent delivery rate in primary PCI (53,54). We still await randomized data in this setting.

Thrombectomy and Embolic Protection

An inherent concern with thrombectomy is the risk of unprotected thrombus disruption and thromboembolism. The combined use of the GuardWire distal occlusion balloon and Export aspiration catheter represent the prototypic system intended to provide both embolic protection and thrombus removal. Use of mechanical thrombectomy in combination with distal protection has also been described (19,55), but minimal data are available. The FLAME trial (56,57) compared embolic protection with aspiration against the EMERALD (46) (embolic protection only) trial. In spite of showing better ST-segment resolution and blush scores, it failed to show a reduction in infarct size or cardiac MACE. Hence, this trial was terminated before the randomization phase.

SUMMARY

Routine use of embolic protection and thrombectomy devices in primary PCI remains an unproven strategy. Selective use of these devices may be appealing and reasonable; however, their routine application cannot be recommended.

COOLING

Rationale

Multiple studies in various animal models of STEMI have shown that reducing myocardial temperature can reduce the extent of myocyte necrosis (58–66). One study, utilizing a swine model, found that for every 1°C reduction in body temperature, there was an approximate 20% decrease in infarct size (60). This reduction in infarct size appeared independent of coronary flow and hypothermia-induced bradycardia (59,66). Delayed cooling of the myocardium, even hours following coronary occlusion, may be beneficial (61,64). This benefit is lessened if initiated after reperfusion has been achieved (65,67).

It is postulated that hypothermia protects myocytes in the setting of STEMI by: (1) decreasing myocardial and whole-body metabolism (60,68), (2) increasing ATP retention and stabilizing the cell membrane (60,64,69), (3) reducing neutrophil infiltration (64,70), and (4) reducing platelet aggregation (71). A role for myocardial cooling in STEMI appears possible if achieved early, ideally prior to reperfusion.

Device Therapies

Surface cooling was utilized in initial animal studies; however, this technique is slow and shivering is problematic. Endovascular cooling techniques have allowed trials of human therapy. Currently, two different endovascular cooling devices with similar basic principles have advanced to clinical trials, the Reprieve® (Radiant Medical Inc., Redwood City, California, U.S.) and Celsius Control™ (Innercool Therapies Inc., San Diego, California, U.S.) systems.

The Reprieve system consists of an expandable heat exchange balloon mounted on a multilumen shaft and attached to an external controller. The device is inserted via a femoral 10F sheath into the inferior vena cava. Cool or warm sterile saline is continuously circulated through the catheter, thereby cooling or warming the blood without perfusion of fluids into the body. Core temperature can be reduced by 2°C to 4°C in 30 minutes. Cooling is initiated as early as possible, ideally in the emergency department or in the catheterization laboratory, prior to angiography. Shivering is suppressed by oral buspirone (a 5HT1A partial agonist) or intravenous meperidine. Following reperfusion the patient is rewarmed at a rate of 1°C per hour.

The Celsius Control system consists of an endovascular catheter and an external console. The distal portion of the catheter incorporates a flexible temperature control element which functions similarly to the multilumen shaft in the Reprieve system.

Trials of Cooling
The first human feasibility study using the Reprieve system was published in 2002 (68). Patients undergoing primary PCI were randomized to endovascular cooling to a target core temperature of 33°C. Cooling and suppression of shivering were successfully achieved in the majority of randomized patients. The therapy appeared safe. SPECT imaging at 30 days revealed a 75% relative risk reduction in the median infarct size, although this was not significant ($p = 0.08$) (68,72,73).

COOL MI was the first large multicenter, prospective, randomized study, enrolling 392 patients (72). Cooling, utilizing the Reprieve system, was not associated with a significant change in infarct size, ejection fraction, or CKMB release (Table 2). However, subgroup analysis of anterior AMI patients who were successfully cooled to below 35°C showed a significant reduction in infarct size at 30 days (9.3% vs. 18.2%, $p = 0.05$) (Table 3). On the basis of these data, the randomized COOL MI II trial is enrolling patients presenting early with large anterior STEMI.

The ICE-IT-1 study randomized 228 patients with anterior or large inferior STEMI (74). Endovascular cooling was achieved using the Celsius Control system

TABLE 2 Reduction in Infarct Size on 30-day SPECT Image in Patients with Anterior and Large Inferior STEMI

Study (Ref.)	Randomized	SPECT done	Relative reduction infarct size	p-Value
COOL MI—feasibility study (68,73)	42	36	58.5%	0.086
COOL MI—pivotal study (72)	392	325	2%	0.834
ICE-IT-1 (74)	228	207	23%	0.14

TABLE 3 Patients with Anterior STEMI < 6 hr

Study (Ref.)	Hypothermia All	<35°C	≥35°C	Normothermia	p-Value
COOL MI—pivotal study (72)	17.9%	9.3%	21.9%	18.2%	0.05
ICE-IT-1 (74)	16.3%	12.9%	17.6%	22.7%	0.09

Note: Percentages represent the infarct size at 30 days assessed by SPECT imaging. p-Values are compared between patients cooled to <35°C and control subjects.

to a target core temperature of 33°C. There was no benefit in terms of 30-day infarct size. However, when 6 of 23 enrolling sites with good protocol compliance were analyzed separately, there appeared to be a 44% relative reduction in infarct size ($p = 0.017$) (Tables 2, 3). It is anticipated that ICE-IT-2 will provide further information with regard to this therapy.

SUPERSATURATED OXYGEN DELIVERY

Rationale

Myocardial hypoxia from coronary occlusion leads to loss of endothelial barrier functions and increased endothelial permeability. This, in turn, increases tissue edema and produces adhesion molecules. Increase in tissue edema further increases myocyte hypoxia, causing a self-propagating vicious cycle (10,75,76). Adhesion molecules also reduce blood flow, causing hypoxia (77). Hypoxia increases leukocyte production, leading to plugging of postcapillary venules and metalloproteinase production, causing adverse LV remodeling (9,12,78).

Supersaturated oxygen is believed to have a favorable effect on myocardial salvage in the setting of STEMI by: (1) antagonizing lipid peroxidation (79), (2) reducing endothelial permeability and conserving the capillary barrier (80,81), (3) reducing leukocyte activation by reducing myeloperoxidase levels (82), and (4) increasing the functional capillary density (81,82).

Device Therapies

Supersaturated oxygen can be delivered using hyperbaric oxygen, an extracorporeal high-flow oxygenator or aqueous oxygen. Early, small human trials with hyperbaric oxygen were inconclusive (83,84), although more recent animal studies of this therapy suggested a reduction in myocardial infarct size (85,86). A more rigorous human study (HOT MI) failed to demonstrate benefit (87,88). Currently, both hyperbaric oxygen and extracorporeal membrane oxygenators are generally thought to be impractical, cumbersome, and potentially dangerous therapies in the setting of STEMI.

Aqueous oxygen is a solution of saline with hyperbaric levels of dissolved oxygen ($pO_2 \sim 30,000$ mmHg, 1ml O_2/ml saline) (89). An investigational system (TherOx®AO, TherOx Inc., Irvine, California, U.S.) mixes standard hospital oxygen with hypoxemic blood. The system permits precise delivery of high concentration oxygen in a bubble-free stable form without the need for large priming volumes, extracorporeal membranes, or a perfusionist (90).

Trials of Supersaturated Aqueous Oxygen

Studies in animal models of reperfusion in STEMI have demonstrated a favorable impact on ST-segment resolution, ejection fraction, infarct size, and microvascular blood flow with intracoronary aqueous oxygen (91–93). A small human pilot study in the setting of primary PCI found the therapy to be well tolerated and safe. An improvement in infarct zone wall motion and left ventricular ejection fraction was suggested (94).

The AMIHOT phase II clinical study (95) randomized 269 patients undergoing successful primary PCI within 24 hours of symptom onset to receive intracoronary aqueous oxygen therapy for 90 minutes. The therapy appeared safe and well tolerated. There was no benefit in terms of the primary end points of ST-segment resolution, infarct size, or wall motion. However, subgroup analysis found a significant improvement in ST-segment resolution and WMSI in patients presenting with anterior AMI. Similarly, in patients presenting early (within 6 hours of symptom onset with either anterior or large inferior STEMI) there was a significant improvement in ST-segment resolution and wall motion score. In this group, infarct size was reduced by 27% ($p = 0.04$). A subsequent study, AMIHOT-II, is specifically designed to look at the benefits of aqueous oxygen therapy in patients presenting within six hours of onset of anterior STEMI.

REFERENCES

1. Weaver WD, Simes RJ, Betriu A, et al. Comparison of primary coronary angioplasty and intravenous thrombolytic therapy for acute myocardial infarction: a quantitative review. JAMA 1997; 278:2093–2098.
2. Keeley EC, Boura JA, Grines CL. Primary angioplasty versus intravenous thrombolytic therapy for acute myocardial infarction: a quantitative review of 23 randomised trials. Lancet 2003; 361:13–20.
3. Ito H, Tomooka T, Sakai N, et al. Lack of myocardial perfusion immediately after successful thrombolysis. A predictor of poor recovery of left ventricular function in anterior myocardial infarction. Circulation 1992; 85:1699–1705.
4. Bolognese L, Carrabba N, Parodi G, et al. Impact of microvascular dysfunction on left ventricular remodeling and long-term clinical outcome after primary coronary angioplasty for acute myocardial infarction. Circulation 2004; 109:1121–1126.
5. Henriques JP, Zijlstra F, Ottervanger JP, et al. Incidence and clinical significance of distal embolization during primary angioplasty for acute myocardial infarction. Eur Heart J 2002; 23:1112–1117.
6. van't Hof AW, Liem A, de Boer MJ, et al. Clinical value of 12-lead electrocardiogram after successful reperfusion therapy for acute myocardial infarction. Zwolle Myocardial infarction Study Group. Lancet 1997; 350:615–619.
7. Kloner RA. Does reperfusion injury exist in humans? J Am Coll Cardiol 1993; 21:537–545.
8. Davies MJ. A macro and micro view of coronary vascular insult in ischemic heart disease. Circulation 1990; 82(suppl 3):II38–II46.
9. Ritter LS, McDonagh PF. Low-flow reperfusion after myocardial ischemia enhances leukocyte accumulation in coronary microcirculation. Am J Physiol 1997; 273(3 pt 2): H1154–H1165.
10. Mazzoni MC, Borgstrom P, Warnke KC, et al. Mechanisms and implications of capillary endothelial swelling and luminal narrowing in low-flow ischemias. Int J Microcirc Clin Exp 1995; 15:265–270.
11. Minyailenko TD, Pozharov VP, Seredenko MM. Severe hypoxia activates lipid peroxidation in the rat brain. Chem Phys Lipids 1990; 55:25–28.
12. Baudry N, Danialou G, Boczkowski J, et al. In vivo study of the effect of systemic hypoxia on leukocyte-endothelium interactions. Am J Respir Crit Care Med 1998; 158:477–483.
13. Rochitte CE, Lima JA, Bluemke DA, et al. Magnitude and time course of microvascular obstruction and tissue injury after acute myocardial infarction. Circulation 1998; 98:1006–1014.
14. Spears JR, Henney C, Prcevski P, et al. Reperfusion microvascular ischemia: attenuation with aqueous oxygen. Circulation 2000; 102:646.
15. Giri S, Mitchel JF, Hirst JA, et al. Synergy between intracoronary stenting and abciximab in improving angiographic and clinical outcomes of primary angioplasty in acute myocardial infarction. Am J Cardiol 2000; 86:269–274.
16. Harjai KJ, Grines C, Stone GW, et al. Frequency, determinants, and clinical implications of residual intracoronary thrombus following primary angioplasty for acute myocardial infarction. Am J Cardiol 2003; 92:377–382.
17. Chow K, Gobin YP, Saver J, et al. Endovascular treatment of dural sinus thrombosis with rheolytic thrombectomy and intra-arterial thrombolysis. Stroke 2000; 31:1420–1425.

18. Garcia LA, Carroza JP. Mechanical thrombectomy in coronary and saphenous vein interventions: a review and case studies. J Invasive Cardiol 2004; 16(suppl 4):S3–S9.
19. Webb J, Chandavimol M, Hamburger JN, et al. Initial experience with a novel coronary rinsing and thrombectomy system: "Rinspiration". J Invasive Cardiol 2006; 18(5):188–192.
20. Silva-Orrego P, Colombo P, Bigi R, et al. Thrombus aspiration before primary angioplasty improves myocardial reperfusion in acute myocardial infarction: the DEAR-MI (Dethrombosis to Enhance Acute Reperfusion in Myocardial Infarction) study. J Am Coll Cardiol 2006; 48(8):1552–1559.
21. Beran G, Lang I, Schreiber W, et al. Intracoronary thrombectomy with the X-sizer catheter system improves epicardial flow and accelerates ST-segment resolution in patients with acute coronary syndrome: a prospective, randomized, controlled study. Circulation 2002; 105:2355–2360.
22. Kuntz RE, Baim DS, Cohen DJ, et al. A trial comparing rheolytic thrombectomy with intracoronary urokinase for coronary and vein graft thrombus (the Vein Graft AngioJet Study [VeGAS 2]). Am J Cardiol 2002; 89:326–330.
23. Napodano M, Pasquetto, G, Sacca, S, et al. Intracoronary thrombectomy improves myocardial reperfusion in patients undergoing direct angioplasty for acute myocardial infarction. J Am Coll Cardiol 2003; 42:1395–1402.
24. Silva JA, Ramee SR, Cohen DJ, et al. Rheolytic thrombectomy for the treatment of acute myocardial infarction in patients with angiographic large thrombus burden: one-year results of the VeGAS 2 acute myocardial infarction registry. J Am Coll Cardiol 2002; 43: A248.
25. Stone GW, Cox DA, Babb J, et al. Prospective, randomized evaluation of thrombectomy prior to percutaneous intervention in diseased saphenous vein grafts and thrombus-containing coronary arteries. J Am Coll Cardiol 2003; 42:2007–2013.
26. Stone GW, Cox DA, Low R, et al. Safety and efficacy of a novel device for treatment of thrombotic and atherosclerotic lesions in native coronary arteries and saphenous vein grafts: results from the multicenter X-Sizer for treatment of thrombus and atherosclerosis in coronary applications trial (X-TRACT) study. Catheter Cardiovasc Interv 2003; 58:419–427.
27. Ali A, Cox D, Dib N, et al. Rheolytic thrombectomy with percutaneous coronary intervention for infarct size reduction in acute myocardial infarction: 30-day results from a multicenter randomized study. J Am Coll Cardiol 2006; 48(2):244–252.
28. Costantini CO, Stone GW, Mehran R, et al. Frequency, correlates, and clinical implications of myocardial perfusion after primary angioplasty and stenting, with and without glycoprotein IIb/IIIa inhibition, in acute myocardial infarction. J Am Coll Cardiol 2004; 44:305–312.
29. Henriques JP, Zijlstra F, van 't Hof AW, et al. Angiographic assessment of reperfusion in acute myocardial infarction by myocardial blush grade. Circulation 2003; 107: 2115–2119.
30. Hoffmann R, Haager P, Arning J, et al. Usefulness of myocardial blush grade early and late after primary coronary angioplasty for acute myocardial infarction in predicting left ventricular function. Am J Cardiol 2003; 92:1015–1019.
31. McLaughlin MG, Stone GW, Aymong E, et al. Prognostic utility of comparative methods for assessment of ST-segment resolution after primary angioplasty for acute myocardial infarction: the Controlled Abciximab and Device Investigation to Lower Late Angioplasty Complications (CADILLAC) trial. J Am Coll Cardiol 2004; 44:1215–1223.
32. Poli A, Fetiveau R, Vandoni P, et al. Integrated analysis of myocardial blush and ST-segment elevation recovery after successful primary angioplasty: Real-time grading of microvascular reperfusion and prediction of early and late recovery of left ventricular function. Circulation 2002; 106:313–318.
33. van 't Hof AW, Liem A, Suryapranata H, et al. Angiographic assessment of myocardial reperfusion in patients treated with primary angioplasty for acute myocardial infarction: myocardial blush grade. Zwolle Myocardial Infarction Study Group. Circulation 1998; 97:2302–2306.
34. Stone GW, Peterson MA, Lansky AJ, et al. Impact of normalized myocardial perfusion after successful angioplasty in acute myocardial infarction. J Am Coll Cardiol 2002; 39:591–597.

35. Topol EJ, Yadav JS. Recognition of the importance of embolization in atherosclerotic vascular disease. Circulation 2000; 101:570–580.
36. Baim DS, Wahr D, George B, et al. Randomized trial of a distal embolic protection device during percutaneous intervention of saphenous vein aorto-coronary bypass grafts. Circulation 2002; 105:1285–1290.
37. Sutsch G, Kiowski W, Bossard A, et al. Use of an emboli containment and retrieval system during percutaneous coronary angioplasty in native coronary arteries. Schweiz Med Wochenschr 2000; 130:1135–1145.
38. Webb JG, Carere RG, Virmani R, et al. Retrieval and analysis of particulate debris after saphenous vein graft intervention. J Am Coll Cardiol 1999; 34:468–475.
39. Huang Z, Katoh O, Nakamura S, et al. Evaluation of the PercuSurge GuardWire plus temporary occlusion and aspiration system during primary angioplasty in acute myocardial infarction. Catheter Cardiovasc Interv 2003; 60:443–451.
40. Kusuyama T, Kataoka T, Lida H, et al. Comparison of temporary occlusion and aspiration system versus the conventional method during coronary stenting for acute myocardial infarction. Am J Cardiol 2004; 94:1041–1043.
41. Nakamura T, Kubo N, Seki Y, et al. Effects of a distal protection device during primary stenting in patients with acute anterior myocardial infarction. Circ J 2004; 68:763–768.
42. Orrego PS, Delgado A, Piccalo G, et al. Distal protection in native coronary arteries during primary angioplasty in acute myocardial infarction: single-center experience. Catheter Cardiovasc Interv 2003; 60:152–158.
43. Pershad A, Cherukiri G, Kirby A. Percusurge guardwire balloon-associated thrombus–a limitation of the Percusurge distal protection system. J Invasive Cardiol 2002; 14:630–632.
44. Yip HK, Wu CJ, Chang HW, et al. Effect of the PercuSurge GuardWire device on the integrity of microvasculature and clinical outcomes during primary transradial coronary intervention in acute myocardial infarction. Am J Cardiol 2003; 92:1331–1335.
45. Amann FW. Revascularization utilizing balloon protection in acute coronary ischemic syndrome [RUBY Registry interim results]. in TCT abstract presentation 2004. Available at: http://www.tctmd.com.
46. Stone GW, Webb JG, Cox D, et al. A randomized, controlled trial of distal micro-circulatory protection during primary angioplasty in acute myocardial infarction. JAMA 2005; (In press).
47. Muramatsu T, Suwa S, Koyama S, et al. Early results from the Japanese Asparagus trial. J Am Coll Cardiol 2004; 43(5 supp2):A285.
48. Muramatsu T. Aspiration of liberated debris in acute MI with GuardWire Plus TM System [ASPARAGUS Trial]. in TCT abstract presentation 2005. Available at: http://www.tctmd.com.
49. Limbruno U, Micheli A, De Carlo M, et al. Mechanical prevention of distal embolization during primary angioplasty: safety, feasibility, and impact on myocardial reperfusion. Circulation 2003; 108:171–176.
50. Popma JJ, Cox N, Hauptmann KE, et al. Initial clinical experience with distal protection using the FilterWire in patients undergoing coronary artery and saphenous vein graft percutaneous intervention. Catheter Cardiovasc Interv 2002; 57:125–134.
51. Gick M, Jander N, Bestehorn HP, et al. Randomized evaluation of the effects of filter-based distal protection on myocardial perfusion and infarct size after primary percu-taneous catheter intervention in myocardial infarction with and without ST-segment elevation. Circulation 2005; 112(10):1462–1469.
52. Mauri L, Cox D, Hermiller J, et al. The PROXIMAL trail: proximal protection during saphenous vein graft intervention using the Proxis Embolic Protection System: a randomized, prospective, multicenter clinical trial. J Am Coll Cardiol 2007; 50(15): 1442–1449.
53. Koch KT, de Winter RJ, Henriques MDJ, et al. Proximal embolic protection and thrombus aspiration in percutaneous coronary intervention of acute myocardial infarction using the Proxis Proxis® device. in TCT abstract presentation 2005. Available at: http://www.tctmd.com.
54. Sutsch G. Early data from pilot studies: progress or more of the same? [PROXIS™ AMI]. in TCT abstract presentation 2004. Available at: http://www.tctmd.com.

55. Ho PC, Leung CY. Rheolytic thrombectomy with distal filter embolic protection as adjunctive therapies to high-risk saphenous vein graft intervention. Catheter Cardiovasc Interv 2004; 61:202–205.
56. Barbeau G. Filter-based distal protection in acute myocardial infarction: first presentation of the Canadian FLAME study. in TCT abstract presentation 2005. Available at http://www.tctmd.com.
57. Hermiller J, Cox D, Barbeau G, et al. Distal filter embolic protection in AMI [The FLAME Registry]. in TCT; 2005. Available at: http://www.tctmd.com.
58. Abendschein DR, Tacker WA Jr., Babbs CF. Protection of ischemic myocardium by whole-body hypothermia after coronary artery occlusion in dogs. Am Heart J 1978; 96:772–780.
59. Chien GL, Wolff RA, Davis RF, et al. "Normothermic range" temperature affects myocardial infarct size. Cardiovasc Res 1994; 28:1014–1017.
60. Duncker DJ, Klassen CL, Ishibashi Y, et al. Effect of temperature on myocardial infarction in swine. Am J Physiol 1996; 270(4 pt 2):H1189–H1199.
61. Miki T, Liu GS, Cohen MV, et al. Mild hypothermia reduces infarct size in the beating rabbit heart: a practical intervention for acute myocardial infarction? Basic Res Cardiol 1998; 93:372–383.
62. van den Doel MA, Gho BC, Duval SY, et al. Hypothermia extends the cardioprotection by ischaemic preconditioning to coronary artery occlusions of longer duration. Cardiovasc Res 1998; 37:76–81.
63. Voorhees WD III, Abendschein DR, Tacker WA Jr. Effect of whole-body hypothermia on myocardial blood flow and infarct salvage during coronary artery occlusion in dogs. Am Heart J 1984; 107(5 pt 1):945–949.
64. Dae MW, Gao DW, Sessler DI, et al. Effect of endovascular cooling on myocardial temperature, infarct size, and cardiac output in human-sized pigs. Am J Physiol Heart Circ Physiol 2002; 282:H1584–H1591.
65. Hale SL, Dave RH, Kloner RA. Regional hypothermia reduces myocardial necrosis even when instituted after the onset of ischemia. Basic Res Cardiol 1997; 92:351–357.
66. Hale SL, Kloner RA. Myocardial temperature in acute myocardial infarction: protection with mild regional hypothermia. Am J Physiol 1997; 273(1 pt 2):H220–H227.
67. Vanden Hoek T, Shao Z, Li C, et al. Do we reperfuse or cool down first to resuscitate ischemic tissue? Circulation 2000; 102(II):570.
68. Dixon SR, Whitbourn RJ, Dae MW, et al. Induction of mild systemic hypothermia with endovascular cooling during primary percutaneous coronary intervention for acute myocardial infarction. J Am Coll Cardiol 2002; 40:1928–1934.
69. Ning XH, Xu CS, Song YC, et al. Hypothermia preserves function and signaling for mitochondrial biogenesis during subsequent ischemia. Am J Physiol 1998; 274(3 pt 2): H786–H793.
70. Toyoda T, Suzuki S, Kassell NF, et al. Intraischemic hypothermia attenuates neutrophil infiltration in the rat neocortex after focal ischemia-reperfusion injury. Neurosurgery 1996; 39:1200–1205.
71. Michelson AD, MacGregor H, Barnard MR, et al. Reversible inhibition of human platelet activation by hypothermia in vivo and in vitro. Thromb Haemost 1994; 71:633–640.
72. O'Neill WW. A prospective randomized trial of mild systemic hypothermia during PCI treatment of ST elevation MI. in TCT. Sep 16. 2003.
73. Rizik DG. Ajunctive therapies inthe treatment of acute MI. in TCT. Dec 21. 2004.
74. Intravascular cooling adjunctive to percutaneous coronary intervention, part 1 (ICE-IT-1). in TCT. Oct, 27. 2004. Washington, DC.
75. Kloner RA, Ganote CE, Jennings RB. The "no-reflow" phenomenon after temporary coronary occlusion in the dog. J Clin Invest 1974; 54:1496–1508.
76. Ogawa S, Gerlach H, Esposito C, et al. Hypoxia modulates the barrier and coagulant function of cultured bovine endothelium. Increased monolayer permeability and induction of procoagulant properties. J Clin Invest 1990; 85:1090–1098.
77. Ginis I, Mentzer SJ, Li X, et al. Characterization of a hypoxia-responsive adhesion molecule for leukocytes on human endothelial cells. J Immunol 1995; 155:802–810.

78. Cha HS, Ahn KS, Jeon CH, et al. Influence of hypoxia on the expression of matrix metalloproteinase-1, -3 and tissue inhibitor of metalloproteinase-1 in rheumatoid synovial fibroblasts. Clin Exp Rheumatol 2003; 21:593–598.
79. Thom SR, Elbuken ME. Oxygen-dependent antagonism of lipid peroxidation. Free Radic Biol Med 1991; 10:413–426.
80. Hills BA. A role for oxygen-induced osmosis in hyperbaric oxygen therapy. Med Hypotheses 1999; 52:259–263.
81. Sirsjo A, Lehr HA, Nolte D, et al. Hyperbaric oxygen treatment enhances the recovery of blood flow and functional capillary density in postischemic striated muscle. Circ Shock 1993; 40:9–13.
82. Zamboni WA, Roth AC, Russell RC, et al. The effect of hyperbaric oxygen on reperfusion of ischemic axial skin flaps: a laser Doppler analysis. Ann Plast Surg 1992; 28:339–341.
83. Thurston JG, Greenwood TW, Bending MR, et al. A controlled investigation into the effects of hyperbaric oxygen on mortality following acute myocardial infarction. Q J Med 1973; 42:751–770.
84. Cameron AJ, Hutton I, Kenmure AC, et al. Haemodynamic and metabolic effects of hyperbaric oxygen in myocardial infarction. Lancet 1966; 2:833–837.
85. Sterling DL, Thornton JD, Swafford A, et al. Hyperbaric oxygen limits infarct size in ischemic rabbit myocardium in vivo. Circulation 1993; 88(4 pt 1):1931–1936.
86. Thomas MP, Brown LA, Sponseller DR, et al. Myocardial infarct size reduction by the synergistic effect of hyperbaric oxygen and recombinant tissue plasminogen activator. Am Heart J 1990; 120:791–800.
87. Shandling AH, Ellestad MH, Hart GB, et al. Hyperbaric oxygen and thrombolysis in myocardial infarction: the "HOT MI" pilot study. Am Heart J 1997; 134:544–550.
88. Stavitsky Y, Shandling AH, Ellestad MH, et al. Hyperbaric oxygen and thrombolysis in myocardial infarction: the 'HOT MI' randomized multicenter study. Cardiology 1998; 90:131–136.
89. Glazier JJ. Attenuation of reperfusion microvascular ischemia by aqueous oxygen: experimental and clinical observations. Am Heart J 2005; 149:580–584.
90. Bartorelli AL. Hyperoxemic perfusion for treatment of reperfusion microvascular ischemia in patients with myocardial infarction. Am J Cardiovasc Drugs 2003; 3:53–63.
91. Spears JR, Wang B, Wu X, et al. Aqueous oxygen: a highly O2-supersaturated infusate for regional correction of hypoxemia and production of hyperoxemia. Circulation 1997; 96:4385–4391.
92. Spears JR, Henney C, Prcevski P, et al. Aqueous oxygen hyperbaric reperfusion in a porcine model of myocardial infarction. J Invasive Cardiol 2002; 14:160–166.
93. Spears JR, Prcevski P, Xu R, et al. Aqueous oxygen attenuation of reperfusion microvascular ischemia in a canine model of myocardial infarction. Asaio J 2003; 49:716–720.
94. Dixon SR, Bartorelli AL, Marcovitz PA, et al. Initial experience with hyperoxemic reperfusion after primary angioplasty for acute myocardial infarction: results of a pilot study utilizing intracoronary aqueous oxygen therapy. J Am Coll Cardiol 2002; 39:387–392.
95. O'Neill WW, Martin JL, Dixon SR, et al. Acute Myocardial Infarction with Hyperoxemic Therapy (AMIHOT): a prospective, randomized trial of intracoronary hyperoxemic reperfusion after percutaneous coronary intervention. J Am Coll Cardiol 2007; 50(5): 397–405.
96. Claeys MJ, Bosmans J, Veenstra L, et al. Determinants and prognostic implications of persistent ST-segment elevation after primary angioplasty for acute myocardial infarction: importance of microvascular reperfusion injury on clinical outcome. Circulation 1999; 99:1972–1977.
97. Schiller NB, Shah PM, Crawford M, et al. Recommendations for quantitation of the left ventricle by two-dimensional echocardiography. American Society of Echocardiography Committee on Standards, Subcommittee on Quantitation of Two-Dimensional Echocardiograms. J Am Soc Echocardiogr 1989; 2:358–367.
98. Ito H, Maruyama A, Iwakura K, et al. Clinical implications of the 'no reflow' phenomenon. A predictor of complications and left ventricular remodeling in reperfused anterior wall myocardial infarction. Circulation 1996; 93:223–228.

99. Keyes JW, Leonard PF, Brody SL, et al. Myocardial infarct quantification in the dog by single photon emission computed tomography. Circulation 1978; 58:227–232.
100. Sciagra R, Bolognese L, Rovai D, et al. Detecting myocardial salvage after primary PTCA: early myocardial contrast echocardiography versus delayed sestamibi perfusion imaging. J Nucl Med 1999; 40:363–370.
101. Wu KC, Zerhouni EA, Judd RM, et al. Prognostic significance of microvascular obstruction by magnetic resonance imaging in patients with acute myocardial infarction. Circulation 1998; 97:765–772.
102. Gibson CM, Cannon CP, Murphy SA, et al. Relationship of TIMI myocardial perfusion grade to mortality after administration of thrombolytic drugs. Circulation 2000; 101:125–130.

16

Optimal Strategies for Prehospital and Emergency Department Evaluation of Patients with STEMI

Judd E. Hollander

Department of Emergency Medicine, Hospital of the University of Pennsylvania, Philadelphia, Pennsylvania, U.S.A.

INTRODUCTION

Potential ischemic heart disease is the third most common cause of Emergency Department (ED) visits, after trauma and upper respiratory infection. There were over 5.8 million ED visits with a primary diagnosis of acute chest pain in 2003 (1). Approximately 18 million electrocardiograms (ECG) are obtained on ED patients in the United States annually (1). This chapter will focus on the specific role of the prehospital provider and the emergency physician in identification, risk stratification, and timely treatment of patients with ST elevation myocardial infarction (STEMI). Because the steps taken by all health care providers who evaluate patients with STEMI are similar, this chapter is organized by the approach to the evaluation and treatment of patients with STEMI, rather than by the location of the health care provider (prehospital or ED).

EARLY IDENTIFICATION OF THE PATIENT WITH STEMI

The care of patients with a potential acute coronary syndrome (ACS) differs from the care of patients with other nonemergent conditions, in that the approach to ACS patients is based most heavily on the ECG. Although standard medical practice typically is to perform a history and physical examination prior to diagnostic testing, this is not ideal in patients with potential ACS. Patients with STEMI are identified by the ECG and, therefore, the ECG is of primary importance and should be obtained either before or concurrent with the history and physical examination.

Electrocardiogram

The standard 12-lead ECG is the single best test to identify patients with acute myocardial infarction (MI) upon ED presentation (2–5). It plays a prominent role in every risk stratification algorithm for MI (6–10). National guidelines call for it to be obtained and interpreted within 10 minutes of presentation (11–14), although this guideline is met in the minority of patients (15).

The addition of V4R-V6R and V7-V9 leads to an 8% increase in sensitivity for MI relative to a standard 12-lead ECG, but at the cost of a 7% decrease in specificity (16,17). Right-sided lead RV4 should be used in the setting of inferior wall MI to assess possible RV involvement (8).

Patients with persistent symptoms and a nondiagnostic initial ECG should receive a repeat ECG to reassess the ST-segments. Continuous 12-lead ST-segment trend monitoring may also be useful in this regard (8). Serial ECGs and continuous 12-lead ST-segment trend monitoring may help identify patients who progress

TABLE 1 Multivariate Significance of the Electrocardiogram in Patients with STEMI Enrolled in GUSTO-1

Electrocardiographic feature	Odds ratio (95% CI)
Sum of ST-segment deviation (19 mm vs. 8 mm)	1.53 (1.38–1.69)
Sum of ST-segment decrease (−1 mm vs. −7 mm)	0.77 (0.72–0.83)
Heart rate (84 bpm vs. 60 bpm)	1.49 (1.41–1.59)
Sum ST-segment increase in II, III, and aVF (6 mm vs. 0 mm)	0.79 (0.71–0.89)
QRS duration 100 msec vs. 80 msec	
Anterior infarct	1.55 (1.43–1.68)
Other location	1.08 (1.03–1.13)
Anterior infarction	
QRS duration 100 msec	1.08 (1.03–1.13)
QRS duration 50 msec	0.61 (0.43–0.86)
Inferior infarction	
No prior AMI	0.67 (0.50–0.90)
Prior AMI	1.41 (0.98–2.02)
Prior infarction	
Inferior infarction	2.47 (2.02–3.00)
Other location	1.17 (0.98–1.41)

Source: From Ref. 3.

from unstable angina to STEMI after the initial ECG. In patients with STEMI, ECG variables not only identify the condition, they also predict the likelihood of 30-day mortality (Table 1) (3).

Prehospital Electrocardiography

Most emergency medical providers still do not have the capability to perform a prehospital 12-lead ECG despite the fact that many studies have shown that both field physicians and specially trained paramedics can implement this technology (18–32). The Milwaukee Prehospital Chest Pain Project, a major U.S. demonstration project, showed the clear feasibility and utility of a 12-lead ECG in the hands of well-trained paramedics (25,28). ECGs were acquired in 95% of patients with chest pain. The prehospital tracings had a high concordance with in-hospital ECGs: 99.3% for MI and 92.8% for angina.

Interpretation of prehospital ECGs can be accomplished by several routes. Historically, 12-lead ECG interpretation was not incorporated into paramedic training, so ECGs were transmitted to a base physician where they were interpreted (33). Alternatively, on-scene computerized interpretation improves sensitivity and specificity of the interpretation (34). When they receive specialized training, paramedics are capable of performing ECG interpretation as well as physicians (35). In 1998, ECG education was added to the emergency medical technician-paramedic curriculum as "enhanced" rather than "core" content (36).

A meta-analysis of five studies that evaluated the utility of the prehospital 12-lead ECG found that "on-scene" time was increased by only 1.2 minutes, while the time to fibrinolytic administration was decreased by 36.1 minutes (37). Only one study examined mortality as an outcome. In the cohort of 199 patients, the mortality was not statistically different (8.4% vs. 15.6%) (38), but that study was underpowered to detect a clinically relevant benefit. Data from the NRMI-2 registry showed that a prehospital ECG was associated with a 10-minute reduction in door-to-needle time and 23-minute reduction in door-to-balloon time, as well as a reduction in mortality (adjusted odds ratio 0.83) (39).

History and Physical Examination

When patients present with acute chest pain syndromes, it is often not clear whether the pain is cardiac or noncardiac in origin. For that reason, most patients with symptoms consistent with an ACS should be considered to have an ACS, until proven otherwise. At the time of presentation, the most immediate concern is the identification of patients who have ACS from the larger cohort of non-ACS chest pain patients. Broad-based ED studies of patients who received an ECG for the evaluation of symptoms consistent with ACS have found that approximately 15% of these patients have an ACS; one-third of whom sustain MI (40–42). Thus, 85% of patients have non-ACS causes for their symptoms. From the ED perspective, it is important to expeditiously distinguish between these two groups of patients.

Although historical features such as substernal location of pain, radiation of pain to the left arm, and history of MI predict a higher likelihood of MI (Table 2), they are not reliable enough to be used to distinguish STEMI from non–ST-segment elevation MI (NSTEMI) from noncardiac chest pain (43–45). Likewise, although traditional cardiac risk factors, derived from population-based cohort studies of asymptomatic patients, are predictive of coronary artery disease in asymptomatic patients, they are poor predictors of MI in patients with symptoms (46). The presence of symptoms outweighs the predictive abilities of cardiac risk factors.

The use of the physical examination to distinguish patients with ACS from patients with noncardiac chest pain is prone to error. Patients with ACS may appear deceptively well without any clinical signs of distress or may be uncomfortable, pale, cyanotic, and in respiratory distress. The first and second heart sounds are often diminished because of poor myocardial contractility. An S3 is present in 15% to 20% of patients with MI. An S4 is common in patients with long-standing hypertension or myocardial dysfunction. The presence of a murmur can be an ominous sign (flail

TABLE 2 Likelihood Ratios for Clinical Features that Increase or Decrease Risk of AMI in Patients Presenting with Chest Pain

Clinical feature	Likelihood ratio (95% CI)
Increased likelihood of AMI	
Pain in chest or left arm	2.7[a]
Chest pain radiation	
To right shoulder	2.9 (1.4–6.0)
To left arm	2.3 (1.7–3.1)
To both left and right arm	7.1 (3.6–14.2)
Chest pain most important symptom	2[a]
History of MI	1.5–3.0[b]
Nausea or vomiting	1.9 (1.7–2.3)
Diaphoresis	2.0 (1.9–2.2)
Third heart sound	3.2 (1.6–6.5)
Hypotension (systolic BP < 80 mmHg)	3.1 (1.8–5.2)
Pulmonary crackles	2.1 (1.4–3.1)
Decreased likelihood of AMI	
Pleuritic chest pain	0.2 (0.2–0.3)
Chest pain sharp or stabbing	0.3 (0.2–0.5)
Positional chest pain	0.3 (0.2–0.4)
Chest pain reproduced by palpation	0.2–0.4[b]

[a]Data not available to calculate confidence intervals.
[b]In heterogeneous studies the likelihood ratios are reported as ranges.
Source: From Ref. 44.

leaflet of the mitral valve or a ventricular septal defect), or it can reflect valvular heart disease. In the ED, knowledge about the patient's baseline condition can help establish which signs and symptoms are chronic; however, this information is often not available, especially in the prehospital setting. Although physical examination findings cannot distinguish between patients with and without ACS with any reasonable degree of reliability, the physical examination still needs to be performed because it can help guide management of patients with STEMI.

Risk Stratification Algorithms
Most risk stratification algorithms for identification of the patient with ACS are designed to distinguish the low-risk patient who can be discharged home or admitted to a non-CCU location from the high-risk patient. All algorithms rely heavily on the ECG. Three algorithms have particular utility for identifying and risk stratifying patients with STEMI: the acute cardiac ischemia-time insensitive predictive instrument (ACI-TIPI), the thrombolytic predictive instrument (TPI), and the thrombolysis in myocardial infarction (TIMI) risk score.

Acute Cardiac Ischemia-Time Insensitive Predictive Instrument
The ACI-TIPI is a computer-generated method to determine the likelihood of ACS at the time of initial clinical evaluation. The ACI-TIPI ECG incorporates age, sex, presence of chest or left arm pain, a chief symptom of chest or left arm pain, pathologic Q waves, and the presence and degree of ST-segment elevation or depression and T-wave elevation or inversion. It reports the percent likelihood of "acute cardiac ischemia" on the ECG record. Four studies including 5496 patients have found that when combined with physician impression, it has a sensitivity of 86% to 95% and a specificity of 78% to 92% for prediction of ACS (47). The ACI-TIPI has not been shown to make a clinically relevant difference in diagnostic accuracy compared with physician judgment alone (48). As a result, it has not been widely incorporated into clinical practice in the ED. It may have more value in the prehospital setting, particularly in settings where paramedics are not trained to interpret the ECG.

Thrombolytic Predictive Instrument
The TPI is a computer-derived estimate of the key outcomes of fibrinolytic therapy (30-day and one-year mortality and bleeding complications including hemorrhagic stroke). At the time of ECG acquisition, age, gender, history of hypertension, diabetes, actual blood pressure, and time since onset of ischemic symptoms are entered into the ECG machine. The ECG is printed along with the TPI predictions. One randomized controlled trial showed an increase in reperfusion therapy in some subsets of patients (females and inferior MI) (49,50). The use of this technology might be beneficial in the prehospital setting.

TIMI Risk Score
A TIMI risk score for STEMI exists. It is a simple integer score (Table 3). The risk score was evaluated in 84,029 patients with STEMI from the National Registry of Myocardial Infarction 3 and correctly predicted risk of death (51). There was a significant graded increase in mortality with higher scores (range, 1.1–30%). The

TABLE 3 Elements of the TIMI Score for ST-segment elevation AMI

Clinical risk indicators	Points
Historical	
Age > 75 yr	3
Age 65–74 yr	2
History of diabetes, hypertension, or angina	1
Physical examination	
Systolic blood pressure < 100 mmHg	3
Heart rate > 100 bpm	2
Killip class II–IV	2
Weight < 67 kg	1
Presentation	
Anterior ST-segment elevation or LBBB	1
Time to reperfusion > 4 hr	1
Total points possible	14

Source: From Ref. 51.

risk score showed strong prognostic capacity overall among patients receiving acute reperfusion therapy whether they were treated with fibrinolytic therapy or primary percutaneous coronary intervention (PCI). However, patients that did not receive reperfusion therapy had a higher mortality rate than that predicted by this risk score (51).

Markers of Myocardial Injury

In the ED, the ideal biomarker will allow early detection of patients with ACS, enable optimal treatment pathways to be initiated, and assist with rapid determination of patient disposition. Biomarkers with high positive predictive values are ideal to mobilize evaluation and treatment for patients at high risk of cardiovascular complications, such as those with STEMI. Decisions regarding reperfusion therapy should not be delayed to obtain results of cardiac biomarkers because up to two-thirds of patients with MI do not have positive biomarkers at the time of initial evaluation (47).

Echocardiography

Echocardiography, when used to assess wall motion, has a sensitivity for detection of an AMI of approximately 93% but a specificity of only 53% to 57% (8). It cannot distinguish old from new MI. As a result, it is more useful in patients without a past history of coronary artery disease. Larger areas of infarction and more depressed left ventricular function predict a higher likelihood of cardiovascular complications and an increased risk for mortality (52). The addition of echocardiography to baseline clinical variables and the initial ECG appears to have independent predictive value (53). The predictive properties of echocardiography and myocardial perfusion imaging were similar with respect to MI, PCI, and presence of coronary artery disease (54). Reperfusion therapy should never be delayed to obtain echocardiography in obvious STEMI patients. On the other hand, echocardiography may help diagnose STEMI in patients where the diagnosis is not clear (patients with left bundle branch block, cocaine-associated chest pain, or patients with ST-segment elevation that might be due to nonischemic conditions such as pericarditis or repolarization abnormalities).

TREATMENT CONSIDERATIONS

Specific Prehospital and ED Treatment Considerations

After demonstration of the safety and efficacy of various treatment strategies, there are other issues that must be considered to optimize incorporation of new treatments into the prehospital and ED setting. These issues focus on the ease of administration, time required for administration, individual institutional and physician preferences, and balancing the needs of multiple patients (ACS and non-ACS patients) simultaneously, since the prioritized care of any one group of patients may have detrimental impact on other patients in the ED (55,56).

From an emergency medicine perspective, the ideal treatment is easily obtained (stored in the ED); rapidly initiated (does not require reconstitution or suspension); administered in a single intravenous bolus (or orally); does not require continued intravenous infusion, titration, or monitoring of therapeutic levels; and is a component of a preestablished multidisciplinary clinical pathway. These treatment characteristics are of paramount importance in the ED, where physicians and nurses are actively caring for multiple critically ill patients simultaneously. Additionally, in the ED, there is the challenge of integrating the care of ACS patients with multiple primary care providers and cardiologists, each of which may have their own personal preferences.

For the treatment of STEMI patients, the decision on which patients will be treated with PCI, fibrinolytic therapy, or facilitated PCI should be protocolized and not addressed anew for each patient who arrives in the ED. Likewise the choice of fibrinolytic agent should be decided in advance and should take into account relative efficacy and safety, ease of administration, and need for concurrent medications. Assuming equivalent efficacy and safety, bolus fibrinolytics would be preferred over agents requiring more complicated intravenous infusions (57). Likewise, concurrent administration of antithrombotic and anti-ischemic agents that can be given in bolus or oral form is preferable.

Deciding the Method of Reperfusion

Reperfusion strategies for STEMI patients are extensively discussed throughout this text. In this section, I will focus on the on clinical decision points relative to the emergency physician in any individual patient. It should be noted, however, that each institution should develop a multidisciplinary committee to reach consensus on the approach to reperfusion therapy at their center. The issues that should be considered on an institutional and individual basis are discussed from the point of view of the emergency physician or prehospital provider.

Each institution, through collaborative development of a clinical pathway, should determine which predominant strategy it will use: primary PCI or fibrinolytic therapy. Which patients will receive which form of reperfusion should be determined taking both individual and institutional characteristics into account.

The choice of reperfusion therapy should take into account the time since symptom onset, risk of complications from STEMI, risk of complications from bleeding, risk of complications from primary PCI, and time required to administer fibrinolytic therapy compared with the time required to transport the patients to a skilled catheterization laboratory (14). Some of these items are patient specific and can best be determined at the bedside. Some of these items are institution specific and quality improvement data can help clinicians determine the best pathway for STEMI patients at their own institution.

The development of the clinical pathway also needs to take institutional strengths and weakness into account. For example, the approach to the patient with STEMI may differ depending upon operator availability, time of day, day of week, or whether it is a holiday (58). It is best to determine reperfusion strategy for all these institution-specific variables in a systematic way rather than when the patient presents to the ED. Clinical pathways should take the consensus guidelines into account, since guideline adherence has been shown to be associated with improved clinical outcomes (59,60).

Prehospital Reperfusion

There are three options for prehospital providers: transport to the closest facility (which will determine method of reperfusion), transport to a primary PCI center, or administer prehospital fibrinolytics.

It has been well established that relatively small delays in initiating reperfusion therapy during the first hours following symptom onset have a negative impact on the likelihood of achieving a favorable outcome (61). One meta-analysis found that treatment 30 minutes earlier while patients were within the first 90 minutes of symptoms decreased the death rate by 10 to 30 lives per 1000 patients (62). The recognition that STEMI patients require time-sensitive reperfusion has traditionally been the argument for ambulance transport to the nearest hospital for fibrinolytic administration (61,62).

Demonstration that a prehospital ECG could improve the time to administration of fibrinolytic therapy, and the astoundingly low 1.2% mortality rate seen in the MITI trial for patients treated within the first 70 minutes, led to several studies evaluating prehospital fibrinolysis (63). A meta-analysis of six randomized controlled trials with a total of 6434 patients found that relative to in-hospital fibrinolysis, prehospital fibrinolysis administered a mean of 58 minutes earlier, reduced all-cause hospital mortality (odds ratio, 0.83; 95% CI, 0.70–0.98) regardless of the training and experience of the provider (64). The improved mortality found with earlier fibrinolytic administration provides the compelling rationale for prehospital treatment of STEMI patients. ER-TIMI 19 demonstrated that a bolus prehospital fibrinolytic reteplase (rPA) improved the time from first medical contact to fibrinolytic administration, particularly in the cohort of patients where door-to-needle time exceeds 20 minutes (65), which is most fibrinolytic-treated patients (66).

Although primary PCI has been shown to provide improved outcomes in an all-comer population (67) of patients presenting to the ED, prehospital fibrinolysis offers a possible advantage, particularly in patients presenting within two to three hours of symptom onset. In the CAPTIM study (68), 840 STEMI patients were randomized to prehospital fibrinolysis versus primary PCI. The patients treated within two hours showed a mortality trend favoring the fibrinolytic treated group (2.2% vs. 5.7%); after two hours, the trend favored primary PCI.

The establishment of a prehospital fibrinolysis program requires a multi-disciplinary approach with significant input from prehospital providers, emergency physicians, and cardiologists both at initiation and continuously (Table 4). Integrated establishment of protocols as well as continuous review and modification are required from providers throughout the region, not just a single institution.

In prehospital systems that are set up to triage STEMI patients to a variety of facilities, time from symptom onset should logically be incorporated into the triage process. Patients with symptom onset of two to three hours or less would be

TABLE 4 Requirements for a Prehospital Fibrinolysis Program

Prehospital provider requirements
Advanced cardiac life support
Training in recognition and management of STEMI
12-lead electrocardiogram capabilities
Reliable lead placement
Reliable transmission (cellular phone in field)
Able to interpret electrocardiogram (either advanced paramedic training or computer assisted)
Reperfusion check list
Ability to establish intravenous access
Ability to store and administer medications
Ability to monitor patient
Regional requirements
Acceptance of program
Method of interpreting 12 lead electrocardiogram
Advanced training
Computerized interpretation
Transmission to central station
Training and quality assurance program

expected to benefit from timely prehospital or ED fibrinolysis in the event that they cannot rapidly receive primary PCI at a skilled center, since the time from symptom onset to reperfusion has more impact on outcome during this critical two to three hour period (69). Patients greater than three hours since symptom onset are expected to have improved outcomes if they are directly triaged to a skilled and available primary PCI center. Patients who are triaged directly from the prehospital setting to the cardiac catheterization laboratory for primary PCI receive expedited care if the cardiac catheterization team is mobilized prior to patient arrival (70).

Transfer Protocols

The clinical data and scientific rationale for establishing transfer protocols are well delineated in chapter 11. The development of transfer protocols and STEMI systems could be modeled after the well-established trauma systems that most emergency physicians are already familiar with. A reasonable strategy includes the following five steps (71):

1. Centralized MI centers with established expertise in primary PCI that are within reasonable proximity to the referral hospitals should be designated.
2. Emergency physicians at referral hospitals should rapidly identify STEMI patients who are candidates for primary PCI, administer initial medications, and rapidly transfer the patient to the MI center.
3. The referral and receiving hospitals should have central administration and coordination of the care.
4. Continuous quality monitoring should assess both processes of care and outcomes of patients that are and are not transferred from the referring hospitals to the centralized MI centers. State trauma foundations perform periodic reviews of this type for trauma centers.
5. Clinical research networks can be formed to extend MI research into the community hospitals.

Waters et al. (71) proposed the following standard measures to evaluate transfer strategies and monitor outcomes: time at referral hospital, transfer time, receiving

TABLE 5   Persons to be Notified with a Single Call for STEMI Transfer

Answering service/hospital operator
Admitting office, patient placement (bed control), and supervisor
Security
House supervisor
Pastoral care
Emergency physician
Emergency department charge nurse
Admitting cardiologist
Interventional cardiologist
Catheterization laboratory manager
Catheterization operations team
Cardiac care unit charge nurse
Cardiology coordinator
STEMI research coordinator/fellow

Source: From Ref. 72.

hospital door-to-balloon time, first medical contact-to-first balloon inflation at PCI hospital, and symptom onset-to-first balloon inflation time. Measurement of these intervals across all systems will allow continuous improvement methodology to determine the area of greatest delays and will facilitate improvement within any single system and allow comparison to successful strategies in other systems.

Using these principles, Henry et al. have demonstrated a 50% reduction in receiving hospital door-to-balloon time for transfer patients (reduction from 192 to 98 minutes) (72). Their system includes prehospital ECGs, immediate ECG acquisition in the community hospital ED, use of hospital specific transfer data sheets, checklists and standing orders, and a level 1 MI kit including all the forms, transfer data sheets, orders, adjunctive medications, and laboratory blood tubes to facilitate an in-the-door to out-the-door time at the referral hospital of under 30 minutes. Communication with the receiving hospital is further facilitated by a single phone call for transfer (Table 5). Clinical information is faxed directly to the receiving cardiac catheterization laboratory. The transfer itself has a predesignated approach depending upon the distance from the primary PCI center and has a designated backup plan accounting for adverse weather conditions and road conditions. On arrival at the primary PCI center, the patient is admitted immediately to the cardiac catheterization laboratory.

Prehospital Triage Protocols

The principles outlined regarding expeditious transfer to a primary PCI hospital could be adapted to the prehospital setting to further reduce the time from symptoms onset to balloon inflation. Rather than making the decision between fibrinolysis and primary PCI in the ED, this decision could be made in the prehospital setting.   Terkelsen et al. demonstrated that prehospital diagnosis and direct referral to a primary PCI center decreased time from first medical contact to first balloon inflation by 81 minutes compared with diagnosis in the ED, and by 40 minutes compared with prehospital diagnosis but transport to a local hospital (73). The demonstration that paramedics can accurately diagnose STEMI in the ambulance and appropriately administer fibrinolytic therapy supports the argument that they could make decisions regarding transfer to a primary PCI center rather than a local hospital. Early PCI laboratory activation, either by the prehospital providers or a telemedicine or emergency medicine physician, further reduces door-to-balloon time (70,73,74).

There is widespread consensus that patients with STEMI should have fibri-nolytic therapy initiated by emergency physicians without delaying care to obtain cardiology consultation (14). Emergency physician initiation of fibrinolytic therapy shortens the door-to-needle time (75–77), improves the likelihood of the patient receiving other appropriate medications, improves the time to ST-segment reso-lution, and decreases cardiovascular complications (75). Protocols to ensure rapid treatment and enable adherence to treatment guidelines require clear a priori definitions of which patients will receive primary PCI, so that the decision regarding method of reperfusion does not delay patient care. The decision on how to manage STEMI patients is best handled via a clinical pathway that requires a minimum of consultation for each new patient.

SPECIAL CONSIDERATIONS IN EMERGENCY MEDICINE

Atypical Presentations

Atypical presentations or silent myocardial ischemia are common. Between 22% and 40% of patients with Q-wave MI identified in large longitudinal studies are clinically unrecognized (78). Women and the elderly are more likely to have atypical presentations. The prognosis for patients who have atypical symptoms at the time of their infarction is worse than that of patients who had more typical symptoms. Multidisciplinary clinical pathways must take into account the volume of patients who present to the ED who have symptoms potentially compatible with ACS, but have atypical presentations. The approach to the initial evaluation of these patients must attempt to identify the STEMI and ACS patients from the multiple other conditions that can present with similar signs and symptoms. A properly interpreted ECG is the best initial test in this cohort and should identify the majority of patients with ACS, requiring time sensitive interventions.

Cocaine-Induced Myocardial Infarction

The risk of MI is increased 24-fold in the hour after cocaine use (79), and 25% of nonfatal MI in patients between the ages of 18 and 45 occurs in patients who have used cocaine (80). Approximately 6% of patients who present to the ED with cocaine-associated chest pain syndromes sustain AMI (81), 44% of which are STEMI (82). Patients with cocaine-associated MI have impaired epicardial and microvascular blood flow (83), and despite initial misconceptions, the majority of patients with cocaine-associated MI have atherosclerotic coronary artery disease (84,85).

Similar to patients with STEMI unrelated to cocaine, patients with cocaine-associated MI should be treated with aspirin, nitroglycerin, and antithombin therapy (11,14,85,86). There are some important treatment differences between patients with STEMI related and unrelated to cocaine (11,14,85,86). Benzodiazepines are also useful in patients with cocaine-associated chest pain; they have been shown to be equivalent to nitroglycerin with respect to symptomatic improvement and they lessen central nervous system toxicity from cocaine (87). Cocaine-associated MI patients have been successfully treated with phentolamine, which is an α-adrenergic antagonist that reverses cocaine-induced coronary artery vasoconstriction (11,85). β-Adrenergic antagonists should be avoided in patients with cocaine-induced STEMI because they worsen coronary artery vasoconstriction and do not improve outcome (11,14,85,86).

Reperfusion is best achieved with PCI in patients with cocaine-associated STEMI (88). Up to 43% of patients with cocaine-associated chest pain without MI meet TIMI criteria for the administration of fibrinolytic agents despite the fact that they are not infarcting (85). The potential administration of fibrinolytic agents to patients who are not infarcting coupled with a very low mortality from cocaine-associated MI limits the utility of fibrinolytic agents (11,85,88). Cardiac catheterization can facilitate diagnosis and allow PCI, if indicated.

REFERENCES

1. McCaig LF, Burt CW. Advance data from vital and health statistics; no. 358. National Hospital Ambulatory Medical Care Survey: 2003 Emergency Department Summary. Hyattsville, MD: National Center for Health Statistics. 2005.
2. Lee T, Cook F, Weisberg M, et al. Acute chest pain in the emergency room: identification and examination of low risk patients. Arch Intern Med 1985; 145:65–69.
3. Hathaway WR, Peterson ED, Wagner GS, et al. Prognostic significance of the initial electrocardiogram in patients with acute myocardial infarction. JAMA 1998; 279:387–391.
4. Slater DK, Hlatky MA, Mark DB, et al. Outcome in suspected acute myocardial infarction with normal or minimally abnormal admission electrocardiographic findings. Am J Cardiol 1987; 60:766–770.
5. Brush JE, Brand DA, Acampora D, et al. Use of the initial electrocardiogram to predict in-hospital complications of acute myocardial infarction. N Engl J Med 1985; 312:1137–1141.
6. Lee TH, Juarez G, Cook EF, et al. Ruling out myocardial infarction. A prospective multicenter validation of a 12-hour strategy for patients at low risk. N Engl J Med 1991; 324:1239–1246.
7. Selker HP, Beshanski JR, Griffith JL, et al. Use of the acute cardiac ischemia time-insensitive predictive instrument (ACI-TIPI) to assist with triage of patients with chest pain or other symptoms suggestive of acute cardiac ischemia: a multicenter, controlled clinical trial. Ann Intern Med 1998; 129:845–845.
8. Selker HP, Zalenski RJ, Antman EM, et al. An evaluation of technologies for identification of acute cardiac ischemia in the emergency department: a report from a National Heart Attack Alert Program Working Group. Ann Emerg Med 1997; 29:13–87.
9. Baxt WG, Shofer FS, Sites FD, et al. A neural computational aid to the diagnosis of acute myocardial infarction. Ann Emerg Med 2002; 39:366–373.
10. Antman EM, Cohen M, Bernink PJ, et al. The TIMI risk score for unstable angina/non-ST elevation MI: A method for prognostication and therapeutic decision making. JAMA 2000; 284:835–834.
11. The American Heart Association in Collaboration with the International Liason Committee on Resuscitation (ILCOR). Guidelines for Cardiopulmonary Resuscitation and Emergency Cardiovascular Care. Circulation 2000; 102:172.
12. Braunwald E, Antman EM, Beasley JW, et al. ACC/AHA guideline update for the management of patients with unstable angina and non–ST-segment elevation myocardial infarction—2002: a report of the American College of Cardiology/American Heart Association Task Force on Practice Guidelines (Committee on the Management of Patients with Unstable Angina). Circulation 2002; 106:1893–1900.
13. Gibler WB, Cannon CP, Blomkalns AL, et al. Practical implementation of the guidelines for unstable angina/non ST segment elevation myocardial infarction in the Emergency Department. Ann Emerg Med 2005; 46:185–197.
14. Antman EM, Anbe DT, Armstrong PW, et al. ACC/AHA guidelines for the management of patients with ST-elevation myocardial infarction: a report of the American College of Cardiology/American Heart Association Task Force on Practice Guidelines (Committee to Revise the 1999 Guidelines for the Management of Patients with Acute Myocardial Infarction). Available at: www.acc.org/clinical/guidelines/stemi/index.pdf.
15. Diercks DB, Peacock WF, Hiestand BC, et al. Frequency and consequences of recording an electrocardiogram >10 minutes after arrival in an emergency room in non-ST-segment elevation acute coronary syndromes. Am J Cardiol 2006; 97:437–442.

16. Zalenski RJ, Cooke D, Rydman R, et al. Assessing the diagnostic value of an ECG containing leads V4R, V8 and V9: The 15 lead ECG. Ann Emerg Med 1993; 22:786–793.

17. Zalenski RJ, Rydman RJ, Sloan EP, et al. Value of posterior and right ventricular leads in comparison to standard 12 lead electrocardiogram in evaluation of ST segment elevation in suspected acute myocardial infarction. Am J Cardiol 1997; 79:1579–1585.

18. Kereiakes DJ, Gibler WB, Martin LH et al. Relative importance of emergency medical transport and the prehospital electrocardiogram on reducing hospital time delay to therapy for acute myocardial infarction: A preliminary report from the Cincinnati Heart Project. Am Heart J 1992; 123:835–840.

19. Castaigne AD, Duval AM, Dubois-Rande JL, et al. Prehospital administration of anisoylated plasminogen streptokinase activator complex in acute myocardial infarction. Drugs 1987; 33(suppl 3):231–234.

20. Villemant D, Barriot P, Bodeman P, et al. At home thrombolysis and myocardial infarction: a real saving of time. Eur Heart J 1987; 8(suppl):103.

21. Weiss AT, Fine DG, Appelbaum D, et al. Prehospital coronary thrombolysis: a new strategy in acute myocardial infarction. Chest 1987; 92:124–128.

22. Bippus PH, Haux R, Schroder R. Prehospital intravenous streptokinase in evolving myocardial infarction: a randomized study about feasibility, safety, and time gain. Eur Heart J 1987; 8(suppl):103.

23. Bossaert LL, Demey HE, Colemont LJ, et al. Prehospital thrombolytic treatment of acute myocardial infarction with anisoylated plasminogen streptokinase activator complex. Crit Care Med 1988; 16:823–830.

24. Castaigne A, Herve C, Duval-Moulin A, et al. Prehospital use of APSAC: results of a placebo-controlled study. Am J Cardiol 1989; 64:A30–A33.

25. Aufderheide TP, Keelan MH, Hendley GE, et al. Milwaukee Chest Pain Project. Phase I. Feasibility and accuracy of prehospital thrombolytic candidate selection. Am J Cardiol 1992; 69:991–996.

26. Weaver WB, Eisenberg MS, Martin JS, et al. Myocardial infarction triage and intervention project. Phase I. Patient characteristics and feasibility of prehospital initiation of thrombolytic therapy. J Am Coll Cardiol 1990; 15:925–931.

27. Gibler WB, Kereiakes DJ, Dean EN, et al. Prehospital diagnosis and treatment of acute myocardial infarction: a north-south perspective. Am Heart J 1991; 121:1–10.

28. Aufderheide TP, Hendley GE, Thakur RK, et al. The diagnostic impact of prehospital 12-lead electrocardiography. Ann Emerg Med 1990; 19:1280–1287.

29. Aufderheide TP, Hendley GE, Woo J, et al. A prospective evaluation of prehospital 12-lead ECG application in chest pain patients. J Electrocardiol 1992; 24(suppl):8–13.

30. Grim P, Feldman T, Childers RW. Evaluation of patients for the need of thrombolytic therapy in the prehospital setting. Ann Emerg Med 1989; 18:483–488.

31. Kereiakes DJ, Weaver WD, Anderson JL. et al. Time delays in the diagnosis and treatment of acute myocardial infarction: A tale of eight cities. Am Heart J 1990; 120:773–780.

32. Karagounis L, Ipsen SK, Jessop MR, et al. Impact of field-transmitted electrocardiography on time to in-hospital thrombolytic therapy in acute myocardial infarction. Am J Cardiol 1990; 66:786–791.

33. Lambrew CT. The experience in telemetry of the electrocardiogram to a base hospital. Heart Lung 1974; 3:756–764.

34. Kudenchuk PJ, Ho MT, Weaver WD, et al. Accuracy of computer interpreted electrocardiography in selecting patients for thrombolytic therapy. MITI project investigators. J Am Coll Cardiol 1991; 17:1486–1491.

35. Feldman JA, Brinsfield K, Bernard S, et al. Real time paramedic compared to blinded physician identification of ST segment elevation myocardial infarction: results of an observational study. Am J Emerg Med 2005; 23:443–448.

36. Garvey JL, MacLeod BA, Sopko G, et al. Prehospital 12-lead electrocardiography programs. J Am Coll Cardiol 2006; 47:485–491.

37. Morrison LJ, Brooks S, Sawadsky B, et al. Prehospital 12 lead electrocardiography impact on acute myocardial infarction treatment times and mortality: a systematic review. Acad Emerg Med 2006; 13:84–89.

38. Millar-Craig MW, Joy AV, Adamowicz M, et al. Reduction in treatment delay by paramedic ECG diagnosis of myocardial infarction with direct CCU admission. Heart 1997; 78:456–461.
39. Canto JG, Rogers WJ, Bowlby IJ, et al. The prehospital electrocardiogram in acute myocardial infarction; is its full potential being realized? J Am Coll Cardiol 1997; 29:498–505.
40. Blomkalns AL, Lindsell CJ, Chandra A, et al. Can electrocardiographic criteria predict adverse cardiac events and positive cardiac markers? Acad Emerg Med 2003; 10:205–210.
41. Miller CD, Lindsell CJ, Khandelwal S, et al. Is the initial diagnostic impression of "noncardiac chest pain" adequate to exclude cardiac disease? Ann Emerg Med 2004; 44:565–574.
42. Pollack CV Jr., Sites FD, Shofer FS, et al. Application of the TIMI risk score for unstable angina and non-ST elevation acute coronary syndrome to an unselected emergency department chest pain population. Acad Emerg Med 2006; 13:13–18.
43. Hickan DH, Sox HC, Sox CH. Systematic bias in recording history in patients with chest pain. J Chronic Dis 1985; 38:91–100.
44. Panju AA, Hemmelgarm BR, Guyatt GH, Simel DL. Is this patient having a myocardial infarction? JAMA 1998; 280:1256–1263.
45. Swap CJ, Nagurney JT. Value and limitations of chest pain history in the evaluation of patients with suspected acute coronary syndromes. JAMA 2005; 294:2623–2629.
46. Jayes RL, Beshansky JR, D'Agostino RB, et al. Do patients' coronary risk factor reports predict acute cardiac ischemia in the emergency department? A multicenter study. J Clin Epidemiol 1992; 45:621–626.
47. Lau J, Ioannidis JPA, Balk EM, et al. Diagnosing acute cardiac ischemia in the Emergency Department: A systematic review of the accuracy and clinical effect of current technologies. Ann Emerg Med 2001; 37:453–460.
48. Sarasin FP, Reymond JM, Griffith JL, et al. Impact of the acute cardiac ischemia time insensitive predictive instrument (ACI-TIPI) on the speed of triage decision making for emergency department patients presenting with chest pain: a controlled clinical trial. J Gen Intern Med 1994; 9:187–194.
49. Selker HP, Griffith JL, Beshansky JR, et al. Patient-specific predictions of outcomes in myocardial infarction for real-time emergency use: a thrombolytic predictive instrument. Ann Intern Med 1997; 127:538–556.
50. Selker HP, Beshansky JR, Griffith JL. Use of the electrocardiograph-based thrombolytic predictive instrument to assist thrombolytic and reperfusion therapy for acute myocardial infarction. A multicenter, randomized, controlled, clinical effectiveness trial. Ann Intern Med 2002; 137:87–95.
51. Morrow DA, Antman EM, Parsons L. et al. Application of the TIMI risk score for ST-elevation MI in the National Registry of Myocardial Infarction 3. JAMA 2001; 286:1356–1359.
52. Fleischmann KE, Lee TH, Come PC, et al. Echocardiographic prediction of complications in patients with chest pain. Am J Cardiol 1997; 79:292–298.
53. Kontos MC, Arrowood JA, Paulsen WHJ, et al. Early echocardiography can predict cardiac events in Emergency Department patients with chest pain. Ann Emerg Med 1998; 31:550–557.
54. Paventi S, Parafati MA, DiLuzio E, et al. Usefulness of two dimensional echocardiography and myocardial perfusion imaging for immediate evaluation of chest pain in the emergency department. Resuscitation 2001; 49:47–51.
55. Chen EH, Mills AM, Lee BY, et al. Impact of concurrent trauma evaluation on time to CT in patients with suspected stroke. Acad Emerg Med 2006; 13:349–352.
56. Fishman PE, Shofer FS, Robey JL, et al. The impact of trauma activations on the care of ED patients with potential acute coronary syndromes. Ann Emerg Med 2006; (in press).
57. Leah V, Clark C, Doyle K, et al. Does a single bolus thrombolytic reduce door to needle time in a district general hospital? Emerg Med J 2004; 21:162–164.
58. Magid DJ, Wang Y, Herrin J, et al. Relationship between time of day, day of week, timeliness of reperfusion, and in-hospital mortality for patients with acute ST-segment elevation myocardial infarction. JAMA 2005; 294:803–812.

59. Mehta BH, Montoye CK, Gallogly M, et al. Improving quality of care for acute myocardial infarction. The guidelines applied in practice (GAP) initiative. JAMA 2002; 287:1269–1276.
60. Eagle KA, Montoye CK, Riba AL, et al. Guideline-based standardized care is associated with substantially lower mortality in medicare patients with acute myocardial infarction. J Am Coll Cardiol 2005; 46:1242–1248.
61. DeLuca G, Suruapranata H, Ottervanger JP, et al. Time delay to treatment and mortality in primary angioplasty for acute myocardial infarction. Circulation 2004; 109:1223–1225.
62. Boersma E, Maas AC, Deckers JW, et al. Early thrombolytic treatment in acute myocardial infarction; reappraisal of the golden hour. Lancet 1996; 348:771–775.
63. Weaver WD, Cerqueria M, Hallstrom AP, et al. Prehospital initiated vs. hospital initiated thrombolytic therapy; the myocardial infarction triage and intervention trial. JAMA 1993; 270:1211–1216.
64. Morrison LJ, Verbeek PR, McDonald AC, et al. Mortality and prehospital thrombolysis for acute myocardial infarction: A meta-analysis. JAMA 2000; 283:2686–2692.
65. Morrow DA, Antman EM, Sayah A, et al. Evaluation of the time saved by pre-hospital initiation of reteplase for ST elevation myocardial infarction: results of the early retevase-thrombolysis in myocardial infarction (ER-TIMI 19) trial. J Am Coll Cardiol 2002; 40:71–77.
66. Fibrinolytic Therapy Trialists (FTT) Collaborative Group. Indications for fibrinolytic therapy in suspected acute myocardial infarction: collaborative overview of early mortality and major morbidity results from all randomized trials of more than 1000 patients. Lancet 1994; 343:311–322.
67. Keeley EC, Boura JA, Grines CL. Primary angioplasty versus intravenous thrombolytic therapy for acute myocardial infarction: a quantitative review of 23 randomised trials. Lancet 2003; 361:13–20.
68. Steg PG, Bonnefoy E, Chabaud S, et al. Impact of time to treatment on mortality after prehospital fibrinolysis or primary angioplasty: data from the CAPTIM randomized clinical trial. Circulation 2003; 108:2851–2856.
69. Gersh BJ, Stone GW, White HD, et al. Pharmacological facilitation of primary percutaneous coronary intervention for acute myocardial infarction: is the slope of the curve the shape of the future? JAMA 2005; 293:979–986.
70. Bradley EH, Roumanis SA, Radford MJ, et al. Achieving door-to-balloon times that meet quality guidelines. How do successful hospitals do it? J Am Coll Cardiol 2005; 46:1236–1241.
71. Waters E, Singh KP, Roe MT, et al. Rationale and strategies for implementing community based transfer protocols for primary percutaneous intervention for acute ST segment elevation myocardial infarction. J Am Coll Cardiol 2004; 43:2153–2159.
72. Henry TD, Unger BT, Sharkey SW, et al. Design of a standardized system for transfer of patients with ST-elevation myocardial infarction for percutaneous coronary intervention. Am Heart J 2005; 150:373–384.
73. Terekelsen CJ, Lassen JF, Noorgard BL, et al. Reduction of treatment delay in patients with ST-elevation myocardial infarction: impact of pre-hospital diagnosis and direct referral to primary percutaneous coronary intervention. Eur Heart J 2005; 26:770–777.
74. Jacoby J, Axelband J, Patterson J, et al. Cardiac cath lab activation by the emergency physician without prior consultation decreases door to balloon time. J Invas Cardiol 2005; 17:154–155.
75. McLean S, O'Reilly M, Doyle M, et al. Improving door to drug time and ST segment resolution in AMI by moving thrombolysis to the emergency department. Accid Emerg Nurs 2004; 12:2–9.
76. Irwani I, Seet CM, Manning PG. Emergency physician versus cardiologist-initiated thrombolysis for acute myocardial infarction: a Singapore experience. Singapore Med J 2004; 45:313–317.
77. Corfield AR, Graham CA, Adams JN, et al. Emergency department thrombolysis improves door to needle times. Emerg Med J 2004; 21:676–680.
78. Sheifer SE, Manolio TA, Gersh BJ. Unrecognized myocardial infarction. Ann Intern Med 2001; 135:801–811.
79. Mittleman MA, Mintzer D, Maclure M, et al. Triggering of myocardial infarction by cocaine. Circulation 1999; 99:2737–2741.

80. Qureshi AI, Suri FK, Guterman LR, et al. Cocaine use and the likelihood of nonfatal myocardial infarction and stroke. Data from the third national health and nutrition examination survey. Circulation 2001; 103:502–506.
81. Hollander JE, Hoffman RS, Gennis P, et al. Prospective multicenter evaluation of cocaine associated chest pain. Acad Emerg Med 1994; 1:330–339.
82. Hollander JE, Hoffman RS, Burstein J, et al. Cocaine associated myocardial infarction. Mortality and complications. Arch Intern Med 1995; 155:1081–1086.
83. Weber JE, Gibson CM, Hynes C, et al. Quantitative comparison of coronary artery flow and myocardial perfusion in patients with acute myocardial infarction in the presence vs. absence of recent cocaine use. Acad Emerg Med 2001; 8:539–540.
84. Hollander JE, Hoffman RS. Cocaine induced myocardial infarction: An analysis and review of the literature. J Emerg Med 1992; 10:169–177.
85. Hollander JE. Management of cocaine associated myocardial ischemia. New Engl J Med 1995; 333:1267–1272.
86. Lange RA, Hillis LD. Cardiovascular complications of cocaine use. N Engl J Med 2001; 345:351–358.
87. Baumann BM, Perrone J, Hornig SE, et al. Randomized controlled double blind placebo controlled trial of diazepam, nitroglycerin or both for treatment of patients with potential cocaine associated acute coronary syndromes. Acad Emerg Med 2000; 7:878–885.
88. Hollander JE, Henry TD. Evaluation and management of the patient who has cocaine associated chest pain. Cardiology Clin 2006; 24:103–14.

17

Management of Complications

Steven M. Hollenberg
*Division of Cardiology, Cooper University Hospital, Camden,
New Jersey, U.S.A.*

INTRODUCTION

Despite significant advances in both reperfusion and adjunctive therapy for acute myocardial infarction (AMI), complications continue to pose significant clinical challenges. These complications can be broken down into two main categories: complications from AMI and complications from the techniques used to achieve reperfusion.

Problems occurring early after AMI include hemodynamic instability, mechanical complications, and arrhythmias. The advent of coronary care units has allowed for more sophisticated means of hemodynamic assessment and monitoring, and equal sophistication is needed in the planning of an approach to diagnosis and management.

MYOCARDIAL INFARCTION COMPLICATIONS

Hemodynamic Instability

Hemodynamic instability can result from hypotension, low cardiac output, pulmonary edema, or cardiogenic shock. Although there is overlap, distinguishing the primary clinical presentation and the pathophysiology of that abnormality has important therapeutic implications. Hypotension resulting from hypovolemia may respond to intravascular fluid repletion alone, whereas hypotension resulting from inadequate cardiac output may require more intensive, supportive measures. Differentiation can be made using a combination of clinical signs, imaging technology, and hemodynamic monitoring.

Evaluation of Patients with Hemodynamic Instability

Initial evaluation entails a focused history, a physical examination, an electrocardiogram (ECG), and laboratory tests. Patients with inadequate perfusion are usually ashen or cyanotic, and can have cool skin and mottled extremities. Cerebral hypoperfusion may cloud the sensorium. Pulses are rapid and faint and may be irregular in the presence of arrhythmias. Clinical signs of congestive heart failure should be sought as well. Jugular venous distention and pulmonary rales are usually present, although their absence does not exclude the diagnosis. A precordial heave resulting from left ventricular (LV) dyskinesis may be palpable. The heart sounds may be distant, and third and/or fourth heart sounds are usually heard. Mechanical complications such as acute mitral regurgitation or ventricular septal defect may be heralded by the presence of a systolic murmur, but these complications may also occur without an audible murmur.

An ECG should be performed immediately to evaluate for recurrence of myocardial ischemia and to assess the rhythm. Other initial diagnostic tests usually include a chest radiograph and measurement of arterial blood gases, electrolytes, complete blood count, and cardiac enzymes.

Echocardiography is an excellent tool for sorting through the differential diagnosis and should be performed as early as possible. Echocardiography allows for expeditious evaluation of overall and regional LV performance, and can rapidly diagnose mechanical causes of shock such as acute mitral regurgitation resulting from papillary muscle rupture, acute ventricular septal defect, and free wall rupture (1). In some cases, echocardiography may reveal findings compatible with right ventricular (RV) infarction, or suggest alternative diagnoses such as pericardial tamponade. Acute right heart failure, manifested by a dilated and hypokinetic right ventricle without hypertrophy suggestive of chronic pulmonary hypertension, can be seen with pulmonary embolism (2). Transthoracic echocardiographic images may be suboptimal due to a poor acoustic window in critically ill patients, particularly those who are obese, have chronic lung disease, or are on positive pressure ventilation. Contrast may be used to improve image quality (3). Transesophageal echocardiography can also provide better visualization, particularly of valvular structures, and can be performed safely at the bedside.

Invasive hemodynamic monitoring may be helpful in the management of patients with AMI and concomitant hemodynamic instability. Intra-arterial pressure monitoring provides a more accurate measurement of intra-arterial pressure and allows beat-to-beat analysis so that decisions regarding therapy can be based on immediate and reproducible blood pressure information (4). Severe hypotension (defined as systolic blood pressure <80 mmHg), therapy with vasopressor/inotropic agents, and cardiogenic shock represent class I indications in the latest ACC/AHA guidelines (5).

Measurements made via pulmonary artery catheterization may be helpful in differentiating inadequate intravascular volume with low left-sided filling pressures from adequate intravascular volume with high left-sided filling pressures due to LV dysfunction (6,7). The hemodynamic profile of RV infarction includes high right-sided filling pressures in the presence of normal or low left-sided pressures (8). Progressive hypotension unresponsive to fluid administration is a class I indication for pulmonary artery catheterization (5). Right heart catheterization is also indicated for suspected mechanical complications if echocardiography is unavailable (5). Invasive hemodynamic monitoring is most useful, however, to optimize therapy in unstable patients, because clinical estimates of filling pressure can be unreliable (9), and because changes in myocardial performance and compliance and therapeutic interventions can change cardiac output and filling pressures precipitously (10).

Hypotension

Hypotension (usually defined as systolic blood pressure <90 mmHg or mean arterial pressure <60 mmHg) can result from hypovolemia, right or LV failure with decreased cardiac output, arrhythmias, mechanical complications, or other conditions such as sepsis or pulmonary embolism.

The initial approach to the hypotensive patient should include fluid resuscitation unless frank pulmonary edema is present. Patients are commonly diaphoretic, and relative hypovolemia may be present. In the original description of hemodynamic subsets in AMI, approximately 20% of patients had low cardiac index and low pulmonary capillary wedge pressure; most had reduced stroke volume and compensatory tachycardia (11). Hemorrhage is an increasingly common problem associated with invasive procedures, fibrinolytic agents, antiplatelet agents, and anticoagulants and merits consideration as well.

Fluid infusion is best initiated with predetermined boluses titrated to clinical end points of heart rate, urine output, and blood pressure. Ischemia produces diastolic as well as systolic dysfunction, and thus elevated filling pressures may be necessary to maintain stroke volume. In patients who do not respond rapidly to initial fluid boluses, echocardiography should be performed to evaluate cardiac function and rule out mechanical complications. Patients with poor physiologic reserve should be considered for invasive hemodynamic monitoring. Optimal filling pressures vary from patient to patient; hemodynamic monitoring can be used to construct a Starling curve at the bedside, identifying the filling pressure at which cardiac output is maximized.

When arterial pressure remains inadequate, therapy with vasopressor agents may be required to maintain coronary perfusion pressure. Maintenance of adequate blood pressure is essential to break the vicious cycle of progressive hypotension with further myocardial ischemia. Dopamine increases both blood pressure and cardiac output, and is usually the first choice in patients with systolic pressures less than 90 mmHg. When hypotension remains refractory, norepinephrine may be necessary to maintain organ perfusion pressure. Phenylephrine, a selective α-1 adrenergic agonist, may be employed to support blood pressure if tachyarrhythmias limit therapy with other vasopressors, although it does not improve cardiac output. Vasopressor infusions need to be titrated carefully in patients with cardiogenic shock to maximize coronary perfusion pressure with the least possible increase in myocardial oxygen demand. Hemodynamic monitoring, with serial measurements of cardiac output, filling pressures, and mixed venous oxygen saturation, may allow for titration of the dosage of vasoactive agents to the minimum dosage required to achieve the chosen therapeutic goals (10).

Pulmonary Congestion

Pulmonary edema may occur acutely on presentation with AMI or may progress over the first several days. The first step in evaluation is to assess the adequacy of perfusion by clinical signs as outlined above. Patients with pulmonary edema and inadequate perfusion have cardiogenic shock and should be treated as such. Patients with pulmonary congestion and adequate cardiac output are hypertensive due to sympathetic stimulation; marginal blood pressure suggests impending cardiogenic shock, and frank hypotension makes the diagnosis.

The cause of pulmonary edema should be investigated by echocardiography, supplemented by invasive monitoring if necessary. Patients with pulmonary edema upon presentation with AMI are at high risk and will benefit from primary percutaneous intervention, if this is feasible (12,13). In patients with heart failure several days after initial presentation, coronary angiography is generally indicated to rule out reocclusion and to perform revascularization. Some patients may not tolerate lying flat for the procedure, and prior intubation and mechanical ventilation may be prudent.

Immediate management goals include assurance of adequate oxygenation and preload reduction to reduce pulmonary congestion. Pulmonary edema in the presence of previous LV dysfunction is often associated with hypervolemia; but without prior LV impairment, pulmonary edema results from acute redistribution of fluid into the lungs. In this setting, the primary effect of the administration of loop diuretics is vasodilation, and overdiuresis can precipitate hypotension (14). Morphine sulfate is very useful because it not only reduces preload, but also decreases anxiety and thus can blunt sympathetic overdrive. Nitroglycerin relieves pulmonary congestion primarily through direct venodilation; at higher doses, coronary artery dilation and increased collateral blood flow may improve ischemia. Nitroglycerin is initially administered sublingually and then should be given by continuous intravenous infusion. The dose should be titrated carefully to avoid hypotension.

Low Output State
Some patients may develop hypoperfusion without frank hypotension, manifested by clinical signs such as cyanosis, cold extremities, oliguria, or altered sensorium (15). Such hypoperfusion may also occur without signs of pulmonary congestion. In an analysis of the clinical profile of patients from the SHOCK trial registry, 28% of patients with cardiogenic shock had no clinical findings of pulmonary congestion, and the mortality for these patients exceeded 70% (15). Such patients should be assessed with echocardiography with or without invasive monitoring and treated as if they had cardiogenic shock.

Cardiogenic Shock
Cardiogenic shock is the most common cause of death in hospitalized patients with AMI. The diagnosis is often made on clinical grounds, by the presence of systemic arterial hypotension along with clinical signs indicative of poor tissue perfusion. A rigorous determination requires hemodynamic confirmation, with sustained systemic hypotension (systolic arterial pressure <90 mmHg or mean arterial pressure $\geq$30 mmHg below basal levels), adequate or elevated LV filling pressures (pulmonary artery wedge pressure >15 mmHg), and a reduced cardiac output (cardiac index <2.2 L/min/m^2) (16). It is important to document myocardial dysfunction and to exclude or correct factors such as hypovolemia, hypoxia, and acidosis.

The predominant cause of cardiogenic shock is LV failure in the setting of AMI (17). Cardiogenic shock usually results from extensive infarction, although a smaller infarction in a patient with previously compromised LV function may also precipitate shock. Cardiogenic shock can also be caused by mechanical complications of infarction such as acute mitral regurgitation, rupture of the interventricular septum, or rupture of the free wall or by a large RV infarction (Fig. 1). Patients may have cardiogenic shock at initial presentation to the hospital, but most do not; shock usually evolves over several hours (17,18), suggesting that early treatment may potentially prevent shock. In fact, some recent data indicate that early fibrinolytic therapy may decrease the incidence of cardiogenic shock (19).

Comparison of patients with early and late shock suggests that shock tends to develop earlier in patients with single-vessel disease than in patients with triple-vessel disease (20). This distinction may have clinical implications, since it suggests that early shock in the setting of AMI may be more amenable to revascularization of the culprit artery by fibrinolysis or angioplasty, whereas shock developing later may require more complete revascularization with multivessel angioplasty or bypass surgery.

Cardiac dysfunction in patients with cardiogenic shock is usually initiated by infarction or ischemia. The myocardial dysfunction resulting from ischemia worsens that ischemia, creating a downward spiral (Fig. 2). Compensatory mechanisms

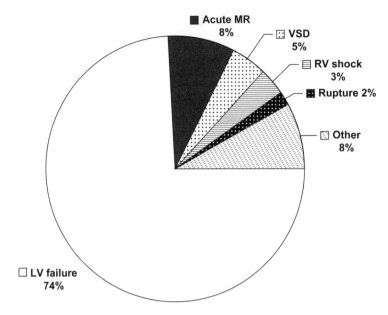

FIGURE 1 Causes of cardiogenic shock in patients with myocardial infarction in the SHOCK trial registry. *Abbreviations*: LV, left ventricular; RV, right ventricular; MR, mitral regurgitation; VSD, ventricular septal defect. *Source*: From Ref. 17.

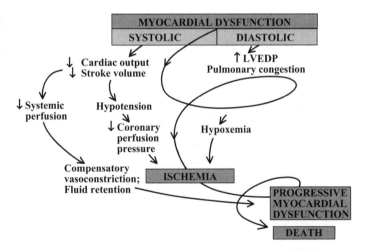

FIGURE 2 The "downward spiral" in cardiogenic shock. Stroke volume and cardiac output fall with left ventricular (LV) dysfunction, producing hypotension and tachycardia that reduce coronary blood flow. Increasing ventricular diastolic pressure reduces coronary blood flow, and increased wall stress elevates myocardial oxygen requirements. All of these factors combine to worsen ischemia. The falling cardiac output also compromises systemic perfusion. Compensatory mechanisms include sympathetic stimulation and fluid retention to increase preload. These mechanisms can actually worsen cardiogenic shock by increasing myocardial oxygen demand and afterload. Thus, a vicious circle can be established. *Abbreviation*: LVEDP, left ventricular end-diastolic pressure. *Source*: From Ref. 16.

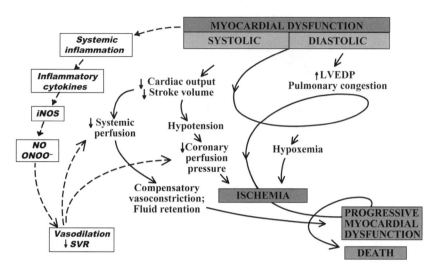

FIGURE 3 Expansion of the pathophysiologic paradigm of cardiogenic shock to include the potential contribution of inflammatory mediators. *Abbreviations*: LVEDP, left ventricular end-diastolic pressure; NO, nitric oxide; iNOS, inducible nitric oxide synthase; ONOO⁻, peroxynitrite; SVR, systemic vascular resistance. *Source*: From Ref. 23.

activated when cardiac output is reduced may become maladaptive and further worsen systolic dysfunction. Increased LV stiffness limits diastolic filling and may result in pulmonary congestion, causing hypoxemia and worsening the imbalance of oxygen delivery and oxygen demand in the myocardium, resulting in further ischemia and myocardial dysfunction (16). The interruption of this cycle of myocardial dysfunction and ischemia forms the basis for the therapeutic regimens for cardiogenic shock.

Recent data suggest that not all patients fit into this classic paradigm. In the SHOCK trial, the average systemic vascular resistance (SVR) was not elevated, and the range of values was wide, suggesting that compensatory vasoconstriction is not universal (21). This has led to an expansion of the classic paradigm to include the possibility of the contribution of inflammatory responses to vasodilation and myocardial stunning, leading clinically to persistence of shock (Fig. 3) (21). Immune activation appears to be common to a number of different forms of shock and production of nitric oxide and peroxynitrite by inducible nitric oxide synthase (iNOS), which has been proposed as one potential mechanism.

Initial Management

Maintenance of adequate oxygenation and ventilation are critical. Many patients require intubation and mechanical ventilation, if only to reduce the work of breathing and facilitate sedation and stabilization before cardiac catheterization. Some small studies have suggested that use of continuous positive airway pressure in patients with cardiogenic pulmonary edema can decrease the need for intubation; but caution is mandated, as noninvasive ventilation failed at least half of the time (22). Electrolyte abnormalities should be corrected, and morphine used to relieve pain and anxiety, thus reducing excessive sympathetic activity. Arrhythmias that impact cardiac output should be corrected promptly with antiarrhythmic drugs, cardioversion, or pacing. Some therapies routinely employed in AMI (such as nitrates, β blockers, and angiotensin-converting enzyme inhibitors) have the potential to exacerbate hypotension in cardiogenic shock, and should be withheld until the patient stabilizes.

The initial approach to the hypotensive patient should include fluid resuscitation unless frank pulmonary edema is present, as relative hypovolemia may be present, and ventricles with decreased compliance may require higher pressures for adequate filling. Patients who do not respond rapidly to initial fluid boluses or those with poor physiologic reserve should be considered for invasive hemodynamic monitoring.

When arterial pressure remains inadequate, therapy with vasopressor agents may be required to maintain adequate coronary perfusion pressure and break the vicious cycle of progressive hypotension with further myocardial ischemia. Dopamine increases both blood pressure and cardiac output, and is usually the first choice in patients with systolic pressures less than 90 mmHg. When hypotension remains refractory, norepinephrine may be necessary to maintain organ perfusion pressure.

Following initial stabilization and restoration of adequate blood pressure, tissue perfusion should be assessed. If tissue perfusion remains inadequate, cardiovascular support with inotropic agent support and/or intra-aortic balloon pumping should be initiated. Dobutamine, a selective β1-adrenergic receptor agonist, can improve myocardial contractility and increase cardiac output, and is the initial agent of choice in patients with systolic pressures greater than 90 mmHg. Dobutamine may exacerbate hypotension in some patients and can precipitate tachyarrhythmias. In some situations, a combination of dopamine and dobutamine can be more effective than either agent alone.

Phosphodiesterase inhibitors, such as milrinone, increase intracellular cyclic AMP (adenosine monophosphate) by mechanisms not involving adrenergic receptors, producing both positive inotropic and vasodilatory actions. Milrinone has fewer chronotropic and arrhythmogenic effects than catecholamines, but has the potential to cause hypotension and has a long half-life; in patients with tenuous clinical status, its use is often reserved for situations in which other agents have proven ineffective (6).

Intra-aortic balloon counterpulsation (IABP) reduces systolic afterload and augments diastolic perfusion pressure, increasing cardiac output and improving coronary blood flow (23). In contrast with inotropic or vasopressor agents, these beneficial effects occur without an increase in oxygen demand. IABP does not, however, produce a significant improvement in blood flow distal to a critical coronary stenosis (24) and has not been shown to improve mortality when used alone without reperfusion therapy or revascularization. In patients with cardiogenic shock and compromised tissue perfusion, IABP can be an essential support mechanism to stabilize patients and allow time for definitive therapeutic measures to be undertaken (23,25). In appropriate settings, more intensive support with mechanical assist devices may also be implemented.

Myocardial Reperfusion

Pathophysiologic considerations favor interventions to restore flow to occluded arteries in patients with cardiogenic shock due to AMI. Although fibrinolytic therapy reduces the likelihood of subsequent development of shock after initial presentation (18,26,27), its role in the management of patients who have already developed shock is less certain. Randomized trials (GISSI, ISIS-2, and GUSTO-1) have not shown decreased mortality with fibrinolytic therapy in patients with established cardiogenic shock (26,28,29). On the other hand, in the SHOCK Registry (30), patients treated with fibrinolytic therapy had a lower in-hospital mortality rate than those who were not in shock (54% vs. 64%, $p = 0.005$), even after adjustment for age and revascularization status.

Fibrinolytic therapy is clearly less effective in patients with cardiogenic shock than in those without. The explanation for this lack of efficacy appears to be the low reperfusion rate achieved in this subset of patients, likely due to a combination of hemodynamic, mechanical, and metabolic factors that prevent achievement and maintenance of infarct-related artery patency (31).

Emergency percutaneous coronary intervention (PCI) is the only intervention that has been shown to consistently reduce mortality rates in patients with cardiogenic shock. Case series have shown results with PCI superior to those with either fibrinolytic therapy or conservative medical management, with mortality rates of approximately 40% to 50%, although these studies are confounded by selection bias (16). Observational studies from registries of randomized trials, most notably the GUSTO-1 trial (32,33), and from the cross-sectional National Registry of Myocardial Infarction–2 (NRMI-2) (34) have also reported improved outcomes in patients with cardiogenic shock selected for revascularization. Two randomized controlled trials have now evaluated revascularization for patients with AMI.

The "Should We Emergently Revascularize Occluded Coronaries for Cardiogenic Shock" (SHOCK) study (35,36) was a randomized, multicenter international trial that assigned patients with cardiogenic shock to receive optimal medical management—including IABP and fibrinolytic therapy—or cardiac catheterization with revascularization using PCI or coronary artery bypass grafting (CABG). The trial enrolled 302 patients and was powered to detect a 20% absolute decrease in 30-day all-cause mortality rates. Mortality at 30 days was 46.7% in patients treated with early intervention and 56% in patients treated with initial medical stabilization, but this difference did not quite reach statistical significance ($p = 0.11$) (35). The control group (patients who received medical management) had a lower mortality rate than in previous studies, likely due to the aggressive use of fibrinolytic therapy (64%) and balloon pumping (86%) in these controls. These data provide indirect evidence that the combination of fibrinolysis and IABP may produce the best outcomes when cardiac catheterization is not immediately available. At six months, mortality in the SHOCK trial was reduced significantly (50.3% compared with 63.1%, $p = 0.027$) (35), and this risk reduction was maintained at 12 months (mortality 53.3% vs. 66.4%, $p < 0.03$) (36). Subgroup analysis showed a substantial improvement in mortality rates in patients younger than 75 years of age at both 30 days (41.4% vs. 56.8%, $p = 0.01$) and six months (44.9% v. 65.0%, $p = 0.003$) (35).

The SMASH (Swiss Multicenter trial of Angioplasty SHOCK) trial was independently conceived and had a very similar design, although a more rigid definition of cardiogenic shock resulted in enrollment of sicker patients and a higher mortality (37). The trial was terminated early because of difficulties in patient recruitment, for two different reasons: early on, several centers declined to participate because it was felt that it would not be ethical to undertake early invasive evaluation in such extremely ill patients, and then, after publication of several encouraging studies documenting the superiority of PCI over fibrinolysis for AMI, many centers felt that it had become unethical not to proceed to early evaluation and revascularization (38). In the SMASH trial, an absolute reduction in 30-day mortality similar to that seen in the SHOCK trial was observed (69%

mortality in the invasive group vs. 78% in the medically managed group, RR = 0.88, 95% CI = 0.6–1.2, p = NS) (37). This benefit was also maintained at one year.

When the results of both the SHOCK and SMASH trials are put into perspective with results from other randomized, controlled trials of patients with AMI, an important point emerges: despite the moderate relative risk reduction (for the SHOCK trial 0.72, CI 0.54–0.95, for the SMASH trial, 0.88, CI, 0.60–1.20) the absolute benefit is important, with nine lives saved for 100 patients treated at 30 days in both trials, and 13.2 lives saved for 100 patients treated at one year in the SHOCK trial.

RV Infarction
RV infarction occurs in up to 30% of patients with inferior MI and is clinically significant in 10% (39). Patients present with hypotension, elevated neck veins, and clear lung fields. Diagnosis is made by identifying ST-segment elevation in right precordial leads or by characteristic hemodynamic findings on right heart catheterization (elevated right atrial and RV end-diastolic pressures with normal to low pulmonary artery occlusion pressure and low cardiac output). Echocardiography may demonstrate RV dilation with depressed contractility (8).

Supportive therapy for patients with RV infarction begins with maintenance of RV preload with fluid administration. Drugs that decrease preload, such as nitrates and diuretics, can induce severe hypotension in patients with RV infarction and should be avoided. In fact, such a response in the presence of an inferior infarction should raise the suspicion of RV involvement. At some point, however, overzealous fluid resuscitation may increase wedge pressure but may not increase cardiac output, and the consequent overdilation of the right ventricle can compromise LV filling and cardiac output (40). Inotropic therapy with dobutamine may be more effective in increasing cardiac output in some patients, and monitoring with serial echocardiograms may also be useful to detect RV overdistention (40). Maintenance of atrioventricular synchrony is also important in these patients to optimize RV filling (8). For patients with continued hemodynamic instability, intra-aortic balloon pumping may be useful, particularly because elevated RV pressures and volumes increase wall stress and oxygen consumption and decrease right coronary perfusion pressure, exacerbating RV ischemia.

Patients with hemodynamic compromise after RV infarction represent a high-risk population (39), and should be considered for PCI. Restoration of normal flow by PCI resulted in dramatic recovery of RV function and a mortality rate of only 2%, whereas unsuccessful reperfusion was associated with persistent hemodynamic compromise and a mortality of 58% (41). On the other hand, surgical intervention is fraught with difficulty, as loss of pericardial constraint can result in acute RV dilation, leading to severe postoperative dysfunction (41). In patients with RV infarction, RV function tends to return to normal over time with supportive therapy, although such therapy may need to be prolonged (39,40).

MECHANICAL COMPLICATIONS

Acute Mitral Regurgitation
Ischemic mitral regurgitation is usually associated with inferior myocardial infarction (MI) and ischemia or infarction of the posterior papillary muscle, which has a single blood supply, usually from the posterior descending branch of a dominant right coronary artery (42). Papillary muscle rupture has a bimodal incidence; either

within 24 hours, or three to seven days after acute infarction. The presentation is dramatic, with the sudden onset of pulmonary edema, hypotension, and cardiogenic shock. When a papillary muscle ruptures, the murmur of acute mitral regurgitation may be limited to early systole because of rapid equalization of pressures in the left atrium and left ventricle. More importantly, the murmur may be soft or inaudible, especially when cardiac output is low (43).

Echocardiography is extremely useful in the differential diagnosis, which includes free wall rupture, ventricular septal rupture, and infarct extension with pump failure. Hemodynamic monitoring with pulmonary artery catheterization may also be helpful. With acute mitral regurgitation, a large "v" wave may be seen on the pulmonary artery wedge tracing, although this is not specific for acute mitral regurgitation and may be seen in acute ventricular septal defect (VSD) or in patients with severe LV dysfunction and decreased compliance (44).

Immediate management includes afterload reduction with nitroprusside and intra-aortic balloon pumping as temporizing measures. Inotropic or vasopressor therapy may also be needed to support cardiac output and blood pressure. Definitive therapy, however, is surgical valve repair or replacement. Although mortality with emergency mitral valve replacement is high, ranging from 20% to 40%, survival and ventricular function are improved after surgery compared with medical therapy (45,46). Surgery, if indicated, should be undertaken as soon as possible, since clinical deterioration can be sudden (43,45).

Ventricular Septal Rupture

The frequency of acute rupture of the interventricular septum has decreased in the reperfusion era to an incidence of less than 1% (47), but this complication still represents about 4% of patients with cardiogenic shock (48). Hypertension, advanced age, and female gender are predisposing factors. The incidence is bimodal, either within 24 hours, or three to five days after AMI. Early ruptures are due to intramural hematomas that dissect into tissue, and the later ruptures are due to ongoing tissue necrosis (47).

Patients with ventricular septal rupture have severe heart failure or cardiogenic shock, with a pansystolic murmur and a parasternal thrill, although both of these findings may be subtle in the presence of a low cardiac output. The hallmark finding is a left-to-right intracardiac shunt ("step-up" in oxygen saturation from right atrium to right ventricle). The diagnosis is most easily made with echocardiography.

Medical therapy consists of mechanical support with an intra-aortic balloon pump and pharmacologic measures, including judicious use of inotropes and afterload reducers. Nitroprusside can be useful to reduce afterload in acute VSD because of its short half-life and titratability. Invasive monitoring is recommended to optimize vasoactive therapy.

Because ventricular septal perforations are exposed to shear forces and removal of tissue by necrosis, the rupture site can expand abruptly, and so operative repair is usually the only viable option for long-term survival. Surgical mortality is quite high (20–50%), especially for inferoposterior ruptures, which tend to be serpiginous and less well circumscribed than anteroapical ruptures, and are harder to repair. The timing of surgery has been controversial (45,49,50), but guidelines now recommend that operative repair should be undertaken early, within 48 hours of the rupture (51). Placement of a septal occluding device may be contemplated in selected patients, but experience is limited.

Free Wall Rupture

Rupture of the ventricular free wall, which should be included in the differential of patients with recurrent chest pain, is uncommon but not entirely rare. In the prefi- brinolytic era, the incidence of cardiac rupture and tamponade was reported at 4% to 6% (5), and in the fibrinolytic era, its incidence is still 0.85% (52). Like the other mechanical complications, its incidence is bimodal, with a peak within the first 24 hours and another at three to five days. The classic patient is elderly, female, and hypertensive. The early use of fibrinolytic therapy reduces the incidence of cardiac rupture, but late use (more than 14 hours after symptom onset) may increase the risk.

Pseudoaneurysm with leakage may be heralded by chest pain, nausea, and restlessness, but frank free wall rupture presents as a catastrophic event with a pulseless rhythm. A pericardial effusion may be visualized by echocardiography, sometimes with layered high-acoustic echoes that suggest thrombous; a myocardial tear may be seen in up to 40% of cases (53). Contrast ventriculography is not a sensitive way to detect a small rupture.

Pericardiocentesis may be necessary to relieve acute tamponade, ideally in the operating room, since the pressure of the pericardial effusion may be tamponading the bleeding. Although mortality after free wall rupture is very high, salvage is possible with expeditious thoracotomy and repair, either with a patch or by direct suturing (54).

ARRHYTHMIAS

Tachycardias

Ventricular tachyarrhythmias after AMI are divided into those occurring in the early phase (first 48 hours) and those in the late phase (after 48 hours). Early phase arrhythmias probably result from micro-reentry, and may be triggered by heightened adrenergic tone, electrolyte disorders, acidosis, or free radical production from myo- cardial reperfusion. The incidence of ventricular fibrillation (VF) is highest in the first four hours after ST-segment elevation myocardial infarction (55), and may be decreasing with increased use of β blockers, earlier reperfusion, and more aggressive correction of electrolyte abnormalities (56). Primary VF is in fact associated with increased in-hospital mortality (contrary to previous teachings), but survivors to hos- pital discharge have the same long-term prognosis as patients without early VF (57).

Accelerated idioventricular rhythm (AIVR) is commonly seen in the first 12 hours after AMI. This is a reperfusion arrhythmia and probably results from increased automaticity of Purkinje fibers. AIVR is relatively specific, but not especially sensitive, for patency of the infarct-related artery, and does not portend an increased risk of VF. AIVR is usually transient and well tolerated, and obser- vation will usually suffice. If patients with LV dysfunction do not tolerate AIVR owing to the loss of atrio-ventricular (AV) synchrony, increasing the atrial rate with atropine or by pacing can suppress the AIVR.

VF and sustained ventricular tachycardia more than 48 hours after AMI in the absence of recurrent ischemia indicates electrical instability and portends a poor prognosis (58). Meta-analyses of patients from the AVID, CASH, and CIDS trials suggest that such patients will benefit from insertion of an implantable cardioverter defibrillator (ICD) (5,59).

Patients with nonsustained ventricular tachycardia, however, represent a more complicated population. Clinical trials have demonstrated that high-risk patients [those with ejection fraction <35% and nonsustained ventricular tachy- cardia (MADIT, MUSST) (60,61), or ejection fraction <30% alone (MADIT-2) (62)] benefit from ICD insertion, but the patients in those trials were enrolled more than one month after AMI (60,62,63). In the recent DINAMIT study, placement of an ICD immediately after AMI did not reduce all-cause mortality (64), and analysis of MADIT-2 demonstrated that patients with a remote MI (at least 18 months previous) benefited greatly from the ICD, whereas those with a more recent MI (less than 18 months) did not (65). Application of ejection fraction criteria in the immediate postinfarction period may not be valid, because some patients may have myocardial stunning with the potential for improved function over time. Thus, what to do in the first month after AMI remains uncertain. Home automated external defibrillators are becoming more affordable, and their efficacy is being tested in clinical trials.

Bradycardias

Conduction abnormalities are a common complication of AMI. These can be transient or permanent. Conduction abnormalities associated with an acute inferior MI usually result from AV nodal ischemia, are transient, and confer a low mortality rate. Conduction abnormalities in association with an acute anterior MI, however, represent extensive necrosis of the infranodal conduction system and the myocardium, and are associated with high in-hospital mortality (66). The ACC/AHA/NASPE recommended guidelines for permanent and temporary implantation of pacemakers in patients with AMI are shown in Table 1.

COMPLICATIONS OF REVASCULARIZATION

Complications of Fibrinolytic Therapy

Bleeding

Bleeding is the primary complication of fibrinolytic therapy, and the most dreaded complication is intracranial hemorrhage (ICH), which occurs primarily on the first day of therapy. The incidence of ICH with fibrinolytics in clinical trials is approximately 0.7% (5), and the rate in a nontrial community registry was similar (67). The ICH rate with streptokinase may be slightly lower than that with alteplase (5). Predictors of the risk of ICH after fibrinolytic therapy differ slightly in different studies but generally include age greater than 75 years, low body weight, hypertension, prior stroke, and use of alteplase (68). Risk scores have been developed to stratify individual patients and facilitate clinical decisions (68).

Therapy of ICH entails discontinuation of fibrinolytic, antiplatelet, and anticoagulation therapies; administration of cryoprecipitate to increase levels of fibrinogen and factor VIII; and administration of fresh frozen plasma to increase factors V and VIII. Protamine, to reverse the effects of heparin, and platelet transfusion may be considered as well, dictated by clinical circumstances.

The incidence of major bleeding after fibrinolytic therapy is highly dependent on how this is defined, but ranges from 1.0% to 1.8%. Bleeding in GUSTO-1 was most often procedure related, occurring in 3.6% of patients after bypass grafting, and at the groin site in 2% of patients undergoing percutaneous intervention (26). The gastrointestinal tract is the most common site of spontaneous bleeding.

Allergic Reactions

Streptokinase is associated with a low incidence of allergic reactions, although most hypotension with infusion is due to activation of vasodilatory proteases and responds to fluids and a decreased infusion rate. Recent (within 1 year) exposure to

TABLE 1 Recommendations for Pacing After an Acute Myocardial Infarction

A. Recommendations for Temporary Transvenous Pacing
   Class I
      1. Asystole
      2. Symptomatic bradycardia
      3. Bilateral bundle branch block (alternating BBB or RBBB with alternating LAFB/LPFB, any age)
      4. New or indeterminate-age bifascicular block (RBBB with LAFB or LPFB, or LBBB) with first-degree AV block
      5. Mobitz type II second-degree AV block
   Class IIA
      1. RBBB and LAFB or LPFB (new or indeterminate)
      2. RBBB with first-degree AV block
      3. LBBB, new or indeterminate
      4. Incessant VT, for atrial or ventricular overdrive pacing
      5. Recurrent sinus pauses (>3 sec) not responsive to atropine
   Class IIB
      1. Bifascicular block of indeterminate age
      2. New or age-indeterminate isolated RBBB
   Class III
      1. First-degree heart block
      2. Type I second-degree AV block with normal hemodynamics
      3. Accelerated idioventricular rhythm
      4. BBB or fascicular block known to exist before AMI

Abbreviations: RBBB: right bundle branch block; LBBB: left bundle branch block; LAFB: left anterior fascicular block; LPFV: left posterior fascicular block; AMI: acute myocardial infarction.
Source: From Ref. 51.

B. Recommendations for Permanent Pacing
   Class I
      1. Persistent second-degree AV block in the His-Purkinje system with bilateral bundle branch block or complete heart block after acute myocardial infarction
      2. Transient advanced (second or third degree) infranodal AV block and associated bundle branch block. If the site of block is uncertain, an electrophysiologic study may be necessary
      3. Persistent and symptomatic second or third degree AV block
   Class IIB
      1. Persistent second- or third-degree AV block at the AV node level
   Class III
      1. Transient AV block in the absence of intraventricular conduction defects
      2. Transient AV block in the presence of isolated left anterior fascicular block
      3. Acquired left anterior fascicular block in the absence of AV block
      4. Persistent first-degree AV block in the presence of bundle branch block that is old or age indeterminate

Source: Adapted from Refs. 81 and 82.

streptokinase produces some degree of antibody-mediated resistance to streptokinase, and such patients should be treated with a different fibrinolytic agent.

Percutaneous Intervention Complications
Procedural Complications
Angiography and PCI in AMI pose the risk of distal embolization of thrombus. In one series, distal embolization was visualized angiographically in 15% (69), which may represent a lower limit of the incidence since not all emboli are detected by angiography. Distal embolization may contribute to the "no-reflow" phenomenon

after intervention. In this series, angiographic success was lower in patients with distal embolization, myocardial blush and resolution of ST-segment elevation were reduced, and long-term mortality was increased (69). Distal protection devices have not been shown to improve ST-segment resolution, infarct size, or major adverse cardiac events in primary PCI, possibly because embolization can occur either before or during placement of the device.

Reflex hypotension, which may be quite severe, can occur in procedures involving occluded right coronary arteries (70). The typical patient is stable until reperfusion of the artery occurs, upon which bradycardia and profound hypotension ensue. Atropine, dopamine, or phenylephrine may be required. The mechanism appears to be a combination of activation of the cardioinhibitory (Bezold–Jarisch) reflex from stimulation of vagal afferents in the ischemic inferoposterior wall and RV ischemia (70).

Coronary artery dissections occur commonly in PCI and increase the risk for abrupt closure. Failed PCI sometimes necessitates emergency CABG, but improvements in catheters, antiplatelet therapy, and particularly the use of stents has decreased the need for emergency CABG from 1% to 2% down to 0.1% to 0.3% (71,72).

Coronary artery perforation may result from guide wires or inflation of oversized balloons. The incidence is 0.2% to 0.6%, and is more common with use of atherectomy devices in complicated lesions. Implantation of polytetrafluoroethylene (PFTE)-covered stents may be successful in sealing the perforation, but emergency CABG is often required, and mortality is high (73).

Vascular Arterial Injury

Bleeding at the vascular access site is a significant and not uncommon complication of PCI. Access site bleeding is related in part to anticoagulation and is more frequent with antiplatelet therapy. Retroperitoneal hematoma may be difficult to diagnose because of concealed bleeding and nonspecific symptoms; it usually becomes apparent only after significant blood loss has occurred. Risk factors for retroperitoneal hematoma in one large series included low body surface area, high femoral artery puncture, and female gender; ST-segment elevation MI as an indication for PCI was not a predictor (74). Most patients can be managed conservatively, but vascular surgical intervention may be required.

Contrast Nephropathy

The incidence of contrast-induced nephropathy varies with the clinical characteristics of the patient population and by the way in which it is defined, but as many as 15% of patients may experience an increase in serum creatinine levels of 25% (75). Risk factors include diabetes, age greater than 75 years, volume depletion, and use of nonsteroidal anti-inflammatory agents as well as preexisting renal disease (75,76). A prediction model for contrast nephropathy after PCI has been developed that includes heart failure, hypertension, balloon pump use, anemia, and contrast volume, in addition to these factors (77). The pathogenesis is not entirely clear, but a combination of ischemia due to effects on renal perfusion and toxic injury to renal tubules is involved. Attempts to minimize the contrast load are clearly advisable.

A host of preventive strategies have been tested, but fluid loading is both the simplest and most effective. Volume expansion with isotonic saline is superior to forced diuresis (76). A small trial suggested that sodium bicarbonate may be superior to sodium chloride, but its size and methodologic concerns prevent it from being regarded as definitive (76). *N*-acetyl-cysteine has been tested in multiple trials and subjected to multiple meta-analyses, but results have been inconsistent for unclear reasons (76). *N*-acetyl-cysteine is inexpensive and well tolerated, and thus it does not seem unreasonable to use it, as long as it is given in addition to rather than in place of other evidence-based measures. In view of the uncertainty about its efficacy, however, its administration should not provide a false sense of security.

Reperfusion Injury
Although early reperfusion after AMI saves lives, animal models of ischemia have shown exacerbation of myocardial injury during reperfusion. Such reperfusion injury contributes to myocardial stunning and postischemic dysfunction that persists despite restoration of normal blood flow. The pathogenesis of stunning has not been conclusively established, but appears to involve a combination of oxidative stress, perturbation of calcium homeostasis, and decreased myofilament responsiveness to calcium (78). The intensity of stunning is determined primarily by the severity of the antecedent ischemic insult (78).

A number of pharmacologic interventions, including free radical scavenging, have been shown to reduce infarct size and improve ventricular function in animal models of ischemia and reperfusion (79). These cardioprotective effects, however, have not been demonstrated to improve outcome in patients with AMI (79). For free radical scavenging, pretreatment appears to be essential, as efficacy is lost with a delay as short at 30 seconds after reperfusion. Other reasons for the failure to translate the promising results of animal studies into clinically applicable therapies include lack of standardized animal models, protocols, and methods of analysis; use of protocols too short to provide meaningful end points; and use of animal models that do not adequately approximate the relevant clinical circumstances (79). In addition, depressed regional systolic function reflects a mixture of necrotic and viable tissue, and separation of stunning from necrosis is challenging.

Some of the preliminary results in clinical trials have been promising. Adenosine treatment in patients receiving fibrinolytic therapy showed some beneficial effects in patients with anterior infarction and at high dose, but the primary outcome was not significantly improved in the treatment group as a whole (80). Sodium-hydrogen exchange inhibitors have improved regional and global ventricular function in early clinical studies, but neurologic side effects were concerning (80).

Adjunctive therapies to limit reperfusion injury might be expected to be most beneficial when delivered at the time of PCI, and this notion has been supported by subgroup analyses in some studies (80). Further testing in adequately powered clinical trials may define a role for inhibition of reperfusion injury in AMI.

REFERENCES

1. Nishimura RA, Tajik AJ, Shub C, et al. Role of two-dimensional echocardiography in the prediction of in-hospital complications after acute myocardial infarction. J Am Coll Cardiol 1984; 4:1080–1087.
2. Ribeiro A, Lindmarker P, Juhlin-Dannfelt A, et al. Echocardiography Doppler in pulmonary embolism: right ventricular dysfunction as a predictor of mortality rate. Am Heart J 1997; 134:479–487.
3. Reilly JP, Tunick PA, Timmermans RJ, et al. Contrast echocardiography clarifies uninterpretable wall motion in intensive care unit patients. J Am Coll Cardiol 2000; 35:485–490.

4. Hollenberg SM, Ahrens TS, Annane D, et al. Practice parameters for hemodynamic support of sepsis in adult patients: 2004 update. Crit Care Med 2004; 32(9):1928–1948.
5. Antman EM, Anbe DT, Armstrong PW, et al. ACC/AHA guidelines for the management of patients with ST-elevation myocardial infarction–executive summary: a report of the American College of Cardiology/American Heart Association Task Force on Practice Guidelines. Circulation 2004; 110:588–636.
6. Califf RM, Bengtson JR. Cardiogenic shock. N Engl J Med 1994; 330:1724–1730.
7. Hollenberg SM, Parrillo JE. Shock. In: Fauci AS, Braunwald E, Isselbacher KJ, et al., eds. Harrison's Principles of Internal Medicine. 14th ed. New York, NY: McGraw-Hill, 1997:214–222.
8. Nedeljkovic ZS, Ryan TJ. Right ventricular infarction. In: Hollenberg SM, Bates ER, eds. Cardiogenic Shock. Armonk, NY: Futura Publishing Company, 2002:161–186.
9. Mimoz O, Rauss A, Rekei N, et al. Pulmonary artery catheterization in critically ill patients: a prospective analysis of outcome changes associated with catheter-prompted changes in therapy. Crit Care Med 1994; 22:573–579.
10. Hollenberg SM, Hoyt JW. Pulmonary artery catheters in cardiovascular disease. New Horiz 1997; 5:207–213.
11. Forrester JS, Diamond G, Chatterjee K, et al. Medical therapy of acute myocardial infarction by application of hemodynamic subsets. N Engl J Med 1976; 295:1404–1413.
12. Spencer FA, Meyer TE, Gore JM, et al. Heterogeneity in the management and outcomes of patients with acute myocardial infarction complicated by heart failure: the National Registry of Myocardial Infarction. Circulation 2002; 105:2605–2610.
13. GUSTO IIb Investigators. A comparison of recombinant hirudin with heparin for the treatment of acute coronary syndromes. N Engl J Med 1996; 335:775–782.
14. Dikshit K, Vyden JK, Forrester JS, et al. Renal and extrarenal hemodynamic effects of furosemide in congestive heart failure after acute myocardial infarction. N Engl J Med 1973; 288:1087–1090.
15. Menon V, Slater JN, White HD, et al. Acute myocardial infarction complicated by systemic hypoperfusion without hypotension: report of the SHOCK trial registry. Am J Med 2000; 108:374–380.
16. Hollenberg SM, Kavinsky CJ, Parrillo JE. Cardiogenic shock. Ann Intern Med 1999; 131:47–59.
17. Hochman JS, Boland J, Sleeper LA, et al. Current spectrum of cardiogenic shock and effect of early revascularization on mortality. Results of an International Registry. Circulation 1995; 91:873–881.
18. Holmes DR, Jr., Bates ER, Kleiman NS, et al. Contemporary reperfusion therapy for cardiogenic shock: the GUSTO-I trial experience. The GUSTO-I Investigators. Global Utilization of Streptokinase and Tissue Plasminogen Activator for Occluded Coronary Arteries. J Am Coll Cardiol 1995; 26:668–674.
19. Bonnefoy E, Lapostolle F, Leizorovicz A, et al. Primary angioplasty versus prehospital fibrinolysis in acute myocardial infarction: a randomised study. Lancet 2002; 360: 825–829.
20. Webb JG, Sleeper LA, Buller CE, et al. Implications of the timing of onset of cardiogenic shock after acute myocardial infarction: a report from the SHOCK Trial Registry. J Am Coll Cardiol 2000; 36(3 suppl A):1084–1090.
21. Hochman JS. Cardiogenic shock complicating acute myocardial infarction: expanding the paradigm. Circulation 2003; 107:2998–3002.
22. Pang D, Keenan SP, Cook DJ, et al. The effect of positive pressure airway support on mortality and the need for intubation in cardiogenic pulmonary edema: a systematic review. Chest 1998; 114:1185–1192.
23. Willerson JT, Curry GC, Watson JT, et al. Intraaortic balloon counterpulsation in patients in cardiogenic shock, medically refractory left ventricular failure and/or recurrent ventricular tachycardia. Am J Med 1975; 58:183–191.
24. Kern MJ, Aguirre F, Bach R, et al. Augmentation of coronary blood flow by intra-aortic balloon pumping in patients after coronary angioplasty. Circulation 1993; 87: 500–511.

25. Bates ER, Stomel RJ, Hochman JS, et al. The use of intraaortic balloon counterpulsation as an adjunct to reperfusion therapy in cardiogenic shock. Int J Cardiol 1998; 65(suppl 1): S37–S42.
26. GUSTO Investigators. An international randomized trial comparing four thrombolytic strategies for acute myocardial infarction. N Engl J Med 1993; 329:673–682.
27. AIMS Trial Study Group. Effect of intravenous APSAC on mortality after acute myocardial infarction: preliminary report of a placebo-controlled clinical trial. Lancet 1988; 1:545–549.
28. Gruppo Italiano per lo Studio Della Streptochinasi Nell'Infarto Miocardico (GISSI). Effectiveness of intravenous thrombolytic treatment in acute myocardial infarction. Lancet 1986; 2:397–402.
29. ISIS-2 Collaborative Group. Randomised trial of intravenous streptokinase, oral aspirin, both, or neither among 17 187 cases of suspected acute myocardial infarction: ISIS-2. Lancet 1988; 2:349–360.
30. Sanborn TA, Sleeper LA, Bates ER, et al. Impact of thrombolysis, intra-aortic balloon pump counterpulsation, and their combination in cardiogenic shock complicating acute myocardial infarction: a report from the SHOCK Trial Registry. J Am Coll Cardiol 2000; 36(3 suppl A):1123–1129.
31. Becker RC. Hemodynamic, mechanical, and metabolic determinants of thrombolytic efficacy: a theoretic framework for assessing the limitations of thrombolysis in patients with cardiogenic shock. Am Heart J 1993; 125:919–929.
32. Berger PB, Holmes DR, Jr., Stebbins AL, et al. Impact of an aggressive invasive catheterization and revascularization strategy on mortality in patients with cardiogenic shock in the Global Utilization of Streptokinase and Tissue Plasminogen Activator for Occluded Coronary Arteries (GUSTO-I) trial: an observational study. Circulation 1997; 96:122–127.
33. Berger PB, Tuttle RH, Holmes DR, Jr., et al. One-year survival among patients with acute myocardial infarction complicated by cardiogenic shock, and its relation to early revascularization: results from the GUSTO-I trial. Circulation 1999; 99:873–878.
34. Rogers WJ, Canto JG, Lambrew CT, et al. Temporal trends in the treatment of over 1.5 million patients with myocardial infarction in the US from 1990 through 1999: the National Registry of Myocardial Infarction 1, 2 and 3. J Am Coll Cardiol 2000; 36:2056–2063.
35. Hochman JS, Sleeper LA, Webb JG, et al. Early revascularization in acute myocardial infarction complicated by cardiogenic shock. N Engl J Med 1999; 341:625–634.
36. Hochman JS, Sleeper LA, White HD, et al. One-year survival following early revascularization for cardiogenic shock. JAMA 2001; 285:190–192.
37. Urban P, Stauffer JC, Bleed D, et al. A randomized evaluation of early revascularization to treat shock complicating acute myocardial infarction. The (Swiss) Multicenter Trial of Angioplasty for Shock-(S)MASH. Eur Heart J 1999; 20:1030–1038.
38. Urban P, Stauffer J-C. Randomized trials of revascularization therapy for cardiogenic shock. In: Hollenberg SM, Bates ER, eds. Cardiogenic Shock. Armonk, NY: Futura Publishing Company, 2002:135–144.
39. Zehender M, Kasper W, Kauder E, et al. Right ventricular infarction as an independent predictor of prognosis after acute inferior myocardial infarction. N Engl J Med 1993; 328:981–988.
40. Dell'Italia LJ, Starling MR, Blumhardt R, et al. Comparative effects of volume loading, dobutamine, and nitroprusside in patients with predominant right ventricular infarction. Circulation 1985; 72:1327–1335.
41. Bowers TR, O'Neill WW, Grines C, et al. Effect of reperfusion on biventricular function and survival after right ventricular infarction. N Engl J Med 1998; 338:933–940.
42. Voci P, Bilotta F, Caretta Q, et al. Papillary muscle perfusion pattern. A hypothesis for ischemic papillary muscle dysfunction. Circulation 1995; 91:1714–1718.
43. Khan SS, Gray RJ. Valvular emergencies. Cardiol Clin 1991; 9:689–709.
44. Fuchs RM, Heuser RR, Yin FC, et al. Limitations of pulmonary wedge V waves in diagnosing mitral regurgitation. Am J Cardiol 1982; 49:849–854.
45. Bolooki H. Emergency cardiac procedures in patients in cardiogenic shock due to complications of coronary artery disease. Circulation 1989; 79:I137–I148.

46. Thompson CR, Buller CE, Sleeper LA, et al. Cardiogenic shock due to acute severe mitral regurgitation complicating acute myocardial infarction: a report from the SHOCK Trial Registry. J Am Coll Cardiol 2000; 36(3 suppl A):1104–1109.

47. Birnbaum Y, Fishbein MC, Blanche C, et al. Ventricular septal rupture after acute myocardial infarction. N Engl J Med 2002; 347:1426–1432.

48. Menon V, Webb JG, Hillis LD, et al. Outcome and profile of ventricular septal rupture with cardiogenic shock after myocardial infarction: a report from the SHOCK Trial Registry. J Am Coll Cardiol 2000; 36(3 suppl A):1110–1116.

49. Chaux A, Blanche C, Matloff JM, et al. Postinfarction ventricular septal defect. Semin Thorac Cardiovasc Surg 1998; 10:93–99.

50. Killen DA, Piehler JM, Borkon AM, et al. Early repair of postinfarction ventricular septal rupture. Ann Thorac Surg 1997; 63:138–142.

51. Ryan TJ, Antman EM, Brooks NH, et al. 1999 update: ACC/AHA guidelines for the management of patients with acute myocardial infarction. A report of the American College of Cardiology/American Heart Association Task Force on Practice Guidelines (Committee on Management of Acute Myocardial Infarction). J Am Coll Cardiol 1999; 34:890–911.

52. Patel MR, Meine TJ, Lindblad L, et al. Cardiac tamponade in the fibrinolytic era: analysis of >100,000 patients with ST-segment elevation myocardial infarction. Am Heart J 2006; 151:316–322.

53. Slater J, Brown RJ, Antonelli TA, et al. Cardiogenic shock due to cardiac free-wall rupture or tamponade after acute myocardial infarction: a report from the SHOCK Trial Registry. J Am Coll Cardiol 2000; 36(3 suppl A):1117–1122.

54. Reardon MJ, Carr CL, Diamond A, et al. Ischemic left ventricular free wall rupture: prediction, diagnosis, and treatment. Ann Thorac Surg 1997; 64:1509–1513.

55. Campbell RW, Murray A, Julian DG. Ventricular arrhythmias in first 12 hours of acute myocardial infarction. Natural history study. Br Heart J 1981; 46:351–357.

56. Antman EM, Berlin JA. Declining incidence of ventricular fibrillation in myocardial infarction. Implications for the prophylactic use of lidocaine. Circulation 1992; 86:764–773.

57. Behar S, Goldbourt U, Reicher-Reiss H, et al. Prognosis of acute myocardial infarction complicated by primary ventricular fibrillation. Principal Investigators of the SPRINT Study. Am J Cardiol 1990; 66:1208–1211.

58. Newby KH, Thompson T, Stebbins A, et al. Sustained ventricular arrhythmias in patients receiving thrombolytic therapy: incidence and outcomes. The GUSTO Investigators. Circulation 1998; 98:2567–2573.

59. Connolly SJ, Gent M, Roberts RS, et al. Canadian implantable defibrillator study (CIDS): a randomized trial of the implantable cardioverter defibrillator against amiodarone. Circulation 2000; 101:1297–1302.

60. Moss AJ, Hall WJ, Cannom DS, et al. Improved survival with an implanted defibrillator in patients with coronary disease at high risk for ventricular arrhythmia. N Engl J Med 1996; 335:1933–1940.

61. Buxton AE, Lee KL, Fisher JD, et al. A randomized study of the prevention of sudden death in patients with coronary artery disease. Multicenter Unsustained Tachycardia Trial Investigators. N Engl J Med 1999; 341:1882–1890.

62. Moss AJ, Zareba W, Hall WJ, et al. Prophylactic implantation of a defibrillator in patients with myocardial infarction and reduced ejection fraction. N Engl J Med 2002; 346:877–883.

63. Buxton AE, Lee KL, DiCarlo L, et al. Electrophysiologic testing to identify patients with coronary artery disease who are at risk for sudden death. Multicenter Unsustained Tachycardia Trial Investigators. N Engl J Med 2000; 342:1937–1945.

64. Hohnloser SH, Kuck KH, Dorian P, et al. Prophylactic use of an implantable cardioverter-defibrillator after acute myocardial infarction. N Engl J Med 2004; 351:2481–2488.

65. Greenberg H, Case RB, Moss AJ, et al. Analysis of mortality events in the Multicenter Automatic Defibrillator Implantation Trial (MADIT-II). J Am Coll Cardiol 2004; 43:1459–1465.

66. Hindman MC, Wagner GS, Jaro M, et al. The clinical significance of bundle branch block complicating acute myocardial infarction. Indications for temporary and permanent pacemaker insertion. Circulation 1978; 58:689–699.

67. Huynh T, Cox JL, Massel D, et al. Predictors of intracranial hemorrhage with fibrinolytic therapy in unselected community patients: a report from the FASTRAK II project. Am Heart J 2004; 48:86–91.
68. Brass LM, Lichtman JH, Wang Y, et al. Intracranial hemorrhage associated with thrombolytic therapy for elderly patients with acute myocardial infarction: results from the Cooperative Cardiovascular Project. Stroke 2000; 31:1802–1811.
69. Henriques JP, Zijlstra F, Ottervanger JP, et al. Incidence and clinical significance of distal embolization during primary angioplasty for acute myocardial infarction. Eur Heart J 2002; 23:1112–1117.
70. Goldstein JA, Lee DT, Pica MC, et al. Patterns of coronary compromise leading to bradyarrhythmias and hypotension in inferior myocardial infarction. Coron Artery Dis 2005; 16:265–274.
71. Yang EH, Gumina RJ, Lennon RJ, et al. Emergency coronary artery bypass surgery for percutaneous coronary interventions: changes in the incidence, clinical characteristics, and indications from 1979 to 2003. J Am Coll Cardiol 2005; 46:2004–2009.
72. Seshadri N, Whitlow PL, Acharya N, et al. Emergency coronary artery bypass surgery in the contemporary percutaneous coronary intervention era. Circulation 2002; 106: 2346–2350.
73. Gruberg L, Pinnow E, Flood R, et al. Incidence, management, and outcome of coronary artery perforation during percutaneous coronary intervention. Am J Cardiol 2000; 86: 680–682.
74. Farouque HM, Tremmel JA, Raissi Shabari F, et al. Risk factors for the development of retroperitoneal hematoma after percutaneous coronary intervention in the era of glyco-protein IIb/IIIa inhibitors and vascular closure devices. J Am Coll Cardiol 2005; 45:363–368.
75. Barrett BJ, Parfrey PS. Clinical practice. Preventing nephropathy induced by contrast medium. N Engl J Med 2006; 354:379–386.
76. Weisbord SD, Palevsky PM. Radiocontrast-induced acute renal failure. J Intensive Care Med 2005; 20:63–75.
77. Mehran R, Aymong ED, Nikolsky E, et al. A simple risk score for prediction of contrast-induced nephropathy after percutaneous coronary intervention: development and initial validation. J Am Coll Cardiol 2004; 44:1393–1399.
78. Bolli R. Basic and clinical aspects of myocardial stunning. Prog Cardiovasc Dis 1998; 40:477–516.
79. Bolli R, Becker L, Gross G, et al. Myocardial protection at a crossroads: the need for translation into clinical therapy. Circ Res 2004; 95:125–134.
80. Cannon RO III. Mechanisms, management and future directions for reperfusion injury after acute myocardial infarction. Nat Clin Pract Cardiovasc Med 2004; 2:88–94.
81. Gregoratos G, Cheitlin MD, Conill A, et al. ACC/AHA Guidelines for Implantation of Cardiac Pacemakers and Antiarrhythmia Devices: Executive Summary: a report of the American College of Cardiology/American Heart Association Task Force on Practice Guidelines (Committee on Pacemaker Implantation). Circulation 1998; 97:1325–1335.
82. Gregoratos G, Abrams J, Epstein AE, Freedman RA, et al. ACC/AHA/NASPE 2002 Guideline Update for Implantation of Cardiac Pacemakers and Antiarrhythmia Devices: A Report of the American College of Cardiology/American Heart Association Task Force on Practice Guideline (ACC/AHA/NASPE Committee on Pacemaker Implantation). J Am Coll Cardiol 2002; 40:1703–1719.

18 Myocyte Regeneration

Eduardo I. de Oliveira
Hospital de Santa Maria and Faculdade de Medicina de Lisboa, Lisbon, Portugal

Stephen G. Ellis
Department of Cardiovascular Medicine, Cleveland Clinic, Cleveland, Ohio, U.S.A.

INTRODUCTION

Despite substantial advances in reperfusion therapy for acute myocardial infarction (AMI), cardiac injury and ventricular dysfunction remain as major consequences with high impact on morbidity and mortality. Perhaps the most innovative and exciting approach lies with the potential to purposefully induce new myocyte formation and/or rescue cardiomyocytes previously destined to die from apoptosis. The endogenous regenerative capacity of the heart is documented (1); however, it appears inadequate to repair injured myocardium in the majority of acute ischemic events. Experiments in animals suggested that the transfer of stem cells could improve cardiac function after infarction through regeneration of the myocardium (2), neovascularization (3), or via paracrine-mediated prevention of ongoing apoptosis (4). In addition, the first clinical studies suggested that this approach was feasible, safe, and potentially effective in humans (5,6). These data generated great enthusiasm in the scientific community and stimulated randomized controlled trials. During 2006–7, several trials provided a more realistic perspective revealing marginal or neutral benefit on this approach. However, there is still opportunity to further develop this technology, leaving room for cautious optimism.

BASIC SCIENCE

Myocardial Self-Regeneration—Cardiac Progenitor Cells

The long-held dogma that cardiomyocytes do not enter the cell cycle after birth, and consequently the heart has no regenerative capacity after injury, has been abandoned in the last decade (1). Like the brain, the heart seems to have reservoirs of progenitor cells that may not be sufficient to replace the acute loss of a large number of cells, but may be able to replace a slow apoptotic loss of cells over a lifetime. Throughout the myocardium, pools of cardiac progenitor cells may participate in the continual replacement of apoptotic cardiomyocytes at a low basal level. Unlike terminally differentiated cardiac cells, these are small cells that do not express cardiac markers and that can self-renew and proliferate (7). Some of them may differentitate into cardiomyocytes in vivo, contributing to repair of the damaged heart after AMI. This potential is limited, in part, by the small number of endogenous progenitor cardiac cells. Attempts to mobilize and to expand endogenous progenitor cells by introducing growth factors hold promise but remain controversial (8). It is likely that the activity of endogenous cardiac progenitor cells will have to be augmented, through knowledge of the mechanisms of normal progenitor expansion and determination during embryonic development, before these cells contribute substantially in the peri- and postinfarction period. Meanwhile, other strategies of myocardial regeneration have been tested.

Myogenic Cell Grafting—Extracardiac Progenitor Cells

Cellular cardiomyoplasty—myogenic cell grafting—involves induced migration or transplantation of stem cells into the myocardium, with further proliferation and differentiation that ultimately would limit the loss of contractile function of the damaged left ventricle. The designation of stem cells is applied to a diversity of cells that can be classified according with their species of origin, development stage (embryonic, fetal, or adult), tissue of origin (hematopoietic, mesenchymal, skeletal, neural), and potential to differentiate into one or more specific types of mature cells (totipotent, pluripotent, multipotent) (9). The use of adequate stem cells subclass and adequate promotion of homing and proliferation seem to be the key factors in this novel approach.

Evidence that primitive cell migration and proliferation can occur spontaneously within the adult myocardium was suggested by posttransplant reports. In one series, hearts from female donors transplanted into male recipients showed a large number of primitive cells originated from the recipient, as established by the presence of a Y chromosome. There was a high degree of differentiation of these cells (myocytes, vessels, etc.) (10). In another study, autopsy results from women after sex-mismatched bone marrow transplantation revealed the presence of a Y chromosome in 0.23% of the cardiomyocytes, suggesting that bone marrow progenitors from male donor marrow populate female recipient myocardium (11). Several techniques were developed to promote this natural mechanism, such as administration of colony stimulating factors [granulocyte colony stimulating factors (G-CSF); granulocyte macrophage colony stimulating factor (GM-CSF)]. However, transdifferentiation of hematopoietic stem cells, i.e., bone marrow–derived cells, into cardiac myocytes is controversial, and several studies have refuted this concept (12–14). One study (13) demonstrated that hematopoietic stem cells do not readily acquire a cardiac phenotype using cardiomyocyte-restricted and ubiquitously expressed reporter transgenes to track the fate of hematopoietic stem cells after transplants into normal and injured adult mouse hearts. No transdifferentiation into cardiomyocytes was detectable, and stem cell–engrafted hearts showed no overt increase in cardiomyocytes compared with sham-engrafted hearts. Another study (14) using the human sex-mismatched (female-to-male) heart transplant model revealed that endothelial (24% ± 8%), Schwann (11% ± 2%), and vascular smooth muscle (3% ± 2%) cells have substantially higher chimerism than cardiomyocytes (0.04% ± 0.05%). Other authors posit that the true mechanism is cell fusion (15), showing that after acute myocardial injury and delivery of transgenically marked bone marrow cells to the injured myocardium, engraftment of infarcted myocardium was transient and hematopoietic in nature, and bone marrow–derived cardiomyocytes were observed outside the infarcted myocardium at a low frequency and were derived exclusively through cell fusion.

Invasive grafting by coronary or intramyocardial injection of neonatal cardiomyocytes, skeletal myoblasts, hematopoietic stem cells, and marrow mesenchymal stem cells in normal or infarcted myocardium has been demonstrated in animal models (16–23). Although the mechanism is uncertain—autologous skeletal myoblasts contract but do not transdifferentiate into new cardiomyocytes (24)—left ventricular remodeling and function were improved in these models (18,20,21,25,26). In a recent study (23), myocardial infarction was created in nude (immune incompetent) rats and 10 days later, rats received in-scar injections of human skeletal myoblasts, CD133$^+$ bone marrow–derived hematopoietic progenitors, or culture medium. One month after transplantation, left ventricular ejection fraction decreased by 8% ± 4% in controls, whereas it increased by 7% ± 3% in CD133$^+$-grafted hearts (p = 0.0015 vs. controls) and by 15% ± 5% in skeletal myoblast-treated hearts (p = 0.008 vs. controls). Engrafted myotubes were identified in all skeletal myoblast-treated hearts by immunofluorescence, whereas in CD133$^+$-grafted hearts, the few human cells were only detected by polymerase chain reaction.

Some authors hypothesize that a paracrine effect may be the explanation for the described benefits. In this theory, the transplanted cells produce growth factors, cytokines (e.g., Pecam-1, P-selectin, β2-integrins (27)), and other signaling molecules that result in improved overall myocardial function such as increased myocardial perfusion due to angiogenesis, prolongation of the survival of myocytes or other cells, or activation of progenitor cells within the myocardium that can differentiate into new cardiomyocytes (4).

Other Strategies

Another important strategy is the appropriate expression of homing factors to promote adequate engraftment of the stem cells. Several specific homing factors have been described such as SDF-1 (28,29), MCP-3 (30), HGF (29), and LIF (29).

A major limitation of the current techniques is the high rate of immediate or rapid stem cell loss. Many factors contribute to the phenomenon, such as cell loss back into the left ventriclular cavity or venous system after direct injection or early cell death after transplantation. Several strategies have been developed to improve the poor cell viability associated with transplantation. In an interesting study (31), rat mesenchymal stem cells where genetically engineered to overexpress the pro-survival gene Akt1 (encoding the Akt protein). These stem cells restored myocardial volume fourfold greater than equal numbers of cells transduced with a reporter gene.

Genetic modulation of ventricular function is another novel strategy that has been evaluated in animal models and in ex vivo human models. Several molecular targets have been identified and tested [phospholamban (32–35), SERCA2a (36,37), β2 adrenergic receptor (38,39), adenylyl cyclase (40), V2 vasopressin receptor (41)]. In vivo delivery of the adenoviral vectors has been achieved by direct injection (42) or the transluminal intracoronary approach (43). Despite the promising results in some of the animal studies, overexpression of the transgenes led to fibrotic cardiomyopathy in others (44). Many technological aspects of delivery and expression of transgenes have still to be improved, and safety issues are still the major concern in the transition to human studies.

CLINICAL SCIENCE—RANDOMIZED TRIALS

Cell Therapy—Randomized Trials

Early, unblinded studies suggested a benefit from stem cell therapy following AMI. However, more recent blinded randomized trials have produced mixed results.

In the Bone Marrow Transfer to Enhance ST-Elevation Infarct Regeneration (BOOST) trial (6,45), after percutaneous coronary intervention with stent implantation in the infarct-related artery, 60 patients were randomized 1:1 to a control group with optimal postinfarction therapy and a bone marrow group that received bone marrow cell harvest and intracoronary single-dose bone marrow cells infusion—approximately 2.5 × 10 (9) unfractioned cells. The intracoronary infusion into the infarct-related artery was performed 4.8 ± 1.3 days after the coronary intervention. Left ventricular ejection fraction was assessed by magnetic resonance imaging (MRI). At six months, left ventricular ejection fraction was 6% greater in the stem cell group than in the control group. However, at 18 months there was no significant difference in left ventricular ejection fraction between the groups. The absolute left ventricular ejection fraction improvement was 6.7% (6 months) and 5.9% (18 months) in the stem cell group compared with 0.7% and 3.1% in the control group, suggesting that the main effect was an acceleration of recovery. Bone marrow cell infusion did not increase the risk of adverse clinical events, in-stent restenosis, or proarrhythmia.

Two additional controlled trials with small cohorts used Ficoll-separated bone marrow cells infusion post percutaneous coronary intervention for AMI. The Autologous Stem-Cell Transplantation in Acute Myocardial Infarction (ASTAMI) trial (46) involved 97 patients and three noninvasive imaging methods (echocardiography, SPECT, MRI) and did not find a significant improvement in left ventricular ejection fraction at six months in the mononuclear bone marrow cell group, as compared with the control group. In the other trial (47) with 67 patients, the authors did not detect an improvement in left ventricular function at four months in the bone marrow cell group compared with the control group, although infarct size was reduced in 28% and regional wall motion was improved. Technical differences in the characteristics and handling of the infused bone marrow cells might be related with the different outcomes (48).

The Reinfusion of Enriched Progenitor Cells and Infarct Remodeling in Acute Myocardial Infarction (REPAIR-AMI) trial (49) was a multicenter, randomized, placebo controlled, double-blind trial where intracoronary infusion of autologous bone marrow cells (2.4×10 (8) Ficoll-separated cells) was administered after three to seven days of successful reperfusion therapy for AMI. At four months, the absolute improvement in left ventricular ejection fraction, measured by angiography, was somewhat greater among patients treated with bone marrow cells than among those given placebo (5.5% vs. 3.0%, $p = 0.01$). Subgroup analysis suggested that the benefit was limited to patients with left ventricular ejection fraction lower then 49% at baseline and to patients treated more than five days after infarction. At one year, there was a significant reduction in combined adverse clinical events (death, recurrence of myocardial infarction, and any revascularization procedure) in the bone marrow group. Data on ventricular function at one year are not available. This is the largest trial (204 patients) and provides the best evidence yet for beneficial effects of bone marrow cell infusion after AMI. It may be challenging to achieve significant improvements in left ventricular ejection fraction in small cohorts of patients who have relatively preserved ventricular function and are receiving state-of-the-art therapy. Even some early trials of reperfusion in patients with AMI demonstrated either no improvement in left ventricular ejection fraction (50) or a modest improvement (51). Validation of cardiac cell therapy will require demonstration of benefit with regard to clinical outcomes, as was the case with reperfusion. Studies performed to date have not been designed or powered to evaluate clinical outcomes.

The use of peripheral blood–derived progenitor cells, instead of mononuclear bone marrow–derived progenitor cells, is another approach to the cardiomyoplasty technique. The Transplantation of Progenitor Cells And Regeneration Enhancement in Acute Myocardial Infarction (TOPCARE-AMI) trial (5,52,53) compared the use of these two populations of cells in the setting of AMI. This trial enrolled

59 patients that were randomly assigned to receive either autologous circulating progenitor cells or autologous bone marrow cells into the infarct artery at 4.9 ± 1.5 days after the coronary event. After four months, left ventricular ejection fraction increased (50% ± 19% to 58% ± 10%, $p < 0.001$) and end-systolic volume decreased (54 ml ± 19 ml to 44 ml ± 20 ml, $p < 0.001$) in both groups. However, there were no differences between groups. Contrast-enhanced MRI after one year revealed increased ejection fraction, reduced infarct size, and absence of reactive hypertrophy. In terms of cardiovascular events, there were no differences between groups and no ventricular arrhythmia or syncope was reported. In a TOPCARE-AMI substudy (54), coronary blood flow reserve was investigated in 40 patients at the time of progenitor cell therapy and at four-month follow-up. At follow-up, improvement of maximal coronary vascular conductance capacity restored coronary flow reserve in the infarct artery.

TOPCARE-AMI seems to indicate that both cell populations are safe and feasible for cardiomyoplasty. However, the results of the Transplantation of Progenitor Cells and Recovery of LV Function in Patients with Chronic Ischemic Heart Disease (TOPCARE-CHD) trial (55) contradict this concept, albeit in a different milieu. TOPCARE-CHD was a randomized, crossover trial that tested the same cell populations of TOPCARE-AMI in patients with chronic ischemic ventricular dysfunction. In this study, the absolute change in left ventricular ejection fraction was significantly greater among patients receiving bone marrow cells than among those receiving circulating progenitor cells. The result was independent of the order in which the cells were given, suggesting that the bone marrow cells effect is somewhat specific. Which quantitative or qualitative differences in the cell populations account for their different effects is currently unknown. Although the benefit observed after bone marrow cells infusion was modest (an increase in left ventricular ejection fraction by 2.9 percentage points), it is remarkable that any benefit was seen in these patients, who were studied on average more than six years after infarction and who were already receiving optimal medical care. Whether repeated infusions would yield additive benefits and whether these benefits would persist will be important questions for future trials.

Colony Stimulating Factors Therapy—Randomized Trials

The use of G-CSF to improve the efficacy of hematopoietic cell cardiomyoplasty is another strategy that has been tested in clinical trials. The Myoblast Autologous Grafting in Ischemic Cardiomyopathy (MAGIC) (56) cell trial evaluated the value of G-CSF in comparison to or in combination with stem cell infusion. Twenty-seven patients with an AMI undergoing bare metal stenting of the culprit lesion were randomly assigned to stem cell mobilization with G-CSF followed by stem cell apheresis and intracoronary reinfusion ($n = 10$), to G-CSF alone ($n = 10$), or to a control group ($n = 7$). Six-month follow-up data in 10 of the study patients demonstrated an improvement in left ventricle ejection fraction with stem cell infusion (48.7–55.1%), but not with G-CSF alone. Stem cell infusion also increased treadmill exercise time and reduced the size of the myocardial perfusion defect. However, administration of G-CSF was associated with an unexpectedly high rate of in-stent restenosis of the culprit lesion (56).

The FIRSTLINE-AMI (57) was an unblinded trial that enrolled 50 patients with AMI treated with successful angioplasty and optimal medical therapy. One to two hours after angioplasty, half of the population was randomly assigned to receive subcutaneous G-CSF (10 μg/kg) for six days. Improvement of left ventricular ejection fraction at rest at four months, and other benefits, including a greater increase in viable myocardium in the infarct territory, were associated with G-CSF therapy. In FIRSTLINE-AMI, there was no evidence of aggravated restenosis with G-CSF therapy (57).

The REVIVAL-2 (58) and STEMMI (59) trials also studied patients with AMI who underwent successful primary angioplasty and five days later were randomly assigned to G-CSF (10 μg/kg) or placebo daily (REVIVAL-2 for five days; STEMMI for six days). REVIVAL-2 (58) and STEMMI (59) enrolled 114 and 78 patients, respectively. In REVIVAL-2 (58), despite a marked increase in circulating stem cells, there was no difference between the groups in the primary end point—a reduction in infarct size at four to six months, as assessed by myocardial perfusion imaging—or in the secondary end points of improvement in left ventricle ejection fraction and angiographic restenosis. In STEMMI (59), at six months, there was no difference between the two groups in the primary end point of change in systolic wall thickening on cardiac MRI, left ventricle ejection fraction, or target vessel revascularization. Another double-blind randomized trial involving patients with large (baseline ejection fraction 20–39%) AMI reperfused (TIMI 3 flow) more than four hours after symptom onset (60). Eighteen patients were randomized in a 2:1 double-blind fashion to G-CSF (two groups of 5 and 10 μg/kg/day subcutaneously for 5 days—6 patients in each group) or matching placebo. Precursor cell mobilization increased by a factor of 5 to 7 in the G-CSF-treated patients, but no significant differences between groups were noted in any measure of left ventricular systolic or diastolic function or major events 30 days after infarction.

The G-CSF-STEMI (61) trial studied the effect of G-CSF treatment in 44 patients undergoing delayed PCI for within seven days of AMI. At three months, there was slight improvement in global and regional myocardial function assessed by MRI in both groups, but G-CSF was not superior to placebo. In both groups, major adverse cardiovascular events occurred and target lesion revascularization from in-stent restenosis occurred in a comparable frequency.

In summary, there is a trend towards lack of benefit in randomized trials of G-CSF alone in patients with an AMI. FIRSTLINE-AMI is the only randomized trial with marginally positive results. Many say that is a small unblinded study that does not change the main stream trend, but others argue that FIRSTLINE-AMI results may be explained by the initiation of therapy in the first hours after PCI (1–2 hours), since animal data showed that efficacy is time dependent (62). In the setting of chronic myocardial ischemia, small unblinded G-CSF trials did not show effect on myocardial perfusion and function. G-CSF did mobilize stem cells of known importance to myocardial regeneration, but there seemed to be a general lack of clinically meaningful homing of the stem cells into the ischemic myocardium (63).

Another approach is to use G-CSF to stimulate the bone marrow and mobilize progenitor cells prior to collection (apheresis) and cardiomyoplasty. MAGIC Cell-3-DES (64) was a randomized placebo controlled trial that studied the value of intracoronary infusion of mobilized peripheral blood stem cells by G-CSF in patients with acute or old myocardial infarction. The acute population underwent successful coronary revascularization with drug-eluting stents and was randomized to cell infusion therapy ($n = 25$) or placebo ($n = 25$). Cell-infusion therapy showed significant additive improvement in left ventricular ejection fraction and end-systolic volume. Cell therapy did not aggravate neointimal growth with drug-eluting stent implantation.

Autologous Skeletal Myoblast Transplantation—Randomized Trials

The MAGIC (65) trial is the only randomized placebo-controlled trial with autologous skeletal myoblast transplantation; however, it involves chronic patients and not acute events. The multicenter phase 2 MAGIC trial compared a placebo injection with either a high-dose (800 million cells) or a low-dose (400 million cells) injection of myoblasts. Eligible patients had to have reduced left ventricular ejection fraction (15–35%), history of myocardial infarction, and planned coronary artery bypass graft surgery. Cells were harvested via muscle biopsy from the patients' thigh muscles, expanded, and delivered via needle injection into the myocardium during surgery. All patients received implantable cardiac defibrillators before hospital discharge. MAGIC was stopped early, after the data safety and monitoring board determined that the study was unlikely to show a benefit of treatment. Only 97 patients were randomized. The co-primary efficacy end point of change in regional wall motion (defined as recovery of infarcted segments) and change in left ventricular ejection fraction (as measured by echocardiography) was not different between the high- or low-dose groups and the placebo group at six-month follow-up. However, measurements of left ventricle volume appeared to decrease in the high-dose group, suggesting a potential benefit in left ventricular remodeling. At six-month follow-up, there were no signals for safety concerns in either of the cell-transfer groups. Major adverse cardiac event rates and ventricular arrhythmias were not different among the groups.

COMPLICATIONS

The safety profile of autologous stem/progenitor cell therapy so far seems to be high overall, although the technique may harbor several adverse effects such as ventricular arrhythmia, acceleration of atherosclerosis or restenosis and induction of ischemic events. Multiple factors may affect the safety of cell infusion into the diseased heart, including the mode of delivery, the type of cells injected, compound characterization, and the heart status, function, and arrhythmogenic potential. Also, any adjunctive treatment used to enhance cellular homing and/or trans-differentiation increases the likelihood of unexpected local or systemic toxicity or side effects (66).

Intracoronary Injection

Several authors reported severe complications with intracoronary injection of stem cells in animal models: augmented myocardial ischemia, as indicated by ST-segment elevation and T-wave changes, frequent ventricular arrhythmia and troponin elevation (67), decreased distal blood flow (68), and histopathologic evidence of microinfarction (69). In human clinical trials, the technique seems to be feasible and safe (5,6,47–49,53,54,69), despite some reported cases of microembolization of the cellular compound (70). Different cell types may explain this disparity. The bone marrow and progenitor cells used in clinical studies have smaller diameters (10 to 12 μm) compared with the mesenchymal stromal cells or umbilical cord blood–derived somatic stem cells (20 μm) that caused microinfarctions in animals (67–69). Also, freshly aspirated cells are smaller than processed cells (67).

Another matter of concern is restenosis of the culprit artery as consequence of cell therapy. Several authors reported the phenomenon of in-stent restenosis and accelerated progression of distal atherosclerosis in the infarct-related artery (56,70,71).

Other studies, however, showed no relationship between intracoronary injection and increased rate of restenosis or accelerated atherosclerosis (6), or between G-CSF administration and restenosis (57,58). However, the fact that circulatory cells are capable of differentiating into vascular structures highlights the need for angiographic follow-up of patients treated with progenitor stem cell infusions. In addition, researchers have found that angiogenesis and inflammation play an important important role in atherosclerotic plaque formation and that lesion expansion may accelerate the coronary atherosclerosis that occurs after infusion of progenitor cells.

Intramyocardial Injection
Intramyocardial delivery can be performed through thoracotomy (transepicardial) or catheter-based techniques (transendocardial). Data derived from animal (72–74) and human (75–78) studies indicate no arrhythmia, infection, myocardial inflammation, increased fibrosis, or perforation caused by catheter-based techniques. The exception is the Euroinject One (79) study, where intramyocardial injection of vascular endothelial growth factor resulted in severe complications in five patients (6.25%) with pericardial tamponade, high-degree atrioventricular block, ST-segment elevation myocardial infarction, embolic events, and sepsis. In fact, endocardial injury may result, varying from microscopic slots with hemorrhagic infiltration (type A), to ecchymosis (type B), to transmyocardial injury (type C) (72,73).

Another aspect, however, is the local effect of the transplanted cells independent of the procedure itself (e.g., arrhythmias related with skeletal myoblasts). In animal studies, myocardial calcification (80) and fibrotic changes (81,82) have been described. Human studies (64,83,84) of local stem cell transplantation during open heart surgery reported an absence of clinically relevant inflammatory responses or myocardial damage or aberrant tissue formation. Other studies, however, raise suspicion about accelerated coronary atherosclerosis and late restenosis (83) and arrhythmias (85,86).

Arrhythmic potential
The biggest concern related with stem cell–based therapy is arrhythmia potential. Most of the candidates are patients with baseline high risk for arrhythmia and sudden death, but some cell-based therapy modalities seem to increase this risk. Studies of intramyocardial skeletal myoblast injection during coronary bypass surgery (86) or by catheter-based technique (87,88) in patients with depressed ischemic cardiomyopathy have shown a high incidence (11–40%) of serious ventricular arrhythmias, whereas studies using bone marrow–derived cells with different modalities of delivery did not (5,6,47,48,53,54,56,76,77,83–85,89–91). It is conceivable that lack of gap junction formation between the myoblasts and cardiomyocytes may serve as a substrate for the formation of a re-entry cycle and resultant ventricular arrhythmia (92). An interesting study (93) characterized the arrhythmogenic profile of cardiomyocytes derived from pluripotent embryonic stem cells and embryonal carcinoma cells. The electrical recordings showed spontaneous activity, low dV/dt, prolonged action potential duration, and easily triggered arrhythmias. These cells had arrhythmogenic potential via the three classic mechanisms: re-entry, automaticity, or triggered activity.

The ex vivo cell-expansion technique seems also to be important. Injection of myoblasts expanded in an autologous medium, rather than fetal bovine medium, resulted in no serious arrhythmia in a series of 20 patients during 14 months of follow-up (94). There is the assumption that trace contamination with xenogeneic proteins induces an immune reaction at the site of injection.

Cytokine treatment

The multisystemic effects of cytokines, particularly their prothrombotic effects on both coagulation proteins and platelets, and the cases of myocardial infarction reported in cancer patients, healthy subjects, and patients with coronary disease receiving G-CSF (95–100), raised concerns about their use in myocyte regeneration therapy.

The safety of G-CSF administration, either as adjunct therapy to cell injection or stand alone therapy, has been examined in several clinical trials, although the findings are still controversial. Particularly in the setting of AMI, aggravated rates of in-stent restenosis with or without mononuclear cell injection (70%) were reported (56). However many others found no association of G-CSF administration and restenosis in patients with AMI who underwent successful PCI (57,58,61). Thus, in the acute setting, G-CSF, did not seem to be associated with increased reinfarction, serious ventricular arrhythmias, or cardiac death (56–61,101). However, in patients with stable severe coronary disease, there are reports of acute coronary syndromes induced by G-CSF (102–104). This may be related to the thrombogenic and inflammatory properties of the cytokine, inducing plaque instability and coronary thrombogenicity. This phenomenon may not occur in the AMI trials as acute stent thrombosis or closure of other lesions/arteries because of concurrent antiplatelet and anticoagulation therapy. The more recent randomized clinical trials that used G-CSF in the acute setting showed a safe profile, however the efficacy was disappointing.

CONCLUSIONS

As recently reported by a task force of the European Society of Cardiology (105), the use of autologous stem/progenitor cell therapy is not at a stage to be used in routine clinical practice. Much of the relevant basic science needs additional study and translation into the clinical arena. The use of intracoronary infusion of autologous stem cells harvested from bone marrow aspirate is the most successful strategy so far, and larger double-blinded, randomized, controlled trials in the setting of AMI should be performed. End points should focus on robust clinical outcomes, as well as major adverse cardiac events and economic gain. Questions concerning optimal cell type or cell combinations, number of cells delivered, timing of delivery, route of delivery, and safety (ventricular arrhythmias and in-stent restenosis) will need to be clarified. Small studies should be designed to explore other alternatives such as laboratory designed cells, paracrine or autocrine mechanisms, cytokine therapy, or catheter-based skeletal myoblast transfer.

REFERENCES

1. Beltrami AP, Urbanek K, Kajstura J, et al. Evidence that human cardiac myocytes divide after myocardial infarction. N Engl J Med 2001; 344:1750–1757.
2. Orlic D, Kajstura J, Chimenti S, et al. Bone marrow cells regenerate infarcted myocardium. Nature 2001; 410:701–705.

3. Kocher AA, Schuster MD, Szabolcs MJ, et al. Neovascularization of ischemic myocardium by human bone-marrow-derived angioblasts prevents cardiomyocyte apoptosis, reduces remodeling and improves cardiac function. Nat Med 2001; 7:430–436.
4. Murry CE, Field LJ, Menasche P. Cell-based cardiac repair: reflections at the 10-year point. Circulation 2005; 112:3174–3183.
5. Assmus B, Schachinger V, Teupe C, et al. Transplantation of Progenitor Cells and Regeneration Enhancement in Acute Myocardial Infarction (TOPCARE-AMI). Circulation 2002; 106:3009–3017.
6. Wollert KC, Meyer GP, Lotz J, et al. Intracoronary autologous bone-marrow cell transfer after myocardial infarction: the BOOST randomised controlled clinical trial. Lancet 2004; 364:141–148.
7. Srivastava D, Ivey KN. Potential of stem-cell-based therapies for heart disease. Nature 2006; 441:1097–1099.
8. Urbanek K, Rota M, Cascapera S, et al. Cardiac stem cells possess growth factor-receptor systems that after activation regenerate the infarcted myocardium, improving ventricular function and long-term survival. Circ Res 2005; 97:663–673.
9. Penn MS, Mal N. Stem cells in cardiovascular disease: methods and protocols. Methods Mol Med 2006; 129:329–351.
10. Quaini F, Urbanek K, Beltrami AP, et al. Chimerism of the transplanted heart. N Engl J Med 2002; 346:5–15.
11. Deb A, Wang S, Skelding KA, et al. Bone marrow-derived cardiomyocytes are present in adult human heart: A study of gender-mismatched bone marrow transplantation patients. Circulation 2003; 107:1247–1249.
12. Chien KR. Stem cells: lost in translation. Nature 2004; 428:607–608.
13. Murry CE, Soonpaa MH, Reinecke H, et al. Haematopoietic stem cells do not transdifferentiate into cardiac myocytes in myocardial infarcts. Nature 2004; 428:664–668.
14. Minami E, Laflamme MA, Saffitz JE, et al. Extracardiac progenitor cells repopulate most major cell types in the transplanted human heart. Circulation 2005; 112:2951–2958.
15. Nygren JM, Jovinge S, Breitbach M, et al. Bone marrow-derived hematopoietic cells generate cardiomyocytes at a low frequency through cell fusion, but not transdifferentiation. Nat Med 2004; 10:494–501.
16. Scorsin M, Marotte F, Sabri A, et al. Can grafted cardiomyocytes colonize peri-infarct myocardial areas? Circulation 1996; 94(suppl 9):II337—II340.
17. Jackson KA, Majka SM, Wang H, et al. Regeneration of ischemic cardiac muscle and vascular endothelium by adult stem cells. J Clin Invest 2001; 107:1395–1402.
18. Scorsin M, Hagege A, Vilquin JT, et al. Comparison of the effects of fetal cardiomyocyte and skeletal myoblast transplantation on postinfarction left ventricular function. J Thorac Cardiovasc Surg 2000; 119:1169–1175.
19. Wang JS, Shum-Tim D, Galipeau J, et al. Marrow stromal cells for cellular cardiomyoplasty: feasibility and potential clinical advantages. J Thorac Cardiovasc Surg 2000; 120:999–1005.
20. Jain M, DerSimonian H, Brenner DA, et al. Cell therapy attenuates deleterious ventricular remodeling and improves cardiac performance after myocardial infarction. Circulation 2001; 103:1920–1927.
21. Ghostine S, Carrion C, Souza LC, et al. Long-term efficacy of myoblast transplantation on regional structure and function after myocardial infarction. Circulation 2002; 106(12 suppl 1):I131–I136.
22. Toma C, Pittenger MF, Cahill KS, et al. Human mesenchymal stem cells differentiate to a cardiomyocyte phenotype in the adult murine heart. Circulation 2002; 105:93–98.
23. Agbulut O, Vandervelde S, Al Attar N, et al. Comparison of human skeletal myoblasts and bone marrow-derived CD133+ progenitors for the repair of infarcted myocardium. J Am Coll Cardiol 2004; 44:458–463.
24. Reinecke H, Poppa V, Murry CE. Skeletal muscle stem cells do not transdifferentiate into cardiomyocytes after cardiac grafting. J Mol Cell Cardiol 2002; 34:241–249.
25. Li RK, Jia ZQ, Weisel RD, et al. Cardiomyocyte transplantation improves heart function. Ann Thorac Surg 1996; 62:654–660; (discussion 60–61).

26. Muller-Ehmsen J, Peterson KL, Kedes L, et al. Rebuilding a damaged heart: long-term survival of transplanted neonatal rat cardiomyocytes after myocardial infarction and effect on cardiac function. Circulation 2002; 105:1720–1726.
27. Sequeira MI, Esch F, Schifferings P, et al. Homing of bone marrow stem cells in ischemic heart tissue is mediated by pecam-1 (cd 31), P-selectin and β2-integrins (abstract). Circulation 2005; 112:II265.
28. Askari AT, Unzek S, Popovic ZB, et al. Effect of stromal-cell-derived factor 1 on stem-cell homing and tissue regeneration in ischaemic cardiomyopathy. Lancet 2003; 362:697–703.
29. Kucia M, Dawn B, Hunt G, et al. Cells expressing early cardiac markers reside in the bone marrow and are mobilized into the peripheral blood after myocardial infarction. Circ Res 2004; 95:1191–1199.
30. Schenk S, Mal N, Finan A, et al. MCP-3 is a myocardial mesenchymal stem cell homing factor. Stem Cells 2007; 25:245–251.
31. Mangi AA, Noiseux N, Kong D, et al. Mesenchymal stem cells modified with Akt prevent remodeling and restore performance of infarcted hearts. Nat Med 2003; 9:1195–1201.
32. Minamisawa S, Hoshijima M, Chu G, et al. Chronic phospholamban-sarcoplasmic reticulum calcium ATPase interaction is the critical calcium cycling defect in dilated cardiomyopathy. Cell 1999; 99:313–322.
33. del Monte F, Harding SE, Dec GW, et al. Targeting phospholamban by gene transfer in human heart failure. Circulation 2002; 105:904–947.
34. Hoshijima M, Ikeda Y, Iwanaga Y, et al. Chronic suppression of heart-failure progression by a pseudophosphorylated mutant of phospholamban via in vivo cardiac rAAV gene delivery. Nat Med 2002; 8:864–871.
35. Iwanaga Y, Hoshijima M, Gu Y, et al. Chronic phospholamban inhibition prevents progressive cardiac dysfunction and pathological remodeling after infarction in rats. J Clin Invest 2004; 113:727–736.
36. del Monte F, Harding SE, Schmidt U, et al. Restoration of contractile function in isolated cardiomyocytes from failing human hearts by gene transfer of SERCA2a. Circulation 1999; 100:2308–2311.
37. del Monte F, Williams E, Lebeche D, et al. Improvement in survival and cardiac metabolism after gene transfer of sarcoplasmic reticulum Ca(2+)-ATPase in a rat model of heart failure. Circulation 2001; 104:1424–1429.
38. Shah AS, Lilly RE, Kypson AP, et al. Intracoronary adenovirus-mediated delivery and overexpression of the beta(2)-adrenergic receptor in the heart : prospects for molecular ventricular assistance. Circulation 2000; 101:408–414.
39. Shah AS, White DC, Emani S, et al. In vivo ventricular gene delivery of a beta-adrenergic receptor kinase inhibitor to the failing heart reverses cardiac dysfunction. Circulation 2001; 103:1311–1316.
40. Lai NC, Roth DM, Gao MH, et al. Intracoronary delivery of adenovirus encoding adenylyl cyclase VI increases left ventricular function and cAMP-generating capacity. Circulation 2000; 102:2396–2401.
41. Weig HJ, Laugwitz KL, Moretti A, et al. Enhanced cardiac contractility after gene transfer of V2 vasopressin receptors In vivo by ultrasound-guided injection or trans-coronary delivery. Circulation 2000; 101:1578–1585.
42. French BA, Mazur W, Geske RS, Bolli R. Direct in vivo gene transfer into porcine myocardium using replication-deficient adenoviral vectors. Circulation 1994; 90:2414–2424.
43. Maurice JP, Hata JA, Shah AS, et al. Enhancement of cardiac function after adenoviral-mediated in vivo intracoronary beta2-adrenergic receptor gene delivery. J Clin Invest 1999; 104:21–29.
44. Liggett SB, Tepe NM, Lorenz JN, et al. Early and delayed consequences of beta(2)-adrenergic receptor overexpression in mouse hearts: critical role for expression level. Circulation 2000; 101:1707–1714.
45. Meyer GP, Wollert KC, Lotz J, et al. Intracoronary bone marrow cell transfer after myocardial infarction: eighteen months' follow-up data from the randomized, controlled BOOST (BOne marrOw transfer to enhance ST-elevation infarct regeneration) trial. Circulation 2006; 113:1287–1294.

46. Lunde K, Solheim S, Aakhus S, et al. Intracoronary injection of mononuclear bone marrow cells in acute myocardial infarction. N Engl J Med 2006; 355:1199–1209.
47. Janssens S, Dubois C, Bogaert J, et al. Autologous bone marrow-derived stemcell transfer in patients with ST-segment elevation myocardial infarction: double-blind, randomised controlled trial. Lancet 2006; 367:113–121.
48. Seeger F, Tonn T, Krzossok N, et al. Cell isolation procedures matter: a comparison of different isolation protocols of bone marrow mononuclear cells used for cell therapy in patients with acute myocardial infarction. Eur Heart J 2007; 28:766–772.
49. Schachinger V, Erbs S, Elsasser A, et al. Intracoronary bone marrow-derived progenitor cells in acute myocardial infarction. N Engl J Med 2006; 355:1210–1221.
50. Khaja F, Walton JA Jr., Brymer JF, et al. Intracoronary fibrinolytic therapy in acute myocardial infarction: report of a prospective randomized trial. N Engl J Med 1983; 308:1305–1311.
51. Anderson JL, Marshall HW, Bray BE, et al. A randomized trial of intracoronary streptokinase in the treatment of acute myocardial infarction. N Engl J Med 1983; 308:1312–1318.
52. Britten MB, Abolmaali ND, Assmus B, et al. Infarct remodeling after intracoronary progenitor cell treatment in patients with acute myocardial infarction (TOPCARE-AMI): mechanistic insights from serial contrast-enhanced magnetic resonance imaging. Circulation 2003; 108:2212–2218.
53. Schachinger V, Assmus B, Britten MB, et al. Transplantation of progenitor cells and regeneration enhancement in acute myocardial infarction: final one-year results of the TOPCARE-AMI Trial. J Am Coll Cardiol 2004; 44:1690–1699.
54. Schachinger V, Assmus B, Honold J, et al. Normalization of coronary blood flow in the infarct-related artery after intracoronary progenitor cell therapy: intracoronary Doppler substudy of the TOPCARE-AMI trial. Clin Res Cardiol 2006; 95:13–22.
55. Assmus B, Honold J, Schachinger V, et al. Transcoronary transplantation of progenitor cells after myocardial infarction. N Engl J Med 2006; 355:1222–1232.
56. Kang HJ, Kim HS, Zhang SY, et al. Effects of intracoronary infusion of peripheral blood stem-cells mobilised with granulocyte-colony stimulating factor on left ventricular systolic function and restenosis after coronary stenting in myocardial infarction: the MAGIC cell randomised clinical trial. Lancet 2004; 363:751–756.
57. Ince H, Petzsch M, Kleine HD, et al. Preservation from left ventricular remodeling by front-integrated revascularization and stem cell liberation in evolving acute myocardial infarction by use of granulocyte-colony-stimulating factor (FIRSTLINE-AMI). Circulation 2005; 112:3097–3106.
58. Zohlnhofer D, Ott I, Mehilli J, et al. Stem cell mobilization by granulocyte colony-stimulating factor in patients with acute myocardial infarction: a randomized controlled trial. JAMA 2006; 295:1003–1010.
59. Ripa RS, Jorgensen E, Wang Y, et al. Stem cell mobilization induced by subcutaneous granulocyte-colony stimulating factor to improve cardiac regeneration after acute ST-elevation myocardial infarction: result of the double-blind, randomized, placebo-controlled stem cells in myocardial infarction (STEMMI) trial. Circulation 2006; 113: 1983–1992.
60. Ellis SG, Penn MS, Bolwell B, et al. Granulocyte colony stimulating factor in patients with large acute myocardial infarction: results of a pilot dose-escalation randomized trial. Am Heart J 2006; 152:1051 E9–E14.
61. Engelmann MG, Theiss HD, Hennig-Theiss C, et al. Autologous bone marrow stem cell mobilization induced by granulocyte colony-stimulating factor after subacute ST-segment elevation myocardial infarction undergoing late revascularization: final results from the G-CSF-STEMI (Granulocyte Colony-Stimulating Factor ST-Segment Elevation Myocardial Infarction) trial. J Am Coll Cardiol 2006; 48:1712–1721.
62. Kastrup J, Ripa RS, Wang Y, et al. Myocardial regeneration induced by granulocyte-colony-stimulating factor mobilization of stem cells in patients with acute or chronic ischaemic heart disease: a non-invasive alternative for clinical stem cell therapy? Eur Heart J 2006; 27:2748–2754.

63. Beohar N, Flaherty JD, Davidson CJ, Vidovich M, Singhal S, Rapp JA, Erdogan A, Lee DC, Rammohan C, Brodsky A, Wu E, Pieper K, Virmani R, Bonow RO, Mehta J. Granulocyte-colony stimulating factor administration after myocardial infarction in a porcine ischemia-reperfusion model: functional and pathological effects of dose timing. Catheter Cardiovasc Interv 2007; 69(2):257–266.

64. Kang HJ, Lee HY, Na SH, et al. Differential effect of intracoronary infusion of mobilized peripheral blood stem cells by granulocyte colony-stimulating factor on left ventricular function and remodeling in patients with acute myocardial infarction versus old myocardial infarction: the MAGIC Cell-3-DES randomized, controlled trial. Circulation 2006; 114(suppl 1):I145–I151.

65. Menasche P. First randomized placebo-controlled Myoblast Autologous Grafting in Ischemic Cardiomyopathy (MAGIC) trial. Chicago, IL: American Heart Association 2006 Scientific Sessions; November 15, 2006 (presentation).

66. Ben-Dor I, Fuchs S, Kornowski R. Potential hazards and technical considerations associated with myocardial cell transplantation protocols for ischemic myocardial syndrome. J Am Coll Cardiol 2006; 48:1519–1526.

67. Vulliet PR, Greeley M, Halloran SM, et al. Intra-coronary arterial injection of mesenchymal stromal cells and microinfarction in dogs. Lancet 2004; 363:783–784.

68. Wilensky RL, Freyman T, Polin GM, et al. A comparison of 3 methods of mesenchymal stem cell delivery following transmural myocardial infarction in porcine model. Eur Heart J 2005; 26:(suppl):219 (abstr).

69. Moelker AD, Spitskovsky D, Baks T, et al. Intracoronary delivery of human umbilical cord derived somatic stem cells does not improve left ventricule function after four weeks in swine with a myocardial infarction. Eur Heart J 2005; 26(suppl):122 (abstr).

70. Blatt A, Cotter G, Leitman M, et al. Intracoronary administration of autologous bone marrow mononuclear cells after induction of short ischemia is safe and may improve hibernation and ischemia in patients with ischemic cardiomyopathy. Am Heart J 2005; 150:986.

71. Bartunek J, Vanderheyden M, Vandekerckhove B, et al. Intracoronary injection of CD133-positive enriched bone marrow progenitor cells promotes cardiac recovery after recent myocardial infarction: feasibility and safety. Circulation 2005; 112(suppl 9):I178–I183.

72. Kornowski R, Fuchs S, Tio FO, et al. Evaluation of the acute and chronic safety of the biosense injection catheter system in porcine hearts. Catheter Cardiovasc Interv 1999; 48:447–53; (discussion 54–55).

73. Fuchs S, Baffour R, Zhou YF, et al. Transendocardial delivery of autologous bone marrow enhances collateral perfusion and regional function in pigs with chronic experimental myocardial ischemia. J Am Coll Cardiol 2001; 37:1726–1732.

74. Kawamoto A, Tkebuchava T, Yamaguchi J, et al. Intramyocardial transplantation of autologous endothelial progenitor cells for therapeutic neovascularization of myocardial ischemia. Circulation 2003; 107:461–468.

75. Fuchs S, Satler LF, Kornowski R, et al. Catheter-based autologous bone marrow myocardial injection in no-option patients with advanced coronary artery disease: a feasibility study. J Am Coll Cardiol 2003; 41:1721–1724.

76. Perin EC, Dohmann HF, Borojevic R, et al. Transendocardial, autologous bone marrow cell transplantation for severe, chronic ischemic heart failure. Circulation 2003; 107:2294–2302.

77. Silva GV, Perin EC, Dohmann HF, et al. Catheter-based transendocardial delivery of autologous bone-marrow-derived mononuclear cells in patients listed for heart transplantation. Tex Heart Inst J 2004; 31:214–219.

78. Dohmann HF, Perin EC, Takiya CM, et al. Transendocardial autologous bone marrow mononuclear cell injection in ischemic heart failure: postmortem anatomicopathologic and immunohistochemical findings. Circulation 2005; 112:521–526.

79. Kastrup J, Jorgensen E, Ruck A, et al. Direct intramyocardial plasmid vascular endothelial growth factor-A165 gene therapy in patients with stable severe angina pectoris A randomized double-blind placebo-controlled study: the Euroinject One trial. J Am Coll Cardiol 2005; 45:982–988.

80. Yoon YS, Park JS, Tkebuchava T, et al. Unexpected severe calcification after transplantation of bone marrow cells in acute myocardial infarction. Circulation 2004; 109: 3154–3157.

81. Wang JS, Shum-Tim D, Chedrawy E, et al. The coronary delivery of marrow stromal cells for myocardial regeneration: pathophysiologic and therapeutic implications. J Thorac Cardiovasc Surg 2001; 122:699–705.
82. Li TS, Hamano K, Hirata K, et al. The safety and feasibility of the local implantation of autologous bone marrow cells for ischemic heart disease. J Card Surg 2003; 18(suppl 2): S69–S75.
83. Ozbaran M, Omay SB, Nalbantgil S, et al. Autologous peripheral stem cell transplantation in patients with congestive heart failure due to ischemic heart disease. Eur J Cardiothorac Surg 2004; 25:342–350; (discussion 50–1).
84. Archundia A, Aceves JL, Lopez-Hernandez M, et al. Direct cardiac injection of G-CSF mobilized bone-marrow stem-cells improves ventricular function in old myocardial infarction. Life Sci 2005; 78:279–283.
85. Stamm C, Westphal B, Kleine HD, et al. Autologous bone-marrow stem-cell transplantation for myocardial regeneration. Lancet 2003; 361:45–46.
86. Menasche P, Hagege AA, Vilquin JT, et al. Autologous skeletal myoblast transplantation for severe postinfarction left ventricular dysfunction. J Am Coll Cardiol 2003; 41:1078–1083.
87. Smits PC, van Geuns RJ, Poldermans D, et al. Catheter-based intramyocardial injection of autologous skeletal myoblasts as a primary treatment of ischemic heart failure: clinical experience with six-month follow-up. J Am Coll Cardiol 2003; 42:2063–2069.
88. Siminiak T, Fiszer D, Jerzykowska O, et al. Percutaneous trans-coronary-venous transplantation of autologous skeletal myoblasts in the treatment of post-infarction myocardial contractility impairment: the POZNAN trial. Eur Heart J 2005; 26:1188–1195.
89. Strauer BE, Brehm M, Zeus T, et al. Repair of infarcted myocardium by autologous intracoronary mononuclear bone marrow cell transplantation in humans. Circulation 2002; 106:1913–1918.
90. Galinanes M, Loubani M, Davies J, et al. Autotransplantation of unmanipulated bone marrow into scarred myocardium is safe and enhances cardiac function in humans. Cell Transplant 2004; 13:7–13.
91. Fuchs S, Kornowski R, Weisz G, et al. Safety and feasibility of transendocardial autologous bone marrow cell transplantation in patients with advanced heart disease. Am J Cardiol 2006; 97:823–829.
92. Hagege AA, Carrion C, Menasche P, et al. Viability and differentiation of autologous skeletal myoblast grafts in ischaemic cardiomyopathy. Lancet 2003; 361:491–492.
93. Zhang YM, Hartzell C, Narlow M, et al. Stem cell-derived cardiomyocytes demonstrate arrhythmic potential. Circulation 2002; 106:1294–1299.
94. Chachques JC, Herreros J, Trainini J, et al. Autologous human serum for cell culture avoids the implantation of cardioverter-defibrillators in cellular cardiomyoplasty. Int J Cardiol 2004; 95(suppl 1):S29–S33.
95. Conti JA, Scher HI. Acute arterial thrombosis after escalated-dose methotrexate, vinblastine, doxorubicin, and cisplatin chemotherapy with recombinant granulocyte colony-stimulating factor. A possible new recombinant granulocyte colony-stimulating factor toxicity. Cancer 1992; 70:2699–2702.
96. Fukumoto Y, Miyamoto T, Okamura T, et al. Angina pectoris occurring during granulocyte colony-stimulating factor-combined preparatory regimen for autologous peripheral blood stem cell transplantation in a patient with acute myelogenous leukaemia. Br J Haematol 1997; 97:666–668.
97. Vij R, Adkins DR, Brown RA, et al. Unstable angina in a peripheral blood stem and progenitor cell donor given granulocyte-colony-stimulating factor. Transfusion 1999; 39:542–543.
98. Anderlini P, Korbling M, Dale D, et al. Allogeneic blood stem cell transplantation: considerations for donors. Blood 1997; 90:903–908.
99. Lindemann A, Rumberger B. Vascular complications in patients treated with granulocyte colony-stimulating factor (G-CSF). Eur J Cancer 1993; 29A:2338–2339.
100. Hill JP, Paul JD, Powell TM, et al. Efficacy and risk of granulocyte colony stimulating factor administration in patients with severe coronary artery disease. Circulation 2003; 108(suppl 4):478.

101. Valgimigli M, Rigolin GM, Cittanti C, et al. Use of granulocyte-colony stimulating factor during acute myocardial infarction to enhance bone marrow stem cell mobilization in humans: clinical and angiographic safety profile. Eur Heart J 2005; 26:1838–1845.
102. Boyle AJ, Whitbourn R, Schlicht S, et al. Intra-coronary high-dose CD34+ stem cells in patients with chronic ischemic heart disease: a 12-month follow-up. Int J Cardiol 2006; 109: 21–27.
103. Hill JM, Syed MA, Arai AE, et al. Outcomes and risks of granulocyte colony-stimulating factor in patients with coronary artery disease. J Am Coll Cardiol 2005; 46:1643–1648.
104. Huttmann A, Duhrsen U, Stypmann J, et al. Granulocyte colony-stimulating factor-induced blood stem cell mobilisation in patients with chronic heart failure–Feasibility, safety and effects on exercise tolerance and cardiac function. Basic Res Cardiol 2006; 101: 78–86.
105. Bartunek J, Dimmeler S, Drexler H, et al. The consensus of the task force of the European Society of Cardiology concerning the clinical investigation of the use of autologous adult stem cells for repair of the heart. Eur Heart J 2006; 27:1338–1340.

The Future of Reperfusion Therapy

Elliott M. Antman
Cardiovascular Division, TIMI Study Group, Brigham and Women's Hospital, Harvard Medical School, Boston, Massachusetts, U.S.A.

INTRODUCTION

Despite compelling evidence that expeditious use of reperfusion therapy improves survival of ST-elevation myocardial infarction (STEMI) patients, this life-saving therapy is often not administered. The future of reperfusion therapy centers around strategies to improve access to timely reperfusion for STEMI and administration of the appropriate ancillary therapy. While a catheter-based approach to reperfusion is becoming increasingly preferred by many clinicians, this form of treatment is not universally available, and for the foreseeable future, fibrinolysis will continue to be an important treatment in the majority of STEMI patients managed worldwide (Fig. 1) (1–3).

LOGISTICS OF CARE

Regardless of the mode of reperfusion, the goal is to minimize total ischemic time, defined as the time from onset of symptoms of STEMI to initiation of reperfusion therapy (2). As stressed in the American College of Cardiology/American Heart Association (ACC/AHA) STEMI Guidelines, several issues should be considered in selecting the type of reperfusion therapy (2).

1. Time from the onset of symptoms to initiation of reperfusion therapy: This is an overarching concept, since it is an important predictor of infarct size and patient outcome (Fig. 2). (4)
2. Risk of the STEMI: The higher the patient's risk of mortality from STEMI, the more percutaneous coronary intervention (PCI) is preferred over fibrinolysis.
3. Risk of bleeding: The higher the risk of bleeding, the greater the preference for a PCI-based reperfusion strategy. For patients who are not candidates for acute reperfusion due to lack of availability of PCI and contraindications to fibrinolysis, antiplatelet and anticoagulant therapy should still be prescribed.
4. Time required for transportation to a skilled PCI center: The delay required for transportation to a skilled PCI center is the greatest operational impediment to routine implementation of a PCI reperfusion strategy. Citing an acceptable delay time (door-to-balloon–door-to-needle) that is applicable to all STEMI patients can only be a rough guide because of the complex decision process involved (Fig. 3A) (5). Pinto et al. have identified the relationships between key patient-level features that influence the decision about an acceptable delay time (Fig. 3B) (6). This underscores the need for the individualization of decision-making, especially when PCI is not readily available.

When PCI capability is available, the best outcomes are achieved by offering this strategy 24 hr/day, 7 days/wk, with a systems goal of a first-medical-contact-to-balloon time within 90 minutes (3). Bradley et al. (7) have identified six key specific

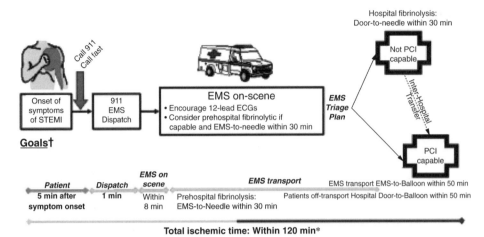

Total ischemic time: Within 120 min*

*Golden Hour = First 60 minutes

FIGURE 1 Options for transportation of STEMI patients and initial reperfusion treatment: goals. Reperfusion in patients with STEMI can be accomplished by the pharmacologic (fibrinolysis) or catheter-based (primary PCI) approaches. The overarching goal is to keep total ischemic time within 120 minutes (ideally within 60 minutes) from symptom onset to initiation of reperfusion treatment. Within this context, the following are goals for the medical system[a] based on the mode of patient transportation and the capabilities at the receiving hospital.

Medical system goals:
EMS transport (recommended):

- If EMS has fibrinolytic capability and the patient qualifies for therapy, prehospital fibrinolysis should be started within 30 minutes of EMS arrival on scene.
- If EMS is not capable of administering prehospital fibrinolysis and the patient is transported to a non-PCI-capable hospital, the door-to-needle time should be within 30 minutes for patients in whom fibrinolysis is indicated.
- If EMS is not capable of administering prehospital fibrinolysis and the patient is transported to a PCI-capable hospital, the EMS-to-balloon time should be within 90 minutes.
- If EMS takes patient to a non-PCI-capable hospital, it is appropriate to consider emergency interhospital transfer of the patient to a PCI-capable hospital for mechanical revascularization if
  - there is a contraindication to fibrinolysis,
  - PCI can be initiated promptly within 90 minutes from EMS arrival-to-balloon time at the PCI-capable hospital, (EMS arrival→transport to non-PCI-capable hospital→arrival at non-PCI-capable hospital to transfer to PCI-capable hospital→arrival at PCI-capable hospital-to-balloon time is 90 minutes), and
  - fibrinolysis is administered and is unsuccessful (i.e., "rescue PCI").

Patient self-transport (discouraged):

- If the patient arrives at a non-PCI capable hospital, the door-to-needle time should be within 30 minutes of arrival at the emergency department.
- If the patient arrives at a PCI-capable hospital, the door-to-balloon time should be within 90 minutes.
- If the patient presents to a non-PCI-capable hospital, it is appropriate to consider emergency interhospital transfer of the patient to a PCI-capable hospital if
  - there is a contraindication to fibrinolysis,

(continued on next page)

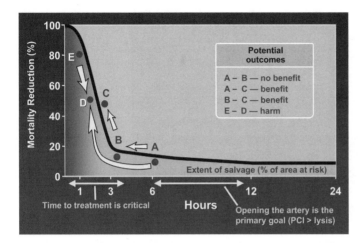

FIGURE 2 Hypothetical construct of the relationship among the duration of symptoms of acute MI before reperfusion therapy, mortality reduction, and extent of myocardial salvage.

Mortality reduction as a benefit of reperfusion therapy is greatest in the first 2 to 3 hours after the onset of symptoms of acute MI, most likely a consequence of myocardial salvage. The exact duration of this critical early period may be modified by several factors, including the presence of functioning collateral coronary arteries, ischemic preconditioning, myocardial oxygen demands, and duration of sustained ischemia. After this early period, the magnitude of the mortality benefit is much reduced, and as the mortality reduction curve flattens, time to reperfusion therapy is less critical. If a treatment strategy, such as facilitated PCI, were able to move patients back up the curve, a benefit would be expected. The magnitude of the benefit will depend on how far up the curve the patient can be shifted. The benefit of a shift from points A or B to point C would be substantial, but the benefit of a shift from point A to point B would be small. A treatment strategy that delays therapy during the early critical period, such as patient transfer for PCI, would be harmful (shift from point D to point C or point B). Between 6 and 12 hours after the onset of symptoms, opening the infarct-related artery is the primary goal of reperfusion therapy, and primary PCI is preferred over fibrinolytic therapy. The possible contribution to mortality reduction of opening the infarct-related artery, independent of myocardial salvage, is not shown. *Abbreviations*: MI, myocardial infarction; PCI, percutaneous coronary intervention. *Source*: Modified from Ref. 4. Copyright © 2005. American Medical Association. All rights reserved.

FIGURE 1 Continued

   o   PCI can be initiated within 90 minutes after the patient presented to the initial receiving hospital or within 60 minutes compared with when fibrinolysis with a fibrin-specific agent could be initiated at the initial receiving hospital, and
   o   fibrinolysis is administered and is unsuccessful (i.e., "rescue PCI").

Note: [a]The medical system goal is to facilitate rapid recognition and treatment of patients with STEMI such that door-to-needle (or medical-contact-to-needle) for initiation of fibrinolytic therapy can be achieved within 30 minutes or door-to-balloon (or medical-contact-to-balloon) for PCI can be achieved within 90 minutes. These goals should not be understood as "ideal" times, but rather the longest times that should be considered acceptable for a given system. Systems that are able to achieve even more rapid times for treatment of patients with STEMI should be encouraged.

Note medical contact is defined as the "time of EMS arrival on scene" after the patient calls EMS/9-1-1 or the "time of arrival at the emergency department door" (whether PCI-capable or non-PCI-capable hospital) when the patient self-transports. *Source*: Modified from Ref. 3.

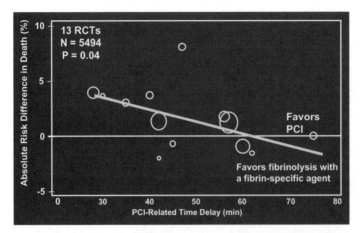

FIGURE 3A Absolute risk reduction in short-term mortality rates with primary PCI as a function of PCI-related time delay in 13 studies involving rtPA. The size of the *circles* reflect the sample sizes of the patient studies. *Solid line*, weighted meta-regression analysis. Values >0 represent benefit with PCI, and values <0 represent harm. *Source*: Modified from Ref. 5

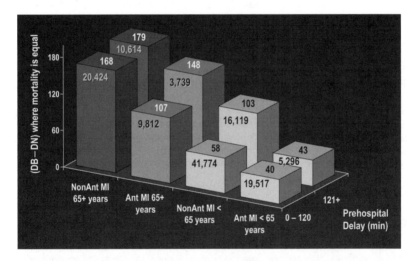

FIGURE 3B Adjusted analysis illustrating significant heterogeneity in the PCI-related delay (DB–DN time) for which the mortality rates with primary PCI and fibrinolysis were comparable after the study population was stratified by prehospital delay, location of infarct, and age. Ant indicates anterior; Non-Ant, nonanterior. To ensure a stable estimate of the mortality difference when primary PCI and fibrinolysis were compared in these subgroups, hospitals were excluded if fewer than 10 STEMI patients were treated with either PCI or fibrinolysis in either category. The DB–DN time at which the mortality benefit was lost was based on multivariate models. Variables included in the model were treatment type (PPCI or fibrinolysis), age, gender, race, diabetes mellitus, hypertension, angina, Killip class 2/3, Killip class 4, previous infarction, current smoking, stroke, pulse, systolic blood pressure, payer, symptom duration, infarct location, and discharge year. Hospital covariates included STEMI volume, PPCI volume, transfer-in rate, rural location, and status as a teaching hospital. *Source*: Modified from Ref. 6.

TABLE 1 Hospital Strategies to Reduce Door-to-Balloon Time

1. Emergency Department activates Catheterization Laboratory while patient is en route to hospital
2. Catheterization Laboratory is activated by Emergency Medicine physician
3. Emergency Department makes a single phone call to active Catheterization Laboratory
4. Arrival time of Catheterization Laboratory personnel <30 min from page
5. Attending cardiologist on call in the hospital
6. Hospital provides real-time feedback to Emergency Department and Catheterization Laboratory

Source: From Ref. 7.

hospital strategies that are associated with a significant reduction in door-to-balloon time (Table 1). An ongoing quality assurance program to identify strategies that will continually improve time-to-treatment and facilitate rapid and appropriate treatment is recommended. An example of such an initiative is the D2B Alliance for Quality launched by the ACC (www.d2balliance.org).

The AHA introduced a multidisciplinary initiative entitled Mission Lifeline, to develop systems and centers of care for STEMI patients (8). In this context, a *system* is defined as an integrated group of separate entities within a region providing specific services for the system that could include emergency medical services (EMS) providers, a community hospital(s), a tertiary center(s), and others. A *center* is defined as an entity such as a community or tertiary hospital that provides patient care services for a specific specialty or service. Movement from the current methods of delivering reperfusion therapy in STEMI to an ideal system requires a rigorous assessment of the needs from the perspectives of the patient (and public at large), the physician [EMS, emergency department (ED), interventional laboratory, coronary care unit (CCU)], the hospital (non-PCI capable and PCI capable), and third-party payers (e.g., commercial insurers, centers for Medicare and Medicaid services). The recommendations for research along the continuum from patient recognition of prodromal symptoms to restoration of flow in the infarct artery are outlined in Table 2 (9) and Figure 4.

INTERFACE OF FIBRINOLYSIS AND PCI

Facilitated PCI refers to a strategy of planned immediate PCI after administration of an initial pharmacologic regimen intended to improve coronary patency before the procedure. These regimens have included high-dose heparin, platelet glycoprotein (GP) IIb/IIIa inhibitors, full-dose or reduced-dose fibrinolytic therapy, and the combination of a GP IIb/IIIa inhibitor with a reduced-dose fibrinolytic agent. Despite the potential advantages, clinical trials of facilitated PCI have not demonstrated any benefit in reducing infarct size or improving outcomes (Fig. 5) (10).

The use of GP IIb/IIIa inhibitors, particularly abciximab, during primary PCI is well established (11). However, facilitated PCI with full-dose fibrinolytic therapy cannot be recommended as a general strategy (3). Nevertheless, selective use of the facilitated strategy with regimens other than full-dose fibrinolytic therapy in high risk subgroups of patients (large MI, hemodynamic or electrical instability) with low bleeding risk who present to hospitals without PCI capability might be performed when transfer delays for primary PCI are anticipated (2-3).

Pharmacologic reperfusion with full-dose fibrinolysis is not uniformly successful in restoring antegrade flow in the infarct artery. In such situations, a

TABLE 2 Recommendations for Research to Improve Timely Access to Reperfusion for STEMI

Recommendation	Level of implementation			Timeframe		
	National/federal	State	Local	Short (<6 mo)	Mid (<12 mo)	Long (>1 yr)
1. Quantify the characteristics, frequency, natural history, and effectiveness of interventions with patients who have early prodromal symptoms of STEMI.	X			X		
2. Conduct patient/family surveys about ways to improve management for STEMI before, during, and after PCI for the acute event.	X	X			X	
3. Conduct research on patient and family preferences regarding transfer to a STEMI Receiving Hospital, i.e., outside of their community.	X				X	X
4. Determine the most effective communication methods to bring about changes in patient/bystander action (decreased delay and appropriate system access).	X					X
5. Evaluate alternate options to EMS; for example, does calling a gatekeeper about symptoms (available 24/7) result in less time delay than calling EMS?	X			X	X	
6. Assess the role of decision support and information technology in the home and its impact on patient/bystander delay and EMS utilization.	X					X
7. Invest in further research and application of information technology to facilitate access to early recognition of symptoms/diagnosis/treatment.	X				X	X
8. Determine the role of health IT in expediting patient consent and transfer of medical records.	X	X				X
9. Study the psychological, medical, logistical, social, financial impacts on patients and families of transfer out of their community (i.e., transfer to a STEMI Receiving Hospital directly by EMS or via inter-hospital transfer).	X					X
10. Determine how realignment of physicians from STEMI Referral Hospitals to STEMI Receiving Hospitals will affect patient care.	X	X	X		X	
11. Determine how STEMI Receiving Hospitals will realign their services to accommodate the added volume of STEMI patients.	X				X	
12. Determine whether direct transport of STEMI patients to a STEMI Receiving Hospital (i.e., not closest hospital) is safe.	X		X		X	
13. Evaluate the feasibility of emergency patient transfer in rural communities.		X	X	X		
14. Determine best approach to use of pre-hospital ECG (i.e., interpreted in field, transmitted to ED, etc).	X	X	X		X	
15. Evaluate 12-lead ECG systems and reliability of data transfer.			X		X	
16. Evaluate the efficacy of extending programs such as "Get With The Guidelines" and "Guidelines Applied to Practice" to include provider, hospitals, and EMS systems in improving adherence to STEMI guidelines.	X					X

Source: From Ref. 9.

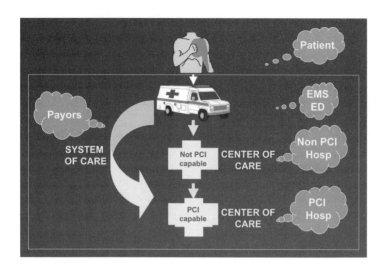

FIGURE 4 Areas requiring consideration in attempts to improve access to timely care for STEMI. Since the total ischemic time (onset of symptoms to reperfusion) is the critical overarching concept in shortening the time to reperfusion in STEMI, consideration should be given to all aspects of the problem along the continuum of care. The patient needs to recognize the onset of symptoms of STEMI and seek medical attention promptly. EMS and ED programs need to rapidly ascertain in the field whether a STEMI is present and efficiently triage the patient to the optimum site for care. Non-PCI capable hospitals need to either rapidly initiate fibrinolysis or expeditiously transfer patients, as indicated, for primary PCI. It is important to avoid compromising the financial viability of non-PCI capable hospitals if STEMI patients are preferentially diverted to PCI capable hospitals. The PCI capable hospital must be configured with equipment and staffing to provide primary PCI on a 24 hour/day seven day/wk basis. Third party payors will need to view the system of care as the unit for reimbursement in order to compensate all STEMI system participants appropriately for care of the STEMI patient. *Source*: Modified from Ref. 3.

strategy of prompt diagnostic angiography with intent to perform PCI is frequently contemplated. In certain patients such as those with cardiogenic shock, severe congestive heart failure/pulmonary edema, or hemodynamically compromising ventricular arrhythmias, a strategy of diagnostic angiography with intent to perform PCI is a useful approach regardless of the time since initiation of fibrinolytic therapy (2). In other situations, given the association between bleeding events and subsequent ischemic events, it would be prudent to select the moderate- and high-risk patients for PCI after fibrinolysis and to treat low-risk patients with medical therapy (2–3). An ECG estimate of potential infarct size in patients with persistent ST-segment elevation and ongoing ischemic pain is useful in selecting patients for rescue PCI (3).] Anterior infarct location or inferior infarct location with right ventricular involvement or precordial ST-segment depression usually predict increased risk. Conversely, patients with symptom resolution, improving ST-segment elevation, or inferior MI localized to 3 ECG leads probably should not be referred for angiography. Likewise, it is doubtful that PCI of a branch artery (diagonal or obtuse marginal branch) will change prognosis.

The philosophy where routine PCI after fibrinolysis is no longer proscribed, but is encouraged, captures the advantage of earlier initiation of reperfusion

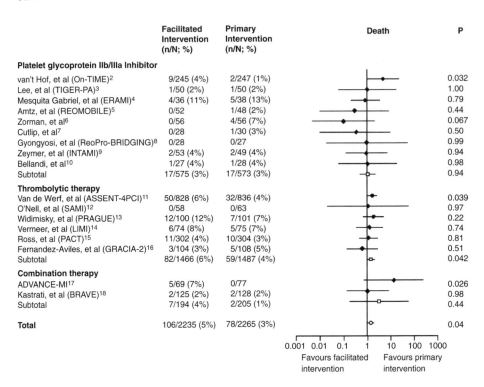

FIGURE 5 Short-term death in patients treated with facilitated or primary PCI. In this meta-analysis mortality was significantly increased (odds ratio 1.38; 95% CI 1.01–1.87; P = 0.04) when STEMI patients were treated with a facilitated PCI regimen compared with primary PCI. Note: Superscripted reference numbers are from the primary source for this figure. *Source*: From Ref. 10.

therapy, beginning with a pharmacologic approach followed by enhancement of flow in the epicardial infarct artery through balloon dilation and stenting, improved myocardial perfusion, and consolidation of the initial benefits of pharmacologic reperfusion by minimizing the risk of recurrent infarction and ischemia. The concept of routine use of PCI after fibrinolysis is referred to as a pharmacoinvasive approach and is supported by the encouraging results of several small-scale trials (12). It is likely that the pharmacoinvasive approach will require a customized initial pharmacologic regimen that integrates several patient features. Potential pharmacologic regimens followed by early PCI that appear worthy of testing include the following:

1. Combination reperfusion therapy with a reduced-dose fibrinolytic agent and a GP IIb/IIIa inhibitor for patients with a large quantity of anterior myocardium at risk and at low risk for bleeding.
2. Fibrinolysis without a GP IIb/IIIa inhibitor, but with a conservative dosing scheme of fibrinolytic and anticoagulant in patients at increased risk of bleeding (e.g., the elderly).
3. GP IIb/IIIa inhibitor therapy alone for patients at the highest risk of bleeding.

ADJUNCTIVE THERAPY

In addition to the fibrinolytic agent, fundamental additional components of the pharmacologic reperfusion regimen include an anticoagulant and antiplatelet agents. Whereas the fibrinolytic agent serves to convert plasminogen to plasmin that digests the fibrin strands in the obstructing thrombus in the infarct artery, adjunctive anticoagulant and antiplatelet therapy serve to prevent rethrombosis of initially successfully reperfused arteries (Fig. 6). A schematic illustration of the coagulation cascade in Figure 7, emphasizing the extrinsic limb (the initial trigger of coagulation with exposure of tissue factor in the disrupted plaque), the intrinsic limb (critical for maintenance of thrombus formation and also activated when the blood comes in contact with foreign substances such as cardiac catheters), and the final common pathway that ultimately leads to fibrin formation. The generation of thrombin during activation of the coagulation cascade not only catalyzes the formation of fibrin, but also networks the coagulation cascade with platelets by activating the thrombin receptor on platelets, ultimately leading to platelet aggregation. Potential sites for inhibition of the coagulation cascade are shown in Figure 7. Some anticoagulants act in more than one position [e.g., unfractionated heparin (UFH), low-molecular-weight heparin (LMWH)], while others act predominantly at a single locus either proximally

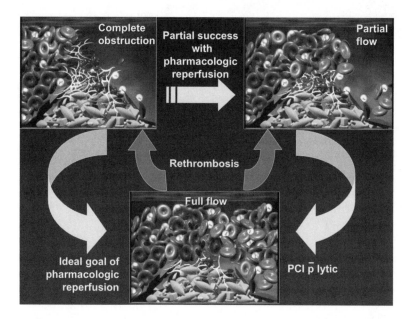

FIGURE 6 Mechanism of benefit of adjunctive pharmacotherapy in patients receiving fibrinolysis for STEMI. In patients with STEMI there is complete cessation of antegrade flow in the infarct artery (TIMI flow grade 0; *top left corner*). The ideal goal of pharmacologic reperfusion (*left curved arrow*) is to achieve full antegrade flow (TIMI grade 3 flow; *bottom center*), the success of which is largely dependent on the ability of the fibrinolytic to achieve lysis of the fibrin strands. In some patients, there is only partial success with pharmacologic reperfusion (TIMI grade 1 or 2; *top right corner*) and PCI is often used after the lytic to achieve full flow (*right curved arrow*). The primary benefit of adjunctive anticoagulant and antiplatelet therapy is to prevent rethrombosis (*upturned curved arrows*) after restoration of flow.

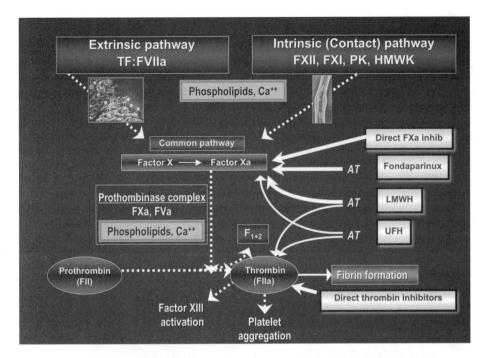

FIGURE 7 Coagulation cascade and anticoagulants. The extrinsic pathway of the coagulation cascade is activated upon exposure of TF in the disrupted plaque responsible for STEMI (*top left*). Factor VII is activated to factor VIIa and the complex of VIIa: TF activates factor X to Xa in the found common pathway, ultimately leading to thrombin generation via the prothrombinase complex. When cardiac catheters come in contact with the blood, the intrinsic (*contact*) pathway (*top right*) is activated, also leading to the activation of factor X. Anticoagulants may act in multiple sites to inhibit the coagulation cascade (e.g., UFH, LMWH, or at single sites proximally (fondaparinux, FXa inhibitors) or distally (direct thrombin inhibitors). When patients make the transition from the medical place of management to the catheterization laboratory, it is important to ensure that there is adequate inhibition of coagulation cascade via the contact pathway. Available data suggest that when fondaparinux is used upstream, it is necessary to add an anticoagulant with anti-IIa activity such as UFH or bivalirudin to minimize the risk of catheter thrombosis. *Abbreviations*: TF, tissue factor; UFH, unfractionated heparin; LMWH, low-molecular-weight heparin; FXa, direct factor Xa.

(fondaparinux, direct and indirect factor Xa inhibitors) or distally (direct thrombin inhibitors) (13).

There is benefit in more prolonged anticoagulant therapy throughout the duration of the index hospitalization in patients receiving fibrinolytics, as seen in the comparisons of reviparin versus placebo (CREATE) (14), fondaparinux versus placebo (stratum I in OASIS-6) (15), and enoxaparin versus UFH (ExTRACT-TIMI 25) (16) (Table 3). The mechanism of the benefit of a more prolonged anticoagulant regimen is probably multifactorial and includes a longer exposure to anticoagulants to prevent rethrombosis of the infarct artery and prevention of the rebound increase in events seen after abrupt discontinuation of UFH infusions (16). When added to prior data, the benefits of anticoagulation therapy started concurrently with non–fibrin-specific fibrinolytic agents (e.g., streptokinase) seen with the LMWHs and fondaparinux makes it reasonable to administer an anticoagulant

TABLE 3 Summary of Observations From Trials of Anticoagulants for STEMI

Anticoagulant	Efficacy (through 30 days)	Safety	Use During PCI
Reviparin	Fibrinolysis: probably superior to placebo. No reperfusion: probably superior to placebo.	Increased risk of serious bleeds[a]	No data on reviparin alone during PCI. Additional anticoagulant with anti-IIa activity, such as UFH or bivalirudin, recommended
Fondaparinux	Fibrinolysis: appears superior to control therapy (placebo/UFH). Relative benefit versus placebo and UFH separately cannot be reliably determined from available data. Primary PCI: when used alone, no advantage over UFH and trend toward worse outcome (see "Use During PCI"). No reperfusion: appears superior to control therapy (placebo/UFH). Relative benefit versus placebo and UFH separately cannot be reliably determined from available data.	Trend toward decreased risk of serious bleeds[a]	Increased risk of catheter thrombosis when fondaparinux is used alone. Additional anticoagulant with anti-IIa activity, such as UFH or bivalirudin, recommended.
Enoxaparin	Fibrinolysis: appears superior to UFH.	Increased risk of serious bleeds[a]	Enoxaparin can be used to support PCI after fibrinolysis. No additional anticoagulant needed.

[a]Definitions of significant bleeds varied among the trials. The original references should be consulted for details.
Source: Modified from Ref. 3.

across the spectrum of fibrinolytic agents in common clinical use [3]. Given the ease of administration and lower risk of heparin-induced thrombocytopenia, the LMWHs and fondaparinux are more attractive options than prolonged infusions of UFH.

When moving to PCI after fibrinolytic therapy, those patients who received upstream UFH or enoxaparin can continue to receive those anticoagulants without crossover to another agent (17). Based on reports of catheter thrombosis with fondaparinux alone during primary PCI in OASIS-6 (15), and the experience with fondaparinux in the OASIS-5 trial (18), fondaparinux should not be used as the sole anticoagulant during PCI but should be coupled with an additional agent that has anti-IIa activity (e.g., UFH or bivalirudin) to ameliorate the risk of catheter complications (Table 3) (15).

The sites of action of antiplatelet agents in contemporary clinical practice are shown in Figure 8 (19). Aspirin (a cyclo-oxygenase inhibitor) is the foundation antiplatelet agent for all patients with STEMI, regardless of the mode of reperfusion. The GP IIb/IIIa inhibitors have established efficacy to support primary PCI for STEMI. The COMMIT-CCS 2 and CLARITY-TIMI 28 trials provide evidence for the benefit of adding the thienopyridine clopidogrel to aspirin in patients

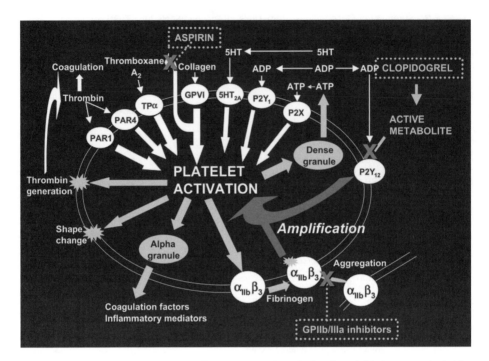

FIGURE 8 Current antiplatelet therapy. Platelets are activated when ligands bind to receptors (*white ovals*) on their surface ultimately leading to the release of contents from the alpha and dense granules. Aspirin is a cyclo-oxygenase inhibitor that decreases the production of thromboxane A2. Clopidogrel is a pro-drug that is converted to an active metabolite in the liver. The active metabolite binds to the $P2Y_{12}$ receptor, minimizing the sustained phase of platelet aggregation. GP IIb/IIIa inhibitors bind to the $\alpha_{IIb}\beta_3$ receptor preventing the cross linking by ligands such as fibrinogen and thereby reducing platelet aggregation. All three types of antiplatelet agents are useful in STEMI patients; see text for further discussion. *Abbreviation*: GP, glycoprotein. *Source*: Modified from Ref. 19.

undergoing fibrinolytic therapy (20,21). While the available data suggest that the oral maintenance dose of clopidogrel should be 75 mg daily, uncertainty exists regarding the efficacy and safety of adding a loading dose to elderly patients (>75 years), especially when they receive a fibrinolytic. On the basis of the CLARITY-TIMI 28 trial, it appears that the administration of clopidogrel at the time of initial fibrinolytic therapy is of benefit when PCI is performed subsequently (3). Extrapolating from experience in patients with UA/NSTEMI as well as those patients undergoing coronary stenting, clopidogrel (for at least one year) can be useful in STEMI patients. Because of variation in response to clopidogrel, several new platelet $P2Y_{12}$ inhibitors are being investigated as shown in Figure 9 (19).

MYOCARDIAL PERFUSION

The advances in reperfusion regimens for STEMI discussed so far have largely focused on efforts to restore flow in the epicardial infarct artery and prevent it from reoccluding. It should be emphasized that the real goal of reperfusion in patients

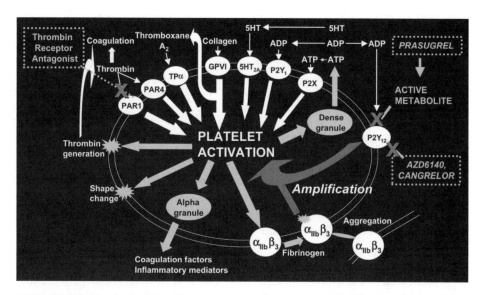

FIGURE 9 Future antiplatelet therapy. Prasugrel is a thienopyridine for which there is more efficient and more rapid generation of the active metabolite than clopidogrel. AZD6140 and Cangrelor are two new direct $P2Y_{12}$ inhibitors available for oral and intravenous administration, respectively. Thrombin receptor antagonists are a new class of antiplatelet agents that block the PAR1 receptor. One or more of the agents shown here may prove to be useful in patients with STEMI. *Source*: Modified from Ref. 19.

with STEMI is to improve myocardial perfusion in the infarct zone. Certainly, myocardial perfusion cannot be improved adequately without restoration of flow in the occluded infarct-related artery. Even patients with TIMI grade 3 flow may not achieve adequate myocardial perfusion (1).

Downstream embolization of platelet aggregates and microvascular spasm from release of vasoactive substances emanating from activated platelets contribute to obstruction of the microvasculature. Potential treatments to ameliorate micro-vasculature obstruction include administration of a GP IIb/IIIa inhibitor either in conjunction with a reduced dose of a fibrinolytic or at the time of PCI; the benefits of GP IIb/IIIa inhibition must be weighed against the increased risk of bleeding (1). Several small trials reported that administration of a vasodilator such as nicorandil, papavarine, or verapamil may help reduce vasospasm. Subsequent efforts have included intracoronary administration of a fibrinolytic after primary PCI for STEMI (22).

Another mechanism of diminished myocardial perfusion is reperfusion injury. Several types of reperfusion injury have been observed in experimental animals. These consist of (1) lethal reperfusion injury—reperfusion-induced death of cells that were still viable at the time of restoration of coronary blood flow; (2) vascular reperfusion injury—progressive damage to the microvasculature so that there is an expanding area of no-reflow and loss of coronary vasodilatory reserve; (3) stunned myocardium—salvaged myocytes displaying a prolonged period of contractile dysfunction following restoration of blood flow; and (4) reperfusion arrhythmias (23). The available evidence suggests that vascular reperfusion injury, stunning, and reperfusion arrhythmias can all occur in patients with STEMI. The concept of lethal reperfusion injury of potentially salvageable myocardium remains controversial, both in experimental animals and in patients.

Several adjunctive pharmacotherapies have been investigated to prevent inflammatory damage in the infarct zone, but so far with limited success only. The effectiveness of such treatments diminishes the later they are started after reperfusion. Trials with antibodies against the CD11/CD18 leukocyte adhesion receptor did not show a reduction in infarct size (24,25). Pexelizumab, a monoclonal antibody against the C5 component of complement, had no effect on mortality in STEMI patients treated with primary PCI (26). Although high-dose adenosine (70 μg/kg/min infusion for 3 hours) was associated with a reduction in infarct size, neither high- nor low-dose adenosine reduced the primary composite clinical end point of death or the development of heart failure at six months compared with placebo (27).

NOVEL MYOCARDIAL THERAPIES

Evidence now exists that human cardiac myocytes divide after STEMI, introducing new avenues for possible treatment of STEMI patients in the future. Two broad approaches have been taken to date (28). The first is myocardial gene therapy directed against oxidative stress-induced injury and protection against apoptosis and inflammation or designed to promote angiogenesis and rescue contractile function. Only a limited number of clinical trials of gene therapy have been reported to date, largely in patients with coronary artery disease that is not amenable to revascularization. While modest increases in surrogate end points such as perfusion imaging have been observed, the relevance of myocardial gene therapy to the future of reperfusion therapy for STEMI remains to be established.

The second approach, myocardial replacement therapy with stem cell therapy, has been attempted in patients with STEMI. Potential sources of donor cells include endothelial progenitor cells, mesenchymal stem cells, skeletal myoblasts, resident cardiac stem cells, or embryonic stem cells (28). The delivery of the donor cells can occur via a transvascular approach or by direct injection into the myocardium. A series of small, mostly uncontrolled studies have shown modest improvements in ejection fraction, but data on hard end points such as mortality and rehospitalization for heart failure or recurrent infarction remain to be evaluated in properly sized trials before the role of myocardial replacement therapy in the future of reperfusion therapy for STEMI can be established (28).

REFERENCES

1. Antman EM. "ST-Elevation Myocardial Infarction: Management." In: Libby P, Bonow RO, Mann DL, Zipes DP (eds.) Braunwald's Heart Disease: A Textbook of Cardiovascular Medicine. 8th ed. Philadelphia, Saunders Elsevier, 2008; 1233–1299.
2. Antman EM, Anbe DT, Armstrong PW, et al. ACC/AHA guidelines for the management of patients with ST-elevation myocardial infarction: a report of the American College of Cardiology/American Heart Association Task Force on Practice Guidelines (Committee to Revise the 1999 Guidelines for the Management of Patients With Acute Myocardial Infarction). Accessed on: April 25, 2007. Available at: www.acc.org/qualityandscience/ clinical/guidelines/stemi/index.pdf.
3. Antman EM, Hand M, Armstrong PW, Bates ER, Green LA, Halasyamani LK, Hochman JS, Krumholz HM, Lamas GA, Mullany CJ, Pearle DL, Sloan MA, Smith SC. Jr. 2007 focused update of the ACC/AHA 2004 Guidelines for the Management of

Patients with ST-Elevation Myocardial Infarction. A report of the American College of Cardiology/American Heart Association Task Force on Practice Guidelines (Writing Group to Review New Evidence and Update the ACC/AHA 2004 Guidelines for the Management of Patients with ST-Elevation Myocardial Infarction). Circulation, published online Dec 10, 2007.

4. Gersh BJ, Stone GW, White HD, et al. Pharmacological facilitation of primary percutaneous coronary intervention for acute myocardial infarction: is the slope of the curve the shape of the future? JAMA 2005; 293:979–986.

5. Nallamothu BK, Antman EM, Bates ER. Primary percutaneous coronary intervention versus fibrinolytic therapy in acute myocardial infarction: Does the choice of fibrinolytic agent impact on the importance of time-to-treatment? Am J Cardiol 2004; 94:772–774.

6. Pinto DS, Kirtane AJ, Nallamothu BK, et al. Hospital delays in reperfusion for ST-elevation myocardial infarction: implications when selecting a reperfusion strategy. Circulation 2006; 114:2019–2025.

7. Bradley EH, Herrin J, Wang Y, et al. Strategies for reducing the door-to-balloon time in acute myocardial infarction. N Engl J Med 2006; 355:2308–2320.

8. Jacobs AK, Antman EM, Ellrodt G, et al. Recommendation to develop strategies to increase the number of ST-segment-elevation myocardial infarction patients with timely access to primary percutaneous coronary intervention. Circulation 2006; 113:2152–2163.

9. Jacobs AK, Antman EM, Faxon DP. Development of systems of care for ST-segment elevation myocardial infarction (STEMI) patients: executive summary. Circulation 2007; 116:217–230.

10. Keeley EC, Boura JA, Grines CL. Comparison of primary and facilitated percutaneous coronary interventions for ST-elevation myocardial infarction: quantitative review of randomised trials. Lancet 2006; 367:579–588.

11. Montalescot G, Antoniucci D, Kastrati A, et al. Abciximab in primary coronary stenting of ST-elevation myocardial infarction: a European meta-analysis on individual patients' data with long-term follow-up. Eur Heart J 2007; 28:443–449.

12. Antman EM, Van de Werf F. Pharmacoinvasive therapy: the future of treatment for ST-elevation myocardial infarction. Circulation 2004; 109:2480–2486.

13. Antman EM. The search for replacements for unfractionated heparin. Circulation 2001; 103:2310–2314.

14. Yusuf S, Mehta SR, Xie C, et al. Effects of reviparin, a low-molecular-weight heparin, on mortality, reinfarction, and strokes in patients with acute myocardial infarction presenting with ST-segment elevation. JAMA 2005; 293:427–435.

15. Yusuf S, Mehta SR, Chrolavicius S, et al. Effects of fondaparinux on mortality and reinfarction in patients with acute ST-segment elevation myocardial infarction: the OASIS-6 randomized trial. JAMA 2006; 295:1519–1530.

16. Antman EM, Morrow DA, McCabe CH, et al. Enoxaparin versus unfractionated heparin with fibrinolysis for ST-elevation myocardial infarction. N Engl J Med 2006; 354:1477–1488.

17. Gibson CM, Murphy SA, Montalescot G, et al. Percutaneous coronary intervention in patients receiving enoxaparin or unfractionated heparin following fibrinolytic therapy for ST-elevation myocardial infarction in the ExTRACT-TIMI 25 trial. J Am Coll Cardiol 2007; 49:2238–2246.

18. Yusuf S, Mehta SR, Chrolavicius S, et al. Comparison of fondaparinux and enoxaparin in acute coronary syndromes. N Engl J Med 2006; 354:1464–1476.

19. Storey RF. Biology and pharmacology of the platelet P2Y12 receptor. Curr Pharm Design 2006; 12(10):1255–1259.

20. Chen ZM, Jiang LX, Chen YP, et al. Addition of clopidogrel to aspirin in 45,852 patients with acute myocardial infarction: randomised placebo-controlled trial. Lancet 2005; 366:1607–1621.

21. Sabatine MS, Cannon CP, Gibson CM, et al. Addition of clopidogrel to aspirin and fibrinolytic therapy for myocardial infarction with ST-segment elevation. N Engl J Med 2005; 352:1179–1189.

22. Sezer M, Oflaz H, Goren T, et al. Intracoronary streptokinase after primary percutaneous coronary intervention. N Engl J Med 2007; 356:1823–1834.

23. Braunwald E, Antman EM. "ST-Elevation Myocardial Infarction: Pathology, Pathophysiology, and Clinical Features." In: Libby P, Bonow RO, Mann DL, Zipes DP (eds.) Braunwald's Heart Disease: A Textbook of Cardiovascular Medicine. 8th ed. Philadelphia, Saunders Elsevier, 2008; 1207–1232.
24. Baran KW, Nguyen M, McKendall GR, et al. Double-blind, randomized trial of an anti-CD18 antibody in conjunction with recombinant tissue plasminogen activator for acute myocardial infarction: limitation of myocardial infarction following thrombolysis in acute myocardial infarction (LIMIT AMI) study. Circulation 2001; 104:2778–2783.
25. Faxon DP, Gibbons RJ, Chronos NA, et al. The effect of blockade of the CD11/CD18 integrin receptor on infarct size in patients with acute myocardial infarction treated with direct angioplasty: the results of the HALT-MI study. J Am Coll Cardiol 2002; 40:1199–1204.
26. Armstrong PW, Granger CB, Adams PX, et al. Pexelizumab for acute ST-elevation myocardial infarction in patients undergoing primary percutaneous coronary intervention: a randomized controlled trial. JAMA 2007; 297:43–51.
27. Kloner RA, Forman MB, Gibbons RJ, et al. Impact of time to therapy and reperfusion modality on the efficacy of adenosine in acute myocardial infarction: the AMISTAD-2 trial. Eur Heart J 2006; 27:2400–2405.
28. Melo L, Ward CA, Dzau VJ, et al. Gene therapies and stem cell therapies. In: Antman EM, ed. Cardiovascular Therapeutics: A Companion to Braunwald's Heart Disease. 3d ed. Philadelphia, PA: WB Saunders, 2007:40–66.

Appendix I   Recommendations from the ACC/AHA Guidelines for the Management of Patients with ST-Elevation Myocardial Infarction[a]

I. CLASSIFICATION OF RECOMMENDATIONS AND LEVEL OF EVIDENCE

A. Classification of Recommendations

Class I: Conditions for which there is evidence and/or general agreement that a given procedure or treatment is beneficial, useful, and effective.

Class II: Conditions for which there is conflicting evidence and/or a divergence of opinion about the usefulness/efficacy of a procedure or treatment.

Class IIa: Weight of evidence/opinion is in favor of usefulness/efficacy

Class IIb: Usefulness/efficacy is less well established by evidence/opinion

Class III: Conditions for which there is evidence and/or general agreement that a procedure/treatment is not useful/effective and in some cases may be harmful.

B. Level of Evidence

Level of Evidence A: Data derived from multiple randomized clinical trials or meta-analyses.

Level of Evidence B: Data derived from a single randomized trial, or nonrandomized studies.

Level of Evidence C: Only consensus opinion of experts, case studies, or standard-of-care.

II. MANAGEMENT BEFORE STEMI

A. Identification of Patients at Risk of STEMI

Class I

1. Primary care providers should evaluate the presence and status of control of major risk factors for coronary heart disease (CHD) for all patients at regular intervals (approximately every 3 to 5 years). (Level of Evidence C)

2. Ten-year risk [National Cholesterol Education Program (NCEP) global risk] of developing symptomatic CHD should be calculated for all patients who have two or more major risk factors to assess the need for primary prevention strategies. (Level of Evidence B)

3. Patients with established CHD should be identified for secondary prevention, and patients with a CHD risk equivalent (e.g., diabetes mellitus, chronic kidney disease, or 10-year risk greater than 20% as calculated by Framingham equations) should receive equally intensive risk factor intervention as those with clinically apparent CHD. (Level of Evidence A)

---

[a]From Refs. 1 and 2.

B. Patient Education for Early Recognition and Response to STEMI

Class I

1. Patients with symptoms of STEMI (chest discomfort with or without radiation to the arms[s], back, neck, jaw, or epigastrium; shortness of breath; weakness; diaphoresis; nausea; lightheadedness) should be transported to the hospital by ambulance rather than by friends or relatives. (Level of Evidence B)
2. Health care providers should actively address the following issues regarding STEMI with patients and their families:
    a. The patient's heart attack risk (Level of Evidence C)
    b. How to recognize symptoms of STEMI (Level of Evidence C)
    c. The advisability of calling 9-1-1 if symptoms are unimproved or worsening after five minutes, despite feelings of uncertainty about the symptoms and fear of potential embarrassment (Level of Evidence C)
    d. A plan for appropriate recognition and response to a potential acute cardiac event that includes the phone number to access emergency medical services (EMS), generally 9-1-1 (Level of Evidence C)
3. Health care providers should instruct patients for whom nitroglycerin has been prescribed previously to take ONE nitroglycerin dose sublingually in response to chest discomfort/pain. If chest discomfort/pain is unimproved or worsening five minutes after one sublingual nitroglycerin dose has been taken, it is recommended that the patient or family member/friend call 9-1-1 immediately to access EMS. (Level of Evidence C)

III. ONSET OF STEMI

A. Out-of-Hospital Cardiac Arrest

Class I

1. All communities should create and maintain a strong "Chain of Survival" for out-of-hospital cardiac arrest that includes early access (recognition of the problem and activation of the EMS system by a bystander), early cardiopulmonary resuscitation (CPR), early defibrillation for patients who need it, and early advanced cardiac life support (ACLS). (Level of Evidence C)
2. Family members of patients experiencing STEMI should be advised to take CPR training and familiarize themselves with the use of an automated external defibrillator (AED). In addition, they should be referred to a CPR training program that has a social support component for family members of post-STEMI patients. (Level of Evidence B)

IV. PREHOSPITAL ISSUES

A. EMS Systems

Class I

1. All EMS first responders who respond to patients with chest pain and/or suspected cardiac arrest should be trained and equipped to provide early defibrillation. (Level of Evidence A)
2. All public safety first responders who respond to patients with chest pain and/or suspected cardiac arrest should be trained and equipped to provide early defibrillation with AEDs. (Provision of early defibrillation with AEDs by nonpublic safety first responders is a promising new strategy, but further study is needed to determine its safety and efficacy.) (Level of Evidence B)

3. Dispatchers staffing 9-1-1 center emergency medical calls should have medical training, should use nationally developed and maintained protocols, and should have a quality-improvement system in place to ensure compliance with protocols. (Level of Evidence C)

B. Prehospital Chest Pain Evaluation and Treatment
Class I
1. Prehospital EMS providers should administer 162 to 325 mg of aspirin (chewed) to chest pain patients suspected of having STEMI unless contraindicated or already taken by patient. Although some trials have used enteric-coated aspirin for initial dosing, more rapid buccal absorption occurs with nonenteric-coated formulations. (Level of Evidence C)

Class IIa
1. It is reasonable for all 9-1-1 dispatchers to advise patients without a history of aspirin allergy who have symptoms of STEMI to chew aspirin (162–325 mg) while awaiting arrival of prehospital EMS providers. Although some trials have used enteric-coated aspirin for initial dosing, more rapid buccal absorption occurs with nonenteric-coated formulations. (Level of Evidence C)
2. It is reasonable that all ACLS providers perform and evaluate 12-lead electro-cardiograms (ECGs) routinely on chest pain patients suspected of STEMI. (Level of Evidence B)
3. If the ECG shows evidence of STEMI, it is reasonable that prehospital ACLS providers review a reperfusion "checklist" and relay the ECG and checklist findings to a predetermined medical control facility and/or receiving hospital. (Level of Evidence C)

C. Prehospital Fibrinolysis
Class IIa
1. Establishment of a prehospital fibrinolysis protocol is reasonable in (1) settings in which physicians are present in the ambulance or in (2) well-organized EMS systems with full-time paramedics who have 12-lead ECGs in the field with transmission capability, paramedic initial and ongoing training in ECG inter-pretation and STEMI treatment, online medical command, a medical director with training/experience in STEMI management, and an ongoing continuous quality-improvement program. (Level of Evidence B)

D. Prehospital Destination Protocols
Class I
1. Patients with STEMI who have cardiogenic shock and are less than 75 years of age should be brought immediately or secondarily transferred to facilities capable of cardiac catheterization and rapid revascularization [percutaneous coronary intervention (PCI) or coronary artery bypass graft surgery (CABG)] if it can be performed within 18 hours of onset of shock. (Level of Evidence A)
2. Patients with STEMI who have contraindications to fibrinolytic therapy should be brought immediately or secondarily transferred promptly (i.e., primary-receiving hospital door-to-departure time less than 30 minutes) to facilities capable of cardiac catheterization and rapid revascularization (PCI or CABG). (Level of Evidence B)
3. Every community should have a written protocol that guides EMS system personnel in determining where to take patients with suspected or confirmed STEMI. (Level of Evidence C)

Class IIa

1. It is reasonable that patients with STEMI who have cardiogenic shock and are 75 years of age or older be considered for immediate or prompt secondary transfer to facilities capable of cardiac catheterization and rapid revascularization (PCI or CABG) if it can be performed within 18 hours of onset of shock. (Level of Evidence B)
2. It is reasonable that patients with STEMI who are at especially high risk of dying, including those with severe congestive heart failure (CHF), be considered for immediate or prompt secondary transfer (i.e., primary-receiving hospital door-to-departure time less than 30 minutes) to facilities capable of cardiac catheterization and rapid revascularization (PCI or CABG). (Level of Evidence B)

V. INITIAL RECOGNITION AND MANAGEMENT IN THE EMERGENCY DEPARTMENT

A. Optimal Strategies for Emergency Department Triage
Class I

1. Hospitals should establish multidisciplinary teams (including primary care physicians, emergency medicine physicians, cardiologists, nurses, and laboratorians) to develop guideline-based, institution-specific written protocols for triaging and managing patients who are seen in the prehospital setting or present to the ED with symptoms suggestive of STEMI. (Level of Evidence B)

B. Initial Patient Evaluation
Class I

1. The delay from patient contact with the health care system (typically, arrival at the ED or contact with paramedics) to initiation of fibrinolytic therapy should be less than 30 minutes. Alternatively, if PCI is chosen, the delay from patient contact with the health care system (typically, arrival at the ED or contact with paramedics) to balloon inflation should be less than 90 minutes. (Level of Evidence B)
2. The choice of initial STEMI treatment should be made by the emergency medicine physician on duty based on a predetermined, institution-specific, written protocol that is a collaborative effort of cardiologists (both those involved in coronary care unit management and intervention lists), emergency physicians, primary care physicians, nurses, and other appropriate personnel. For cases in which the initial diagnosis and treatment plan is unclear to the emergency physician or is not covered directly by the agreed-on protocol, immediate cardiology consultation is advisable. (Level of Evidence C)

1. History
Class I

1. The targeted history of STEMI patients taken in the ED should ascertain whether the patient has had prior episodes of myocardial ischemia such as stable or unstable angina, MI, CABG, or PCI. Evaluation of the patient's complaints should focus on chest discomfort, associated symptoms, sex- and age-related differences in presentation, hypertension, diabetes mellitus, possibility of aortic dissection, risk of bleeding, and clinical cerebrovascular disease (amaurosis fugax, face/limb weakness or clumsiness, face/limb numbness or sensory loss, ataxia, or vertigo). (Level of Evidence C)

2. Physical Examination
Class I
1. A physical examination should be performed to aid in the diagnosis and assessment of the extent, location, and presence of complications of STEMI. (Level of Evidence C)
2. A brief, focused, and limited neurological examination to look for evidence of prior stroke or cognitive deficits should be performed on STEMI patients before administration of fibrinolytic therapy. (Level of Evidence C)

3. Electrocardiogram
Class I
1. A 12-lead ECG should be performed and shown to an experienced emergency physician within 10 minutes of ED arrival for all patients with chest discomfort (or anginal equivalent) or other symptoms suggestive of STEMI. (Level of Evidence C)
2. If the initial ECG is not diagnostic of STEMI but the patient remains symptomatic, and there is a high clinical suspicion for STEMI, serial ECGs at 5- to 10-minute intervals or continuous 12-lead ST-segment monitoring should be performed to detect the potential development of ST elevation. (Level of Evidence C)
3. In patients with inferior STEMI, right-sided ECG leads should be obtained to screen for ST elevation suggestive of right ventricular (RV) infarction. (Level of Evidence B)

4. Laboratory Examinations
Class I
1. Laboratory examinations should be performed as part of the management of STEMI patients but should not delay the implementation of reperfusion therapy. (Level of Evidence C)

5. Biomarkers of Cardiac Damage
Class I
1. Cardiac-specific troponins should be used as the optimum biomarkers for the evaluation of patients with STEMI who have coexistent skeletal muscle injury. (Level of Evidence C)
2. For patients with ST elevation on the 12-lead ECG and symptoms of STEMI, reperfusion therapy should be initiated as soon as possible and is not contingent on a biomarker assay. (Level of Evidence C)

Class IIa
1. Serial biomarker measurements can be useful to provide supportive non-invasive evidence of reperfusion of the infarct artery after fibrinolytic therapy in patients not undergoing angiography within the first 24 hours after fibrinolytic therapy. (Level of Evidence B)

Class III
1. Serial biomarker measurements should not be relied on to diagnose reinfarction within the first 18 hours after the onset of STEMI. (Level of Evidence C)

a. Bedside testing for serum cardiac biomarkers
Class I
1. Although handheld bedside (point-of-care) assays may be used for a qualitative assessment of the presence of an elevated level of a serum cardiac biomarker, subsequent measurements of cardiac biomarker levels should be performed with a quantitative test. (Level of Evidence B)
2. For patients with ST elevation on the 12-lead ECG and symptoms of STEMI, reperfusion therapy should be initiated as soon as possible and is not contingent on a bedside biomarker assay. (Level of Evidence C)

6. Imaging
Class I
1. Patients with STEMI should have a portable chest X-ray, but this should not delay implementation of reperfusion therapy (unless a potential contraindication, such as aortic dissection, is suspected). (Level of Evidence C)
2. Imaging studies such as a high-quality portable chest X-ray, transthoracic and/ or transesophageal echocardiography, and a contrast chest computed tomographic scan or a MRI scan should be used to differentiate STEMI from aortic dissection in patients for whom this distinction is initially unclear. (Level of Evidence B)

Class IIa
1. Portable echocardiography is reasonable to clarify the diagnosis of STEMI and allow risk stratification of patients with chest pain on arrival at the ED, especially if the diagnosis of STEMI is confounded by left bundle-branch block (LBBB) or pacing, or there is suspicion of posterior STEMI with anterior ST depressions. (Level of Evidence B)

Class III
1. Single-photon emission computed tomography (SPECT) radionuclide imaging should not be performed to diagnose STEMI in patients for whom the diagnosis of STEMI is evident on the ECG. (Level of Evidence B)

C. Management
1. Routine Measures
a. Oxygen
Class I
1. Supplemental oxygen should be administered to patients with arterial oxygen desaturation (SaO_2 less than 90%). (Level of Evidence B)

Class IIa
1. It is reasonable to administer supplemental oxygen to all patients with uncomplicated STEMI during the first six hours. (Level of Evidence C)

b. Nitroglycerin
Class I
1. Patients with ongoing ischemic discomfort should receive sublingual nitroglycerin (0.4 mg) every five minutes for a total of three doses, after which an assessment should be made about the need for intravenous nitroglycerin. (Level of Evidence C)

2. Intravenous nitroglycerin is indicated for relief of ongoing ischemic discomfort, control of hypertension, or management of pulmonary congestion. (Level of Evidence C)

Class III
1. Nitrates should not be administered to patients with systolic blood pressure less than 90 mm Hg or greater than or equal to 30 mm Hg below baseline, severe bradycardia (less than 50 bpm), tachycardia (more than 100 bpm), or suspected RV infarction. (Level of Evidence C)
2. Nitrates should not be administered to patients who have received a phosphodiesterase inhibitor for erectile dysfunction within the last 24 hours (48 hours for tadalafil). (Level of Evidence B)

c. Analgesia
Class I
1. Morphine sulfate (2 to 4 mg IV with increments of 2 to 8 mg IV repeated at 5- to 15-minute intervals) is the analgesic of choice for management of pain associated with STEMI. (Level of Evidence C)
2. Patients routinely taking NSAIDs (except for aspirin), both nonselective as well as COX-2 selective agents, prior to STEMI should have those agents discontinued at the time of presentation with STEMI because of the increased risks of mortality, reinfarction, hypertension, heart failure, and myocardial rupture associated with their use. (Level of Evidence C)

Class III
1. NSAIDs (except for aspirin), both nonselective as well as COX-2 selective agents, should not be administered during hospitalization for STEMI because of the increased risks of mortality, reinfarction, hypertension, heart failure, and myocardial rupture associated with their use. (Level of Evidence C)

d. Aspirin
Class I
1. Aspirin should be chewed by patients who have not taken aspirin before presentation with STEMI. The initial dose should be 162 mg (Level of Evidence A) to 325 mg (Level of Evidence C). Although some trials have used enteric-coated aspirin for initial dosing, more rapid buccal absorption occurs with nonenteric-coated aspirin formulations.

e. β-blockers
Class I
1. Oral β-blocker therapy should be initiated in the first 24 hours for patients who do not have any of the following: (1) signs of heart failure, (2) evidence of a low output state, (3) increased risk for cardiogenic shock, or (4) other relative contraindications to β-blockade (PR interval greater than 0.24 seconds, second or third degree heart block, active asthma or reactive airway disease). (Level of Evidence B)

Class IIa
1. It is reasonable to administer an intravenous β-blocker at the time of presentation to STEMI patients who are hypertensive and who do not have any of the

following: 1) signs of heart failure, 2) evidence of low output state, 3) increased risk for cardiogenic shock, or 4) other relative contraindications to β-blockade (PR interval greater than 0.24 seconds, second or third degree heart block, active asthma or reactive airway disease) (Level of Evidence B). Patients with early contraindications within the first 24 hours of STEMI should be reevaluated for candidacy for β-blocker therapy as secondary prevention (Level of Evidence B). Patients with moderate or severe LV failure should receive β-blocker therapy as secondary prevention with a gradual titration scheme (Level of Evidence B).

Class III
1. Intravenous β-blockers should not be administered to STEMI patients who have any of the following: (1) signs of heart failure, (2) evidence of low output state, (3) increased risk for cardiogenic shock, or (4) other relative contradictions to β-blockade (PR interval greater than 0.24 seconds, second or third degree heart block, active asthma or reactive airway disease). (Level of Evidence A)

2. Reperfusion
Class I
1. All STEMI patients should undergo rapid evaluation for reperfusion therapy and have a reperfusion strategy implemented promptly after contact with the medical system. (Level of Evidence A)
2. STEMI patients presenting to a hospital with PCI capability should be treated with primary PCI within 90 minutes of first medical contact as a systems goal. (Level of Evidence A)
3. STEMI patients presenting to a hospital without PCI capability, and who cannot be transferred to a PCI center and undergo PCI within 90 minutes of first medical contact, should be treated with fibrinolytic therapy within 30 minutes of hospital presentation as a systems goal unless fibrinolytic therapy is contraindicated (Level of Evidence B)

3. Pharmacological Reperfusion
a. Indications for fibrinolytic therapy
Class I
1. In the absence of contraindications, fibrinolytic therapy should be administered to STEMI patients with symptom onset within the prior 12 hours and ST elevation greater than 0.1 mV in at least two contiguous precordial leads or at least two adjacent limb leads. (Level of Evidence A)
2. In the absence of contraindications, fibrinolytic therapy should be administered to STEMI patients with symptom onset within the prior 12 hours and new or presumably new LBBB. (Level of Evidence A)

Class IIa
1. In the absence of contraindications, it is reasonable to administer fibrinolytic therapy to STEMI patients with symptom onset within the prior 12 hours and 12-lead ECG findings consistent with a true posterior MI. (Level of Evidence C)
2. In the absence of contraindications, it is reasonable to administer fibrinolytic therapy to patients with symptoms of STEMI beginning within the prior 12 to 24 hours who have continuing ischemic symptoms and ST elevation greater

than 0.1 mV in at least two contiguous precordial leads or at least two adjacent limb leads. (Level of Evidence B)

Class III
1. Fibrinolytic therapy should not be administered to asymptomatic patients whose initial symptoms of STEMI began more than 24 hours earlier. (Level of Evidence C)
2. Fibrinolytic therapy should not be administered to patients whose 12-lead ECG shows only ST-segment depression except if a true posterior MI is suspected. (Level of Evidence A)

b. Contraindications/cautions
Class I
1. Health care providers should ascertain whether the patient has neurological contraindications to fibrinolytic therapy, including any history of intracranial hemorrhage (ICH), significant closed head or facial trauma within the past three months, uncontrolled hypertension, or ischemic stroke within the past three months. (Level of Evidence A)
2. STEMI patients at substantial (greater than or equal to 4%) risk of ICH should be treated with PCI rather than with fibrinolytic therapy. (Level of Evidence A)

c. Complications of fibrinolytic therapy: Neurological and other
Class I
1. The occurrence of a change in neurological status during or after reperfusion therapy, particularly within the first 24 hours after initiation of treatment, is considered to be due to ICH until proven otherwise. Fibrinolytic, antiplatelet, and anticoagulant therapies should be discontinued until brain imaging scan shows no evidence of ICH. (Level of Evidence A)
2. Neurology and/or neurosurgery or hematology consultations should be obtained for STEMI patients who have ICH as dictated by clinical circumstances. (Level of Evidence C)
3. In patients with ICH, infusions of cryoprecipitate, fresh frozen plasma, protamine, and platelets should be given, as dictated by clinical circumstances. (Level of Evidence C)

Class IIa
1. In patients with ICH, it is reasonable to:
   a. Optimize blood pressure and blood glucose levels. (Level of Evidence C)
   b. Reduce intracranial pressure with an infusion of mannitol, endotracheal intubation, and hyperventilation. (Level of Evidence C)
   c. Consider neurosurgical evacuation of ICH. (Level of Evidence C)

d. Combination therapy with glycoprotein IIb/IIIa inhibitors
Class IIb
1. Combination pharmacological reperfusion with abciximab and half-dose reteplase or tenecteplase may be considered for prevention of reinfarction (Level of Evidence A) and other complications of STEMI in selected patients: anterior location of MI, age less than 75 years, and no risk factors for bleeding. In two clinical trials of combination reperfusion, the prevention of reinfarction did not translate into a survival benefit at either 30 days or one year. (Level of Evidence B)

2. Combination pharmacological reperfusion with abciximab and half-dose reteplase or tenecteplase may be considered for prevention of reinfarction and other complications of STEMI in selected patients (anterior location of MI, age less than 75 years, and no risk factors for bleeding) in whom an early referral for angiography and PCI (i.e., facilitated PCI) is planned. (Level of Evidence C)

Class III
1. Combination pharmacological reperfusion with abciximab and half-dose reteplase or tenecteplase should not be given to patients aged greater than 75 years because of an increased risk of ICH. (Level of Evidence B)

4. Percutaneous Coronary Intervention
a. Coronary angiography
Class I
1. Diagnostic coronary angiography should be performed:
   a. In candidates for primary or rescue PCI. (Level of Evidence A)
   b. In patients with cardiogenic shock who are candidates for revascularization. (Level of Evidence A)
   c. In candidates for surgical repair of ventricular septal rupture (VSR) or severe mitral regurgitation (MR). (Level of Evidence B)
   d. In patients with persistent hemodynamic and/or electrical instability. (Level of Evidence C)

Class III
1. Coronary angiography should not be performed in patients with extensive comorbidities in whom the risks of revascularization are likely to outweigh the benefits. (Level of Evidence C)

b. Primary PCI
Class I
1. General considerations: If immediately available, primary PCI should be performed in patients with STEMI (including true posterior MI) or MI with new or presumably new LBBB who can undergo PCI of the infarct artery within 12 hours of symptom onset, if performed in a timely fashion (balloon inflation within 90 minutes of presentation) by persons skilled in the procedure (individuals who perform more than 75 PCI procedures per year). The procedure should be supported by experienced personnel in an appropriate laboratory environment (performs more than 200 PCI procedures per year of which at least 36 are primary PCI for STEMI, and has cardiac surgery capability). (Level of Evidence A)
2. Specific considerations:
   a. Primary PCI should be performed as quickly as possible, with a goal of a medical contact-to-balloon or door-to-balloon time of within 90 minutes. (Level of Evidence B)
   b. If the symptom duration is within three hours and the expected door-to-balloon time minus the expected door-to-needle time is:
      i. within one hour, primary PCI is generally preferred. (Level of Evidence B)
      ii. greater than one hour, fibrinolytic therapy (fibrin-specific agents) is generally preferred. (Level of Evidence B)
   c. If symptom duration is greater than three hours, primary PCI is generally preferred and should be performed with a medical contact-to-balloon or

door-to-balloon time as brief as possible, with a goal of within 90 minutes. (Level of Evidence B)

d. Primary PCI should be performed for patients younger than 75 years old with ST elevation or LBBB who develop shock within 36 hours of MI and are suitable for revascularization that can be performed within 18 hours of shock, unless further support is futile because of the patient's wishes or contra-indications/unsuitability for further invasive care. (Level of Evidence A)

e. Primary PCI should be performed in patients with severe CHF and/or pulmonary edema (Killip class 3) and onset of symptoms within 12 hours. The medical contact-to-balloon or door-to-balloon time should be as short as possible (i.e., goal within 90 min). (Level of Evidence B)

Class IIa

1. Primary PCI is reasonable for selected patients 75 years or older with ST elevation or LBBB or who develop shock within 36 hours of MI and are suitable for revascularization that can be performed within 18 hours of shock. Patients with good prior functional status who are suitable for revascularization and agree to invasive care may be selected for such an invasive strategy. (Level of Evidence B)

2. It is reasonable to perform primary PCI for patients with onset of symptoms within the prior 12 to 24 hours and one or more of the following:
   a. Severe CHF (Level of Evidence C)
   b. Hemodynamic or electrical instability (Level of Evidence C)
   c. Persistent ischemic symptoms. (Level of Evidence C)

Class IIb

1. The benefit of primary PCI for STEMI patients eligible for fibrinolysis is not well established when performed by an operator who performs fewer than 75 PCI procedures per year. (Level of Evidence C)

Class III

1. PCI should not be performed in a noninfarct artery at the time of primary PCI in patients without hemodynamic compromise. (Level of Evidence C)

2. Primary PCI should not be performed in asymptomatic patients more than 12 hours after onset of STEMI if they are hemodynamically and electrically stable. (Level of Evidence C)

c. Primary PCI in fibrinolytic-ineligible patients
Class I

1. Primary PCI should be performed in fibrinolytic-ineligible patients who present with STEMI within 12 hours of symptom onset. (Level of Evidence C)

Class IIa

1. It is reasonable to perform primary PCI for fibrinolytic-ineligible patients with onset of symptoms within the prior 12 to 24 hours and one or more of the following:
   a. Severe CHF (Level of Evidence C)
   b. Hemodynamic or electrical instability (Level of Evidence C)
   c. Persistent ischemic symptoms (Level of Evidence C)

d. Primary PCI without on-site cardiac surgery
Class IIb

1. Primary PCI might be considered in hospitals without on-site cardiac surgery, provided that there exists a proven plan for rapid transport to a cardiac surgery

operating room in a nearby hospital with appropriate hemodynamic support capability for transfer. The procedure should be limited to patients with STEMI or MI with new, or presumably new, LBBB on ECG and should be done in a timely fashion (balloon inflation within 90 minutes of presentation) by persons skilled in the procedure (at least 75 PCIs per year) and at hospitals that perform a minimum of 36 primary PCI procedures per year. (Level of Evidence B)

Class III
1. Primary PCI should not be performed in hospitals without on-site cardiac surgery and without a proven plan for rapid transport to a cardiac surgery operating room in a nearby hospital or without appropriate hemodynamic support capability for transfer. (Level of Evidence C)

e. Facilitated PCI
Class IIb
1. Facilitated PCI using regimens other than full-dose fibrinolytic therapy might be considered as a reperfusion strategy when all of the following are present: (a) patients are at high risk, (b) PCI is not immediately available within 90 minutes, and (c) bleeding risk is low (younger age, absence of poorly controlled hypertension, normal body weight). (Level of Evidence C)

Class III
1. A planned reperfusion strategy using full-dose fibrinolytic therapy followed by PCI is not recommended and may be harmful. (Level of Evidence B)

f. Immediate (or emergency) invasive strategy and rescue PCI
Class I
1. A strategy of coronary angiography with intent to perform PCI (or emergency CABG) is recommended in patients who have received fibrinolytic therapy and have: (a) shock in patients less than 75 years of age who are suitable candidates for revascularization (Level of Evidence B), (b) severe congestive heart failure and/or pulmonary edema (Killip class III) (Level of Evidence B), or (c) hemodynamically compromising ventricular arrhythmias (Level of Evidence C)

Class IIa
1. A strategy of coronary angiography with intent to perform PCI (or emergency CABG) is reasonable in patients 75 years or older who have received fibrinolytic therapy, and are in shock, provided they are suitable candidates for revascularization. (Level of Evidence B)
2. It is reasonable to perform rescue PCI for patients with one or more of the following: (a) hemodynamic or electrical instability. (Level of Evidence C), or (b) persistent ischemic symptoms. (Level of Evidence C)
3. A strategy of coronary angiography with intent to perform rescue PCI is reasonable for patients in whom fibrinolytic therapy has failed (ST-segment elevation less than 50% resolved after 90 minutes following initiation of fibrinolytic therapy in the lead showing the worst initial elevation) and a moderate or large area of myocardium at risk [anterior MI, inferior MI with RV involvement or precordial-segment depression] (unless further invasive management is futile because of the patient's wishes or contraindications/unsuitability for further invasive care). (Level of Evidence B)

Class IIb

1. A strategy of coronary angiography with intent to perform PCI in the absence of any of the above Class I or IIa indications might be reasonable but its benefits and risks are not well established. The benefits of rescue PCI are greater the earlier it is initiated after the onset of ischemic discomfort. (Level of Evidence C)

Class III

1. A strategy of coronary angiography with intent to perform PCI (or emergency CABG) is not recommended in patients who have received fibrinolytic therapy if invasive management is futile because of the patient's wishes or contra-indication/unsuitability for further invasive care. (Level of Evidence C)

g. PCI for cardiogenic shock
Class I

1. Primary PCI is recommended for patients less than 75 years old with ST elevation or LBBB who develop shock within 36 hours of MI and are suitable for revascularization that can be performed within 18 hours of shock, unless further support is futile because of the patient's wishes or contraindications/unsuitability for further invasive care. (Level of Evidence A)

Class IIa

1. Primary PCI is reasonable for selected patients aged 75 years or older with ST elevation or LBBB who develop shock within 36 hours of MI and who are suitable for revascularization that can be performed within 18 hours of shock. Patients with good prior functional status who are suitable for revascularization and agree to invasive care may be selected for such an invasive strategy. (Level of Evidence B)

h. Percutaneous coronary intervention after fibrinolysis or for patients
not undergoing primary reperfusion
Class I

1. In patients whose anatomy is suitable, PCI should be performed when there is objective evidence of recurrent MI. (Level of Evidence C)
2. In patients whose anatomy is suitable, PCI should be performed for moderate or severe spontaneous or provocable myocardial ischemia during recovery from STEMI. (Level of Evidence B)
3. In patients whose anatomy is suitable, PCI should be performed for cardiogenic shock or hemodynamic instability (section V.C.4.g., PCI for Cardiogenic). (Level of Evidence B)

Class IIa

1. It is reasonable to perform routine PCI in patients with LV ejection fraction (LVEF) less than or equal to 0.40, CHF, or serious ventricular arrhythmias. (Level of Evidence C)
2. It is reasonable to perform PCI when there is documented clinical heart failure during the acute episode, even though subsequent evaluation shows preserved LV function (LVEF greater than 0.40). (Level of Evidence C)

Class IIb

1. PCI of hemodynamically significant stenosis in a patent infarct artery >24 hours after STEMI may be considered as part of a routine invasive strategy. (Level of Evidence B)

Class III
1. PCI of an occluded infarct artery >24 hours after STEMI is not recommended in asymptomatic patients with one- or two- vessel disease if they are hemodynamically and electrically stable and do not have evidence of severe ischemia. (Level of Evidence B)

5. Acute Surgical Reperfusion
Class I
1. Emergency or urgent CABG in patients with STEMI should be undertaken in the following circumstances:

   a. Failed PCI with persistent pain or hemodynamic instability in patients with coronary anatomy suitable for surgery. (Level of Evidence B)
   b. Persistent or recurrent ischemia refractory to medical therapy in patients who have coronary anatomy suitable for surgery, have a significant area of myocardium at risk, and are not candidates for PCI or fibrinolytic therapy. (Level of Evidence B)
   c. At the time of surgical repair of postinfarction VSR or mitral valve insufficiency. (Level of Evidence B)
   d. Cardiogenic shock in patients less than 75 years old with ST elevation, LBBB, or posterior MI who develop shock within 36 hours of STEMI, have severe multivessel or left main disease, and are suitable for revascularization that can be performed within 18 hours of shock, unless further support is futile because of the patient's wishes or contraindications/unsuitability for further invasive care. (Level of Evidence A)
   e. Life-threatening ventricular arrhythmias in the presence of greater than or equal to 50% left main stenosis and/or triple-vessel disease. (Level of Evidence B)

Class IIa
1. Emergency CABG can be useful as the primary reperfusion strategy in patients who have suitable anatomy, who are not candidates for fibrinolysis or PCI, and who are in the early hours (6–12 hours) of an evolving STEMI, especially if severe multivessel or left main disease is present. (Level of Evidence B)
2. Emergency CABG can be effective in selected patients 75 years or older with ST elevation, LBBB, or posterior MI who develop shock within 36 hours of STEMI, have severe triple-vessel or left main disease, and are suitable for revascularization that can be performed within 18 hours of shock. Patients with good prior functional status who are suitable for revascularization and agree to invasive care may be selected for such an invasive strategy. (Level of Evidence B)

Class III
1. Emergency CABG should not be performed in patients with persistent angina and a small area of risk if they are hemodynamically stable. (Level of Evidence C)
2. Emergency CABG should not be performed in patients with successful epicardial reperfusion but unsuccessful microvascular reperfusion. (Level of Evidence C)

6. Assessment of Reperfusion
Class IIa
1. It is reasonable to monitor the pattern of ST elevation, cardiac rhythm, and clinical symptoms over the 60 to 180 minutes after initiation of fibrinolytic therapy.

Noninvasive findings suggestive of reperfusion include relief of symptoms, maintenance or restoration of hemodynamic and/or electrical stability, and a reduction of at least 50% of the initial ST-segment elevation injury pattern on a follow-up ECG 60 to 90 minutes after initiation of therapy. (Level of Evidence B)

7. Ancillary Therapy
a. Anticoagulants as ancillary therapy to reperfusion therapy
Class I
1. Patients undergoing percutaneous or surgical revascularization should be given unfractionated heparin_ (UFH). (Level of Evidence C)
2. Platelet counts should be monitored daily in patients given UFH. (Level of Evidence C)
3. Patients undergoing reperfusion with fibrinolytics should receive anticoagulant therapy for a minimum of 48 hours (Level of Evidence C), and preferably for the duration of the index hospitalization, up to eight days (using a regimen other that UFH). (Level of Evidence A)
   Anticoagulant regimens with established efficacy include:
   a. UFH [initial intravenous bolus 60 U/kg (maximum 4000U)] followed by an intravenous infusion of 12 U/kg/hr (maximum 1000 U/hr) initially, adjusted to maintain the activated partial thromboplastin time (aPTT) at 1.5 to 2.0 time control (approximately 50 to 70 seconds) (Level of Evidence C). (Note: the available data do not suggest a benefit of prolonging the duration of the infusion of UFH beyond 48 hours in the absence of ongoing indications for anticoagulation; more prolonged infusions of UFH increase the risk of development of heparin-induce thrombocytopenia.)
   b. Enoxaparin (provided the serum creatinine is less than 2.5g/dL in men and 2.0 mg/dL in women): for patients less than 75 years of age, an initial 30 mg intravenous bolus is given, followed 15 minutes later by subcutaneous injections of 1.0 mg/kg every 12 hours; for patients at least 75 years of age, the initial intravenous bolus is eliminated and the subcutaneous regimen is 0.75 mg/kg every 12 hours. Regardless of age, if the creatinine clearance (using the Cockroft-Gault formula) during the course of treatment is estimated to be less than 30 mL/min, the subcutaneous regimen is 1.0 mg/kg every 24 hours. Maintenance dosing with enoxaparin should be continued for the duration of the index hospitalization, up to eight days. (Level of Evidence A)
   c. Fondaparinux (provided the serum creatinine is less that 3.0 mg/dL): subcutaneous injections of 2.5 mg once daily. Maintenance dosing with fondaparinux should be continued for the duration of the index hospitalization, up to eight days. (Level of Evidence B)

For patients undergoing PCI after having received an anticoagulant regimen, the following dosing recommendations should be followed:

a. For prior treatment with UFH: measure the activated clotting time (ACT) and administer boluses of UFH to achieve a target of 250 to 300 seconds with the HemoTec device or 300 to 350 seconds with the Hemochron device if no GP IIb/IIIa inhibitor is to be administered; if GP IIb/IIIa inhibitors are administered, the ACT target is 200 seconds with either device (Level of Evidence C). Bivalirudin may also be sued in patients treated previously with UFH.

b. For prior treatment with enoxaparin: if the last subcutaneous dose was administered within the prior eight hours, no additional enoxaparin should be given; if the last subcutaneous dose was administered at least 8 to 12 hours earlier, an intravenous dose of 0.3 mg/kg of enoxaparin should be given. (Level of Evidence B)

c. For prior treatment with fondaparinux: measure the ACT and administer boluses of UFH or bivalirudin to achieve a target of 250 to 300 seconds with the HemoTec device or 300 to 350 seconds with the Hemochron device if no GP IIb/IIa inhibitor is to be administered; if GP IIb/IIa inhibitors are administered, the ACT target is 200 seconds with either device. (Level of Evidence C)

Class IIa

1. In patients with known heparin-induced thrombocytopenia, it is reasonable to consider bivalirudin as a useful alternative to heparin to be used in conjunction with streptokinase. Dosing according to the HERO (Hirulog and Early Reperfusion or Occlusion)-2 regimen (a bolus of 0.25 mg/kg followed by an intravenous infusion of 0.5 mg/kg/hr for the first 12 hours and 0.25 mg/kg/hr for the subsequent 36 hours) is recommended but with a reduction in the infusion rate if the PTT is above 75 seconds within the first 12 hours. (Level of Evidence B)

Class III

1. Because of the risk of catheter thrombosis, fondaparinux should not be used as the sole anticoagulant to support PCI. An additional anticoagulant with anti-IIa activity should be administered. (Level of Evidence C)

b. Aspirin
Class I

1. A daily dose of aspirin (initial dose of 162 to 325 mg orally; maintenance dose of 75 to 162 mg) should be given indefinitely after STEMI to all patients without a true aspirin allergy. (Level of Evidence A)

c. Thienopyridines
Class I

1. Clopidogrel 75 mg per day orally should be added to aspirin in patients with STEMI regardless of whether they undergo reperfusion with fibrinolytic therapy or do not receive reperfusion therapy (Level of Evidence A). Treatment with clopidogrel should continue for at least 14 days (Level of Evidence B).

2. In patients who have undergone diagnostic cardiac catheterization and for whom PCI is planned, clopidogrel should be started and continued for at least one month after bare metal stent implantation, for several months after drug-eluting stent implantation (three months for sirolimus, six months for paclitaxel), and for up to 12 months in patients who are not at high risk for bleeding. (Level of Evidence B)

3. In patients taking clopidogrel in whom CABG is planned, the drug should be withheld for at least five days, and preferably for seven unless the urgency for revascularization outweighs the risks of excess bleeding. (Level of Evidence B)

Class IIa

1. Clopidogrel is probably indicated in patients receiving fibrinolytic therapy who are unable to take aspirin because of hypersensitivity or major gastrointestinal intolerance. (Level of Evidence C)

2. In patients less than age 75 years who received fibrinolytic therapy or who do not receive reperfusion therapy, it is reasonable to administer an oral clopidogrel loading dose of 300 mg. (No data are available to guide decision making regarding an oral loading dose in patients greater than or equal to 75 years of age.) (Level of Evidence C)
3. Long-term maintenance therapy (e.g., 1 year) with clopidogrel (75 mg/day orally) is reasonable in STEMI patients regardless of whether they undergo reperfusion with fibrinolytic therapy or do not receive reperfusion therapy. (Level of Evidence C)

d. Glycoprotein IIb/IIIa inhibitors
Class IIa
1. It is reasonable to start treatment with abciximab as early as possible before primary PCI (with or without stenting) in patients with STEMI. (Level of Evidence B)

Class IIb
1. Treatment with tirofiban or eptifibatide may be considered before primary PCI (with or without stenting) in patients with STEMI. (Level of Evidence C)

e. Inhibition of renin-angiotensin-aldosterone system
Class I
1. An angiotensin converting enzyme (ACE) inhibitor should be administered orally within the first 24 hours of STEMI to patients with anterior infarction, pulmonary congestion, or LVEF less than 0.40, in the absence of hypotension (systolic blood pressure less than 100 mm Hg or less than 30 mm Hg below baseline) or known contraindications to that class of medications. (Level of Evidence A)
2. An angiotensin receptor blocker (ARB) should be administered to STEMI patients who are intolerant of ACE inhibitors and who have either clinical or radiological signs of heart failure or LVEF less than 0.40. Valsartan and candesartan have established efficacy for this recommendation. (Level of Evidence C)

Class IIa
1. An ACE inhibitor administered orally within the first 24 hours of STEMI can be useful in patients without anterior infarction, pulmonary congestion, or LVEF less than 0.40 in the absence of hypotension (systolic blood pressure less than 100 mm Hg or less than 30 mm Hg below baseline) or known contraindications to that class of medications. The expected treatment benefit in such patients is less (5 lives saved per 1000 patients treated) than for patients with LV dysfunction. (Level of Evidence B)

Class III
1. An intravenous ACE inhibitor should not be given to patients within the first 24 hours of STEMI because of the risk of hypotension. (A possible exception may be patients with refractory hypertension.) (Level of Evidence B)

f. Strict glucose control during STEMI
Class I
1. An insulin infusion to normalize blood glucose is recommended for patients with STEMI and complicated courses. (Level of Evidence B)

Class IIa
1. During the acute phase (first 24–48 hours) of the management of STEMI in patients with hyperglycemia, it is reasonable to administer an insulin infusion

to normalize blood glucose, even in patients with an uncomplicated course. (Level of Evidence B)
2. After the acute phase of STEMI, it is reasonable to individualize treatment of diabetics, selecting from a combination of insulin, insulin analogs, and oral hypoglycemic agents that achieve the best glycemic control and are well tolerated. (Level of Evidence C)

g. Magnesium
Class IIa
1. It is reasonable that documented magnesium deficits be corrected, especially in patients receiving diuretics before the onset of STEMI. (Level of Evidence C)
2. It is reasonable that episodes of torsade de pointes-type ventricular tachycardia (VT) associated with a prolonged QT interval be treated with 1 to 2 g of magnesium administered as an intravenous bolus over five minutes. (Level of Evidence C)

Class III
1. In the absence of documented electrolyte deficits or torsade de pointes-type VT, routine intravenous magnesium should not be administered to STEMI patients at any level of risk. (Level of Evidence A)

h. Calcium channel blockers
Class IIa
1. It is reasonable to give verapamil or diltiazem to patients in whom β-blockers are ineffective or contraindicated (e.g., bronchospastic disease) for relief of ongoing ischemia or control of a rapid ventricular response with atrial fibrillation or flutter after STEMI in the absence of CHF, LV dysfunction, or atrioventricular (AV) block. (Level of Evidence C)

Class III
1. Diltiazem and verapamil are contraindicated in patients with STEMI and associated systolic LV dysfunction and CHF. (Level of Evidence A)
2. Nifedipine (immediate-release form) is contraindicated in treatment of STEMI because of the reflex sympathetic activation, tachycardia, and hypotension associated with its use. (Level of Evidence B)

VI. HOSPITAL MANAGEMENT

A. Location
1. Coronary Care Unit
Class I
1. STEMI patients should be admitted to a quiet and comfortable environment that provides for continuous monitoring of the ECG and pulse oximetry and has ready access to facilities for hemodynamic monitoring and defibrillation. (Level of Evidence C)
2. The patient's medication regimen should be reviewed to confirm the administration of aspirin and β-blockers in an adequate dose to control heart rate and to assess the need for intravenous nitroglycerin for control of angina, hypertension, or heart failure. (Level of Evidence A)
3. The ongoing need for supplemental oxygen should be assessed by monitoring arterial oxygen saturation. When stable for six hours, the patient should be reassessed for oxygen need (i.e., O2 saturation of less than 90%), and discontinuation of supplemental oxygen should be considered. (Level of Evidence C)

4. Nursing care should be provided by individuals certified in critical care, with staffing based on the specific needs of patients and provider competencies, as well as organizational priorities. (Level of Evidence C)
5. Care of STEMI patients in the critical care unit (CCU) should be structured around protocols derived from practice guidelines. (Level of Evidence C)
6. Electrocardiographic monitoring leads should be based on the location and rhythm to optimize detection of ST deviation, axis shift, conduction defects, and dysrhythmias. (Level of Evidence B)

Class III
1. It is not an effective use of the CCU environment to admit terminally ill, "do not resuscitate" patients with STEMI, because clinical and comfort needs can be provided outside of a critical care environment. (Level of Evidence C)

2. Stepdown Unit
Class I
1. It is a useful triage strategy to admit low-risk STEMI patients who have undergone successful PCI directly to the stepdown unit for post-PCI care rather than to the CCU. (Level of Evidence C)
2. STEMI patients originally admitted to the CCU who demonstrate 12 to 24 hours of clinical stability (absence of recurrent ischemia, heart failure, or hemodynamically compromising dysrhythmias) should be transferred to the stepdown unit. (Level of Evidence C)

Class IIa
1. It is reasonable for patients recovering from STEMI who have clinically symptomatic heart failure to be managed on the stepdown unit, provided that facilities for continuous monitoring of pulse oximetry and appropriately skilled nurses are available. (Level of Evidence C)
2. It is reasonable for patients recovering from STEMI who have arrhythmias that are hemodynamically well tolerated (e.g., atrial fibrillation with a controlled ventricular response; paroxysms of nonsustained VT lasting less than 30 seconds) to be managed on the stepdown unit, provided that facilities for continuous monitoring of the ECG, defibrillators, and appropriately skilled nurses are available. (Level of Evidence C)

Class IIb
1. Patients recovering from STEMI who have clinically-significant pulmonary disease requiring high-flow supplemental oxygen or noninvasive mask ventilation/bilevel positive airway pressure (BIPAP)/continuous positive airway pressure (CPAP) may be considered for care on a stepdown unit provided that facilities for continuous monitoring of pulse oximetry and appropriately skilled nurses with a sufficient nurse:patient ratio are available. (Level of Evidence C)

B. Early General Measures
1. Level of Activity
Class IIa
1. After 12 to 24 hours, it is reasonable to allow patients with hemodynamic instability or continued ischemia to have bedside commode privileges. (Level of Evidence C)

Class III
1. Patients with STEMI who are free of recurrent ischemic discomfort, symptoms of heart failure, or serious disturbances of heart rhythm should not be on bed rest for more than 12 to 24 hours. (Level of Evidence C)

2. Diet
Class I
1. Patients with STEMI should be prescribed the NCEP Adult Treatment Panel III (ATP III) Therapeutic Lifestyle Changes (TLC) diet, which focuses on reduced intake of fats and cholesterol, less than 7% of total calories as saturated fats, less than 200 mg of cholesterol per day, increased consumption of omega-3 fatty acids, and appropriate caloric intake for energy needs. (Level of Evidence C)
2. Diabetic patients with STEMI should have an appropriate food group balance and caloric intake. (Level of Evidence B)
3. Sodium intake should be restricted in STEMI patients with hypertension or heart failure. (Level of Evidence B)

3. Patient Education in the Hospital Setting
Class I
1. Patient counseling to maximize adherence to evidence-based post-STEMI treatments (e.g., compliance with taking medication, exercise prescription, and smoking cessation) should begin during the early phase of hospitalization, occur intensively at discharge, and continue at follow-up visits with providers and through cardiac rehabilitation programs and community support groups, as appropriate. (Level of Evidence C)
2. Critical pathways and protocols and other quality-improvement tools (e.g., the ACC "Guidelines Applied in Practice" and the AHA's "Get with the Guidelines") should be used to improve the application of evidence-based treatments by patients with STEMI, caregivers, and institutions. (Level of Evidence C)

4. Analgesia/Anxiolytics
Class IIa
1. It is reasonable to use anxiolytic medications in STEMI patients to alleviate short-term anxiety or altered behavior related to hospitalization for STEMI. (Level of Evidence C)
2. It is reasonable to routinely assess the patient's anxiety level and manage it with behavioral interventions and referral for counseling. (Level of Evidence C)

C. Medication Assessment
1. β-Blockers
Class I
1. Patients receiving β-blockers within the first 24 hours of STEMI without adverse effects should continue to receive them during the early convalescent phase of STEMI. (Level of Evidence A)
2. Patients without contraindications to β-blockers who did not receive them within the first 24 hours after STEMI should have them started in the early convalescent phase. (Level of Evidence A)

3. Patients with early contraindications within the first 24 hours of STEMI should be reevaluated for candidacy for β-blocker therapy. (Level of Evidence C)

2. Nitroglycerin
Class I
1. Intravenous nitroglycerin is indicated in the first 48 hours after STEMI for treatment of persistent ischemia, CHF, or hypertension. The decision to administer intravenous nitroglycerin and the dose used should not preclude therapy with other proven mortality-reducing interventions, such as β-blockers or ACE inhibitors. (Level of Evidence B)
2. Intravenous, oral, or topical nitrates are useful beyond the first 48 hours after STEMI for treatment of recurrent angina or persistent CHF if their use does not preclude therapy with β-blockers or ACE inhibitors. (Level of Evidence B)

Class IIb
1. The continued use of nitrate therapy beyond the first 24 to 48 hours in the absence of continued or recurrent angina or CHF may be helpful, although the benefit is likely to be small and is not well established in contemporary practice. (Level of Evidence B)

Class III
1. Nitrates should not be administered to patients with systolic pressure less than 90 mm Hg or greater than or equal to 30 mm Hg below baseline, severe bradycardia (less than 50 bpm), tachycardia (more than 100 bpm), or RV infarction. (Level of Evidence C)

3. Inhibition of the renin-angiotensin-aldosterone system
Class I
1. An ACE inhibitor should be administered orally during convalescence from STEMI in patients who tolerate this class of medication, and it should be continued over the long term. (Level of Evidence A)
2. An ARB should be administered to STEMI patients who are intolerant of ACE inhibitors and have either clinical or radiological signs of heart failure or LVEF less than 0.40. Valsartan and candesartan have demonstrated efficacy for this recommendation. (Level of Evidence B)
3. Long-term aldosterone blockade should be prescribed for post-STEMI patients without significant renal dysfunction (creatinine should be less than or equal to 2.5 mg/dL in men and less than or equal to 2.0 mg/dL in women) or hyperkalemia (potassium should be less than or equal to 5.0 mEq/L) who are already receiving therapeutic doses of an ACE inhibitor, have an LVEF less than or equal to 0.40, and have either symptomatic heart failure or diabetes. (Level of Evidence A)

Class IIa
1. In STEMI patients who tolerate ACE inhibitors, an ARB can be useful as an alternative to ACE inhibitors, provided there are either clinical or radiological signs of heart failure or LVEF is less than 0.40. Valsartan and candesartan have established efficacy for this recommendation. (Level of Evidence B)

4. Antiplatelets
Class I
1. Aspirin 162 to 325 mg should be given on day one of STEMI and in the absence of contraindications should be continued indefinitely on a daily basis thereafter at a dose of 75 to 162 mg. (Level of Evidence A)
2. A thienopyridine (preferably clopidogrel) should be administered to patients who are unable to take aspirin because of hypersensitivity or major gastrointestinal intolerance. (Level of Evidence C)
3. For patients taking clopidogrel for whom CABG is planned, if possible, the drug should be withheld for at least five days, and preferably for seven unless the urgency for revascularization outweighs the risks of bleeding. (Level of Evidence B)
4. For patients who have undergone diagnostic cardiac catheterization and for whom PCI is planned, clopidogrel should be started and continued for at least one month after bare metal stent implantation and for several months after drug-eluting stent implantation (3 months for sirolimus, 6 months for paclitaxel) and up to 12 months in patients who are not at high risk for bleeding. (Level of Evidence B)

5. Anticoagulants
Class I
1. Intravenous UFH (bolus of 60 U/kg, maximum 4000 U IV; initial infusion 12 U/kg/hr, maximum of 1000 U/h) or LMWH should be used in patients after STEMI who are at high risk for systemic emboli (large or anterior MI, atrial fibrillation, previous embolus, known LV thrombus, or cardiogenic shock). (Level of Evidence C)

Class IIa
1. Patients with STEMI who do not undergo reperfusion therapy should be treated with anticoagulant therapy (non-UFH regimen) for the duration of the index hospitalization, up to eight days (Level of Evidence B). Convenient strategies that can be used include those with LMWH (Level of Evidence C) or fondaparinux (Level of Evidence B) using the same dosing regimens as for patients who receive fibrinolytic therapy.

Class IIb
1. Prophylaxis for deep venous thrombosis (DVT) with subcutaneous LMWH (dosed appropriately for specific agent) or with subcutaneous UFH, 7500 U to 12 500 U twice per day until completely ambulatory, may be useful, but the effectiveness of such a strategy is not well established in the contemporary era of routine aspirin use and early mobilization. (Level of Evidence C)

6. Oxygen
Class I
1. Supplemental oxygen therapy should be continued beyond the first six hours in STEMI patients with arterial oxygen desaturation (SaO_2 less than 90%) or overt pulmonary congestion. (Level of Evidence C)

D. Estimation of Infarct Size
1. Electrocardiographic Techniques
Class I
1. All patients with STEMI should have follow-up ECGs at 24 hours and at hospital discharge to assess the success of reperfusion and/or the extent of infarction defined in part by the presence or absence of new Q waves. (Level of Evidence B)

E. Hemodynamic Disturbances
1. Hemodynamic Assessment
Class I
1. Pulmonary artery catheter monitoring should be performed for the following:
   a. Progressive hypotension, when unresponsive to fluid administration or when fluid administration may be contraindicated. (Level of Evidence C)
   b. Suspected mechanical complications of STEMI, (i.e., VSR, papillary muscle rupture, or free wall rupture with pericardial tamponade) if an echocardiogram has not been performed. (Level of Evidence C)
2. Intra-arterial pressure monitoring should be performed for the following:
   a. Patients with severe hypotension (systolic arterial pressure less than 80 mm Hg). (Level of Evidence C)
   b. Patients receiving vasopressor/inotropic agents. (Level of Evidence C)
   c. Cardiogenic shock. (Level of Evidence C)

Class IIa
1. Pulmonary artery catheter monitoring can be useful for the following:
   a. Hypotension in a patient without pulmonary congestion who has not responded to an initial trial of fluid administration. (Level of Evidence C)
   b. Cardiogenic shock. (Level of Evidence C)
   c. Severe or progressive CHF or pulmonary edema that does not respond rapidly to therapy. (Level of Evidence C)
   d. Persistent signs of hypoperfusion without hypotension or pulmonary congestion. (Level of Evidence C)
   e. Patients receiving vasopressor/inotropic agents. (Level of Evidence C)
2. Intra-arterial pressure monitoring can be useful for patients receiving intravenous sodium nitroprusside or other potent vasodilators. (Level of Evidence C)

Class IIb
1. Intra-arterial pressure monitoring might be considered in patients receiving intravenous inotropic agents. (Level of Evidence C)

Class III
1. Pulmonary artery catheter monitoring is not recommended in patients with STEMI without evidence of hemodynamic instability or respiratory compromise. (Level of Evidence C)
2. Intra-arterial pressure monitoring is not recommended for patients with STEMI who have no pulmonary congestion and have adequate tissue perfusion without use of circulatory support measures. (Level of Evidence C)

2. Hypotension
Class I
1. Rapid volume loading with an IV infusion should be administered to patients without clinical evidence for volume overload. (Level of Evidence C)
2. Rhythm disturbances or conduction abnormalities causing hypotension should be corrected. (Level of Evidence C)
3. Intra-aortic balloon counterpulsation should be performed in patients who do not respond to other interventions, unless further support is futile because of the patient's wishes or contraindications/unsuitability for further invasive care. (Level of Evidence B)

4. Vasopressor support should be given for hypotension that does not resolve after volume loading. (Level of Evidence C)
5. Echocardiography should be used to evaluate mechanical complications unless these are assessed by invasive measures. (Level of Evidence C)

3. Low-Output State
Class I
1. LV function and potential presence of a mechanical complication should be assessed by echocardiography if these have not been evaluated by invasive measures. (Level of Evidence C)
2. Recommended treatments for low-output states include:
    a. Inotropic support (Level of Evidence B)
    b. Intra-aortic counterpulsation (Level of Evidence B)
    c. Mechanical reperfusion with PCI or CABG (Level of Evidence B)
    d. Surgical correction of mechanical complications (Level of Evidence B)

Class III
1. β-blockers or calcium channel antagonists should not be administered to patients in a low-output state due to pump failure. (Level of Evidence B)

4. Pulmonary Congestion
Class I
1. Oxygen supplementation to arterial saturation greater than 90% is recommended for patients with pulmonary congestion. (Level of Evidence C)
2. Morphine sulfate should be given to patients with pulmonary congestion. (Level of Evidence C)
3. ACE inhibitors, beginning with titration of a short-acting ACE inhibitor with a low initial dose (e.g., 1 to 6.25 mg of captopril) should be given to patients with pulmonary edema unless the systolic blood pressure is less than 100 mm Hg or more than 30 mm Hg below baseline. Patients with pulmonary congestion and marginal or low blood pressure often need circulatory support with inotropic and vasopressor agents and/or intra-aortic balloon counterpulsation to relieve pulmonary congestion and maintain adequate perfusion. (Level of Evidence A)
4. Nitrates should be administered to patients with pulmonary congestion unless the systolic blood pressure is less than 100 mm Hg or more than 30 mm Hg below baseline. Patients with pulmonary congestion and marginal or low blood pressure often need circulatory support with inotropic and vasopressor agents and/or intra-aortic balloon counterpulsation to relieve pulmonary congestion and maintain adequate perfusion. (Level of Evidence C)
5. A diuretic (low- to intermediate-dose furosemide, or torsemide or bumetanide) should be administered to patients with pulmonary congestion if there is associated volume overload. Caution is advised for patients who have not received volume expansion. (Level of Evidence C)
6. β-blockade should be initiated before discharge for secondary prevention. For those who remain in heart failure throughout the hospitalization, low doses should be initiated, with gradual titration on an outpatient basis. (Level of Evidence B)
7. Long-term aldosterone blockade should be prescribed for post-STEMI patients without significant renal dysfunction (creatinine should be less than or equal to 2.5 mg/dL in men and less than or equal to 2.0 mg/dL in women) or hyperkalemia (potassium should be less than or equal to 5.0 mEq/L) who are already receiving therapeutic doses of an ACE inhibitor, have an LVEF less than or equal to 0.40, and have either symptomatic heart failure or diabetes. (Level of Evidence A)

8. Echocardiography should be performed urgently to estimate LV and RV function and to exclude a mechanical complication. (Level of Evidence C)

Class IIb
1. It may be reasonable to insert an intra-aortic balloon pump (IABP) for the management of patients with refractory pulmonary congestion. (Level of Evidence C)

Class III
1. β-blockers or calcium channel blockers should not be administered acutely to STEMI patients with frank cardiac failure evidenced by pulmonary congestion or signs of a low-output state. (Level of Evidence B)

5. Cardiogenic Shock
Class I
1. Intra-aortic balloon counterpulsation is recommended for STEMI patients when cardiogenic shock is not quickly reversed with pharmacological therapy. The IABP is a stabilizing measure for angiography and prompt revascularization. (Level of Evidence B)
2. Intra-arterial monitoring is recommended for the management of STEMI patients with cardiogenic shock. (Level of Evidence C)
3. Early revascularization, either PCI or CABG, is recommended for patients less than 75 years old with ST elevation or LBBB who develop shock within 36 hours of MI and are suitable for revascularization that can be performed within 18 hours of shock, unless further support is futile because of the patient's wishes or contraindications/unsuitability for further invasive care. (Level of Evidence A)
4. Fibrinolytic therapy should be administered to STEMI patients with cardiogenic shock who are unsuitable for further invasive care and do not have contraindications to fibrinolysis. (Level of Evidence B)
5. Echocardiography should be used to evaluate mechanical complications unless these are assessed by invasive measures. (Level of Evidence C)

Class IIa
1. Pulmonary artery catheter monitoring can be useful for the management of STEMI patients with cardiogenic shock. (Level of Evidence C)
2. Early revascularization, either PCI or CABG, is reasonable for selected patients 75 years or older with ST elevation or LBBB who develop shock within 36 hours of MI and are suitable for revascularization that can be performed within 18 hours of shock. Patients with good prior functional status who agree to invasive care may be selected for such an invasive strategy. (Level of Evidence B)

6. RV Infarction
Class I
1. Patients with inferior STEMI and hemodynamic compromise should be assessed with a right precordial V4R lead to detect ST-segment elevation and an echocardiogram to screen for RV infarction. (Level of Evidence B)
2. The following principles apply to therapy of patients with STEMI and RV infarction and ischemic dysfunction:
   a. Early reperfusion should be achieved if possible. (Level of Evidence C)
   b. AV synchrony should be achieved, and bradycardia should be corrected. (Level of Evidence C)
   c. RV preload should be optimized, which usually requires initial volume challenge in patients with hemodynamic instability, provided the jugular venous pressure is normal or low. (Level of Evidence C)

d. RV afterload should be optimized, which usually requires therapy for concomitant LV dysfunction. (Level of Evidence C)

e. Inotropic support should be used for hemodynamic instability not responsive to volume challenge. (Level of Evidence C)

Class IIa

1. After infarction that leads to clinically significant RV dysfunction, it is reasonable to delay CABG surgery for four weeks to allow recovery of contractile performance. (Level of Evidence C)

7. Mechanical Causes of Heart Failure/Low-Output Syndrome

a. Mitral valve regurgitation
Class I

1. Patients with acute papillary muscle rupture should be considered for urgent cardiac surgical repair, unless further support is considered futile because of the patient's wishes or contraindications/unsuitability for further invasive care. (Level of Evidence B)

2. CABG surgery should be undertaken at the same time as mitral valve surgery. (Level of Evidence B)

b. VSR after STEMI
Class I

1. Patients with STEMI complicated by the development of a VSR should be considered for urgent cardiac surgical repair, unless further support is considered futile because of the patient's wishes or contraindications/unsuitability for further invasive care. (Level of Evidence B)

2. CABG should be undertaken at the same time as repair of the VSR. (Level of Evidence B)

c. Left ventricular free-wall rupture
Class I

1. Patients with free-wall rupture should be considered for urgent cardiac surgical repair, unless further support is considered futile because of the patient's wishes or contraindications/unsuitability for further invasive care. (Level of Evidence B)

2. CABG should be undertaken at the same time as repair of free-wall rupture. (Level of Evidence C)

d. Left ventricular aneurysm
Class IIa

1. It is reasonable that patients with STEMI who develop a ventricular aneurysm associated with intractable ventricular tachyarrhythmias and/or pump failure unresponsive to medical and catheter-based therapy be considered for LV aneurysmectomy and CABG surgery. (Level of Evidence B)

8. Intra-Aortic Balloon Counterpulsation

Class I

1. Intra-aortic balloon counterpulsation should be used in STEMI patients with hypotension (systolic blood pressure less than 90 mm Hg or 30 mm Hg below

baseline mean arterial pressure) who do not respond to other interventions, unless further support is futile because of the patient's wishes or contra-indications/ unsuitability for further invasive care. (Level of Evidence B)
2. Intra-aortic balloon counterpulsation is recommended for STEMI patients with low-output state. (Level of Evidence B)
3. Intra-aortic balloon counterpulsation is recommended for STEMI patients when cardiogenic shock is not quickly reversed with pharmacological therapy. IABP is a stabilizing measure for angiography and prompt revascularization. (Level of Evidence B)
4. Intra-aortic balloon counterpulsation should be used in addition to medical therapy for STEMI patients with recurrent ischemic-type chest discomfort and signs of hemodynamic instability, poor LV function, or a large area of myocardium at risk. Such patients should be referred urgently for cardiac catheterization and should undergo revascularization as needed. (Level of Evidence C)

Class IIa
1. It is reasonable to manage STEMI patients with refractory polymorphic VT with intra-aortic balloon counterpulsation to reduce myocardial ischemia. (Level of Evidence B)

Class IIb
1. It may be reasonable to use intra-aortic balloon counterpulsation in the management of STEMI patients with refractory pulmonary congestion. (Level of Evidence C)

F. Arrhythmias After STEMI
1. Ventricular Arrhythmias
a. Ventricular fibrillation
Class I
1. Ventricular fibrillation (VF) or pulseless VT should be treated with an unsynchronized electric shock with an initial monophasic shock energy of 200 J; if unsuccessful, a second shock of 200 to 300 J should be given, and then, if necessary, a third shock of 360 J. (Level of Evidence B)

Class IIa
1. It is reasonable that VF or pulseless VT that is refractory to electrical shock be treated with amiodarone (300 mg or 5 mg/kg, IV bolus) followed by a repeat unsynchronized electric shock. (Level of Evidence B)
2. It is reasonable to correct electrolyte and acid-base disturbances (potassium greater than 4.0 mEq/L and magnesium greater than 2.0 mg/dL) to prevent recurrent episodes of VF once an initial episode of VF has been treated. (Level of Evidence C)

Class IIb
1. It may be reasonable to treat VT or shock-refractory VF with boluses of intravenous procainamide. However, this has limited value owing to the length of time required for administration. (Level of Evidence C)

Class III
1. Prophylactic administration of antiarrhythmic therapy is not recommended when using fibrinolytic agents. (Level of Evidence B)

b. Ventricular tachycardia
Class I

1. Sustained (more than 30 seconds or causing hemodynamic collapse) polymorphic VT should be treated with an unsynchronized electric shock with an initial monophasic shock energy of 200 J; if unsuccessful, a second shock of 200 to 300 J should be given, and, if necessary, a third shock of 360 J. (Level of Evidence B)
2. Episodes of sustained monomorphic VT associated with angina, pulmonary edema, or hypotension (blood pressure less than 90 mm Hg) should be treated with a synchronized electric shock of 100 J initial monophasic shock energy. Increasing energies may be used if not initially successful. Brief anesthesia is desirable if hemodynamically tolerable. (Level of Evidence B)
3. Sustained monomorphic VT not associated with angina, pulmonary edema, or hypotension (blood pressure less than 90 mm Hg) should be treated with:
    a. Amiodarone: 150 mg infused over 10 minutes (alternative dose 5 mg/kg); repeat 150 mg every 10 to 15 minutes as needed. Alternative infusion: 360 mg over six hours (1 mg/min), then 540 mg over the next 18 hours (0.5 mg/min). The total cumulative dose, including additional doses given during cardiac arrest, must not exceed 2.2 g over 24 hours. (Level of Evidence B)
    b. Synchronized electrical cardioversion starting at monophasic energies of 50 J (brief anesthesia is necessary). (Level of Evidence B)

Class IIa

1. It is reasonable to manage refractory polymorphic VT by:
    a. Aggressive attempts to reduce myocardial ischemia and adrenergic stimulation, including therapies such as β-adrenoceptor blockade, IABP use, and consideration of emergency PCI/CABG surgery. (Level of Evidence B)
    b. Aggressive normalization of serum potassium greater than 4.0 mEq/L and of magnesium greater than 2.0 mg/dL. (Level of Evidence C)
    c. If the patient has bradycardia to a rate less than 60 beats per minute or long QTc, temporary pacing at a higher rate may be instituted. (Level of Evidence C)

Class IIb

1. It is may be useful to treat sustained monomorphic VT not associated with angina, pulmonary edema, or hypotension (blood pressure less than 90 mm Hg) with a procainamide bolus and infusion. (Level of Evidence C)

Class III

1. The routine use of prophylactic antiarrhythmic drugs (i.e., lidocaine) is not indicated for suppression of isolated ventricular premature beats, couplets, runs of accelerated idioventricular rhythm, or nonsustained VT. (Level of Evidence B)
2. The routine use of prophylactic antiarrhythmic therapy is not indicated when fibrinolytic agents are administered. (Level of Evidence B)

c. Ventricular premature beats
Class III

1. Treatment of isolated ventricular premature beats, couplets, and nonsustained VT is not recommended unless they lead to hemodynamic compromise. (Level of Evidence A)

d. Accelerated idioventricular rhythms and accelerated junctional rhythms
Class III
1. Antiarrhythmic therapy is not indicated for accelerated idioventricular rhythm. (Level of Evidence C)
2. Antiarrhythmic therapy is not indicated for accelerated junctional rhythm. (Level of Evidence C)

e. Implantable cardioverter defibrillator implantation in patients after STEMI
Class I
1. An implantable cardioverter-defibrillator (ICD) is indicated for patients with VF or hemodynamically significant sustained VT more than two days after STEMI, provided the arrhythmia is not judged to be due to transient or reversible ischemia or reinfarction. (Level of Evidence A)
2. An ICD is indicated for patients without spontaneous VF or sustained VT more than 48 hours after STEMI whose STEMI occurred at least one month previously, who have an LVEF between 0.31 and 0.40, demonstrate additional evidence of electrical instability (e.g., nonsustained VT), and have inducible VF or sustained VT on electrophysiological testing. (Level of Evidence B)
Class IIa
1. If there is reduced LVEF (0.30 or less), at least one month after STEMI and three months after coronary artery revascularization, it is reasonable to implant an ICD in post-STEMI patients without spontaneous VF or sustained VT more than 48 hours after STEMI. (Level of Evidence B)

Class IIb
1. The usefulness of an ICD is not well established in STEMI patients without spontaneous VF or sustained VT more than 48 hours after STEMI who have a reduced LVEF (0.31–0.40) at least one month after STEMI but who have no additional evidence of electrical instability (e.g., nonsustained VT). (Level of Evidence B)
2. The usefulness of an ICD is not well established in STEMI patients without spontaneous VF or sustained VT more than 48 hours after STEMI who have a reduced LVEF (0.31–0.40) at least one month after STEMI and additional evidence of electrical instability (e.g., nonsustained VT) but who do not have inducible VF or sustained VT on electrophysiological testing. (Level of Evidence B)

Class III
1. An ICD is not indicated in STEMI patients who do not experience spontaneous VF or sustained VT more than 48 hours after STEMI and in whom the LVEF is greater than 0.40 at least one month after STEMI. (Level of Evidence C)

2. Supraventricular Arrhythmias/Atrial Fibrillation
Class I
1. Sustained atrial fibrillation and atrial flutter in patients with hemodynamic compromise or ongoing ischemia should be treated with one or more of the following:
   a. Synchronized cardioversion with an initial monophasic shock of 200 J for atrial fibrillation and 50 J for flutter preceded by brief general anesthesia or conscious sedation whenever possible. (Level of Evidence C)

b. For episodes of atrial fibrillation that do not respond to electrical cardioversion or recur after a brief period of sinus rhythm, the use of antiarrhythmic therapy aimed at slowing the ventricular response is indicated. One or more of these pharmacological agents may be used:
   i. Intravenous amiodarone. (Level of Evidence C)
   ii. Intravenous digoxin for rate control principally for patients with severe LV dysfunction and heart failure. (Level of Evidence C)
2. Sustained atrial fibrillation and atrial flutter in patients with ongoing ischemia but without hemodynamic compromise should be treated with one or more of the following:
   a. β-adrenergic blockade is preferred unless contraindicated. (Level of Evidence C)
   b. Intravenous diltiazem or verapamil. (Level of Evidence C)
   c. Synchronized cardioversion with an initial monophasic shock of 200 J for atrial fibrillation and 50 J for flutter preceded by brief general anesthesia or conscious sedation whenever possible. (Level of Evidence C)
3. For episodes of sustained atrial fibrillation or flutter without hemodynamic compromise or ischemia, rate control is indicated. In addition, patients with sustained atrial fibrillation or flutter should be given anticoagulant therapy. Consideration should be given to cardioversion to sinus rhythm in patients with a history of atrial fibrillation or flutter prior to STEMI. (Level of Evidence C)
4. Reentrant paroxysmal supraventricular tachycardia, because of its rapid rate, should be treated with the following in the sequence shown:
   a. Carotid sinus massage. (Level of Evidence C)
   b. Intravenous adenosine (6 mg × 1 over 1 to 2 seconds; if no response, 12 mg IV after 1 to 2 minutes may be given; repeat 12 mg dose if needed. (Level of Evidence C)
   c. Intravenous β-adrenergic blockade with metoprolol (2.5 to 5.0 mg every 2 to 5 minutes to a total of 15 mg over 10 to 15 minutes) or atenolol (2.5 to 5.0 mg over 2 minutes to a total of 10 mg in 10 to 15 minutes). (Level of Evidence C)
   d. Intravenous diltiazem [20 mg (0.25 mg/kg)] over two minutes followed by an infusion of 10 mg/h). (Level of Evidence C)
   e. Intravenous digoxin, recognizing that there may be a delay of at least one hour before pharmacological effects appear [8 to 15 μg/kg (0.6 to 1.0 mg in a person weighing 70 kg)]. (Level of Evidence C)

Class III
1. Treatment of atrial premature beats is not indicated. (Level of Evidence C)

3. Bradyarrhythmias
a. Ventricular asystole
Class I
1. Prompt resuscitative measures, including chest compressions, atropine, vasopressin, epinephrine, and temporary pacing, should be administered to treat ventricular asystole. (Level of Evidence B)

G. Use of Permanent Pacemakers
1. Permanent Pacing for Bradycardia or Conduction Blocks Associated with STEMI
Class I
1. Permanent ventricular pacing is indicated for persistent second-degree AV block in the His-Purkinje system with bilateral bundle-branch block or third-degree AV block within or below the His-Purkinje system after STEMI. (Level of Evidence B)

2. Permanent ventricular pacing is indicated for transient advanced second- or third-degree infranodal AV block and associated bundle-branch block. If the site of block is uncertain, an electrophysiological study may be necessary. (Level of Evidence B)
3. Permanent ventricular pacing is indicated for persistent and symptomatic second- or third-degree AV block. (Level of Evidence C)

Class IIb
1. Permanent ventricular pacing may be considered for persistent second- or third-degree AV block at the AV node level. (Level of Evidence B)

Class III
1. Permanent ventricular pacing is not recommended for transient AV block in the absence of intraventricular conduction defects. (Level of Evidence B)
2. Permanent ventricular pacing is not recommended for transient AV block in the presence of isolated left anterior fascicular block. (Level of Evidence B)
3. Permanent ventricular pacing is not recommended for acquired left anterior fascicular block in the absence of AV block. (Level of Evidence B)
4. Permanent ventricular pacing is not recommended for persistent first-degree AV block in the presence of bundle-branch block that is old or of indeterminate age. (Level of Evidence B)

2. Sinus Node Dysfunction After STEMI
Class I
1. Symptomatic sinus bradycardia, sinus pauses greater than three seconds, or sinus bradycardia with a heart rate less than 40 bpm and associated hypotension or signs of systemic hemodynamic compromise should be treated with an intravenous bolus of atropine 0.6 to 1.0 mg. If bradycardia is persistent and maximal (2 mg) doses of atropine have been used, transcutaneous or transvenous (preferably atrial) temporary pacing should be instituted. (Level of Evidence C)

3. Pacing Mode Selection in STEMI Patients
Class I
1. All patients who have an indication for permanent pacing after STEMI should be evaluated for ICD indications. (Level of Evidence C)

Class IIa
1. It is reasonable to implant a permanent dual-chamber pacing system in STEMI patients who need permanent pacing and are in sinus rhythm. It is reasonable that patients in permanent atrial fibrillation or flutter receive a single-chamber ventricular device. (Level of Evidence C)
2. It is reasonable to evaluate all patients who have an indication for permanent pacing after STEMI for biventricular pacing (cardiac resynchronization therapy). (Level of Evidence C)

H. Recurrent Chest Pain After STEMI
1. Pericarditis
Class I
1. Aspirin is recommended for treatment of pericarditis after STEMI. Doses as high as 650 mg orally (enteric) every four to six hours may be needed. (Level of Evidence B)

2. Anticoagulation should be immediately discontinued if pericardial effusion develops or increases. (Level of Evidence C)

Class IIa

1. For episodes of pericarditis after STEMI that are not adequately controlled with aspirin, it is reasonable to administer one or more of the following:
   a. Colchicine 0.6 mg every 12 hours orally. (Level of Evidence B)
   b. Acetaminophen 500 mg orally every six hours. (Level of Evidence C)

Class IIb

1. Nonsteroidal anti-inflammatory drugs may be considered for pain relief; however, they should not be used for extended periods because of their continuous effect on platelet function, an increased risk of myocardial scar thinning, and infarct expansion. (Level of Evidence B)
2. Corticosteroids might be considered only as a last resort in patients with pericarditis refractory to aspirin or nonsteroidal drugs. Although corticosteroids are effective for pain relief, their use is associated with an increased risk of scar thinning and myocardial rupture. (Level of Evidence C)

Class III

1. Ibuprofen should not be used for pain relief because it blocks the antiplatelet effect of aspirin and can cause myocardial scar thinning and infarct expansion. (Level of Evidence B)

2. Recurrent Ischemia/Infarction

Class I

1. Patients with recurrent ischemic-type chest discomfort after initial reperfusion therapy for STEMI should undergo escalation of medical therapy with nitrates and β-blockers to decrease myocardial oxygen demand and reduce ischemia. Intravenous anticoagulation should be initiated if not already accomplished. (Level of Evidence B)
2. In addition to escalation of medical therapy, patients with recurrent ischemic-type chest discomfort and signs of hemodynamic instability, poor LV function, or a large area of myocardium at risk should be referred urgently for cardiac catheterization and undergo revascularization as needed. Insertion of an IABP should also be considered. (Level of Evidence C)
3. Patients with recurrent ischemic-type chest discomfort who are considered candidates for revascularization should undergo coronary arteriography and PCI or CABG as dictated by coronary anatomy. (Level of Evidence B)

Class IIa

1. It is reasonable to (re)administer fibrinolytic therapy to patients with recurrent ST elevation and ischemic-type chest discomfort who are not considered candidates for revascularization or for whom coronary angiography and PCI cannot be rapidly (ideally within 60 minutes from the onset of recurrent discomfort) implemented. (Level of Evidence C)

Class III

1. Streptokinase should not be readministered to treat recurrent ischemia/ infarction in patients who received a nonfibrin-specific fibrinolytic agent more than five days previously to treat the acute STEMI event. (Level of Evidence C)

I. Other Complications
1. Ischemic Stroke
Class I
1. Neurological consultation should be obtained in STEMI patients who have an acute ischemic stroke. (Level of Evidence C)
2. STEMI patients who have an acute ischemic stroke should be evaluated with echocardiography, neuroimaging, and vascular imaging studies to determine the cause of the stroke. (Level of Evidence C)
3. STEMI patients with acute ischemic stroke and persistent atrial fibrillation should receive lifelong moderate intensity [international normalized ratio (INR) 2 to 3] warfarin therapy. (Level of Evidence A)
4. STEMI patients with or without acute ischemic stroke who have a cardiac source of embolism (atrial fibrillation, mural thrombus, or akinetic segment) should receive moderate-intensity (INR 2 to 3) warfarin therapy (in addition to aspirin). The duration of warfarin therapy should be dictated by clinical circumstances (e.g., at least 3 months for patients with an LV mural thrombus or akinetic segment and indefinitely in patients with persistent atrial fibrillation). The patient should receive LMWH or UFH until adequately anticoagulated with warfarin. (Level of Evidence B)

Class IIa
1. It is reasonable to assess the risk of ischemic stroke in patients with STEMI. (Level of Evidence A)
2. It is reasonable that STEMI patients with nonfatal acute ischemic stroke receive supportive care to minimize complications and maximize functional outcome. (Level of Evidence C)

Class IIb
1. Carotid angioplasty/stenting, four to six weeks after ischemic stroke, might be considered in STEMI patients who have an acute ischemic stroke attributable to an internal carotid artery—origin stenosis of at least 50% and who have a high surgical risk of morbidity/mortality early after STEMI. (Level of Evidence C)

2. DVT and Pulmonary Embolism
Class I
1. DVT or pulmonary embolism after STEMI should be treated with full-dose LMWH for a minimum of five days and until the patient is adequately anticoagulated with warfarin. Start warfarin concurrently with LMWH and titrate to INR of 2 to 3. (Level of Evidence A)
2. Patients with CHF after STEMI who are hospitalized for prolonged periods, unable to ambulate, or considered at high risk for DVT and are not otherwise anticoagulated should receive low-dose heparin prophylaxis, preferably with LMWH. (Level of Evidence A)

J. CABG Surgery After STEMI
1. Timing of Surgery
Class IIa
1. In patients who have had a STEMI, CABG mortality is elevated for the first three to seven days after infarction, and the benefit of revascularization must be balanced against this increased risk. Patients who have been stabilized

(no ongoing ischemia, hemodynamic compromise, or life-threatening arrhythmia) after STEMI and who have incurred a significant fall in LV function should have their surgery delayed to allow myocardial recovery to occur. If critical anatomy exists, revascularization should be undertaken during the index hospitalization. (Level of Evidence B)

2. Arterial Grafting
Class I
1. An internal mammary artery graft to a significantly stenosed left anterior descending coronary artery should be used whenever possible in patients undergoing CABG after STEMI. (Level of Evidence B)

3. CABG for Recurrent Ischemia After STEMI
Class I
1. Urgent CABG is indicated if the coronary angiogram reveals anatomy that is unsuitable for PCI. (Level of Evidence B)

4. Elective CABG Surgery After STEMI in Patients With Angina
Class I
1. CABG is recommended for patients with stable angina who have significant left main coronary artery stenosis. (Level of Evidence A)
2. CABG is recommended for patients with stable angina who have left main equivalent disease: significant (at least 70%) stenosis of the proximal left anterior descending coronary artery and proximal left circumflex artery. (Level of Evidence A)
3. CABG is recommended for patients with stable angina who have 3-vessel disease (Survival benefit is greater when LVEF is less than 0.50). (Level of Evidence A)
4. CABG is beneficial for patients with stable angina who have 1- or 2-vessel coronary disease without significant proximal left anterior descending coronary artery stenosis but with a large area of viable myocardium and high-risk criteria on noninvasive testing. (Level of Evidence B)
5. CABG is recommended in patients with stable angina who have 2-vessel disease with significant proximal left anterior descending coronary artery stenosis and either ejection fraction less than 0.50 or demonstrable ischemia on noninvasive testing. (Level of Evidence A)

5. CABG Surgery After STEMI and Antiplatelet Agents
Class I
1. Aspirin should not be withheld before elective or nonelective CABG after STEMI. (Level of Evidence C)
2. Aspirin (75–325 mg daily) should be prescribed as soon as possible (within 24 hours) after CABG unless contraindicated. (Level of Evidence B)
3. In patients taking clopidogrel in whom elective CABG is planned, the drug should be withheld for five to seven days. (Level of Evidence B)

K. Convalescence, Discharge, and Post-MI Care

1. Risk Stratification at Hospital Discharge

a. Role of exercise testing

Class I

1. Exercise testing should be performed either in the hospital or early after discharge in STEMI patients not selected for cardiac catheterization and without high-risk features to assess the presence and extent of inducible ischemia. (Level of Evidence B)
2. In patients with baseline abnormalities that compromise ECG interpretation, echocardiography or myocardial perfusion imaging should be added to standard exercise testing. (Level of Evidence B)

Class IIb

1. Exercise testing might be considered before discharge of patients recovering from STEMI to guide the postdischarge exercise prescription or to evaluate the functional significance of a coronary lesion previously identified at angiography. (Level of Evidence C)

Class III

1. Exercise testing should not be performed within two to three days of STEMI in patients who have not undergone successful reperfusion. (Level of Evidence C)
2. Exercise testing should not be performed to evaluate patients with STEMI who have unstable postinfarction angina, decompensated CHF, life-threatening cardiac arrhythmias, noncardiac conditions that severely limit their ability to exercise, or other absolute contraindications to exercise testing. (Level of Evidence C)
3. Exercise testing should not be used for risk stratification in patients with STEMI who have already been selected for cardiac catheterization. (Level of Evidence C)

b. Role of echocardiography

Class I

1. Echocardiography should be used in patients with STEMI not undergoing LV angiography to assess baseline LV function, especially if the patient is hemodynamically unstable. (Level of Evidence C)
2. Echocardiography should be used to evaluate patients with inferior STEMI, clinical instability, and clinical suspicion of RV infarction. (Level of Evidence C)
3. Echocardiography should be used in patients with STEMI to evaluate suspected complications, including acute MR, cardiogenic shock, infarct expansion, VSR, intracardiac thrombus, and pericardial effusion. (Level of Evidence C)
4. Stress echocardiography (or myocardial perfusion imaging) should be used in patients with STEMI for inhospital or early postdischarge assessment for inducible ischemia when baseline abnormalities are expected to compromise ECG interpretation. (Level of Evidence C)

Class IIa

1. Echocardiography is reasonable in patients with STEMI to re-evaluate ventricular function during recovery when results are used to guide therapy. (Level of Evidence C)
2. Dobutamine echocardiography (or myocardial perfusion imaging) is reasonable in hemodynamically and electrically stable patients four or more days after

STEMI to assess myocardial viability when required to define the potential efficacy of revascularization. (Level of Evidence C)

3. In STEMI patients who have not undergone contrast ventriculography, echocardiography is reasonable to assess ventricular function after revascularization. (Level of Evidence C)

Class III

1. Echocardiography should not be used for early routine reevaluation in patients with STEMI in the absence of any change in clinical status or revascularization procedure. Reassessment of LV function 30 to 90 days later may be reasonable. (Level of Evidence C)

c. Exercise myocardial perfusion imaging
Class I

1. Dipyridamole or adenosine stress perfusion nuclear scintigraphy or dobutamine echocardiography before or early after discharge should be used in patients with STEMI who are not undergoing cardiac catheterization to look for inducible ischemia in patients judged to be unable to exercise. (Level of Evidence B)

Class IIa

1. Myocardial perfusion imaging or dobutamine echocardiography is reasonable in hemodynamically and electrically stable patients 4 to 10 days after STEMI to assess myocardial viability when required to define the potential efficacy of revascularization. (Level of Evidence C)

d. LV function
Class I

1. LVEF should be measured in all STEMI patients. (Level of Evidence B)

e. Invasive evaluation
Class I

1. Coronary arteriography should be performed in patients with spontaneous episodes of myocardial ischemia or episodes of myocardial ischemia provoked by minimal exertion during recovery from STEMI. (Level of Evidence A)

2. Coronary arteriography should be performed for intermediate- or high-risk findings on noninvasive testing after STEMI. (Level of Evidence B)

3. Coronary arteriography should be performed if the patient is sufficiently stable before definitive therapy of a mechanical complication of STEMI, such as acute MR, VSR, pseudoaneurysm, or LV aneurysm. (Level of Evidence B)

4. Coronary arteriography should be performed in patients with persistent hemodynamic instability. (Level of Evidence B)

5. Coronary arteriography should be performed in survivors of STEMI who had clinical heart failure during the acute episode but subsequently demonstrated well-preserved LV function. (Level of Evidence C)

Class IIa

1. It is reasonable to perform coronary arteriography when STEMI is suspected to have occurred by a mechanism other than thrombotic occlusion of an atherosclerotic plaque. This would include coronary embolism, certain metabolic or hematological diseases, or coronary artery spasm. (Level of Evidence C)

2. Coronary arteriography is reasonable in STEMI patients with any of the following: diabetes mellitus, LVEF less than 0.40, CHF, prior revascularization, or life-threatening ventricular arrhythmias. (Level of Evidence C)

Class IIb
1. Coronary arteriography may be considered as part of an invasive strategy for risk assessment after fibrinolytic therapy (Level of Evidence B) or for patients not undergoing primary reperfusion. (Level of Evidence C)

Class III
1. Coronary arteriography should not be performed in survivors of STEMI who are thought not to be candidates for coronary revascularization. (Level of Evidence A)

f. Assessment of ventricular arrhythmias
Class IIb
1. Noninvasive assessment of the risk of ventricular arrhythmias may be considered (including signal-averaged ECG, 24-hour ambulatory monitoring, heart rate variability, micro T-wave alternans, and T-wave variability) in patients recovering from STEMI. (Level of Evidence B)

L. Secondary Prevention
Class I
1. Patients who survive the acute phase of STEMI should have plans initiated for secondary prevention therapies. (Level of Evidence A)

1. Patient Education Before Discharge
Class I
1. Before hospital discharge, all STEMI patients should be educated about and actively involved in planning for adherence to the lifestyle changes and drug therapies that are important for the secondary prevention of cardiovascular disease. (Level of Evidence B)
2. Post-STEMI patients and their family members should receive discharge instructions about recognizing acute cardiac symptoms and appropriate actions to take in response (i.e., calling 9-1-1 if symptoms are unimproved or worsening five minutes after onset, or if symptoms are unimproved or worsening five minutes after one sublingual nitroglycerin dose) to ensure early evaluation and treatment should symptoms recur. (Level of Evidence C)
3. Family members of STEMI patients should be advised to learn about AEDs and CPR and be referred to a CPR training program. Ideally, such training programs would have a social support component targeting family members of high-risk patients. (Level of Evidence C)

2. Lipid Management
Class I
1. Dietary therapy that is low in saturated fat and cholesterol (less than 7% of total calories as saturated fat and less than 200 mg/day cholesterol) should be started on discharge after recovery from STEMI. Increased consumption of the following should be encouraged: omega-3 fatty acids, fruits, vegetables, soluble

(viscous) fiber, and whole grains. Calorie intake should be balanced with energy output to achieve and maintain a healthy weight. (Level of Evidence A)
2. A lipid profile should be obtained from past records, if not available, it should be performed in all patients with STEMI, preferably after they have fasted and within 24 hours of admission. (Level of Evidence C)
3. The target LDL-C level after STEMI should be substantially less than 100 mg/dL. (Level of Evidence A)
    a. Patients with LDL-C 100 mg/dL or above should be prescribed drug therapy on hospital discharge, with preference given to statins. (Level of Evidence A)
    b. Patients with LDL-C less than 100 mg/dL or unknown LDL-C levels should be prescribed statin therapy on hospital discharge. (Level of Evidence B)
4. Patients with nonhigh-density lipoprotein cholesterol (non-HDL-C) levels less than 130 mg/dL who have an HDL-C level less than 40 mg/dL should receive special emphasis on nonpharmacological therapy (e.g., exercise, weight loss, and smoking cessation) to increase HDL-C. (Level of Evidence B)

Class IIa
1. It is reasonable to prescribe drug therapy at discharge to patients with non-HDL-C greater than or equal to 130 mg/dL, with a goal of reducing non-HDL-C to substantially less than 130 mg/dL. (Level of Evidence B)
2. It is reasonable to prescribe drug therapy such as niacin or fibrate therapy to raise HDL-C levels in patients with LDL-C less than 100 mg/dL and non-HDL-C less than 130 mg/dL but HDL-C less than 40 mg/dL despite dietary and other nonpharmacological therapy (Level of Evidence B). Dietary-supplement niacin must not be used as a substitute for prescription niacin, and over-the-counter niacin should be used only if approved and monitored by a physician.
3. It is reasonable to add drug therapy with either niacin or a fibrate to diet regardless of LDL-C and HDL-C levels when triglyceride levels are greater than 500 mg/dL. In this setting, non-HDL-C (goal substantially less than 130 mg/dL) should be the cholesterol target rather than LDL-C (Level of Evidence B). Dietary supplement niacin must not be used as a substitute for prescription niacin, and over-the-counter niacin should be used only if approved and monitored by a physician.

3. Weight Management
Class I
1. Measurement of waist circumference and calculation of body mass index are recommended. Desirable body mass index range is 18.5 to 24.9 kg/m2. A waist circumference greater than 40 inches in men and 35 inches in women would result in evaluation for metabolic syndrome and implementation of weight-reduction strategies. (Level of Evidence B)
2. Patients should be advised about appropriate strategies for weight management and physical activity (usually accomplished in conjunction with cardiac rehabilitation). (Level of Evidence B)
3. A plan should be established to monitor the response of body mass index and waist circumference to therapy (usually accomplished in conjunction with cardiac rehabilitation). (Level of Evidence B)

4. Smoking Cessation
Class I
1. Patients recovering from STEMI who have a history of cigarette smoking should be strongly encouraged to stop smoking and to avoid secondhand smoke. Counseling should be provided to the patient and family along with pharmacological therapy (including nicotine replacement and bupropion) and formal smoking-cessation programs as appropriate. (Level of Evidence B)
2. All STEMI patients should be assessed for a history of cigarette smoking. (Level of Evidence A)

5. Antiplatelet Therapy
Class I
1. A daily dose of aspirin 75 to 162 mg orally should be given indefinitely to patients recovering from STEMI. (Level of Evidence A)
2. If true aspirin allergy is present, preferably clopidogrel (75 mg orally per day), or alternatively, ticlopidine (250 mg orally twice daily) should be substituted. (Level of Evidence C)
3. If true aspirin allergy is present, warfarin therapy with a target INR of 2.5 to 3.5 is a useful alternative to clopidogrel in patients less than 75 years of age who are at low risk for bleeding and who can be monitored adequately for dose adjustment to maintain a target INR range. (Level of Evidence C)
4. At the time of preparation for hospital discharge, the patient's need for treatment of chronic musculoskeletal discomfort should be assessed and a stepped-care approach to pain management should be used for selection of treatments. Pain relief should begin with acetaminophen or aspirin, small doses of narcotics, or nonacetylated salicylates. (Level of Evidence C)

Class IIa
1. It is reasonable to use nonselective NSAIDs such as naproxen if initial therapy with acetaminophen, small doses of narcotics, or nonacetylated salicylates is insufficient. (Level of Evidence C)

Class IIb
1. NSAIDs with increasing degrees of relative COX-2 selectivity may be considered for pain relief only for situations where intolerable discomfort persists despite attempts at stepped care therapy with acetaminophen, small doses of narcotics, nonacetylated salicylates, or nonselective NSAIDs. In all cases, the lowest effective doses should be used for the shortest possible time. (Level of Evidence C)

Class III
1. NSAIDs with increasing degrees of relative COX-2 selectivity should not be administered to STEMI patients with chronic musculoskeletal discomfort when therapy with acetaminophen, small doses of narcotics, nonacetylated salicylates, or nonselective NSAIDs provides acceptable levels of pain relief. (Level of Evidence C)

6. Inhibition of Renin-Angiotensin-Aldosterone System
Class I
1. An ACE inhibitor should be prescribed at discharge for all patients without contraindications after STEMI. (Level of Evidence A)

2. Long-term aldosterone blockade should be prescribed for post-STEMI patients without significant renal dysfunction (creatinine should be less than or equal to 2.5 mg/dL in men and less than or equal to 2.0 mg/dL in women) or hyperkalemia (potassium should be less than or equal to 5.0 mEq/L) who are already receiving therapeutic doses of an ACE inhibitor, have an LVEF less than or equal to 0.40, and have either symptomatic heart failure or diabetes. (Level of Evidence A)
3. An ARB should be prescribed at discharge in those STEMI patients who are intolerant of an ACE inhibitor and have either clinical or radiological signs of heart failure and LVEF less than 0.40. Valsartan and candesartan have established efficacy for this recommendation. (Level of Evidence B)

Class IIa
1. In STEMI patients who tolerate ACE inhibitors, an ARB can be useful as an alternative to ACE inhibitors in the long-term management of STEMI patients, provided there are either clinical or radiological signs of heart failure or LVEF less than 0.40. Valsartan and candesartan have established efficacy for this recommendation. (Level of Evidence B)

Class IIb
1. The combination of an ACE inhibitor and an ARB may be considered in the long-term management of STEMI patients with persistent symptomatic heart failure and LVEF less than 0.40. (Level of Evidence B)

7. β-Blockers
Class I
1. All patients after STEMI except those at low risk (normal or near-normal ventricular function, successful reperfusion, and absence of significant ventricular arrhythmias) and those with contraindications should receive β-blocker therapy. Treatment should begin within a few days of the event, if not initiated acutely, and continue indefinitely. (Level of Evidence A)
2. Patients with moderate or severe LV failure should receive β-blocker therapy with a gradual titration scheme. (Level of Evidence B)

Class IIa
1. It is reasonable to prescribe β-blockers to low-risk patients after STEMI who have no contraindications to that class of medications. (Level of Evidence A)

8. Blood Pressure Control
Class I
1. Blood pressure should be treated with drug therapy to a target level of less than 140/90 mm Hg and to less than 130/80 mm Hg for patients with diabetes or chronic kidney disease. (Level of Evidence B)
2. Lifestyle modification (weight control, dietary changes, physical activity, and sodium restriction) should be initiated in all patients with blood pressure greater than or equal to 120/80 mm Hg. (Level of Evidence B)

Class IIb
1. A target blood pressure goal of 120/80 mm Hg for post-STEMI patients may be reasonable. (Level of Evidence C)

Class III
1. Short-acting dihydropyridine calcium channel blocking agents should not be used for the treatment of hypertension. (Level of Evidence B)

9. Diabetes Management
Class I
1. Hypoglycemic therapy should be initiated to achieve HbA1c less than 7%. (Level of Evidence B)

Class III
1. Thiazolidinediones should not be used in patients recovering from STEMI who have New York Heart Association class III or IV heart failure. (Level of Evidence B)

10. Hormone Therapy
Class III
1. Hormone therapy with estrogen plus progestin should not be given de novo to postmenopausal women after STEMI for secondary prevention of coronary events. (Level of Evidence A)
2. Postmenopausal women who are already taking estrogen plus progestin at the time of a STEMI should not continue hormone therapy. However, women who are beyond one to two years after initiation of hormone therapy who wish to continue hormone therapy for another compelling indication should weigh the risks and benefits, recognizing a greater risk of cardiovascular events. However, hormone therapy should not be continued while patients are on bedrest in the hospital. (Level of Evidence B)

11. Warfarin Therapy
Class I
1. Warfarin should be given to aspirin-allergic post-STEMI patients with indications for anticoagulation as follows:
   a. Without stent implanted (INR 2.5 to 3.5). (Level of Evidence B)
   b. With stent implanted and clopidogrel 75 mg/day administered concurrently (INR 2.0 to 3.0). (Level of Evidence C)
2. Warfarin (INR 2.5 to 3.5) is a useful alternative to clopidogrel in aspirin-allergic patients after STEMI who do not have a stent implanted. (Level of Evidence B)
3. Warfarin (INR 2.0 to 3.0) should be prescribed for post-STEMI patients with either persistent or paroxysmal atrial fibrillation. (Level of Evidence A)
4. In post-STEMI patients with LV thrombus noted on an imaging study, warfarin should be prescribed for at least three months (Level of Evidence B) and indefinitely in patients without an increased risk of bleeding (Level of Evidence C).
5. Warfarin alone (INR 2.5 to 3.5) or warfarin (INR 2.0 to 3.0) in combination with aspirin (75–162 mg) should be prescribed in post-STEMI patients who have no stent implanted and who have indications for anticoagulation. (Level of Evidence B)

Class IIa
1. In post-STEMI patients less than 75 years of age without specific indications for anticoagulation who can have their level of anticoagulation monitored reliably, warfarin alone (INR 2.5 to 3.5) or warfarin (INR 2.0 to 3.0) in combination with aspirin (75–162 mg) can be useful for secondary prevention. (Level of Evidence B)

2. It is reasonable to prescribe warfarin to post-STEMI patients with LV dysfunction and extensive regional wall-motion abnormalities. (Level of Evidence A)

Class IIb

1. Warfarin may be considered in patients with severe LV dysfunction, with or without CHF. (Level of Evidence C)

12. Physical Activity
Class I

1. On the basis of assessment of risk, ideally with an exercise test to guide the prescription, all patients recovering from STEMI should be encouraged to exercise for a minimum of 30 minutes, preferably daily but at least three or four times per week (walking, jogging, cycling, or other aerobic activity), supplemented by an increase in daily lifestyle activities (e.g., walking breaks at work, gardening, and household work). (Level of Evidence B)
2. Cardiac rehabilitation/secondary prevention programs, when available, are recommended for patients with STEMI, particularly those with multiple modifiable risk factors and/or those moderate- to high-risk patients in whom supervised exercise training is warranted. (Level of Evidence C)

13. Antioxidants
Class III

1. Antioxidant vitamins such as vitamin E and/or vitamin C supplements should not be prescribed to patients recovering from STEMI to prevent cardiovascular disease. (Level of Evidence A)

VII. LONG-TERM MANAGEMENT

A. Psychosocial Impact of STEMI
Class I

1. The psychosocial status of the patient should be evaluated, including inquiries regarding symptoms of depression, anxiety, or sleep disorders and the social support environment. (Level of Evidence C)

Class IIa

1. Treatment with cognitive-behavioral therapy and selective serotonin reuptake inhibitors can be useful for STEMI patients with depression that occurs in the year after hospital discharge. (Level of Evidence A)

B. Cardiac Rehabilitation
Class IIa

1. Cardiac rehabilitation/secondary prevention programs, when available, are recommended for patients with STEMI, particularly those with multiple modifiable risk factors and/or those moderate- to high-risk patients in whom supervised exercise training is warranted. (Level of Evidence C)

C. Follow-Up Visit with Medical Provider
Class I

1. A follow-up visit should delineate the presence or absence of cardiovascular symptoms and functional class. (Level of Evidence C)

2. The patient's list of current medications should be reevaluated in a follow-up visit, and appropriate titration of ACE inhibitors, β-blockers, and statins should be undertaken. (Level of Evidence C)
3. The predischarge risk assessment and planned workup should be reviewed and continued. This should include a check of LV function and possibly Holter monitoring for those patients whose early post-STEMI ejection fraction was 0.31 to 0.40 or lower, in consideration of possible ICD use. (Level of Evidence C)
4. The health care provider should review and emphasize the principles of secondary prevention with the patient and family members. (Level of Evidence C)
5. The psychosocial status of the patient should be evaluated in follow-up, including inquiries regarding symptoms of depression, anxiety, or sleep disorders and the social support environment. (Level of Evidence C)
6. In a follow-up visit, the health care provider should discuss in detail issues of physical activity, return to work, resumption of sexual activity, and travel, including driving and flying. (Level of Evidence C)
7. Patients and their families should be asked if they are interested in CPR training after the patient is discharged from the hospital. (Level of Evidence C)
8. Providers should actively review the following issues with patients and their families:
   a. The patient's heart attack risk. (Level of Evidence C)
   b. How to recognize symptoms of STEMI. (Level of Evidence C)
   c. The advisability of calling 9-1-1 if symptoms are unimproved or worsening after five minutes, despite feelings of uncertainty about the symptoms and fear of potential embarrassment. (Level of Evidence C)
   d. A plan for appropriate recognition and response to a potential acute cardiac event, including the phone number to access EMS, generally 9-1-1. (Level of Evidence C)
9. Cardiac rehabilitation/secondary prevention programs, when available, are recommended for patients with STEMI, particularly those with multiple modifiable risk factors and/or those moderate- to high-risk patients in whom supervised exercise training is warranted. (Level of Evidence C)

REFERENCES

1. Antman EM, Anbe DT, Armstrong PW, et al. ACC/AHA guidelines for the management of patients with ST-elevation myocardial infarction: a report of the American College of Cardiology/American Heart Association Task Force on Practice Guidelines (Committee to Revise the 1999 Guidelines for the Management of Patients With Acute Myocardial Infarction. 2004). Available at: http://www.acc.org/clinical/guidelines/stemi/index.pdf.
2. Antman EM, Hand M, Armstrong PW, et al. July 2007 focused update of the ACC/AHA 2004 Guidelines for the Management of Patients With ST-Elevation Myocardial Infarction: a report of the American College of Cardiology/American Heart Association Task Force on Practice Guidelines: Writing Group To Review New Evidence and Update the ACC/AHA 2004 Guidelines for the Management of Patients With ST-Elevation Myocardial Infarction, Writing on Behalf of the 2004 STEMI Writing Committee. Circulation. J Am Coll Cardiol 2008; 51:210–247.

Appendix II   ESC STEMI Guidelines

Reperfusion Therapy

Recommendations	Class I	IIa	IIb	III	Level of evidence
Reperfusion therapy is indicated in all patients with history of chest pain/discomfort of <12 h and associated with ST-segment elevation of (presumed) new bundle-branch block on the ECG	X				A
Primary PCI					
• preferred treatment if performed by experienced team <90 min after first medical contact	X				A
• indicated for patients in shock and those with contraindication to fibrinolytic therapy	X				C
• GP IIb/IIIa antagonist and primary PCI					
No stenting	X				A
With stenting		X			A
Rescue PCI					
• after failed thrombolysis in patient with large infarcts		X			B
Fibrinolytic treatment					
In the absence of contraindications (see Table 1) and if primary PCI cannot be performed within 90 min after first medical contact by an experienced team, pharmacological reperfusion should be initiated as soon as possible.	X				A
• choice of fibrinolytic agent depends on individual assessment of benefit and risk, availability and cost					
In patients presenting late (>4 h after symptom onset) a more fibrin-specific agent such as tenecteplase or alteplase is preferred		X			B
For dosages of fibrinolytic and antithrombin agents see Tables 2 and 3					
• pre-hospital initiation of fibrinolytic therapy if appropriate facilities exist	X				B
• readministration of a non-immunogenic lytic agent if evidence of reocclusion and medical reperfusion not available		X			B
• if not already on aspirin 150–325 mg chewable aspirin (no enteric-coated tablets)	X				A
• with alteplase and reteplase, a weight-adjusted dose of heparin should be given with early and frequent adjustments according to the aPTT	X				B
• with streptokinase heparin is optional		X			B

Routine Prophylactic Therapies in the Acute Phase

Recommendations	Class I	IIa	IIb	III	Level of evidence
• Aspirin: 150–325 mg (no enteric-coated formulation)	X				A
• Intravenous beta-blocker: for all patient in whom it is not contraindicated Oral beta-blocker: cfr. Infra			X		A
• ACE inhibitors: oral formulation on first day					
to all patients in whom it is not contraindicated		X			A
to high-risk patients	X				A
• Nitrates			X		A
• Calcium antagonists				X	B
• Magnesium				X	A
• Lidocaine				X	B

Secondary Prevention

Recommendations	Class I	IIa	IIb	III	Level of evidence
• Stop smoking	X				C
• Optimal glycemic control in diabetic patients	X				B
• Blood pressure control in hypertensive patients	X				C
• Mediterranean-type diet	X				B
• Supplementation with 1 g fish oil n-3 poly-unsaturated fatty acid	X				B
• Aspirin: 75 to 160 mg daily	X				A
if aspirin is not tolerated					
clopidogrel (75 mg daily)			X		C
oral anticoagulant		X			B
• Oral beta-blockers: to all patients if no contraindications	X				A
• Continuation of ACE-inhibition started on the first day (cfr. supra)	X				A
• Statins:					
if in spite of dietary measures total cholesterol >190 mg/dL and/or LDL cholesterol >115 mg/dL	X				A
• Fibrates:					
if HDL cholesterol ≤45 mg/dL and triglycerides ≥200 mg/dL		X			A
• Calcium antagonists (diltiazem or verapamil) if contraindication to β blockers and no heart failure			X		B
• Nitrates in the absence of angina				X	A

Index